TYPE 2 DIABETES

Edited by **Kazuko Masuo**

Type 2 Diabetes
http://dx.doi.org/10.5772/46238
Edited by Kazuko Masuo

Contributors

Dhastagir Sultan Sheriff, Elshaari Fa, Sachu Philips, Naruemon Leelayuwat, Hong Yang, Rashid Muhammad Ansari, John Dixon, Colette Browning, Maria Mota, Simona Popa, Arturo A. Arce-Esquivel, Catherine Mikus, Aaron Bunker, M. Harold Laughlin, Catalano, Giovanni Scandale, Katia Cristina Portero McLellan, Lance Sloan, Roberto Burini, Reuven Zimlichman, Valeria Hirschler, Shaker A Mousa, Fernando Grover, Jarrod Shapiro, Diane Koshimune, Rebecca Moellmer, Subhashini Yaturu, Daniela Seelenfreund, Rodrigo Gonzalez, Pilar Durruty, Sergio Lobos, Nicolas Palou, Nigel Turner, Nadine Montemarano, Andrzej Kokoszka, Marcin Obrębski, Joanna Ostasz, Aleksandra Jodko, Rafał Radzio, Louis Ragolia, Raymond Lau, Roberto Pontarolo, Gina Agarwal, Kazuko Masuo

Published by InTech

Janeza Trdine 9, 51000 Rijeka, Croatia

Publishing Process Manager Danijela Duric
Technical Editor InTech DTP team
Cover InTech Design team

Additional hard copies can be obtained from orders@intechopen.com

Type 2 Diabetes, Edited by Kazuko Masuo
p. cm.
ISBN 978-953-51-1171-9

For EU product safety concerns:
IN TECH d.o.o., Prolaz Marije Krucifikse Kozulić 3, 51000 Rijeka, Croatia, info@intechopen.com or visit our website at intechopen.com.

Meet the editor

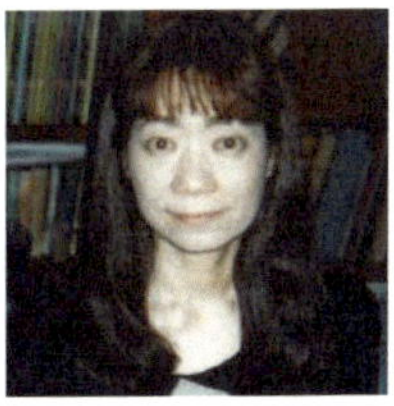

Associate Professor Kazuko Masuo, MD., PhD. is currently working as an Associate Medical Director in the Nucleus Network Ltd., Baker IDI Heart & Diabetes Institute, and an Academic Fellow in the Baker IDI Heart & Diabetes Institute, in Melbourne, Victoria, Australia. She graduated as MD and received PhD at the Department of Geriatric Medicine and the Department of Pharmacology in Osaka University Postgraduate School of Medicine, Osaka, Japan, under supervision of Professors Kumahara and Ogihara. She conducted a series of longitudinal studies over 10 years investigating weight change and neurohormonal changes, and these studies were a mile stone research to understand how obesity impacts on hypertension, diabetes, and cardiac- and renal-complications, and how to manage these conditions. She is a certificated specialist in cardiology, endocrinology, nephrology and gerontology, and in several editorial boards for medical journals. She has 100 publications in international, peer reviewed medical journals on obesity, hypertension, diabetes, genetics and renal dysfunction, 15 book chapters, and has edited 6 books.

Contents

Preface

The epidemic like rise in the prevalence of obesity constitutes an undoubted global serious, health problem. Importantly, type 2 diabetes is frequently associated with obesity and, together, constitute a significant burden in terms of patients morbidity and escalating health care costs. Patients with type 2 diabetes have 2-4 times higher risk of cardiovascular risk and renal complications than those without diabetes and their relative risk for cardiovascular disease, mortality and morbidity is twice as high. In addition, the elevated cardiovascular risk affecting with type 2 diabetes may be attributed to dyslipidemia hypertension, coronary heart disease, renal injury, and cancer. Importantly, when taken in isolation, obesity, hypertension, diabetes and dyslipidemia are all associated with increased risk of the development of cardiovascular and renal complications; however, the coexistence of this triumvirate generates a substantial elevation in disease risk. The driving forces linking obesity and type 2 diabetes remain to be clarified due, in part, to the complex and multifactorial nature of the conditions that involve environmental, genetic, life style and behavioural confounders. Additionally, it is recognized that insulin resistance, beta-cell function in the pancreas, epigenetic and molecular mechanisms are also involved.

This book on "Type 2 diabetes" includes three separate parts separated, consisting of **(1) Pathophysiology** understanding the pathogenesis and mechanisms of the onset and development of type 2 diabetes; **(2) Complications** of type 2 diabetes; including proteinuria as a marker of renal complication, and foot ulcers, which are frequently experienced in medical practice as type 2 diabetes progress; and **(3) Prevention and Treatments** for type 2 diabetes, including effective screening for type 2 diabetes, non-pharmacological treatments by lifestyle modification, surgical treatments, pharmacological treatments, insulin therapy, and a development of psycho-diabetic Kit for support to diagnose psychological status.

"Pathophysiology" section: Insulin resistance plays an important role in type 2 diabetes and obesity-related diseases. Dr Arce-Esquivel et al. contributed to this book with an excellent review titled **(i) "insulin resistance, endothelial dysfunction"**. The relationship between insulin resistance and endothelial dysfunction and the interaction between insulin and its vascular and metabolic effects from the signalling pathway to target tissues (i.e. vessels) are discussed. In addition, they reviewed the effects of exercise, as a part of lifestyle modification, on vascular insulin resistance. **(ii) "Beta-cell function under physiological conditions and the potential beta-cell failure mechanisms"** was written by Dr. Popa and Prof. Mota. They highlighted the importance of a long-term glucolipotoxixity for the onset of type 2 diabetes. To understand the mechanisms of beta-cell dysfunction helps in the implication for treatment of beta-cell dysfunction. The next 2 chapters focused on the molecular mechanisms on insulin resistance and type 2 diabetes, and both chapters were excellently written for readers to understand molecular basis on type 2 diabetes. Dr. Kata et al. reviewed the chapter with **(iii) "epigenetic regulation and mechanisms in type 2 diabetes"** with the thrifty phenotype hypothesis by Halas et al. Epigenetic and molecular mechanisms in intra-uterine growth retardation (IUGR) were covered. Epigenetic modifications affecting glucose regulation and insulin secretion in the IUGR organs (i.e. liver, pancreas beta-cells, and muscles) can contribute to the onset of type 2 diabetes along with the genetic and environmental influences. Environmental effects such as lifestyle modifications (i.e. exercise, nutrients, and diet) can also induce epigenetic alterations. Dr. Turner showed the chapter **(iv) "Mitochondrial metabolism and insulin action"** to understand the molecular mechanism of glucose metabolisms, insulin resistance and possible mechanisms to cause type 2 diabetes with precise figures.

The next three chapters showed the characteristics of type 2 diabetes in brainstem focusing on sympathovagal system and thyrotropin releasing hormone (TRH), vessels, renal function and lipid metabolisms. The chapter **(v) "Sympathovagal imbalance in type 2 diabetes: Role of brainstem Thyrotoropin-releasing hormone"** by Dr Yang showed the importance of brainstem and sympathovagal regulation in regulation on glucose metabolisms in type 2 diabetes, especially focusing on TRH. The chapter **(vi) "Arterial stiffness" by Dr. Catalano** discussed that arterial stiffness is worse with aging, diabetes, dyslipidemia and cardiovascular and coronary artery diseases, and it can be a marker for cardiovascular risks and complications. Pulse-wave velocity (PWV) is currently considered the "gold standard" in aortic compliance. This chapter reviewed the importance of arterial stiffness in type 2 diabetes, the mechanisms of arterial stiffness, the relationships between glucose levels and arterial stiffness, and how to reduce it in type 2 diabetes. The inverse association between body mass index (BMI) and glomerular filtration rate and between insulin resistance and renal function were observed in Argentinian healthy boys with post-pubertal age in the chapter **(vii) "Association between creatinine clearance and insulin-resistance in healthy adolescent boys"** by Dr. Hirschler, et al. In this study, creatinine clearance was calculated with Modification of Diet in Renal Disease and quadratic equation (MDRD). Prof. Dhstagir et al. presented their own data including the comparisons of the lipids parameters in patients with coronary artery disease with and without diabetes in the chapter **(viii) "HDL, apo B/apo A1 ratio, diabetes mellitus and cardiovascular disease".** He concluded the accelerated atherosclerosis associated with insulin resistance is strongly related to abnormal lipids metabolisms, and it contributes to high incidence of cardiovascular disease in type 2 diabetes.

"Complications" section includes the chapter **(ix) "Diabetes mellitus type 2 and proteinuria".** Proteinuria is very frequently observed in patients with type 2 diabetes at diabetes clinic, and is a good predictor for future renal failure and cardiovascular morbidity and mortality. Prof. Zimlichman and Dr. Cernes et al. excellently reviewed this from the pathogenesis to clinical implications. In the very interesting chapter **(x) "Diabetes and Cancer"**, many epidemiological studies have shown frequent co-occurrence of diabetes, obesity and cancer. Dr. Yaturu discussed possible mechanisms of coexistence, such as hyperinsulinemia as a mitogenic effects, increased bioability insulin-like growth factor-1 (IGF-1) with corresponding receptor (IGFR), decreased level of adiponectin in obesity and type 2 diabetes, and increased oxidative stress. In the chapter **(xi) "Anemia in diabetic kidney disease"**, Dr. Montemarano, et al. showed the potential mechanisms of anemia in chronic kidney disease. Both chapters of (xi) and (xii), focus on foot ulcer. Chapter titled with **(xii) "Diabetic Foot Ulcers: Treatment and Prevention"** by Prof. Jarrod, et al. covered a very wide range of a medical conditions on foot ulcer including pathophysiology, risk factors, clinical symptoms, treatment, complications, and Charcot neuroarthropathy, which is independently reviewed very well by Dr. Paez et al. in the next chapter **(xiii) "The diabetic Charcot foot: New insights on treatment"** . These chapters are very helpful for diabetes practice clinics.

"Prevention and Treatments" section: The chapter, **(xiv) "Screening for diabetes in family practice"** by Dr. Agarwal discussed the importance of the early detection of diabetes/pre-diabetes/diabetic complications and the benefits of "Family Health Networks in Ontario", a new family practitioners' network system. This chapter is very helpful for family physicians (general practitioners) to screen diabetes/pre-diabetes. The next four chapters, consisting of **(xv) "Socio-ecological approach to self-management"** by Dr. Ansari, et al., **(xvi) "Lifestyle modification is the first line treatment for type 2 diabetes"** by A/Prof. Masuo, **(xvii) "Control and prevention of obesity and diabetes type 2 through non-pharmacological treatments"** by Dr. Seelenfreund et al. and **(xviii) "Beneficial effects of alternative exercise in patients with diabetes type 2"** by A/Prof. Leelayuwat, highlighted the importance and benefits of lifestyle modification including diet and exercise on better control for diabetes with different approaches. The chapter (xviii) discussed on the benefits of marine deriving products is interesting.

Long-term medical therapy for obesity and obesity-related diseases such as type 2 diabetes is often unsuccessful for the majority of patients in clinical practice. Bariatric weight loss surgery has remained the most effective means achieving and maintaining weight loss. The chapter, **(xix) "Understanding the effects of Roux-en-Y gastric bypass (RYGB) surgery on type 2 diabetes"** by Drs. Lau and Rogolia, et al. is an excellent chapter to understand the mechanisms, effects on insulin resistance, central nervous system, and other neurohormonal changes, benefits, and side effects in significant weight loss achieved by Roux-en-Y gastric bypass surgery.

On the other hand, Drs. Sanches and Pontarolo, et al. discussed pharmacological treatments for type 2 diabetes in the chapter **(xx) "Advances in treatments and therapeutic intervention in type 2 diabetes mellitus: Pharmacological treatments for type 2 diabetes"** and Dr. Azad and Prof. Mousa, et al. reviewed insulin therapy in the chapter **(xxi) "Insulin therapy for diabetes"**. Both chapters are very practical for diabetic patients and medical practitioners.

The chapter **(xxii) "Hypolipidemic and antioxidant activity of Cassia Tora seed extract"** investigated by Dr. Kumar, et al. is a unique chapter. They found Casia Tora seed contained antioxidant enzymes and lipases reactivating activity, and it would be helpful to treat for dyslipidemia caused by inhibition of hepatic cholesterol biosynthesis, activation of tissue lipase, SOD, and CAT. Casia Tora seed extract is also known for its effectiveness for many diseases.

Diabetes is observed in higher prevalence in patients with depression, and depression is observed in higher prevalence in diabetic patients. Psychological factors impact strongly on the management of diabetes and the prognosis of the disease. The chapter **(xxiii) "Psychodiabetic Kit and its application in clinical practice and research"** by Prof. Kokoszka et al. highlighted on the importance of psychological factors on the management of diabetes, especially in diabetes self-control and they developed more simple psychotherapeutic Kit than previous ones (WHO-5, MIND, PAID). This Kit may be a useful and beneficial for psychotherapeutic diagnoses and education of patients dealing with coping with diabetes related stressor.

This book coveres a wide range of material with a focus on type 2 diabetes. Articles included pathophysiology, mechanisms, characteristics, complications, screening, prevention and treatments for type 2 diabetes. In summary, this book directed that i) insulin resistance and beta-cell dysfunction in the pancreas area major mechanisms for the onset and development of type 2 diabetes and its complications; ii) epigenetic of glucose metabolism and mitochondrial metabolisms are strongly related to glucose metabolisms; iii) renal dysfunction including proteinuria, cancer, anemia, diabetic foot ulcers, dyslipidemia; iv) weight loss with lifestyle modification including diet and/or exercise and nutritional factors is an important aspect in treating type 2 diabetes, and help the efficacy of anti-diabetic medications; v) pharmacological treatments and insulin therapy are discussed. I believe that this book covers all current hot, but unique, topics in type 2 diabetes. Further investigations on mechanisms and genetics will be needed, because more knowledge may prevent obesity and resultant type 2 diabetes, and help to control diabetes. .

The editor thanks the authors of all submissions, our nurse, Mr. Tracy Mallett for reviewing manuscripts and discussion, and the publishing process manager, Ms. Iva Simcic, for her tireless assistance. I, the editor, enjoyed the variety of articles and hope that this book is useful for your clinical practice, and research and hope that the content of this book facilitates the reduction of the global burden of type 2 diabetes and obesity-related diseases.

Associate Professor Kazuko Masuo, MD, PhD, FAHA
Nucleus Network Ltd.,
Baker IDI Heart & Diabetes Institute

Academic Fellow, Baker IDI Heart & Diabetes Institute.,
Melbourne, Australia

Section 1

Pathophysiology

Chapter 1

Insulin Resistance and Endothelial Dysfunction: Macro and Microangiopathy

Arturo A. Arce-Esquivel, Aaron K. Bunker,
Catherine R. Mikus and M. Harold Laughlin

Additional information is available at the end of the chapter

http://dx.doi.org/10.5772/56475

1. Introduction

Insulin has classically been considered a hormone that acts primarily on skeletal muscle, adipose tissue and the liver in the control of glucose homeostasis. However, recent evidence indicates that insulin is also a vascular hormone that has an essential role in both regulating glucose homeostasis through influencing blood flow (e.g. glucose uptake in skeletal muscle and adipose tissue) and in maintaining vascular health.

Among the most important cardiovascular actions of insulin is to stimulate production of the potent vasodilator nitric oxide (NO) from vascular endothelium, increasing blood flow to skeletal muscle and other target tissues. These actions take place not only on conduit arteries (i.e. macrovasculature), but also on resistance and terminal arterioles (i.e. microvasculature). Abnormally high insulin concentrations (i.e. early stage of type 2 diabetes) and/or insulin resistance (i.e. tissues do not respond to insulin normally) have a profound impact on vascular homeostasis that manifests as impaired endothelial function, vasodilation, microvessel disease (i.e. retinopathy and nephropathy), and enhanced vascular inflammation and atherosclerotic lesion formation.

Approximately 90-95% of patients with diabetes mellitus have type 2 diabetes, which is characterized by insulin resistance or the inability of insulin to exert its metabolic actions. Indeed, early in the disease the pancreas produces more and more insulin to compensate for insulin resistance in target tissues. Eventually the pancreas may 'wear out' and the patient may no longer be able to produce insulin. Furthermore, there is good support for the notion that insulin resistance is itself an important risk factor for cardiovascular disease.

Thus, this chapter is intended to summarize the current available literature describing the physiologic and pathophysiologic role of insulin in the vasculature, and the mechanisms underlying the development of vascular insulin resistance from three standpoints. First, the role of insulin in the vasculature will be discussed with a specific focus on the interactions between the vascular and metabolic effects of insulin. Second, the role that vascular insulin resistance may play in the pathogenesis of vascular disease will be explored. Finally, this chapter will present evidence for the beneficial effects of exercise and physical activity in managing insulin resistance (i.e. improved insulin sensitivity) and improving endothelial function.

2. Physiological role of insulin in the vasculature

2.1. Signaling pathways

It has been more than 90 years since the role of insulin in glucose homeostasis was first discovered. Since that time, it has been established that insulin receptors are expressed on nearly every cell surface in the body, and great strides have been made in understanding insulin signal transduction pathways. In the endothelium, insulin simultaneously stimulates the production of the vasodilator NO and the vasoconstrictor endothelin-1 (ET-1) through signaling pathways that closely parallel the insulin signaling pathways which regulate glucose uptake and cell growth and differentiation in skeletal muscle, adipose, and other tissues.

Typically, the net result of insulin stimulation in the vasculature is vasodilation, which serves to distribute blood flow to target tissues for glucose uptake. The hemodynamic effects of insulin typically account for up to 40% of insulin-stimulated skeletal muscle glucose uptake [1-10]. However, in insulin resistant states, the balance between the production of vasodilator and vasoconstrictor substances shifts, impairing insulin-stimulated vasodilation and contributing to reductions in insulin-stimulated glucose uptake [1, 2, 11-14].

2.1.1. Insulin signaling in the endothelium — Vasodilation

The insulin receptor is a cell-surface heterotetrameric protein comprised of two extracellular α subunits and two transmembrane β subunits joined by disulfide bonds. The binding of insulin to the extracellular α subunits initiates conformational changes that activate intrinsic tyrosine kinase activity on the intracellular portion of the transmembrane β subunits. Activation of the receptor tyrosine kinase promotes trans-autophosphorylation of the β subunits as well as the tyrosine phosphorylation of multiple docking proteins, including insulin receptor substrates 1 (IRS-1) and 2 (IRS-2). IRS-1 is necessary for insulin-stimulated production of NO in the endothelium [15], whereas IRS-2 is primarily implicated in delivery of insulin to the skeletal muscle interstitium [16] but may also contribute to NO production [17].

The src homology 2 (SH2) domain of the p85 regulatory subunit of phosphoinosiditde 3-kinase (PI-3K) binds to the tyrosine phosphorylated IRS-1, activating catalytic p110 subunit of PI-3K. PI-3K then converts the membrane phospholipid phosphatidylinositol 4,5-bisphosphate (PIP_2)

to phosphatidylinositol 3,4,5-trisphosphate (PIP_3), which recruits 3-phosphoinositide-dependent protein kinase-1 (PDK1) and protein kinase B (PKB) to the plasma membrane where PDK1 activates PKB, also known as Akt. Finally, Akt directly phosphorylates endothelial nitric oxide synthase (eNOS) at Ser1177, catalyzing the conversion of L-arginine to L-citrulline and NO. Insulin may also stimulate the production of the vasodilator prostacyclin (PGI_2) from the vascular endothelium [18, 19]. Although the signaling mechanism appears to be independent of insulin-stimulated NO production, it has yet to be elucidated.

2.1.2. Insulin signaling in the endothelium — Vasoconstriction

In addition to stimulating the production of NO through the PI-3K/Akt pathway, insulin also stimulates the production of the potent vasoconstrictor ET-1 through a separate mitogen-activated protein kinase (MAPK) pathway [20-22]. The divergence of the two pathways originates at IRS-1 where the binding of PI3-K differentiates the NO pathway and the binding of growth factor receptor bound protein 2 (Grb2) initiates the ET-1 pathway.

As described above, the binding of insulin to the insulin receptor initiates a cascade of autophosphorylation events including the activation of the docking proteins IRS-1 and IRS-2. Concurrently, the Src homology containing (Shc) protein is also activated by the insulin receptor. Binding of the SH2 domain of Grb2 to the phosphorylated tyrosine residues of IRS-1 or Shc activates the preassociated guanosine triphosphate (GTP) exchange factor Sos (son of sevenless). Sos activates Ras (rat sarcoma), a small GTP binding protein, that subsequently binds and activates the serine-threonine protein kinase Raf (rapidly growing fibrosarcoma). Raf activates MAPK/extra-cellular signal-regulated kinase (MEK) which then activates ERK1/2, also known as p44/42 mitogen-activated protein kinase (MAPK). Activation of MAPK ultimately leads to insulin-stimulated production of ET-1 [20]. However, the specific cell signaling events linking the activation of MAPK and ET-1 production are poorly understood.

2.1.3. Insulin signaling in the endothelium — Opposing pahways

The branches of the insulin signaling pathway yielding NO and ET-1 are widely viewed as distinct. However, inhibition of the MAPK pathway augments activation of eNOS, and, conversely, blockade of the PI3K pathway enhances expression of vascular adhesion molecules downstream of MAPK [23], indicating that there is likely some interaction between the two branches of the insulin signaling cascade.

2.1.4. Anti-inflammatory and atheroprotective effects of insulin

The primary atheroprotective effects of insulin are exerted through the production of NO. In addition to being a vasodilator, NO also exhibits antithrombic, antifibrinolytic, and antiatherogenic properties, including mitigation of cell growth and proliferation and inhibition of platelet and leukocyte adhesion. NO also stimulates arteriogenesis (reviewed [24]) and mitochondrial biogenesis [25] and positively modulates mitochondrial function [26].

Additionally, insulin prevents tumor necrosis factor (TNF) α-induced apoptosis of endothelial cells by inhibiting caspase-9 activity [27] and increases the expression of antioxidant enzymes, including heme oxygenase-1 (HO-1) through the PI-3K/Akt pathway [28].

Activation of the insulin receptor creates a 'burst' of intracellular reactive oxygen species (ROS), including hydrogen peroxide (H_2O_2). At normal physiological concentrations, H_2O_2 transiently inactivates negative regulators of insulin signaling, including protein tyrosine phosphatase 1B (PTP1B), protein phosphatase 2A (PP2A), and phosphatase and tensin homolog (PTEN). Thus, when the insulin receptor is activated, the resulting burst of H_2O_2, in effect, removes inhibition of signal transduction through the insulin signaling cascade.

In summary, insulin stimulates two pathways in the endothelium. One leads to the production of the vasodilator NO through PI3K and Akt, whereas the other mediates production of the vasoconstrictor ET-1 through MAPK (Figure 1).

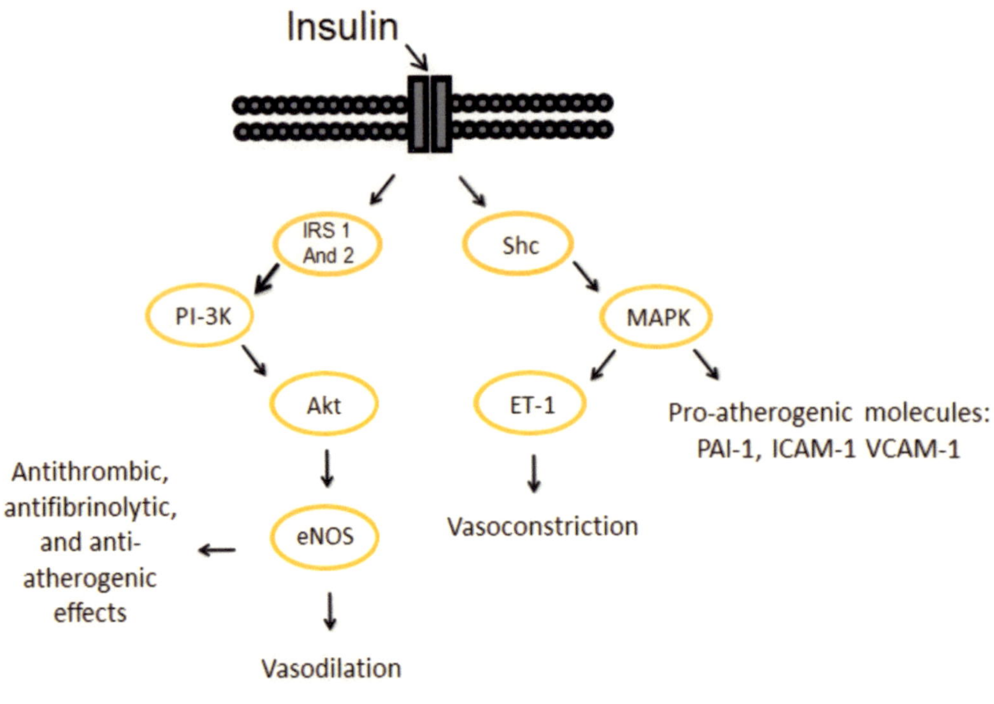

Figure 1. Insulin, vasodilation and vasoconstriction, pathways in the endothelium. IRS-1 and 2, insulin receptor substrate-1 and -2; PI-3K, phosphoinosiditde 3-kinase; Akt or PKB, protein kinase B; eNOS, endothelial nitric oxide synthase; Shc, Src homology containing; MAPK, mitogen-activated protein kinase pathway; PAI-1, plasminogen activator inhibitor type-1; ICAM-1, intracellular adhesion molecule; VCAM-1, vascular cell adhesion molecule; ET-1, endothelin-1.

2.2. Vascular effects

Insulin-stimulated production of NO from endothelium leads to capillary recruitment, vasodilation, increased blood flow to target tissues (e.g., skeletal muscle), and subsequent augmentation of glucose disposal. Removal of the endothelium or inhibition of NOS ablates insulin-stimulated vasodilation *in vitro* [29-34], and insulin-mediated blood flow is abolished by co-administration of the NOS inhibitor L-N^{G}-monomethyl-L-arginine (L-NMMA) *in vivo* [35, 36], establishing the critical role of NO in insulin-stimulated vasodilation.

Increases in circulating insulin that accompany ingestion of a mixed meal or a glucose challenge increase limb blood flow and decrease vascular resistance [9, 37]. Insulin-stimulated production of NO from the vascular endothelium leads to increases in skeletal muscle blood flow *in vivo*, and these increases have been proposed to occur in two phases [8]. The first occurs within five minutes of insulin stimulation and involves the dilation of terminal arterioles that increase the number of perfused capillaries (i.e., capillary recruitment) without concomitant changes in total limb blood flow [38]. Subsequently, there is a relaxation of larger resistance vessels, which increases overall limb blood flow; this effect can be observed within 30 minutes of insulin stimulation, while peak flow is reached after two hours [39].

As previously described, PI-3K-dependent insulin-signaling pathways regulate vasodilator actions of insulin, while the MAPK-dependent insulin-signaling pathways promote vasoconstrictor actions of insulin. Nevertheless, in the absence of disease, the opposing cardiovascular actions of insulin exist in a balance that support cardiovascular and metabolic homeostasis.

Baron [40] was the first to theorize that the ability of insulin to increase limb/muscle blood flow might be a critical component of insulin-stimulated glucose uptake. Indeed, a number of studies have demonstrated a strong correlation between limb blood flow and glucose uptake across a broad range of insulin infusion rates [1, 2, 12-14, 41, 42]. Intravenous infusion of insulin is reported to increase total limb blood flow in the majority [2, 5, 40, 43-46] but not all [47-50] human studies. There are a number of theories to explain why an insulin-stimulated increase in blood flow is not always observed. Discrepancies among studies could be the result of differences in subject selection as well as differences in physical fitness, muscularity, endothelial function, and capillary density of study subjects. Technical limitations or differences in sensitivity of various experimental approaches for estimating limb blood flow (e.g., plethysmography, thermodilution, dye dilution, Doppler ultrasound) may also contribute to contradictory reports. It has been suggested that while an increase in total blood flow is not always observed, insulin can re-distribute blood flow by influencing which vessels are perfused without affecting total blood flow [51, 52].

Insulin modulates microvascular perfusion through the relaxation of terminal arteries and through capillary recruitment [38, 40, 44, 46, 53-55]. Strong correlations between measures of insulin-mediated capillary recruitment and skeletal muscle glucose uptake [14, 54] have been viewed by some as evidence of insulin regulating 'nutritive' blood flow[5, 52-54]. In other words, insulin may promote the dilation of specific terminal arterioles to increase perfusion of capillary beds that experience little or no perfusion under basal conditions [52]. Support for this notion comes from a number of studies demonstrating that increases in capillary recruitment and microvascular blood flow precede increases in glucose uptake in response to insulin, whereas changes in bulk limb blood flow are typically observed after the onset of changes in glucose disposal [44]. Together, these data suggest that changes in bulk flow may be secondary to changes in capillary recruitment.

In addition to stimulating vasodilation, insulin promotes opposing mechanisms which lead to vasoconstriction, including activation of the sympathetic nervous system and secretion of the vasoconstrictor ET-1 from the endothelium [56, 57]. Increases in sympathetic nerve activity and circulating catecholamines are observed following insulin infusion or meal ingestion [58-60]. The sympatho-excitatory effects of insulin are thought to function primarily to maintain blood pressure by offsetting peripheral vasodilation [58]. In support of this theory, insulin decreases blood pressure in persons with autonomic failure [61], and, in patients who have undergone regional sympathectomy, increases in blood flow in the denervated limb precede changes in blood flow in the innervated limb [62]. Although there is evidence of cholinergic involvement in hemodynamic responses to insulin in rats [63], neither cholinergic nor β-adrenergic systems appear to be involved in humans [64].

3. Insulin resistance and endothelial dysfunction

3.1. Signaling pathways

3.1.1. Changes in insulin signaling in the endothelium in insulin resistance

Lipotoxicity, glucotoxicity, and inflammation disrupt insulin signaling in the endothelium and lead to reduced insulin-stimulated blood flow in obesity and type 2 diabetes.

3.1.2. Reactive oxygen species

In type 2 diabetes, glucotoxicity and lipotoxicity, stimulate the production of ROS. Elevations in ROS contribute to the development and progression of vascular complications associated with type 2 diabetes by directly interfering with insulin signaling and limiting NO bioavailability.

Hyperglycemia activates the polyol pathway, converting excess glucose to sorbitol and finally fructose [65]. When fructose reacts with proteins, lipids, and nucleic acids, advanced glycation end products (AGE) are formed, which, in turn, stimulate ROS production [66]. Hyperglycemia further contributes to ROS by inducing peroxidation of circulating glucose and lipoproteins and interfering with auto-oxidation processes [67]. Neurohormonal over-activation and inflammation also contribute to ROS (superoxide) formation via stimulation of NADPH oxidase activity and expression [68]. ROS generation is further compounded by reductions in superoxide dismutase, catalase, and glutathione peroxidase, which impair antioxidant capacity in type 2 diabetes [69].

When generated in excess, ROS impairs insulin signaling by impairing insulin-stimulated activation of Akt and eNOS [70, 71] and limiting NO bioavailability [72]. Typically, the production of NO occurs in a sequence of tightly coupled reactions involving eNOS, tetrahydrobiopterin (BH_4), and several other co-factors [73]. ROS limits BH_4 availability, resulting in eNOS uncoupling and superoxide production [73]. Additionally, ROS may interact directly with NO to form the powerful oxidant peroxynitrite (ONOO-), which may contribute to further uncoupling of eNOS. In other words, excess oxidative stress diverts NO to inactivate free radicals, thereby limiting the amount of NO available for vasoregulatory processes. Finally, eNOS expression is reduced in type 2 diabetes, putatively as a result of reduced or altered shear stress patterns.

3.1.3. Alternative mechanisms by which lipotoxicity and glucotoxicity interfere with insulin signaling in the endothelium

Lipotoxicity (dyslipidemia) contributes to endothelial insulin resistance by impairing the PI3K/Akt/eNOS branch of the insulin signaling pathway while augmenting the MAPK/ET-1 branch [6]. Elevated free fatty acids (FFAs) and lipid metabolites (diacylglycerols, ceramides, acyl coenzyme As) activate protein kinase C (PKC), IkB kinase β (IKKB), and nuclear factor-κB (NF-κB), which serine phosphorylate IRS-1 [23, 74, 75]. Unlike tyrosine phosphorylation, which activates IRS-1, serine phosphorylation deactivates IRS-1 and effectively blunts insulin-stimulated production of NO.

Glucotoxicity activates the hexosamine biosynthetic pathway, promoting the production of *O*-linked β-N-acetylglucosamine (*O*-GlcNAc). Insulin signaling is impaired when O-linked glycosylation obstructs key phosphorylation sites on IRS-1 and eNOS [70, 76]. AGEs generated as a result of hyperglycemia activate PKC, which inhibits activation of PI-3K/Akt via serine phosphorylation of IRS-1/2 [77], as well as NF-κB, which increases the expression of ET-1 [78]. AGEs also accelerate the degradation of eNOS mRNA [79].

3.1.4. Cytokines, hormones, and other proteins

Elevated cytokines are associated with insulin resistance and contribute to endothelial dysfunction. Increases in cytokines, including TNF-α, C-reactive protein (CRP), and interleukin-6 (IL-6), inhibit insulin-stimulated NO production by decreasing eNOS expression and by activating serine kinases which serine phosphorylate and inactivate IRS-1/2, thereby inhibiting the PI3K/Akt/eNOS pathway [8, 31, 80, 81]. Moreover, TNF-α and CRP enhance ET-1 production [82, 83].

Obesity and type 2 diabetes are associated with elevations in leptin and resistin, which contribute to increases in TNF-α, IL-6, ROS, and ET-1 [84-87]. Leptin also enhances serine phosphorylation of IRS-1, thereby impairing insulin signaling through the PI-3K/Akt pathway [88]. Resistin, on the other hand, reduces eNOS expression [89]. Conversely, although adiponectin and ghrelin stimulate NO production through PI-3K/Akt signaling pathways and enhance NO bioavailability [90-92], both are reduced in individuals who are obese or have type 2 diabetes.

3.1.5. Proatherogenic effects of insulin

Insulin also stimulates the expression of pro-atherogenic molecules in the endothelium through MAPK-dependent pathways [93], including, plasminogen activator inhibitor type-1 (PAI-1) [94], intracellular adhesion molecule (ICAM-1) [95], vascular cell adhesion molecule (VCAM-1) [95], and E-selectin [95]. Inhibition of PI-3K or Akt results in increased expression of these pro-atherogenic molecules, indicating that the PI-3K/Akt pathway may inhibit the expression of atherothrombic factors in addition to stimulating the production of protective molecules, including NO [95].

3.2. Vascular effects

The vascular actions of insulin are altered in insulin resistant states owing to impairments in the PI3K/Akt/eNOS pathway, over-activation of the MAPK/ET-1 pathway, and/or altered bioavailability of or sensitivity to NO and/or ET-1. Furthermore, impairments in vascular responses to insulin are proportional to the degree of metabolic insulin resistance [43, 96]. Shared causal factors such as glucotoxicity, lipotoxicity, inflammation, and oxidative stress interact at multiple levels to create reciprocal relationships between insulin resistance and endothelial dysfunction that may help explain the frequent clustering of metabolic and cardiovascular disorders [8].

There is a strong association between insulin resistance and endothelial dysfunction, measured in terms of impaired endothelium-dependent vasodilatation [97, 98]. For instance, in healthy volunteers there is a close correlation between insulin sensitivity and basal NO production [99]. In addition, insulin-resistant humans have impaired endothelium-dependent vasodilator responses, measured using a variety of techniques [97, 100]. Endothelial dysfunction is also detectable in healthy first-degree relatives of patients with type 2 diabetes, who are themselves at increased risk of developing diabetes [101].

Furthermore, reduced efficacy of insulin to stimulate blood flow has been demonstrated in obesity, type 2 diabetes, and polycystic ovarian syndrome [45, 102]. The relationship between insulin resistance and endothelial dysfunction is independent of traditional cardiovascular risk factors (including blood pressure, plasma cholesterol, and triglycerides), yet a potential contribution of other confounding factors cannot be ruled out. Animal studies have also described similar findings [103-105]. Winters et al. reported impaired endothelium-dependent vasodilatation in mice with obesity and insulin resistance secondary to a naturally occurring gene mutation [103]. Transgenic mice with perturbations of the insulin-signaling pathway causing insulin resistance exhibit impairment of endothelium-dependent vasodilatation, whilst the response to exogenous NO donors remains intact [105].

Insulin resistance results in a selective impairment of the vasodilating and anti-atherogenic PI3-K/Akt pathway, whereas MAPK pathway remains unaffected [6, 106]. As a result, the compensatory hyperinsulinaemia occurring in insulin resistant states overactivates the MAPK pathway, favoring vasoconstriction. Insulin resistance and hyperinsulinemia transpire concurrently, rendering the deleterious consequences on endothelial function more severe than the sum of each alone.

Clinical studies have shown that high free fatty acid concentrations are associated with impairment of endothelium-dependent vasodilation and increased blood pressure [4, 107], putatively as a consequence of decreased NO availability. As previously mentioned, one of the characteristics of insulin resistance is the presence of chronic low grade inflammation along with increased circulating levels of cytokines and of inflammatory markers, including TNF-

α[108, 109]. Interestingly, TNF-α concentrations are negatively associated with capillary recruitment, perhaps explaining, at least in part, its relationship with insulin resistance [110]. ET-1 plays a pivotal role in insulin resistance and vascular dysfunction [111], as shown by experiments carried out both *in vitro* and *in vivo*. *In vitro*, sustained exposure of insulin-responsive cells to ET-1 impairs insulin sensitivity [112, 113]. Similarly, ET-1 causes insulin resistance *in vivo*, which may be prevented by administration of drugs which interfere with the ET-1 receptor type A [114].

The loss of skeletal muscle capillary density is observed in insulin resistance and type 2 diabetes, and insulin action is positively correlated with capillary density [115]. Furthermore, vasodilation in skeletal muscle in response to insulin infusion is reduced in obese subjects in comparison with lean controls [43]. Insulin-mediated capillary recruitment is blunted in cases of insulin resistance and obesity and is tightly linked to impairments in glucose uptake [52, 116]. Under conditions of insulin resistance, the balance of insulin action shifts toward vasoconstriction. This further exacerbates insulin resistance by limiting the delivery of insulin and nutrients to myocytes by decreasing nutritive flow and available capillary surface area.

4. Vascular insulin resistance and the role of exercise

Physical activity may be beneficial in slowing the initiation and progression of insulin resistance and cardiovascular disease through favorable effects on body weight, insulin sensitivity, glycemic control, blood pressure, lipid profiles, fibrinolysis, inflammatory defense systems, and endothelial function [117]. For instance, exercise exerts many of the same effects in the muscle vasculature as insulin [118]. Exercise efficiently increases muscle capillary recruitment, as well as total muscle blood flow [119]. Furthermore, exercise effects are thought to be mediated by intermittent shear stress (tangential force of blood flowing on the endothelial surface), an established physiological stimulus for NO [120]. Extensive comprehensive reviews regarding the global beneficial effects and/or recommendations of exercise/physical activity in patients with insulin resistance have been previously published elsewhere [117, 121-123]. The following section is intended to present the available evidence of the beneficial effects of exercise/physical activity on endothelial function.

4.1. Acute effects of exercise

Studies examining the acute effects of aerobic exercise training on endothelial function in insulin resistance subjects with few or no other major comorbidities are limited. One study examined blood ET-1 (a powerful endogenous vasoconstrictor) levels and leg blood flow during insulin infusions in healthy older subjects (non-diabetic and physically active, ~70 years of age) that were assigned into exercise training and control groups. The exercise training group treadmill exercised for 45-min at 70% of maximum heart rate. Only in the exercise training group did leg blood flow at baseline tend to increase while ET-1 blood plasma levels declined [124].

Other studies demonstrating declines in insulin sensitivity in response to acute physical inactivity in healthy populations [125-127] are corroborated by evidence that reducing sedentary time in order to improve metabolic health is equally if not more important than the benefits associated with a physically active lifestyle [128, 129]. Importantly, unfavorable changes in insulin sensitivity with the bed rest [125] were associated with decreases in forearm and calf flow-mediated dilation (FMD), an index of vascular endothelial function. Basal arterial tone also increased with bed rest as evidenced by decreased brachial artery diameter and increased systolic blood pressure.

4.2. Chronic effects of exercise training

Although studies examining the chronic effects of aerobic exercise training on endothelial function in persons with insulin resistance or type 2 diabetes range widely in their experimental design, the results of these studies indicate that exercise training improves endothelial function. For instance, in obese insulin resistant males and females, exercising three times per week (30-min each time using an unspecified modality) at 60- 80% of maximal heart rate under supervision and at home for at least 150-min/week for 6 months improved brachial FMD [130]. Conversely, microvascular reactivity did not improve following the exercise program in the same subjects. Furthermore, in hemodialysis patients, a 3-month aerobic exercise training program improved arterial stiffness (assessed using artery pressure waveform analysis) [131].

Exercise training also improves/maintains endothelial function in the obese Zucker rats (OZ), a model of insulin resistance and obesity, relative to non-exercising OZ. A treadmill exercise program (24 m/min, 30-min/day, 5 days/wk for 4-6wks) was shown to improve functional hyperemia and endothelial-dependent vasodilation in the spinotrapezius microvasculature when measured using intravital microscopy [132]. The same exercise program improved microvascular endothelial function in OZ due to decreased thromboxane receptor-mediated vasoconstriction [133], and not due to increased blood pressure [132]. It should be noted that these OZ studies were conducted at single time-points while the rats were developing and/or had already developed insulin resistance. See the "OLETF" studies described below for a summary of the effects of exercise on endothelial function during insulin resistance time-course studies.

Similar to the effects of acute physical inactivity, chronic physical inactivity (~6 years) led to the development of insulin resistance and reduced FMD in lean adult male rhesus monkeys [127]. Furthermore, insulin-mediated changes in capillary blood volume were inversely correlated with the degree of insulin resistance and directly with physical activity levels.

Studies using the Otsuka Long-Evans Tokushima Fatty (OLETF) rat model of insulin resistance and obesity have revealed that chronic aerobic physical activity alone (i.e. free access to running wheels from 12-40 weeks of age) maintains/improves endothelial function in conduit [134] and resistance arteries [34, 135-137]. These studies established that the maintained/improved endothelial function in the OLETFs was mediated by improvements in NO signaling and/or attenuated ET-1 sensitivity and/or production. Additionally, insulin resistance manifested prior to significant progressive declines (20-35%) in endothelial function [134]. Other OLETF studies demonstrating the positive effect of exercise training (i.e. a training program on a treadmill) as an interventional measure for endothelial function were conducted at single time-points while the rats were developing and/or had developed insulin resistance [138, 139].

It deserves mention that the experimental design of the OZ [132, 133] and several OLETF [34, 134-137] studies that were described above were such that the chronic aerobic exercise training/ physical activity served as a *preventative* measure for endothelial dysfunction associated with insulin resistance. Additionally, all human (for both acute and chronic studies) and some of the OLETF studies [138, 139] discussed above the exercise training also served as an interventional measure for endothelial dysfunction associated with insulin resistance.

Although there is evidence that resistance training improves insulin-stimulated glucose uptake, there have been few studies specifically examining the effects of resistance training on insulin-mediated blood flow. Juel *et al.* [140] compared the effects of six weeks of progressive single-leg strength training (3 days/wk, 3 sets of 10 repetitions at 70-80% of one repetition maximum; leg press, knee extension, and hamstring curl) on leg flow determined by thermodilution during a two-stage hyperinsulinemic-euglycemic clamp in the trained and untrained legs of ten patients with type 2 diabetes and seven male controls. Prior to the intervention, insulin-stimulated leg blood flow was greater in controls. Following the intervention, basal blood flow was similar between the trained and untrained legs in both groups, and leg blood flow was higher in the trained leg during the second stage of insulin infusion in healthy controls and during both stages in patients with type 2 diabetes. These findings seem to suggest that resistance training may enhance insulin-mediated blood flow in healthy individuals as well as those with type 2 diabetes. However, it is unclear whether changes in capillarity may contribute to this response.

Chronic exercise training produces increases in the expression and activity of proteins involved in insulin signaling and glucose uptake as well as increases in mitochondrial biogenesis and fatty acid oxidation [141, 142]. Chronic exercise training also increases eNOS expression in vessels experiencing increases in blood flow during exercise [143] and up-regulates antioxidant enzymes including, superoxide dismutase and glutathione peroxidase [144]. Finally, chronic exercise also reverses factors known to stimulate ROS formation, including, inflammation, glucotoxicity, and lipotoxicity [144]. Together, these adaptations likely contribute to improvements in endothelial function associated with exercise training.

5. Final conclusions

In summary, insulin stimulates two pathways in the endothelium. One pathway leads to the production of the vasodilator NO through PI3K and Akt, while the other mediates production of the vasoconstrictor ET-1 through MAPK [6, 31, 145]. Insulin-mediated glucose disposal is largely dependent upon the vasodilatory effects of insulin, which enhance blood flow and, thus, delivery of glucose and insulin to target tissues. Typically, insulin-stimulated vasodilation is responsible for up to 40% of insulin-stimulated glucose disposal following a meal [8].

The glucotoxicity, lipotoxicity, and inflammation associated with insulin resistance work in concert to alter insulin signaling, leading to an imbalance in the production of vasodilator and vasoconstrictor substances in response to insulin. Resulting impairments in the PI3K/Akt/

eNOS pathway concomitant with enhanced stimulation of the MAPK/ET-1 pathway precipitate hypertension, reduced blood flow, and impaired delivery of glucose and insulin to target tissues [7, 8, 52, 146]. Similar perturbations are observed in skeletal muscle insulin signaling in obesity and type 2 diabetes [8, 52], indicating that the metabolic and vascular insulin resistance associated with obesity and type 2 diabetes may develop in tandem.

Alterations in vascular NO bioavailability and/or attenuated ET-1 or attenuated thromboxane sensitivity/production appear to contribute to endothelial dysfunction associated with insulin resistance. These studies also collectively suggest that endothelial dysfunction can be improved/maintained with acute or chronic aerobic exercise training/physical activity when used either thru interventional or preventative measures. The beneficial effect of exercise on vascular insulin action was consistent across studies of conduit artery blood flow *in vivo* and microvascular reactivity to insulin *in vitro*, in both humans and rodents, and in response to both short-term and chronic exercise training. Clearly, even in cases of prolonged disease progression, exercise training might be able to remedy some of the effects of insulin resistance on the vasculature.

Acknowledgements

The authors thank Berit Hansen for the illustration and J. Matt McMcrary and Kristen Roles for their technical assistance.

Author details

Arturo A. Arce-Esquivel[1,2], Aaron K. Bunker[3], Catherine R. Mikus[4] and M. Harold Laughlin[1]

1 Department of Biomedical Sciences, University of Missouri, Columbia, Missouri, USA

2 Department of Health and Kinesiology, The University of Texas at Tyler, Tyler, Texas, USA

3 Department of Biology and Chemistry, Morningside College, Sioux City, Iowa, USA

4 Duke University Medical Center, Division of Cardiology, Durham, North Carolina, USA

References

[1] Baron AD, Laakso M, Brechtel G, Hoit B, Watt C, Edelman SV. Reduced postprandial skeletal muscle blood flow contributes to glucose intolerance in human obesity. J Clin Endocrinol Metab 1990;70(6) 1525-33. Epub 1990/06/01.

[2] Laakso M, Edelman SV, Brechtel G, Baron AD. Impaired insulin-mediated skeletal muscle blood flow in patients with NIDDM. Diabetes 1992;41(9) 1076-83. Epub 1992/09/01.

[3] Cleland SJ, Petrie JR, Ueda S, Elliott HL, Connell JM. Insulin-mediated vasodilation and glucose uptake are functionally linked in humans. Hypertension 1999;33(1 Pt 2) 554-8. Epub 1999/02/04.

[4] Clerk LH, Rattigan S, Clark MG. Lipid infusion impairs physiologic insulin-mediated capillary recruitment and muscle glucose uptake in vivo. Diabetes 2002;51(4) 1138-45. Epub 2002/03/28.

[5] Clark MG, Wallis MG, Barrett EJ, Vincent MA, Richards SM, Clerk LH, et al. Blood flow and muscle metabolism: a focus on insulin action. Am J Physiol Endocrinol Metab 2003;284(2) E241-58. Epub 2003/01/18.

[6] Muniyappa R, Montagnani M, Koh KK, Quon MJ. Cardiovascular actions of insulin. Endocr Rev 2007;28(5) 463-91. Epub 2007/05/26.

[7] Muniyappa R, Quon MJ. Insulin action and insulin resistance in vascular endothelium. Curr Opin Clin Nutr Metab Care 2007;10(4) 523-30. Epub 2007/06/15.

[8] Kim JA, Montagnani M, Koh KK, Quon MJ. Reciprocal relationships between insulin resistance and endothelial dysfunction: molecular and pathophysiological mechanisms. Circulation 2006;113(15) 1888-904. Epub 2006/04/19.

[9] Fugmann A, Millgard J, Sarabi M, Berne C, Lind L. Central and peripheral haemodynamic effects of hyperglycaemia, hyperinsulinaemia, hyperlipidaemia or a mixed meal. Clin Sci (Lond) 2003;105(6) 715-21. Epub 2003/07/29.

[10] Colberg SR, Sigal RJ, Fernhall B, Regensteiner JG, Blissmer BJ, Rubin RR, et al. Exercise and type 2 diabetes: the American College of Sports Medicine and the American Diabetes Association: joint position statement. Diabetes Care 2010;33(12) e147-67. Epub 2010/12/01.

[11] Baron AD, Laakso M, Brechtel G, Edelman SV. Mechanism of insulin resistance in insulin-dependent diabetes mellitus: a major role for reduced skeletal muscle blood flow. J Clin Endocrinol Metab 1991;73(3) 637-43. Epub 1991/09/01.

[12] Baron AD, Brechtel-Hook G, Johnson A, Hardin D. Skeletal muscle blood flow. A possible link between insulin resistance and blood pressure. Hypertension 1993;21(2) 129-35. Epub 1993/02/01.

[13] Baron AD, Steinberg HO, Chaker H, Leaming R, Johnson A, Brechtel G. Insulin-mediated skeletal muscle vasodilation contributes to both insulin sensitivity and responsiveness in lean humans. J Clin Invest 1995;96(2) 786-92. Epub 1995/08/01.

[14] Baron AD, Tarshoby M, Hook G, Lazaridis EN, Cronin J, Johnson A, et al. Interaction between insulin sensitivity and muscle perfusion on glucose uptake in human skele-

tal muscle: evidence for capillary recruitment. Diabetes 2000;49(5) 768-74. Epub 2000/07/25.

[15] Montagnani M, Ravichandran LV, Chen H, Esposito DL, Quon MJ. Insulin receptor substrate-1 and phosphoinositide-dependent kinase-1 are required for insulin-stimulated production of nitric oxide in endothelial cells. Mol Endocrinol 2002;16(8) 1931-42. Epub 2002/07/30.

[16] Kubota T, Kubota N, Moroi M, Terauchi Y, Kobayashi T, Kamata K, et al. Lack of insulin receptor substrate-2 causes progressive neointima formation in response to vessel injury. Circulation 2003;107(24) 3073-80. Epub 2003/06/18.

[17] Kubota T, Kubota N, Kumagai H, Yamaguchi S, Kozono H, Takahashi T, et al. Impaired insulin signaling in endothelial cells reduces insulin-induced glucose uptake by skeletal muscle. Cell Metab 2011;13(3) 294-307. Epub 2011/03/02.

[18] Kahn NN, Bauman WA, Hatcher VB, Sinha AK. Inhibition of platelet aggregation and the stimulation of prostacyclin synthesis by insulin in humans. Am J Physiol 1993;265(6 Pt 2) H2160-7. Epub 1993/12/01.

[19] Sobrevia L, Nadal A, Yudilevich DL, Mann GE. Activation of L-arginine transport (system y+) and nitric oxide synthase by elevated glucose and insulin in human endothelial cells. J Physiol 1996;490 (Pt 3) 775-81. Epub 1996/02/01.

[20] Potenza MA, Marasciulo FL, Chieppa DM, Brigiani GS, Formoso G, Quon MJ, et al. Insulin resistance in spontaneously hypertensive rats is associated with endothelial dysfunction characterized by imbalance between NO and ET-1 production. Am J Physiol Heart Circ Physiol 2005;289(2) H813-22. Epub 2005/03/29.

[21] Formoso G, Chen H, Kim JA, Montagnani M, Consoli A, Quon MJ. Dehydroepiandrosterone mimics acute actions of insulin to stimulate production of both nitric oxide and endothelin 1 via distinct phosphatidylinositol 3-kinase- and mitogen-activated protein kinase-dependent pathways in vascular endothelium. Mol Endocrinol 2006;20(5) 1153-63. Epub 2005/12/24.

[22] Potenza MA, Marasciulo FL, Tarquinio M, Quon MJ, Montagnani M. Treatment of spontaneously hypertensive rats with rosiglitazone and/or enalapril restores balance between vasodilator and vasoconstrictor actions of insulin with simultaneous improvement in hypertension and insulin resistance. Diabetes 2006;55(12) 3594-603. Epub 2006/11/30.

[23] Taniguchi CM, Emanuelli B, Kahn CR. Critical nodes in signalling pathways: insights into insulin action. Nat Rev Mol Cell Biol 2006;7(2) 85-96. Epub 2006/02/24.

[24] Maiorana A, O'Driscoll G, Taylor R, Green D. Exercise and the nitric oxide vasodilator system. Sports Med 2003;33(14) 1013-35. Epub 2003/11/06.

[25] Nisoli E, Clementi E, Paolucci C, Cozzi V, Tonello C, Sciorati C, et al. Mitochondrial biogenesis in mammals: the role of endogenous nitric oxide. Science 2003;299(5608) 896-9. Epub 2003/02/08.

[26] Nisoli E, Falcone S, Tonello C, Cozzi V, Palomba L, Fiorani M, et al. Mitochondrial biogenesis by NO yields functionally active mitochondria in mammals. Proc Natl Acad Sci U S A 2004;101(47) 16507-12. Epub 2004/11/17.

[27] Hermann C, Assmus B, Urbich C, Zeiher AM, Dimmeler S. Insulin-mediated stimulation of protein kinase Akt: A potent survival signaling cascade for endothelial cells. Arterioscler Thromb Vasc Biol 2000;20(2) 402-9. Epub 2000/02/17.

[28] Geraldes P, Yagi K, Ohshiro Y, He Z, Maeno Y, Yamamoto-Hiraoka J, et al. Selective regulation of heme oxygenase-1 expression and function by insulin through IRS1/ phosphoinositide 3-kinase/Akt-2 pathway. J Biol Chem 2008;283(49) 34327-36. Epub 2008/10/16.

[29] Chen YL, Messina EJ. Dilation of isolated skeletal muscle arterioles by insulin is endothelium dependent and nitric oxide mediated. Am J Physiol 1996;270(6 Pt 2) H2120-4. Epub 1996/06/01.

[30] Schroeder CA, Jr., Chen YL, Messina EJ. Inhibition of NO synthesis or endothelium removal reveals a vasoconstrictor effect of insulin on isolated arterioles. Am J Physiol 1999;276(3 Pt 2) H815-20. Epub 1999/03/10.

[31] Eringa EC, Stehouwer CD, Merlijn T, Westerhof N, Sipkema P. Physiological concentrations of insulin induce endothelin-mediated vasoconstriction during inhibition of NOS or PI3-kinase in skeletal muscle arterioles. Cardiovasc Res 2002;56(3) 464-71. Epub 2002/11/26.

[32] Eringa EC, Stehouwer CD, van Nieuw Amerongen GP, Ouwehand L, Westerhof N, Sipkema P. Vasoconstrictor effects of insulin in skeletal muscle arterioles are mediated by ERK1/2 activation in endothelium. Am J Physiol Heart Circ Physiol 2004;287(5) H2043-8. Epub 2004/04/03.

[33] Eringa EC, Stehouwer CD, Walburg K, Clark AD, van Nieuw Amerongen GP, Westerhof N, et al. Physiological concentrations of insulin induce endothelin-dependent vasoconstriction of skeletal muscle resistance arteries in the presence of tumor necrosis factor-alpha dependence on c-Jun N-terminal kinase. Arterioscler Thromb Vasc Biol 2006;26(2) 274-80. Epub 2005/12/03.

[34] Mikus CR, Rector RS, Arce-Esquivel AA, Libla JL, Booth FW, Ibdah JA, et al. Daily physical activity enhances reactivity to insulin in skeletal muscle arterioles of hyperphagic Otsuka Long-Evans Tokushima Fatty rats. J Appl Physiol 2010;109(4) 1203-10. Epub 2010/07/17.

[35] Scherrer U, Randin D, Tappy L, Vollenweider P, Jequier E, Nicod P. Body fat and sympathetic nerve activity in healthy subjects. Circulation 1994;89(6) 2634-40. Epub 1994/06/01.

[36] Steinberg HO, Brechtel G, Johnson A, Fineberg N, Baron AD. Insulin-mediated skeletal muscle vasodilation is nitric oxide dependent. A novel action of insulin to increase nitric oxide release. J Clin Invest 1994;94(3) 1172-9. Epub 1994/09/01.

[37] Straznicky NE, Lambert GW, Masuo K, Dawood T, Eikelis N, Nestel PJ, et al. Blunted sympathetic neural response to oral glucose in obese subjects with the insulin-resistant metabolic syndrome. Am J Clin Nutr 2009;89(1) 27-36. Epub 2008/12/06.

[38] Vincent MA, Dawson D, Clark AD, Lindner JR, Rattigan S, Clark MG, et al. Skeletal muscle microvascular recruitment by physiological hyperinsulinemia precedes increases in total blood flow. Diabetes 2002;51(1) 42-8. Epub 2002/01/05.

[39] Baron AD, Brechtel-Hook G, Johnson A, Cronin J, Leaming R, Steinberg HO. Effect of perfusion rate on the time course of insulin-mediated skeletal muscle glucose uptake. Am J Physiol 1996;271(6 Pt 1) E1067-72. Epub 1996/12/01.

[40] Baron AD. Hemodynamic actions of insulin. Am J Physiol 1994;267(2 Pt 1) E187-202. Epub 1994/08/01.

[41] Ebeling P, Bourey R, Koranyi L, Tuominen JA, Groop LC, Henriksson J, et al. Mechanism of enhanced insulin sensitivity in athletes. Increased blood flow, muscle glucose transport protein (GLUT-4) concentration, and glycogen synthase activity. J Clin Invest 1993;92(4) 1623-31. Epub 1993/10/01.

[42] Fugmann A, Sarabi M, Karlstrom B, Berne C, Lithell H, Lind L. Blood flow is an important determinant of forearm glucose uptake following a mixed meal. Acta Diabetol 2003;40(3) 113-7. Epub 2003/11/08.

[43] Laakso M, Edelman SV, Brechtel G, Baron AD. Decreased effect of insulin to stimulate skeletal muscle blood flow in obese man. A novel mechanism for insulin resistance. J Clin Invest 1990;85(6) 1844-52. Epub 1990/06/01.

[44] Coggins M, Lindner J, Rattigan S, Jahn L, Fasy E, Kaul S, et al. Physiologic hyperinsulinemia enhances human skeletal muscle perfusion by capillary recruitment. Diabetes 2001;50(12) 2682-90. Epub 2001/11/28.

[45] Clerk LH, Vincent MA, Jahn LA, Liu Z, Lindner JR, Barrett EJ. Obesity blunts insulin-mediated microvascular recruitment in human forearm muscle. Diabetes 2006;55(5) 1436-42.

[46] Muniyappa R, Karne RJ, Hall G, Crandon SK, Bronstein JA, Ver MR, et al. Oral glucosamine for 6 weeks at standard doses does not cause or worsen insulin resistance or endothelial dysfunction in lean or obese subjects. Diabetes 2006;55(11) 3142-50.

[47] DeFronzo RA, Gunnarsson R, Bjorkman O, Olsson M, Wahren J. Effects of insulin on peripheral and splanchnic glucose metabolism in noninsulin-dependent (type II) diabetes mellitus. J Clin Invest 1985;76(1) 149-55.

[48] Kelley DE, Reilly JP, Veneman T, Mandarino LJ. Effects of insulin on skeletal muscle glucose storage, oxidation, and glycolysis in humans. Am J Physiol 1990;258(6 Pt 1) E923-9.

[49] Lembo G, Napoli R, Capaldo B, Rendina V, Iaccarino G, Volpe M, et al. Abnormal sympathetic overactivity evoked by insulin in the skeletal muscle of patients with essential hypertension. J Clin Invest 1992;90(1) 24-9.

[50] Sakai K, Imaizumi T, Masaki H, Takeshita A. Intra-arterial infusion of insulin attenuates vasoreactivity in human forearm. Hypertension 1993;22(1) 67-73.

[51] Barrett EJ, Eggleston EM, Inyard AC, Wang H, Li G, Chai W, et al. The vascular actions of insulin control its delivery to muscle and regulate the rate-limiting step in skeletal muscle insulin action. Diabetologia 2009;52(5) 752-64. Epub 2009/03/14.

[52] Clark MG. Impaired microvascular perfusion: a consequence of vascular dysfunction and a potential cause of insulin resistance in muscle. Am J Physiol Endocrinol Metab 2008;295(4) E732-50.

[53] Rattigan S, Clark MG, Barrett EJ. Hemodynamic actions of insulin in rat skeletal muscle: evidence for capillary recruitment. Diabetes 1997;46(9) 1381-8. Epub 1997/09/01.

[54] Vincent MA, Clerk LH, Lindner JR, Klibanov AL, Clark MG, Rattigan S, et al. Microvascular recruitment is an early insulin effect that regulates skeletal muscle glucose uptake in vivo. Diabetes 2004;53(6) 1418-23. Epub 2004/05/27.

[55] Vincent MA, Clerk LH, Lindner JR, Price WJ, Jahn LA, Leong-Poi H, et al. Mixed meal and light exercise each recruit muscle capillaries in healthy humans. Am J Physiol Endocrinol Metab 2006;290(6) E1191-7.

[56] Ferri C, De Mattia G. The effect of insulin on endothelin-1 (ET-1) secretion in human cultured endothelial cell. Metabolism 1995;44(5) 689-90. Epub 1995/05/01.

[57] Ferri C, Pittoni V, Piccoli A, Laurenti O, Cassone MR, Bellini C, et al. Insulin stimulates endothelin-1 secretion from human endothelial cells and modulates its circulating levels in vivo. J Clin Endocrinol Metab 1995;80(3) 829-35. Epub 1995/03/01.

[58] Fagius J, Berne C. Increase in muscle nerve sympathetic activity in humans after food intake. Clin Sci (Lond) 1994;86(2) 159-67. Epub 1994/02/01.

[59] Fagius J. Sympathetic nerve activity in metabolic control--some basic concepts. Acta Physiol Scand 2003;177(3) 337-43. Epub 2003/03/01.

[60] Young CN, Deo SH, Chaudhary K, Thyfault JP, Fadel PJ. Insulin enhances the gain of arterial baroreflex control of muscle sympathetic nerve activity in humans. J Physiol 2010;588(Pt 18) 3593-603. Epub 2010/07/21.

[61] Mathias CJ, da Costa DF, Fosbraey P, Christensen NJ, Bannister R. Hypotensive and sedative effects of insulin in autonomic failure. Br Med J (Clin Res Ed) 1987;295(6591) 161-3. Epub 1987/07/18.

[62] Sartori C, Trueb L, Nicod P, Scherrer U. Effects of sympathectomy and nitric oxide synthase inhibition on vascular actions of insulin in humans. Hypertension 1999;34(4 Pt 1) 586-9. Epub 1999/10/16.

[63] Levesque M, Santure M, Pitre M, Nadeau A, Bachelard H. Cholinergic involvement in vascular and glucoregulatory actions of insulin in rats. Diabetes 2006;55(2) 398-404. Epub 2006/01/31.

[64] Randin D, Vollenweider P, Tappy L, Jequier E, Nicod P, Scherrer U. Effects of adrenergic and cholinergic blockade on insulin-induced stimulation of calf blood flow in humans. Am J Physiol 1994;266(3 Pt 2) R809-16. Epub 1994/03/01.

[65] Singleton JR, Smith AG, Russell JW, Feldman EL. Microvascular complications of impaired glucose tolerance. Diabetes 2003;52(12) 2867-73. Epub 2003/11/25.

[66] Singh R, Barden A, Mori T, Beilin L. Advanced glycation end-products: a review. Diabetologia 2001;44(2) 129-46. Epub 2001/03/29.

[67] Cameron NE, Eaton SE, Cotter MA, Tesfaye S. Vascular factors and metabolic interactions in the pathogenesis of diabetic neuropathy. Diabetologia 2001;44(11) 1973-88. Epub 2001/11/24.

[68] Bauersachs J, Bouloumie A, Fraccarollo D, Hu K, Busse R, Ertl G. Endothelial dysfunction in chronic myocardial infarction despite increased vascular endothelial nitric oxide synthase and soluble guanylate cyclase expression: role of enhanced vascular superoxide production. Circulation 1999;100(3) 292-8. Epub 1999/07/21.

[69] Hey-Mogensen M, Hojlund K, Vind BF, Wang L, Dela F, Beck-Nielsen H, et al. Effect of physical training on mitochondrial respiration and reactive oxygen species release in skeletal muscle in patients with obesity and type 2 diabetes. Diabetologia 2010;53(9) 1976-85. Epub 2010/06/08.

[70] Du XL, Edelstein D, Dimmeler S, Ju Q, Sui C, Brownlee M. Hyperglycemia inhibits endothelial nitric oxide synthase activity by posttranslational modification at the Akt site. J Clin Invest 2001;108(9) 1341-8. Epub 2001/11/07.

[71] Goldin A, Beckman JA, Schmidt AM, Creager MA. Advanced glycation end products: sparking the development of diabetic vascular injury. Circulation 2006;114(6) 597-605. Epub 2006/08/09.

[72] Schiffrin EL. Oxidative stress, nitric oxide synthase, and superoxide dismutase: a matter of imbalance underlies endothelial dysfunction in the human coronary circulation. Hypertension 2008;51(1) 31-2. Epub 2007/12/12.

[73] Raman CS, Li H, Martasek P, Kral V, Masters BS, Poulos TL. Crystal structure of constitutive endothelial nitric oxide synthase: a paradigm for pterin function involving a novel metal center. Cell 1998;95(7) 939-50. Epub 1999/01/06.

[74] Kim F, Tysseling KA, Rice J, Pham M, Haji L, Gallis BM, et al. Free fatty acid impairment of nitric oxide production in endothelial cells is mediated by IKKbeta. Arterioscler Thromb Vasc Biol 2005;25(5) 989-94. Epub 2005/02/26.

[75] Du X, Edelstein D, Obici S, Higham N, Zou MH, Brownlee M. Insulin resistance reduces arterial prostacyclin synthase and eNOS activities by increasing endothelial fatty acid oxidation. J Clin Invest 2006;116(4) 1071-80. Epub 2006/03/11.

[76] Ball LE, Berkaw MN, Buse MG. Identification of the major site of O-linked beta-N-acetylglucosamine modification in the C terminus of insulin receptor substrate-1. Mol Cell Proteomics 2006;5(2) 313-23. Epub 2005/10/26.

[77] Miele C, Riboulet A, Maitan MA, Oriente F, Romano C, Formisano P, et al. Human glycated albumin affects glucose metabolism in L6 skeletal muscle cells by impairing insulin-induced insulin receptor substrate (IRS) signaling through a protein kinase C alpha-mediated mechanism. J Biol Chem 2003;278(48) 47376-87. Epub 2003/09/13.

[78] Quehenberger P, Bierhaus A, Fasching P, Muellner C, Klevesath M, Hong M, et al. Endothelin 1 transcription is controlled by nuclear factor-kappaB in AGE-stimulated cultured endothelial cells. Diabetes 2000;49(9) 1561-70. Epub 2000/09/02.

[79] Chakravarthy U, Hayes RG, Stitt AW, McAuley E, Archer DB. Constitutive nitric oxide synthase expression in retinal vascular endothelial cells is suppressed by high glucose and advanced glycation end products. Diabetes 1998;47(6) 945-52. Epub 1998/05/30.

[80] Anderson HD, Rahmutula D, Gardner DG. Tumor necrosis factor-alpha inhibits endothelial nitric-oxide synthase gene promoter activity in bovine aortic endothelial cells. J Biol Chem 2004;279(2) 963-9. Epub 2003/10/29.

[81] Zhang L, Wheatley CM, Richards SM, Barrett EJ, Clark MG, Rattigan S. TNF-alpha acutely inhibits vascular effects of physiological but not high insulin or contraction. Am J Physiol Endocrinol Metab 2003;285(3) E654-60. Epub 2003/05/22.

[82] Sury MD, Frese-Schaper M, Muhlemann MK, Schulthess FT, Blasig IE, Tauber MG, et al. Evidence that N-acetylcysteine inhibits TNF-alpha-induced cerebrovascular endothelin-1 upregulation via inhibition of mitogen- and stress-activated protein kinase. Free Radic Biol Med 2006;41(9) 1372-83. Epub 2006/10/07.

[83] Xu JW, Morita I, Ikeda K, Miki T, Yamori Y. C-reactive protein suppresses insulin signaling in endothelial cells: role of spleen tyrosine kinase. Mol Endocrinol 2007;21(2) 564-73. Epub 2006/11/11.

[84] Loffreda S, Yang SQ, Lin HZ, Karp CL, Brengman ML, Wang DJ, et al. Leptin regulates proinflammatory immune responses. FASEB J 1998;12(1) 57-65. Epub 1998/01/23.

[85] Yamagishi SI, Edelstein D, Du XL, Kaneda Y, Guzman M, Brownlee M. Leptin induces mitochondrial superoxide production and monocyte chemoattractant protein-1 expression in aortic endothelial cells by increasing fatty acid oxidation via protein kinase A. J Biol Chem 2001;276(27) 25096-100. Epub 2001/05/09.

[86] Quehenberger P, Exner M, Sunder-Plassmann R, Ruzicka K, Bieglmayer C, Endler G, et al. Leptin induces endothelin-1 in endothelial cells in vitro. Circ Res 2002;90(6) 711-8. Epub 2002/04/06.

[87] Kougias P, Chai H, Lin PH, Lumsden AB, Yao Q, Chen C. Adipocyte-derived cytokine resistin causes endothelial dysfunction of porcine coronary arteries. J Vasc Surg 2005;41(4) 691-8. Epub 2005/05/06.

[88] Hennige AM, Stefan N, Kapp K, Lehmann R, Weigert C, Beck A, et al. Leptin down-regulates insulin action through phosphorylation of serine-318 in insulin receptor substrate 1. FASEB J 2006;20(8) 1206-8. Epub 2006/04/14.

[89] Verma S, Li SH, Wang CH, Fedak PW, Li RK, Weisel RD, et al. Resistin promotes endothelial cell activation: further evidence of adipokine-endothelial interaction. Circulation 2003;108(6) 736-40. Epub 2003/07/23.

[90] Chen H, Montagnani M, Funahashi T, Shimomura I, Quon MJ. Adiponectin stimulates production of nitric oxide in vascular endothelial cells. J Biol Chem 2003;278(45) 45021-6. Epub 2003/08/29.

[91] Hattori Y, Suzuki M, Hattori S, Kasai K. Globular adiponectin upregulates nitric oxide production in vascular endothelial cells. Diabetologia 2003;46(11) 1543-9. Epub 2003/10/11.

[92] Tesauro M, Schinzari F, Iantorno M, Rizza S, Melina D, Lauro D, et al. Ghrelin improves endothelial function in patients with metabolic syndrome. Circulation 2005;112(19) 2986-92. Epub 2005/11/02.

[93] Bonetti PO, Lerman LO, Lerman A. Endothelial dysfunction: a marker of atherosclerotic risk. Arterioscler Thromb Vasc Biol 2003;23(2) 168-75. Epub 2003/02/18.

[94] Mukai Y, Wang CY, Rikitake Y, Liao JK. Phosphatidylinositol 3-kinase/protein kinase Akt negatively regulates plasminogen activator inhibitor type 1 expression in vascular endothelial cells. Am J Physiol Heart Circ Physiol 2007;292(4) H1937-42. Epub 2006/12/19.

[95] Montagnani M, Golovchenko I, Kim I, Koh GY, Goalstone ML, Mundhekar AN, et al. Inhibition of phosphatidylinositol 3-kinase enhances mitogenic actions of insulin in endothelial cells. J Biol Chem 2002;277(3) 1794-9. Epub 2001/11/15.

[96] Baron AD. Insulin resistance and vascular function. J Diabetes Complications 2002;16(1) 92-102. Epub 2002/03/02.

[97] Steinberg HO, Chaker H, Leaming R, Johnson A, Brechtel G, Baron AD. Obesity/ insulin resistance is associated with endothelial dysfunction. Implications for the syndrome of insulin resistance. J Clin Invest 1996;97(11) 2601-10.

[98] Williams SB, Cusco JA, Roddy MA, Johnstone MT, Creager MA. Impaired nitric oxide-mediated vasodilation in patients with non-insulin-dependent diabetes mellitus. J Am Coll Cardiol 1996;27(3) 567-74. Epub 1996/03/01.

[99] Petrie JR, Ueda S, Webb DJ, Elliott HL, Connell JM. Endothelial nitric oxide production and insulin sensitivity. A physiological link with implications for pathogenesis of cardiovascular disease. Circulation 1996;93(7) 1331-3.

[100] Laine H, Yki-Jarvinen H, Kirvela O, Tolvanen T, Raitakari M, Solin O, et al. Insulin resistance of glucose uptake in skeletal muscle cannot be ameliorated by enhancing endothelium-dependent blood flow in obesity. J Clin Invest 1998;101(5) 1156-62.

[101] Balletshofer BM, Rittig K, Enderle MD, Volk A, Maerker E, Jacob S, et al. Endothelial dysfunction is detectable in young normotensive first-degree relatives of subjects with type 2 diabetes in association with insulin resistance. Circulation 2000;101(15) 1780-4.

[102] Hermann TS, Li W, Dominguez H, Ihlemann N, Rask-Madsen C, Major-Pedersen A, et al. Quinapril treatment increases insulin-stimulated endothelial function and adiponectin gene expression in patients with type 2 diabetes. J Clin Endocrinol Metab 2006;91(3) 1001-8.

[103] Winters B, Mo Z, Brooks-Asplund E, Kim S, Shoukas A, Li D, et al. Reduction of obesity, as induced by leptin, reverses endothelial dysfunction in obese (Lep(ob)) mice. J Appl Physiol 2000;89(6) 2382-90.

[104] Katakam PV, Ujhelyi MR, Hoenig ME, Miller AW. Endothelial dysfunction precedes hypertension in diet-induced insulin resistance. Am J Physiol 1998;275(3 Pt 2) R788-92.

[105] Abe H, Yamada N, Kamata K, Kuwaki T, Shimada M, Osuga J, et al. Hypertension, hypertriglyceridemia, and impaired endothelium-dependent vascular relaxation in mice lacking insulin receptor substrate-1. J Clin Invest 1998;101(8) 1784-8.

[106] Cusi K, Maezono K, Osman A, Pendergrass M, Patti ME, Pratipanawatr T, et al. Insulin resistance differentially affects the PI 3-kinase- and MAP kinase-mediated signaling in human muscle. J Clin Invest 2000;105(3) 311-20. Epub 2000/02/17.

[107] Egan BM, Greene EL, Goodfriend TL. Nonesterified fatty acids in blood pressure control and cardiovascular complications. Curr Hypertens Rep 2001;3(2) 107-16. Epub 2001/03/29.

[108] Hotamisligil GS, Arner P, Caro JF, Atkinson RL, Spiegelman BM. Increased adipose tissue expression of tumor necrosis factor-alpha in human obesity and insulin resistance. J Clin Invest 1995;95(5) 2409-15. Epub 1995/05/01.

[109] Miyazaki Y, Pipek R, Mandarino LJ, DeFronzo RA. Tumor necrosis factor alpha and insulin resistance in obese type 2 diabetic patients. Int J Obes Relat Metab Disord 2003;27(1) 88-94. Epub 2003/01/18.

[110] Ijzerman RG, Voordouw JJ, Van Weissenbruch MM, Yudkin JS, Serne EH, Delemarre-van de Waal HA, et al. TNF-alpha levels are associated with skin capillary recruitment in humans: a potential explanation for the relationship between TNF-alpha and insulin resistance. Clin Sci (Lond) 2006;110(3) 361-8. Epub 2005/12/01.

[111] Marasciulo FL, Montagnani M, Potenza MA. Endothelin-1: the yin and yang on vascular function. Curr Med Chem 2006;13(14) 1655-65. Epub 2006/06/22.

[112] Ishibashi KI, Imamura T, Sharma PM, Huang J, Ugi S, Olefsky JM. Chronic endothelin-1 treatment leads to heterologous desensitization of insulin signaling in 3T3-L1 adipocytes. J Clin Invest 2001;107(9) 1193-202. Epub 2001/05/09.

[113] Wilkes JJ, Hevener A, Olefsky J. Chronic endothelin-1 treatment leads to insulin resistance in vivo. Diabetes 2003;52(8) 1904-9. Epub 2003/07/29.

[114] Ottosson-Seeberger A, Lundberg JM, Alvestrand A, Ahlborg G. Exogenous endothelin-1 causes peripheral insulin resistance in healthy humans. Acta Physiol Scand 1997;161(2) 211-20. Epub 1997/11/21.

[115] Lillioja S, Young AA, Culter CL, Ivy JL, Abbott WG, Zawadzki JK, et al. Skeletal muscle capillary density and fiber type are possible determinants of in vivo insulin resistance in man. J Clin Invest 1987;80(2) 415-24. Epub 1987/08/01.

[116] Sjostrand M, Gudbjornsdottir S, Holmang A, Lonn L, Strindberg L, Lonnroth P. Delayed transcapillary transport of insulin to muscle interstitial fluid in obese subjects. Diabetes 2002;51(9) 2742-8. Epub 2002/08/28.

[117] Marwick TH, Hordern MD, Miller T, Chyun DA, Bertoni AG, Blumenthal RS, et al. Exercise training for type 2 diabetes mellitus: impact on cardiovascular risk: a scientific statement from the American Heart Association. Circulation 2009;119(25) 3244-62. Epub 2009/06/10.

[118] Clifford PS. Skeletal muscle vasodilatation at the onset of exercise. J Physiol 2007;583(Pt 3) 825-33. Epub 2007/07/07.

[119] Rattigan S, Wheatley C, Richards SM, Barrett EJ, Clark MG. Exercise and insulin-mediated capillary recruitment in muscle. Exerc Sport Sci Rev 2005;33(1) 43-8. Epub 2005/01/11.

[120] Miller VM, Vanhoutte PM. Enhanced release of endothelium-derived factor(s) by chronic increases in blood flow. Am J Physiol 1988;255(3 Pt 2) H446-51. Epub 1988/09/01.

[121] Goodyear LJ, Kahn BB. Exercise, glucose transport, and insulin sensitivity. Annu Rev Med 1998;49 235-61. Epub 1998/03/24.

[122] Henriksen EJ. Invited review: Effects of acute exercise and exercise training on insulin resistance. J Appl Physiol 2002;93(2) 788-96. Epub 2002/07/23.

[123] Frosig C, Richter EA. Improved insulin sensitivity after exercise: focus on insulin signaling. Obesity (Silver Spring) 2009;17 Suppl 3 S15-20. Epub 2009/11/21.

[124] Fujita S, Rasmussen BB, Cadenas JG, Drummond MJ, Glynn EL, Sattler FR, et al. Aerobic exercise overcomes the age-related insulin resistance of muscle protein metabolism by improving endothelial function and Akt/mammalian target of rapamycin signaling. Diabetes 2007;56(6) 1615-22. Epub 2007/03/14.

[125] Hamburg NM, McMackin CJ, Huang AL, Shenouda SM, Widlansky ME, Schulz E, et al. Physical inactivity rapidly induces insulin resistance and microvascular dysfunction in healthy volunteers. Arterioscler Thromb Vasc Biol 2007;27(12) 2650-6. Epub 2007/10/13.

[126] Kim K, Valentine RJ, Shin Y, Gong K. Associations of visceral adiposity and exercise participation with C-reactive protein, insulin resistance, and endothelial dysfunction in Korean healthy adults. Metabolism 2008;57(9) 1181-9. Epub 2008/08/16.

[127] Chadderdon SM, Belcik JT, Smith E, Pranger L, Kievit P, Grove KL, et al. Activity restriction, impaired capillary function, and the development of insulin resistance in lean primates. Am J Physiol Endocrinol Metab 2012;303(5) E607-13. Epub 2012/06/29.

[128] Helmerhorst HJ, Wijndaele K, Brage S, Wareham NJ, Ekelund U. Objectively measured sedentary time may predict insulin resistance independent of moderate- and vigorous-intensity physical activity. Diabetes 2009;58(8) 1776-9. Epub 2009/05/28.

[129] Katzmarzyk PT. Physical activity, sedentary behavior, and health: paradigm paralysis or paradigm shift? Diabetes 2010;59(11) 2717-25. Epub 2010/10/29.

[130] Hamdy O, Ledbury S, Mullooly C, Jarema C, Porter S, Ovalle K, et al. Lifestyle modification improves endothelial function in obese subjects with the insulin resistance syndrome. Diabetes Care 2003;26(7) 2119-25. Epub 2003/07/02.

[131] Mustata S, Chan C, Lai V, Miller JA. Impact of an exercise program on arterial stiffness and insulin resistance in hemodialysis patients. J Am Soc Nephrol 2004;15(10) 2713-8. Epub 2004/10/07.

[132] Xiang L, Naik J, Hester RL. Exercise-induced increase in skeletal muscle vasodilatory responses in obese Zucker rats. Am J Physiol Regul Integr Comp Physiol 2005;288(4) R987-91. Epub 2004/12/18.

[133] Sebai M, Lu S, Xiang L, Hester RL. Improved functional vasodilation in obese Zucker rats following exercise training. Am J Physiol Heart Circ Physiol 2011;301(3) H1090-6. Epub 2011/06/21.

[134] Bunker AK, Arce-Esquivel AA, Rector RS, Booth FW, Ibdah JA, Laughlin MH. Physical activity maintains aortic endothelium-dependent relaxation in the obese type 2 diabetic OLETF rat. Am J Physiol Heart Circ Physiol 2010;298(6) H1889-901. Epub 2010/03/23.

[135] Bender SB, Newcomer SC, Harold Laughlin M. Differential vulnerability of skeletal muscle feed arteries to dysfunction in insulin resistance: impact of fiber type and daily activity. Am J Physiol Heart Circ Physiol 2011;300(4) H1434-41. Epub 2011/02/15.

[136] Martin JS, Padilla J, Jenkins NT, Crissey JM, Bender SB, Rector RS, et al. Functional adaptations in the skeletal muscle microvasculature to endurance and interval sprint training in the type 2 diabetic OLETF rat. J Appl Physiol 2012;113(8) 1223-32. Epub 2012/08/28.

[137] Mikus CR, Roseguini BT, Uptergrove GM, Morris EM, Rector RS, Libla JL, et al. Voluntary wheel running selectively augments insulin-stimulated vasodilation in arterioles from white skeletal muscle of insulin-resistant rats. Microcirculation 2012;19(8) 729-38. Epub 2012/07/19.

[138] Minami A, Ishimura N, Harada N, Sakamoto S, Niwa Y, Nakaya Y. Exercise training improves acetylcholine-induced endothelium-dependent hyperpolarization in type 2 diabetic rats, Otsuka Long-Evans Tokushima fatty rats. Atherosclerosis 2002;162(1) 85-92. Epub 2002/04/12.

[139] Sakamoto S, Minami K, Niwa Y, Ohnaka M, Nakaya Y, Mizuno A, et al. Effect of exercise training and food restriction on endothelium-dependent relaxation in the Otsuka Long-Evans Tokushima Fatty rat, a model of spontaneous NIDDM. Diabetes 1998;47(1) 82-6. Epub 1998/01/08.

[140] Juel C, Holten MK, Dela F. Effects of strength training on muscle lactate release and MCT1 and MCT4 content in healthy and type 2 diabetic humans. J Physiol 2004;556(Pt 1) 297-304. Epub 2004/01/16.

[141] Muoio DM, Koves TR. Skeletal muscle adaptation to fatty acid depends on coordinated actions of the PPARs and PGC1 alpha: implications for metabolic disease. Appl Physiol Nutr Metab 2007;32(5) 874-83. Epub 2007/12/07.

[142] Thyfault JP, Cree MG, Zheng D, Zwetsloot JJ, Tapscott EB, Koves TR, et al. Contraction of insulin-resistant muscle normalizes insulin action in association with in-

creased mitochondrial activity and fatty acid catabolism. Am J Physiol Cell Physiol 2007;292(2) C729-39. Epub 2006/10/20.

[143] McAllister RM, Newcomer SC, Pope ER, Turk JR, Laughlin MH. Effects of chronic nitric oxide synthase inhibition on responses to acute exercise in swine. J Appl Physiol 2008;104(1) 186-97. Epub 2007/11/03.

[144] Kojda G, Hambrecht R. Molecular mechanisms of vascular adaptations to exercise. Physical activity as an effective antioxidant therapy? Cardiovasc Res 2005;67(2) 187-97.

[145] Montagnani M, Quon MJ. Insulin action in vascular endothelium: potential mechanisms linking insulin resistance with hypertension. Diabetes Obes Metab 2000;2(5) 285-92. Epub 2001/02/28.

[146] Vincent MA, Clerk LH, Rattigan S, Clark MG, Barrett EJ. Active role for the vasculature in the delivery of insulin to skeletal muscle. Clin Exp Pharmacol Physiol 2005;32(4) 302-7. Epub 2005/04/07.

Chapter 2

Beta-Cell Function and Failure in Type 2 Diabetes

Simona Popa and Maria Mota

Additional information is available at the end of the chapter

http://dx.doi.org/10.5772/56467

1. Introduction

Type 2 diabetes mellitus (T2DM) results from a combination of genetic and environmental factors that induces tissue insulin resistance and beta-cell failure.

The purpose of the present chapter is to focus on beta-cell function under physiological conditions and to review the potential beta-cell failure mechanisms, the place in natural history of T2DM and implication for treatment of beta-cell dysfunction.

2. Normal beta-cell function

The main role of beta-cell is to synthesize and secrete insulin in order to maintain circulating glucose levels within physiological range. Although there exist several triggers of insulin secretion like nutrients (amino acids such as leucine, glutamine in combination with leucine, nonesterified fatty acid), hormones, neurotransmitters and drugs (sulfonylurea, glinides), glucose represents the main physiological insulin secretagogue [1].

According to the most widely accepted hypothesis, insulin secretion is a multistep process initiated with glucose transport into beta-cell through specific transporters (GLUT1 and GLUT2 in particular) and phosphorylation by glucokinase, which directs metabolic flux through glycolysis, producing pyruvate as the terminal product of the pathway [2]. Pyruvate then enters the mitochondria and is decarboxylated to acetyl-CoA, which enters the tricarboxylic acid cycle.

The tricarboxylic acid cycle proper begins with a condensation of acetyl-CoA and oxaloacetate, to form citrate, a reaction catalysed by citrate synthase. Aconitase catalyses the convertion of citrate to isocitrate. NAD-linked isocitrate dehydrogenase then oxidatively decarboxylates isocitrate to form α-ketoglutarate. The α-ketoglutarate is oxidised to succinyl-CoA in a reaction catalysed by α-ketoglutarate dehydrogenase. Succinyl-CoA synthase then catalyses the conversion of succinyl-CoA to succinate, with the concomitant phosphorylation of GDP to GTP. Succinate dehydrogenase catalyses the oxidation of succinate to fumarate. Fumarase catalyses the conversion of fumarate to malate and after that malate dehydrogenase catalyses the final step of the tricarboxylic acid cycle, oxidising malate to oxaloacetate and producing NADH.

Three pathways enable the recycling of the tricarboxylic acid cycle intermediates into and out of mitochondrion, allowing a continuous production of intracellular messengers [3-5]. These three cycles share, as a common terminal step, the conversion of malate to pyruvate concomitant with the production of cytosolic NADPH.

- Pyruvate/malate shuttle,

The oxaloacetate produced by pyruvate carboxylase is converted to malate by mitochondrial malate dehydrogenase. Malate exits the mitochondria to the cytoplasm where it is subsequently oxidised to pyruvate concomitant with the production of NADPH by cytosolic malic enzyme. Pyruvate then re-enters mitochondria for the next round of carboxylation by pyruvate carboxylase [3-5].

- Pyruvate/citrate shuttle,

The oxaloacetate condenses with acetyl-CoA to form citrate, mediated by citrate synthase. Citrate then exits the mitochondrion to the cytoplasm where it is converted back to oxaloacetate and acetyl-CoA by ATP-citrate lyase. Oxaloacetate is converted by cytosolic malate dehydrogenase to malate before being converted to pyruvate by malic enzyme. Acetyl-CoA is subsequently carboxylated by acetyl-CoA carboxylase to form malonyl-CoA for conversion to long-chain acyl-CoA by fatty acid synthase. Malonyl-CoA inhibits carnitine palmitoyl transferase-1, which transports fatty acyl-CoA into mitochondria where it is oxidised, leading to increase in long-chain acyl-CoAs in the cytosol [3-5].

- Pyruvate/isocitrate shuttle

The oxaloacetate condenses with acetyl-CoA to form citrate, mediated by citrate synthase before being converted to isocitrate. Isocitrate then exits the mitochondrion to the cytoplasm via the citrate/isocitrate transporter and is converted to α-ketoglutarate by the cytosolic NADPdependent isocitrate dehydrogenase. α-Ketoglutarate is further converted to oxaloacetate via the malate/aspartate shuttle as mentioned earlier in the NADH shuttle system [3-5].

The sequences of the tricarboxylic acid cycle and of shuttle pathways are followed by synthesis of reducing equivalents (NADH, NADPH, FADH2) in the mitochondria and transfer them to the electron transport chain [6]. The NADPH oxidase complex in the plasma membrane is also activated through protein kinase C, which is activated by fatty acid derived signalling molecules.

These events result in an enhanced ratio of ATP to ADP in the cytoplasm, which determines the closure of the ATP-sensitive K^+ channels, depolarization of the plasma membrane, influx of extracellular Ca^{2+} and activation of exocytosis which takes place in several stages including recruitment, docking, priming, and fusion of insulin granules to the beta-cell plasma membrane [1,6,7].

Two independent studies, using diazoxide for maintaining the ATP-sensitive K^+ channels in the open state or mice in which the ATP-sensitive K^+ channels were disrupted, indicated that glucose –stimulated insulin secretion can also occur independently of ATP-sensitive K^+ channels activity [8].

Under physiological conditions, there is a hyperbolic relation between insulin secretion and insulin sensitivity. Classically, glucose-stimulated insulin secretion is characterized by a first phase, which ends within a few minutes, and prevents or decreases glucose concentration and a more prolonged second phase in which insulin is released proportionally to the plasma glucose [9].

In addition, it has been demonstrated that the release of insulin is oscillatory, with relatively stable rapid pulses occurring at every 8-10 minutes which are superimposed on low-frequency oscillations [10]. In humans the amplitude of insulin oscillations is 100-fold higher in the portal vein than in the systemic circulation implying preferential hepatic extraction of insulin pulses.

Research to further understand the roles of these pathways may provide strategies for future therapies of T2DM.

3. Place of beta-cell dysfunction in natural history of type 2 diabetes

T2DM is a progressive condition caused by genetic and environmental factors that induce tissue insulin resistance and beta-cell dysfunction.

Based on the United Kingdom Prospective Diabetes Study (UKPDS) and on the Belfast Diabetes Study, it is estimated that at diagnosis of T2DM, beta-cell function is already reduced by 50-60% and that this reduction of beta-cell function seems to start with 10-12 years before the appearance of hyperglycemia [11,12].

Several lines of evidence indicated that there is no hyperglycemia without beta-cell dysfunction [13,14].

In most subjects with obesity-induced insulin resistance developing increased insulin secretion, insulin gene expression and beta-cell mass, these compensatory mechanisms can succeed to maintain glucose homeostasis and avoidance of diabetes mellitus [13-15]. Progression from beta-cell compensation to failure in the face of obesity-induced insulin resistance occurs in a subset of genetically predisposed individuals who fail to adequately compensate for the increased insulin demand, leading to glucolipotoxicity.

In this phase insulin secretion (in relation to the degree of insulin resistance), insulin gene expression and beta-cell mass are reduced, causing increased levels of glucose and free fatty acids [13,14].

In T2DM, the typical beta-cell functional alterations are represented by:

- change of threshold for insulin secretion triggering with relatively selective loss of responsivity to glucose compared to other insulin secretagogues like arginin or glibenclamide
- alteration of insulin secretion oscillatory patterns with impairment of both high frequency and ultradian oscillations
- reduced or absent first phase insulin secretion initially to intravenous glucose and then to mixed meal ingestion
- prolongation of second phase of insulin secretion
- gradual, time-dependent irreversible damage to cellular components of insulin production [9,13-18].

Longitudinal studies in humans have clearly demonstrated that beta-cell function deteriorates during the years. In the phase which precedes overt diabetes the decline of beta-cell function is slow but constant (2% per year) [19]. After the development of overt hyperglycemia there appears a significant acceleration (18% per year) in beta-cell failure, and the beta-cell function deteriorates regardless of the therapeutic regimen [11,19,20]. The accelerated beta-cell dysfunction is the consequence of glucolipotoxicity. Consequent deterioration in metabolic equilibrium with increasing levels of glucose and free fatty acids, enhance and accelerate beta-cell dysfunction, lead to beta-cell apoptosis that does not seems to be adequately compensated by regenerative process and subsequent decrease of beta-cell mass.

4. Potential mechanism and modulators of beta-cell failure

The main focus of the present chapter is on potential beta-cell failure mechanisms in T2DM.

The initial alterations in beta-cell function are likely to reflect intrinsic defects, whereas the accelerated beta-cell dysfunction which mainly occurs after the development of overt hyperglycemia is the consequence of glucolipotoxicity [21]. This reflects a genetic predisposition for beta-cell defect, whereas the subsequent beta-cell failure may be a consequence of concomitant environmental conditions.

Schematic representation of the role of cellular dysfunction in the natural history of T2DM is included in Figure 1.

5. Genetic factors

Several genes associated with increased risk of developing T2DM have been identified in genome-wide association studies [22]. There were detected several genetic variants of genes that confer risk of diabetes by interfering with next three mechanisms:

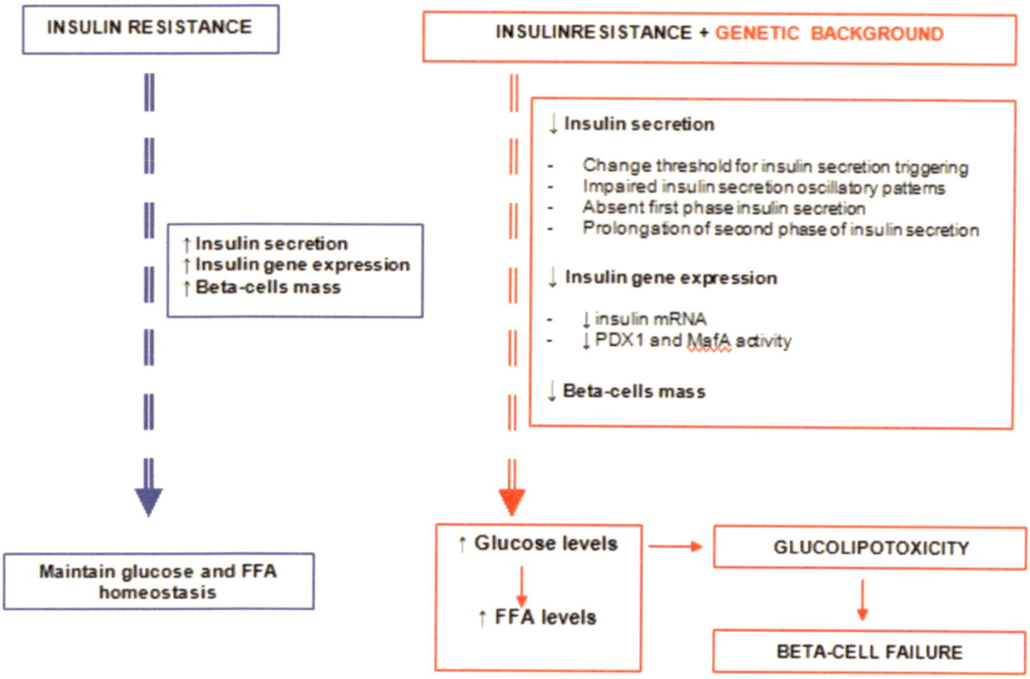

Figure 1. Place of beta-cell dysfunction in natural history of type 2 diabetes

- **reduction of insulin secretion**: KCNJ11 [23], HHEX [24-26], SLC30A8 [25,27], CAPN10 [28], CDKAL1 [29,30], IGF2BP2 [30,31], CDKN2A/B [24], MTNR1B [32-36], CDC123/CAMK1D [35,37], JAZF1 [37] and TSPAN8/LGR5 [37]
- **impairment in incretin release**: TCF7L2 [38], WFS1 [39], KCNQ1 [40,41]
- **impaired proinsulin-to-insulin conversion**: CAPN10 [28], TCF7L2 [42-45], SLC30A8 [42], and CDKAL1 [42]

The most important so far type 2 diabetes risk gene, *TCF7L2*, interferes with all three mechanisms.

TCF7L2 encodes for the transcription factor TCF7L2, which induces the expression of a number of genes including the insulin gene [46], the gene coding for intestinal proglucagon [47], genes coding for proprotein convertases 1 and 2 [43] and for proteins important in insulin exocytosis and genes critical for beta-cell proliferation [48].

The *KCNJ11* encodes the Kir6.2 subunit of the ATP-sensitive K channel of beta-cells. Genetic variation in this gene obviously affects the beta-cell excitability and insulin secretion [23].

HHEX encodes a transcription factor necessary for the organogenesis of the ventral pancreas [49] and two SNPs (rs1111875, rs7923837) in *HHEX* were found to be associated with reduced insulin secretion [24-26].

SLC30A8 encodes the protein zinc transporter 8, which provide zinc for maturation, storage and exocytosis of the insulin granules [50]. Variants in this gene show to be associated with reduced glucose-stimulated insulin secretion [25,27] and alterations in proinsulin to insulin conversion [42].

A number of SNPs, and particularly the rs10830963 C>G SNP in *MTNR1B* enhances the melatonin-induced inhibition of insulin secretion, leading to higher fasting blood glucose and an increased T2DM risk [32-36].

The molecular mechanisms by which loci or SNPs in the other genes affect glucose-stimulated insulin secretion, proinsulin to insulin conversion and incretin-induced insulin secretion are currently poorly understood.

These observations suggest that a genetic predisposition is associated with an initially beta-cell intrinsic defect which, in case of increased demand as it is in obesity and insulin resistance, leads to beta-cell failure.

6. Glucolipotoxicity

Growing evidence indicated that long-term elevated plasma levels of glucose and fatty acids contribute to beta-cell function decline, a phenomenon known as glucolipotoxicity. Glucolipotoxicity differs from beta-cell exhaustion, which is a reversible phenomenon characterized by depletion of insulin granules due to prolonged exposure to secretagogues. Unlike glucolipotoxicity, beta-cell exhaustion is associated with normal production of insulin [51].

A multitude of clinical and preclinical studies have shown deleterious effects of beta-cells chronic exposure to elevated glucose levels.

Given the existence of insulin resistance and a predisposing genetic background, there occurs the elevation of glucose levels, which lead to progressively decreases of insulin secretion, insulin gene expression and insulin promoter activity (PDX-1 and MAFA) [52,53].

Chronic exposure of beta-cells to hyperglycemia can also induce beta-cells apoptosis by increasing proapoptotic genes expression (Bad, Bid, Bik) while antiapoptotic gene expression Bcl-2 remains unaffected [54].

There is a strong relationship between glucotoxicity and lipotoxicity. Thus, hyperglycemia increases malonyl-CoA levels, leading to the inhibition of carnitine palmitoyl transferase-1 and subsequently to decreased oxidation of fatty acids and lipotoxicity [52].

Increased fatty acids in the pancreas leads to intrapancreatic accumulation of triglycerides [55]. Lim E et al showed that the intrapancreatic fat is associated with beta-cell dysfunction and that sustained negative energy balance induces restoration of beta-cellular function [56].

Elevated levels of glucose and saturated fatty acids in beta cells, stimulates AMP-activated protein kinase, which contributes to increased expression of sterolregulatory-element-binding-protein-1c (SREBP1c), leading to increased lipogenesis [57]. Glucose also increases the expression of liver X receptor which then contributes to enhancing SREBP1c expression [58].

Several studies provide evidence that prolonged exposure of beta cells to elevated levels of free fatty acids can have many deleterious effects, such as:

- **Decreased glucose-stimulated insulin secretion** [52,59]. Activation of the isoform of protein kinase C (PKCε) by free fatty acids which has been suggested as a possible candidate signaling molecule underlying the decrease in insulin secretion [60].
- **Impaired insulin gene exepression** by down-regulation of PDX-1 and MafA insulin gene promoter activity [61]. PDX-1 is affected in its ability to translocate to the nucleus, whereas MafA is affected at the level of its expression [61]. Free fatty acid impairs insulin gene expression only in the presence of hyperglycemia [62]. Palmitate affects both insulin gene expression and insulin secretion, unlike oleate which affects only insulin secretion [63]. Extracellular-regulated kinase (ERK) 1/2 phosphorylation, JNK activation, PKB phosphorylation, and Per- Arnt-Sim kinase (PASK) signalling pathways mediate the palmitate-induced inhibition of insulin gene expression [64,65].
- **Increased synthesis of ceramides** from palmitic acid only, which impairs insulin gene expression, induces cell death by inhibition of anti-apoptotic protein Bcl2, without affecting insulin secretion [62,66,67].
- **Up regulation of UCP2**, leading to reduction of glucose-stimulated ATP generation [68].
- **Activation** of the **oxidative stress** [69].
- **Activation** of the **unfolded protein response** [70].
- **Increased beta-cells inflammation** by stimulations of NF-kB, Il-1β and IFN-γ production [71].
- **Beta-cell apoptosis** mediated by several mechanism including increased ceramides, caspases activation, decreased Bcl2 expression, inflammation response, ROS production, unfolded protein response [66,72-74]. Saturated fatty acids are involved in beta-cell apoptosis, whereas unsaturated fatty acids are usually protective [75,76].
- **Increased islet amyloid polypeptide** [77].

Recent studies suggest that deleterious effect of free fatty acids are expressed mostly in the presence of hyperglycemia which inhibits fatty acid oxidation and lead to accumulation of cytosolic long-chain acyl-CoA esters, generation of ceramide and lipid partitioning.

Increased intracellular cholesterol content may also lead to glucolipotoxicity. ATP-binding cassette transporter subfamily A member 1 (ABCA1) appears to mediate intracellular cholesterol accumulation and impaired insulin secretion, probably at the level of insulin exocytosis [78].

Several mechanisms have been proposed for glucolipotoxicity induced beta-cell dysfunction and death, such as: endoplasmic reticulum stress, mitochondrial dysfunction and reactive oxygen species production, islet inflammation and islet amyloid polypeptide increasing.

There is a significant relationship between the mechanisms triggered by glucolipotoxicy, creating thus a vicious cycle that eventually leads to beta-cell failure (Figure 2.).

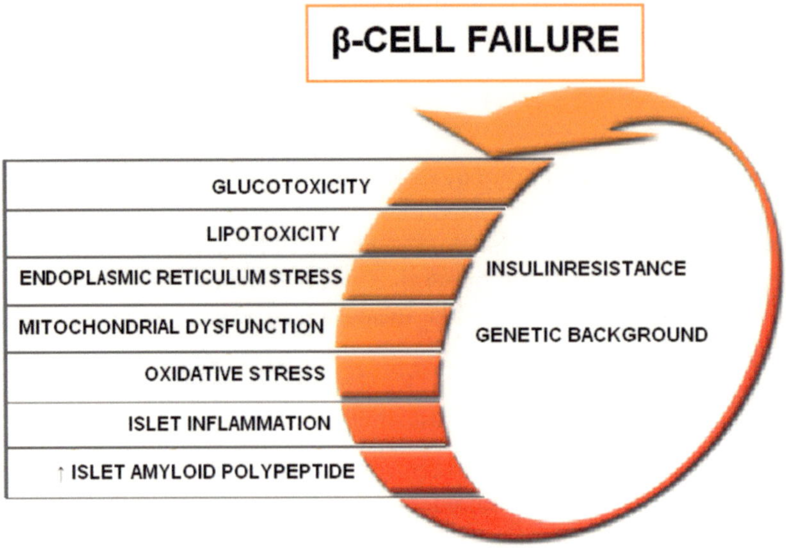

Figure 2. Potential mechanism of beta-cell failure

7. Endoplasmic reticulum stress

The endoplasmic reticulum is responsible for the protein synthesis, being involved in protein translation, folding and assessing quality before protein secretion. Chronic hyperglycemia, elevated levels of saturated free fatty acid in beta-cell lead to sustained increased demand for insulin biosynthesis via increasing both insulin transcription and translation, and to increased proinsulin biosynthesis, which generates a heavy load of unfolded/misfolded proteins in the endoplasmic reticulum lumen. Accumulation of unfolded and misfolded protein in the endoplasmic reticulum lumen may impose endoplasmic reticulum stress [79,80]. Inflammatory cytokines such as IL-1β and IFN-γ, can also cause endoplasmic reticulum stress [72].

Endoplasmic reticulum stress induced beta-cell activation of an adaptive system named unfolded protein response by which it attenuates protein translation, increases protein folding and promotes misfolded protein degradation [81,82].

The unfolded protein response is mediated by activation of three transmembrane endoplasmic reticulum proteins:

- protein-kinase-RNA-(PKR-) like ER kinase/ eukaryotic translation initiation factor 2 alpha (PERK/eIF2α)
- inositol-requiring 1/X-box- bindingprotein-1 (IRE1/XBP-1)

- activating transcription factor 6 (ATF6) [83,84].

The unfolded protein response alleviates endoplasmic reticulum stress by inducing a number of downstream responses:

- decrease new proteins arrival into the endoplasmic reticulum by attenuation of further translation of mRNAs via PERK/eIF2α activation. Thus, it prevents additional protein misfolding and further accumulation of unfolded protein;
- increase the folding capacity of the endoplasmic reticulum to deal with misfolded proteins via the induction of endoplasmic reticulum chaperones. This response is mediated by IRE1/XBP-1 and ATF6;
- increase in the extrusion of misfolded proteins from the endoplasmic reticulum and subsequently endoplasmic reticulum-associated protein degradation (ERAD);
- triggering apoptosis by the activation of CCAAT/enhancendoplasmic reticulum-binding homologous protein (CHOP) [81-85].

Among the three different signaling pathways of the endoplasmic reticulum stress response (ATF6, IRE1/XBP-1, and PERK/eIF2α), only ATF6 down-regulated PDX-1 and MafA insulin gene promote activity [86].

Extensive studies have indicated that IRE1/XBP-1 activation leads to increases of proinsulin biosynthesis under transient high glucose conditions like postprandial hyperglycemia and, by contrast, causes suppression of insulin mRNA expression and increases insulin mRNA degradation under chronic high glucose exposure [87,88].

Given these data it can be asserted that the appearance of endoplasmic reticulum stress, due to glucolipotoxicity and inflammatory cytokines, can lead to beta-cell dysfunction and death.

8. Mitochondrial dysfunction and ROS production

Beta cell mitochondria play a key role in the insulin secretion process, not only by providing energy in the form of ATP to support insulin secretion, but also by synthesising metabolites that can act as factors that couple glucose sensing to insulin granule exocytosis [3].

Mitochondrial dysfunction and abnormal morphology occur before the onset of hyperglycemia and play an important role in beta-cell failure [89]. In diabetic state, the proteins from the mitochondrial inner membrane are decreased, and also may exist transcriptional changes of the mitochondrial proteins [89].

Mitochondrial dysfunction, induced by glucolipotoxicity, plays a pivotal role in beta-cell failure and leads to increased ROS production as a result of metabolic stress.

Under conditions of normoglycemia production of ROS - superoxide anion (O2 • -) and hydrogen peroxide (H2O2) - is performed during mitochondrial electron transport or through several oxidoreductases and metal-catalyzed oxidation of metabolites [90].

In the presence of hyperglycemia, hexosamine, sorbitol, PCK activations and Shiff reaction pathways, may represent sources of oxidative stress along with oxidative phosphorylation and auto-oxidation of glucose in mitochondria [91].

ROS effects can be reduced by activation of antioxidant enzymes including: superoxide dismutase, which converts O2 • - to H2O2 and also catalase, glutathione peroxide and peroxiredoxin that convert H2O2 into oxygen and water. Levels of antioxidant enzymes in beta cells are very low (catalase and glutathione peroxide levels were much lower than those of superoxide dismutase), making beta cells be vulnerable to oxidative stress [92].

Low concentrations of ROS contribute to increased glucose-stimulated insulin secretion, but only in the presence of glucose-induced elevations in ATP [93].

Li N. et al indicated that transient oxidative stress can cause impaired glucose-induced ATP generation, decreased glucose-stimulated insulin secretion, down-regulation of the respiratory chain and increased mitochondrial ROS production [94]. All these effects are reversible in time after transient increase ROS.

Chronic and significant elevation of ROS, resulted from an imbalance between ROS production and scavenging by endogenous antioxidants, may lead to beta-cell failure [95,96].

Persistent oxidative stress mediates beta-cell failure through several different mechanisms, including:

- **Decreased insulin secretion**. Oxidative stress inhibits the respiratory chain, allowing the transfer of electrons to molecular oxygen to form superoxide, and also inhibits the enzymes involved in glucose metabolism (glyceraldehyde-3-phosphate-dehydrogenase from glycolytic pathway and aconitase from Krebs cycle), leading to reduced ATP / ADP ratio and to impaired insulin release [97-100].
- **Decreased insulin gene expression** via activation of JNK pathway, also by posttranscriptional loss of PDX-1 and posttranslational loss of MafA [21,52,101].
- **Islet inflammation** due to activation of NF-kB pathway [102].
- **Mitochondrial dysfunction** by promoting DNA fragmentation, the peroxidation of membrane phospholipids such as cardiolipin [16,103].
- **Increased islet amyloid polypeptide and endoplasmic reticulum stress** [104-106].
- **Beta-cells apoptosis** by activating uncoupling protein-2 which results in proton leak leading to reduced ATP synthesis [107].
- **Beta-cells lipid accumulation** via SREBP1c [108].

The antioxidant effect varies depending on the type of exposure of beta cells to ROS. Thus, under beta-cells exposure to low concentrations of ROS, antioxidants lower the insulin secretion [109,110]. Instead, under the glucolipotoxicity, antioxidants increase the insulin secretion and reduce beta cell apoptosis [108].

9. Islet inflammation

Several studies indicated that prolonged exposure of pancreatic islet to chronic hyperglycemia, increased levels of saturated fatty acids and increased ROS may trigger the production of inflammatory cytokines such as nuclear transcription factor kB (NF-κB), interleukin-1β (IL-1β) and γ-interferon (IFN-γ), TNF-α, leading to beta-cells dysfunction and apoptosis [71]. Additionally, beta-cells dysfunction and apoptosis may also be triggered by pro-inflammatory signals from other organs, such as adipose tissue [111,112].

Transient activation of **NF-κB** may be beneficial to insulin secretion [113], but persistent activation of NF-kB may induce cell dysfunction, due to the reduction of beta-cell protein expression including insulin, GLUT-2, and PDX-1 concomitant with an increase in iNOS expression [113].

There is good evidence that NF-kB mediates direct or through Il-1β, the activation of inducible nitric oxide synthase (iNOS) in pancreatic beta-cells which, in turn, induces the expression of proinflammatory genes, interferes with electron transfer and inhibits ATP synthesis in mitochondria, leading to decreased insulin secretion and beta-cell dysfunction [114].

Chronic exposure of beta-cell to inflammatory cytokines, like **Il-1β, IFN-γ or TNF-α**, can cause endoplasmic reticulum stress and the unfolded protein response activation in beta-cells, and also beta-cells apoptosis [72,115]. Because, as indicated by Donath *et al*, the apoptotic beta-cells can provoke, in turn, an immune response, a vicious cycle may develop [115].

Another cytokine involved in beta-cells dysfunction is the PANcreatic DERived factor (PANDER). PANDER is a novel cytokine that is highly expressed in pancreatic islets [116]. Because PANDER protein is cosecreted with insulin from pancreatic beta-cells [117] it is reasonable to speculate that PANDER may regulate the insulin secretion process [117, 118].

The adipocytokines released by adipocytes, including adiponectin, leptin, resistin, visfatin, TNF-α and IL-6, may also modulate the beta-cell function and survival.

Adiponectin receptors were found in human and rat pancreatic beta-cells and their expression can be upregulated by unsaturated fatty acid but not by saturated fatty acid [116].

In beta-cells, adiponectin may induce phosphorylation of acetyl coenzyme A carboxylase, leading to inhibition of fatty acids synthesis and preventing of lipid accumulation in beta-cells [112]. There have not been revealed significant effects of adiponectin on basal or glucose-stimulated insulin secretion [112].

Leptin is another adipocytokine that may interfere with beta-cell function and survival. In studies on animal model, leptin has been shown to inhibit insulin secretion via activation of ATP-regulated potassium channels and reduction in cellular cAMP level [116], inhibit insulin biosynthesis by activating suppressor of cytokine signalling 3 (SOCS3) [119], suppress acetylcholine-induced insulin secretion [116] and induce the expression of inflammatory genes [120].

Studies performed on human islets indicated that chronic exposure to leptin stimulates the release of IL-1β and inhibits UCP2 expression, leading to beta-cell dysfunction and apoptosis [111].

Other adipocytokines including TNF-α, IL-6, resistin, visfatin may also modulate beta-cell function and survival, although it is unclear whether the amount released into the circulation is sufficient to affect beta-cells [111].

10. Islet amyloid polypeptide

Human islet amyloid polypeptide (amylin) is expressed almost exclusively in beta-cells and is costored and coreleased with insulin in response to beta-cells secretagogues. Glucolipotoxicity causes increased insulin requirement and those lead to increased production of both insulin and amylin. High concentrations of amyloid are toxic to beta-cells and have been implicated in beta-cell dysfunction and apoptosis [121,122].

The effect of Islet amyloid polypeptide on beta-cell function is not fully elucidated.

Studies *in vivo* have shown that the islet amyloid polypeptide inhibits the first and second phase of glucose-stimulated insulin secretion, but this occurs only at concentrations of islet amyloid polypeptide above physiological range [77].

In vitro studies, however, have yielded contradictory results. Several studies have indicated an inhibitory effect of islet amyloid polypeptide physiological concentration on insulin secretion [123], but other studies have reported no inhibitory effect of islet amyloid polypeptide on insulin release [77].

One possible explanation for these inconsistent results may be that there was not taken into consideration the islet amyloid polypeptide increased tendency to aggregate in amyloid-like fibrils and thus the effects of early islet amyloid polypeptide preparations may be questioned [77].

Studies performed on islet amyloid polypeptide knock-out or transgenic mice, using pure and fully active islet amyloid polypeptide, suggest that islet amyloid polypeptide limits glucose-induced insulin secretion [124].

11. Beta-cell failure — Implication for treatment

Understanding the causes for beta-cell failure is of capital importance to develop new and more effective therapeutic strategies.

Taking into consideration the existence of early beta-cell dysfunction and the significant reduction of beta-cell mass in the natural history of T2DM as well as the progressive character of these pathophysiological modifications, **insulin therapy** could be an important option for obtaining and maintaining an optimal glycemic control.

Li Y. et al indicated that short term intensive insulin therapy of newly diagnosed T2DM may improve cell function, by restoring the first-phase insulin secretion and by decreased proinsulin/insulin ratio [125].

Increasing insulin levels by exogenous insulin administration for the control of hyperglycemia may appear initially contraindicated in patients with evidence of insulin resistance, so it is imperative to simultaneously address insulin resistance with metformin.

Several lines of evidence indicated that **metformin** could improve beta-cell function and survival. Incubation of T2DM islets with metformin was associated with increased insulin content, insulin mRNA expression and glucose responsiveness, and also with reduced cell apoptosis by normalization of caspase 3 and caspase 8 activities [103].

It has been shown that metformin, and also the **PPAR gamma agonists** can protect beta-cell from deleterious effects of glucolipotoxicity [126,127].

Other therapeutic options for beta-cell protection, such as **incretins** are actually under debate. Recent studies have shown that effects of incretins vary depending on the time of exposure of beta-cells to GLP-1 or GLP-1R agonists.

Thus, acute exposure of cells to the incretins, determine stimulation of glucose-dependent insulin secretion, the subacute exposure leads to increased insulin biosynthesis and insulin gene transcription, whereas the chronic exposure induces beta-cell mass increase by stimulation of cell proliferation, neogenesis and inhibition of cell apoptosis [21].

Changing profile of cytokines secretion from pancreatic beta-cells and also of adipocytokines may be promising therapeutic options for beta-cellular dysfunction [116].

Future advances in the area of beta-cell failure mechanism and modulators may lead to the identification of possible novel therapeutic strategies.

Author details

Simona Popa and Maria Mota*

*Address all correspondence to: mmota53@yahoo.com

Department of Diabetes, Nutrition and Metabolic Diseases; University of Medicine and Pharmacy, Craiova, Romania

References

[1] MacDonald MJ, et al. Perspective: emerging evidence for signaling roles of mitochondrial anaplerotic products in insulin secretion. Am J Physiol Endocrinol Metab 2005;288:E1–15

[2] Matschinsky FM. Glucokinase as glucose sensor and metabolic signal generator in pancreatic betacells and hepatocytes. Diabetes 1990;39:647–652.

[3] Jitrapakdee S, et al. Regulation of insulin secretion: role of mitochondrial signalling. Diabetologia. 2010;53(6):1019-32.

[4] Farfari S, et al. Glucose-regulated anaplerosis and cataplerosis in pancreatic beta-cells: possible implication of a pyruvate/citrate shuttle in insulin secretion. Diabetes 2000;49:718–726.

[5] MacDonald MJ. Feasibility of a mitochondrial pyruvate malate shuttle in pancreatic islets. Further implication of cytosolic NADPH in insulin secretion. J Biol Chem 1995;270:20051–20058.

[6] MacDonald MJ, et al. Pyruvate dehydrogenase and pyruvate carboxylase. Sites of pretranslational regulation by glucose of glucose-induced insulin release in pancreatic islets. J Biol Chem 1991;266:22392–22397.

[7] Seino S, et al. Pancreatic beta-cell signaling: toward better understanding of diabetes and its treatment. Proc Jpn Acad Ser B Phys Biol Sci. 2010;86(6):563-77

[8] Gembal M, et al. Evidence that glucose can control insulin release independently from its action on ATP-sensitive K+ channels in mouse B cells. J Clin Invest 1992;89:1288–1295.

[9] Del Prato S, et al. Phasic insulin release and metabolic regulation in type 2 diabetes. Diabetes 2002;51(suppl 1):S109–16.

[10] Porksen N. The in vivo regulation of pulsatile insulin secretion. Diabetologia 2002;45:3–20.

[11] U.K. prospective diabetes study 16. Overview of 6 years' therapy of type II diabetes: a progressive disease. U.K. Prospective Diabetes Study Group. Diabetes 1995, 19: 125– 129.

[12] Levy J, et al. Beta-cell deterioration determines the onset and rate of progression of secondary dietary failure in type 2 diabetes mellitus: the 10-year followup of the Belfast Diet Study. Diabet Med 1998, 15: 290– 296.

[13] Kahn SE. The relative contribution of insulin resistance and beta-cell dysfunction to the pathophysiology of type 2 diabetes.Diabetologia 2003;46:3–19.

[14] Marchetti P, et al. An overview of pancreatic beta-cell defects in human type 2 diabetes: Implications for treatment. Regul Pept. 2008.7;146(1-3):4-11.

[15] Buchanan TA. Pancreatic beta-cell loss and preservation in type 2 diabetes. Clin Ther 2003;25(suppl B):32–46.

[16] Del Guerra S., et al. Functional and molecular defects of pancreatic islets in human type 2 diabetes. Diabetes, 2005;54(3):727–735.

[17] Ma ZA, et al. Mitochondrial Dysfunction and ?-Cell Failure in Type 2 DiabetesMellitus. Exp Diabetes Res. 2012;2012:703538.

[18] Marchetti P, et al. The pancreatic beta-cell in human type 2 diabetes. Nutr Metab Cardiovasc Dis 2006;16(suppl 1):S3–6.

[19] Lencioni C, et al. Beta-cell failure in type 2 diabetes mellitus. Curr Diab Rep. 2008;8(3):179-84.

[20] Poitout V, et al. Glucolipotoxicity of the pancreatic beta cell. Biochim Biophys Acta. 2010 Mar;1801(3):289-98.

[21] Wajchenberg BL. Beta-cell failure in diabetes and preservation by clinical treatment.Endocr Rev. 2007;28(2):187-218.

[22] Schäfer SA, et al. New type 2 diabetes risk genes provide new insights in insulin secretion mechanisms. Diabetes Res Clin Pract. 2011;93 Suppl 1:S9-24.

[23] Villareal DT, et al. Kir6.2 variant E23K increases ATP-sensitive K+ channel activity and is associated with impaired insulin release and enhanced insulin sensitivity in adults with normal glucose tolerance. Diabetes 2009;58(8):1869–78.

[24] Grarup N, et al. Studies of association of variants near the HHEX, CDKN2A/B, and IGF2BP2 genes with type 2 diabetes and impaired insulin release in 10,705 Danish subjects: validation and extension of genome-wide association studies. Diabetes 2007;56(12):3105–11.

[25] Staiger H, et al. Polymorphisms within novel risk loci for type 2 diabetes determine beta-cell function. PLoS ONE 2007;2(9):e832.

[26] Staiger H, et al. A candidate type 2 diabetes polymorphism near the HHEX locus affects acute glucose-stimulated insulin release in European populations: results from the EUGENE2 study. Diabetes 2008;57(2):514–7.

[27] Boesgaard TW, et al. The common SLC30A8 Arg325Trp variant is associated with reduced first-phase insulin release in 846 non-diabetic offspring of type 2 diabetes patients – the EUGENE2 study. Diabetologia 2008; 51(5):816–20.

[28] Turner MD, et al. Calpain facilitates actin reorganization during glucose-stimulated insulin secretion. Biochem Biophys Res Commun 2007;352(3):650–5.

[29] Stancakova A, et al. Single-nucleotide polymorphism rs7754840 of CDKAL1 is associated with impaired insulin secretion in nondiabetic offspring of type 2 diabetic subjects and in a large sample of men with normal glucose tolerance. J Clin Endocrinol Metab 2008;93(5):1924–30.

[30] Groenewoud MJ, et al. Variants of CDKAL1 and IGF2BP2 affect first-phase insulin secretion during hyperglycaemic clamps. Diabetologia 2008;51(9):1659–63.

[31] Palmer ND, et al. Quantitative trait analysis of type 2 diabetes susceptibility loci identified from whole genome association studies in the Insulin Resistance Atherosclerosis Family Study. Diabetes 2008;57(4):1093–100.

[32] Lyssenko V, et al. Common variant in MTNR1B associated with increased risk of type 2 diabetes and impaired early insulin secretion. Nat Genet 2009;41(1):82–8.

[33] Mulder H, et al. Melatonin receptors in pancreatic islets: good morning to a novel type 2 diabetes gene. Diabetologia 2009;52(7):1240–9.

[34] Langenberg C, et al. Common genetic variation in the melatonin receptor 1B gene (MTNR1B) is associated with decreased early-phase insulin response Diabetologia 2009; 52(8):1537–42.

[35] Simonis-Bik AM, et al. Gene variants in the novel type 2 diabetes loci CDC123/CAMK1D, THADA, ADAMTS9, BCL11A, and MTNR1B affect different aspects of pancreatic beta-cell function. Diabetes 2010; 59(1):293–301.

[36] Stancakova A, et al. Association of 18 confirmed susceptibility loci for type 2 diabetes with indices of insulin release, proinsulin conversion, and insulin sensitivity in 5,327 nondiabetic Finnishmen. Diabetes 2009;58(9):2129–36.

[37] Grarup N, et al. Association testing of novel type 2 diabetes risk alleles in the JAZF1, CDC123/CAMK1D, TSPAN8, THADA, ADAMTS9, and NOTCH2 loci with insulin release, insulin sensitivity, and obesity in a population-based sample of 4,516 glucose-tolerant middle-aged Danes. Diabetes 2008;57(9):2534–40.

[38] Shu L, et al. Decreased TCF7L2 protein levels in type 2 diabetes mellitus correlate with downregulation of GIPand GLP-1 receptors and impaired beta- cell function. Hum Mol Genet 2009;18(13):2388–99.

[39] Sparso T, et al. Impact of polymorphisms in WFS1 on prediabetic phenotypes in a population-based sample of middle-aged people with normal and abnormal glucose regulation. Diabetologia 2008;51(9):1646–52.

[40] Mussig K, et al. Association of type 2 diabetes candidate polymorphisms in KCNQ1 with incretin and insulin secretion. Diabetes 2009;58(7):1715– 20.

[41] Jonsson A, et al. A variant in the KCNQ1 gene predicts future type 2 diabetes and mediates impaired insulin secretion. Diabetes 2009;58(10):2409–13.

[42] Kirchhoff K, et al. Polymorphisms in the TCF7L2, CDKAL1 and SLC30A8 genes are associated with impaired proinsulin conversion. Diabetologia 2008;51(4):597–601.

[43] Loos RJ, et al. TCF7L2 polymorphisms modulate proinsulin levels and beta-cell function in a British Europid population. Diabetes 2007;56(7):1943–7.

[44] Stolerman ES, et al. TCF7L2 variants are associated with increased proinsulin/insulin ratios but not obesity traits in the Framingham Heart Study. Diabetologia 2009; 52(4): 614–20.

[45] Da Silva X, et al. TCF7L2 regulates late events in insulin secretion from pancreatic islet beta-cells. Diabetes 2009;58(4):894–905.

[46] Loder MK, et al. TCF7L2 controls insulin gene expression and insulin secretion in mature pancreatic beta-cells. Biochem Soc Trans 2008;36(Pt 3):357–9.

[47] Yi F, et al. TCF-4 mediates cell type-specific regulation of proglucagon gene expression by beta-catenin and glycogen synthase kinase-3beta. J Biol Chem 2005; 280(2): 1457–64.

[48] Rulifson IC, et al. Wnt signaling regulates pancreatic beta cell proliferation. Proc Natl Acad Sci U S A 2007;104(15):6247–52.

[49] Bort R, et al. Hex homeobox gene-dependent tissue positioning is required for organogenesis of the ventral pancreas. Development 2004;131(4):797–806.

[50] Chimienti F, et al. In vivo expression and functional characterization of the zinc transporter ZnT8 in glucose-induced insulin secretion. J Cell Sci 2006;119(Pt 20):4199–4206.

[51] Van Raalte DH, et al. Glucolipotoxicity and beta cells in type 2 diabetes mellitus: Target for durable therapy? Diabetes Res Clin Pract. 2011;93 S 1:S37-46.

[52] Poitout V, et al. Glucolipotoxicity: fuel excess and beta-cell dysfunction. Endocr Rev 2008;29(3):351–66.

[53] Khaldi MZ, et al. Increased glucose sensitivity of both triggering and amplifying pathways of insulin secretion in rat islets cultured for 1 wk in high glucose. Am J Physiol Endocrinol Metab 2004;287:E207–17.

[54] Patane G, et al. Role of ATP production and uncoupling protein-2 in the insulin secretory defect induced by chronic exposure to high glucose or free fatty acids and effects of peroxisome proliferator-activated receptor-gamma inhibition. Diabetes 2002;51:2749–56.

[55] Gastaldelli A. Role of beta-cell dysfunction, ectopic fat accumulation and insulin resistance in the pathogenesis of type 2 diabetes mellitus. Diabetes Res Clin Pract. 2011;93 Suppl 1:S60-5

[56] Lim EL, et al. Reversal of type 2 diabetes: normalisation of beta cell function in association with decreased pancreas and liver triacylglycerol. Diabetologia. 2011;54(10): 2506-14.

[57] Wang X, et al. Palmitate activates AMPactivated protein kinase and regulates insulin secretion from beta cells. Biochem Biophys Res Commun 2007;352:463–468.

[58] Choe SS, et al. Chronic activation of liver X receptor induces beta-cell apoptosis through hyperactivation of lipogenesis: liver X receptor-mediated lipotoxicity in pancreatic beta-cells. Diabetes 2007;56:1534-543.

[59] Gravena C, et al. Acute effects of fatty acids on insulin secretion from rat and human islets of Langerhans. J Endocrinol 2002, 173: 73– 80.

[60] Schmitz-Peiffer C, et al. Inhibition of PKCepsilon improves glucose-stimulated insulin secretion and reduces insulin clearance. Cell Metab 2007;6:320–328.

[61] Hagman DK, et al. Palmitate inhibits insulin gene expression by altering PDX-1 nuclear localization and reducing MafA expression in isolated rat islets of Langerhans. J Biol Chem 2005;280:32413–8.

[62] Kelpe CL, et al. Palmitate inhibition of insulin gene expression is mediated at the transcriptional level via ceramide synthesis. J Biol Chem 2003;278:30015–30021

[63] Moore PC, et al. Evidence against the involvement of oxidative stress in fatty acid inhibition of insulin secretion. Diabetes. 2004;53:2610–2616

[64] Solinas G, et al. Saturated fatty acids inhibit induction of insulin gene transcription by JNK-mediated phosphorylation of insulin-receptor substrates. Proc Natl AcadSciUSA 2006;103:16454–9.

[65] Fontes G, et al. Involvement of Per-Arnt-Sim knase and extracellular-regulated kinases- ? in palmitate inhibition of insulin gene expression in pancreatic b-cells. Diabetes 2009;58:2048–58.

[66] Lupi R, et al. Prolonged exposure to free fatty acids has cytostatic and pro-apoptotic effects on human pancreatic islets: evidence that beta-cell death is caspase mediated, partially dependent on ceramide pathway, and Bcl-2 regulated. Diabetes 2002;51:1437–42.

[67] Maedler K, et al. Monounsaturated fatty acids prevent the deleterious effects of palmitate and high glucose on human pancreatic beta-cell turnover and function. Diabetes 2003;52:726-33.

[68] Joseph JW, et al. Free fatty acid-induced beta-cell defects are dependent on uncoupling protein 2 expression. J Biol Chem 2004;279:51049-56.

[69] Kim JW, et al. Glucolipotoxicity in Pancreatic ?-Cells. Diabetes Metab J 2011;35:444-450

[70] Laybutt DR, et al. Endoplasmic reticulum stress contributes to beta cell apoptosis in type 2 diabetes. Diabetologia 2007;50:752-63.

[71] Haopeng Yang, et al. The role of fatty acid metabolism and lipotoxicity in pancreatic beta-cell injury: identification of potential therapeutic targets. Acta Pharmaceutica Sinica B 2012;2(4):396–402

[72] Cunha DA, et al. Initiation and execution of lipotoxic ER stress in pancreatic betacells. J Cell Sci 2008;121:2308–2318.

[73] Bachar E, et al. Glucose amplifies fatty acid-induced endoplasmic reticulum stress in pancreatic beta-cells via activation of mTORC1. PloS One 2009;4:e4954.

[74] Gwiazda KS, et al. Effects of palmitate on ER and cytosolic Ca2+ homeostasis in beta-cells. Am J Physiol Endocrinol Metab 2009;296:E690–701.

[75] Cnop M, et al. Inverse relationship between cytotoxicity of free fatty acids in pancreatic islet cells and cellular triglyceride accumulation. Diabetes 2001;50:1771–1777.

[76] El-Assaad W, et al. Saturated fatty acids synergize with elevated glucose to cause pancreatic beta-cell death. Endocrinology 2003;144:4154–4163.

[77] Westermark P, et al. Islet amyloid polypeptide, islet amyloid, and diabetes mellitus. Physiol Rev 91: 795–826, 2011

[78] Brunham LR, et al. Beta-Cell ABCA1 influences insulin secretion, glucose homeostasis and response to thiazolidinedione treatment. Nat Med 2007;13:340–347

[79] Fonseca SG, et al. Endoplasmic reticulum stress and pancreatic ?-cell death. Trends Endocrinol Metab. 2011; 22(7): 266–274

[80] Scheuner D, et al. Control of mRNA translation preserves endoplasmic reticulum function in beta cells and maintains glucose homeostasis. Nat Med. 2005; 11:757–764.

[81] Zhang K, et al. Protein folding in the endoplasmic reticulum and the unfolded protein response. Handb Exp Pharmacol. 2006;(172):69-91.

[82] Ron D, et al. Signal integration in the endoplasmic reticulum unfolded protein response. Nat Rev Mol Cell Biol. 2007;8(7):519-29.

[83] Eizirik DL, et al. The Role for Endoplasmic Reticulum Stress in Diabetes Mellitus. Endocr Rev. 2008;29(1):42-61.

[84] Kaufman RJ, et al. The unfolded protein response in nutrient sensing and differentiation. Nat Rev Mol Cell Biol. 2002;3(6):411-21.

[85] Karunakaran U, et al. Guards and Culprits in the Endoplasmic Reticulum: Glucolipotoxicity and ?-Cell Failure in Type II Diabetes. Exp Diabetes Res. 2012;2012:639762.

[86] Seo HY, et al. Endoplasmic reticulum stress-induced activation of activating transcription factor 6 decreases insulin gene expression via up-regulation of orphan nuclear receptor small heterodimer partner. Endocrinology. 2008;149(8):3832-41.

[87] Kim MK, et al. Endoplasmic reticulum stress and insulin biosynthesis: a review. Exp Diabetes Res. 2012;2012:509437.

[88] Lipson KL, et al. Regulation of insulin biosynthesis in pancreatic beta cells by an endoplasmic reticulum-resident protein kinase IRE1. Cell Metab. 2006;4(3):245-54.

[89] Lu H, et al. Molecular and Metabolic Evidence for Mitochondrial Defects Associated With ?-Cell Dysfunction in a Mouse Model of Type 2 Diabetes. Diabetes. 2010;59(2): 448-59

[90] Forman HJ, et al. Reactive oxygen species and cell signaling: respiratory burst in macrophage signaling. Am J Respir Crit Care Med. 2002;15;166(12 Pt 2):S4-8.

[91] Kowluru A. Regulatory roles for small G proteins in the pancreatic beta-cell: lessons from models of impaired insulin secretion. Am J Physiol Endocrinol Metab. 2003;285(4):E669-84.

[92] Prentki M, et al. Islet beta cell failure in type 2 diabetes. J Clin Invest 2006;116:1802–12.

[93] Wollheim CB, et al. Beta-cell mitochondria and insulin secretion: messenger role of nucleotides and metabolites. Diabetes. 2002;51 Suppl 1:S37-42.

[94] Li N, et al. Transient oxidative stress damages mitochondrial machinery inducing persistent beta-cell dysfunction. J Biol Chem. 2009;28;284(35):23602-12.

[95] Pi J, et al. ROS signaling, oxidative stress and Nrf2 in pancreatic beta-cell function. Toxicol Appl Pharmacol. 2010;1;244(1):77-83.

[96] Evans JL, et al. Are oxidative stress-activated signaling pathways mediators of insulin resistance and beta-cell dysfunction?. Diabetes. 2003;52(1):1-8.

[97] Rebelato E, et al. Control of the intracellular redox state by glucose participates in the insulin secretion mechanism. PLoS One. 2011;6(8):e24507.

[98] Gier B, et al. Suppression of KATP channel activity protects murine pancreatic beta cells against oxidative stress. J Clin Invest. 2009;119(11):3246-56.

[99] Rebelato E, et al. Low doses of hydrogen peroxide impair glucose-stimulated insulin secretion via inhibition of glucose metabolism and intracellular calcium oscillations. Metabolism. 2010;59(3):409-13.

[100] Delgado EH, et al. Mitochondrial respiratory dysfunction and oxidative stress after chronic malathion exposure. Neurochem Res. 2006;31(8):1021-5.

[101] Harmon JS, et al. Oxidative stress-mediated, post-translational loss of MafA protein as a contributing mechanism to loss of insulin gene expression in glucotoxic beta-cells. J Biol Chem 2005;280:11107-1113

[102] Robertson RP, et al. Beta-Cell glucose toxicity, lipotoxicity, and chronic oxidative stress in type 2 diabetes. Diabetes. 2004;53(Suppl 1):S119–S124

[103] Marchetti P, et al. Pancreatic islets from type 2 diabetic patients have functional defects and increased apoptosis that are ameliorated by metformin. J Clin Endocrinol Metab 2004;89:5535–41.

[104] Rieusset J. Mitochondria and endoplasmic reticulum: mitochondria-endoplasmic reticulum interplay in type 2 diabetes pathophysiology. Int J Biochem Cell Biol. 2011;43(9):1257-62.

[105] Leem J, et al. Interaction between mitochondria and the endoplasmic reticulum: implications for the pathogenesis of type 2 diabetes mellitus. Exp Diabetes Res. 2012;2012:242984

[106] Li XL, et al. Involvement of mitochondrial dysfunction in human islet amyloid polypeptide-induced apoptosis in INS-1E pancreatic beta cells: An effect attenuated by phycocyanin. Int J Biochem Cell Biol. 2011;43(4):525-34.

[107] Pi J, et al. Persistent oxidative stress due to absence of uncoupling protein 2 associated with impaired pancreatic beta-cell function. Endocrinology. 2009;150(7):3040-8.

[108] Lim S, et al. Mitochondria-targeted Antioxidants Protect Pancreatic Beta- cells against Oxidative Stress and Improve Insulin Secretion in Glucotoxicity and Glucolipotoxicity. Cell Physiol Biochem. 2011;28(5):873-86.

[109] Pi J, et al. Reactive oxygen species as a signal in glucose-stimulated insulin secretion. Diabetes. 2007;56(7):1783-91.

[110] Leloup C, et al. Mitochondrial reactive oxygen species are obligatory signals for glucose-induced insulin secretion. Diabetes. 2009;58(3):673-81.

[111] Maedler K, et al. Leptin modulates beta-cell expression of IL-1 receptor antagonist and release of IL-1beta in human islets. Proc Natl Acad Sci USA. 2004;101:8138–8143

[112] Staiger K, et al. Adiponectin is functionally active in human islets but does not affect insulin secretory function or beta-cell lipoapoptosis. J Clin Endocrinol Metab. 2005;90(12):6707-13.

[113] Papaccio G, et al. A biphasic role of nuclear transcription factor (NF)-kappaB in the islet beta-cell apoptosis induced by interleukin (IL)-1beta. J Cell Physiol. 2005;204(1): 124-30.

[114] Yang J, et al. Leucine metabolism in regulation of insulin secretion from pancreatic beta cells. Nutr Rev. 2010;68(5):270-9.

[115] Donath MY, et al. Inflammatory mediators and islet beta-cell failure: a link between type 1 and type 2 diabetes. J Mol Med. 2003;81:455–470

[116] Wang C, et al. Cytokines in the Progression of Pancreatic ?-Cell Dysfunction. Int J Endocrinol. 2010;2010:515136.

[117] Burkhardt BR, et al. PDX-1 interaction and regulation of the Pancreatic Derived Factor (PANDER, FAM3B) promoter. Biochim Biophys Acta. 2008;1779(10):645-51

[118] Robert-Cooperman CE, et al. Targeted disruption of pancreatic-derived factor (PANDER, FAM3B) impairs pancreatic beta-cell function. Diabetes. 2010;59(9):2209-18.

[119] Laubner K, et al. Inhibition of preproinsulin gene expression by leptin induction of suppressor of cytokine signaling 3 in pancreatic beta-cells. Diabetes. 2005;54(12): 3410-7.

[120] Hekerman P, et al. Leptin induces inflammation-related genes in RINm5F insulinoma cells. BMC Mol Biol. 2007;23;8:41.

[121] Hoppener JWM, et al. Role of amyloid in type 2 diabetes mellitus. Int J Biochem Cell Biol 2006;38:726–36.

[122] Ritzel RA, et al. Human islet amyloid polypeptide oligomers disrupt cell coupling, induce apoptosis, and impair insulin secretion in isolated human islets. Diabetes 2007;56:65–71.

[123] Zhu T, et al. Islet amyloid polypeptide acts on glucose-stimulated beta cells to reduce voltage-gated calcium channel activation, intracellular Ca2_ concentration, and insulin secretion. Diabetes Metab Res Rev. 2011;27(1):28-34

[124] Cluck MW, et al. The regulation of amylin and insulin gene expression and secretion. Pancreas 30: 1–14, 2005.

[125] Li Y, et al. Induction of long-term glycemic control in newly diagnosed type 2 diabetic patients is associated with improvement of beta-cell function. Diabetes Care. 2004;27:2597–2602

[126] Lupi R, et al. Lipotoxicity in human pancreatic islets and the protective effect of metformin. Diabetes 2002;51 (Suppl 1):S134–7.

[127] Lupi R, et al. Rosiglitazone prevents the impairment of human islet function induced by fatty-acids. Evidence for a role PPAR-{gamma}2 in the modulation of insulin secretion. Am J Physiol Endocrinol Metab 2004;286:E560–7.

Chapter 3

Epigenetics of Glucose Metabolism and the Basis for T2DM Interventions

Katia Cristina Portero McLellan,
Rodrigo Minoro Manda, Lance A. Sloan and
Roberto Carlos Burini

Additional information is available at the end of the chapter

http://dx.doi.org/10.5772/56507

1. Introduction

1.1. Epigenetic regulation

Type 2 Diabetes Mellitus (T2DM) is a disorder caused by genetic interactions between susceptible loci and environmental influences. Simple Mendelian inheritance patterns have failed to describe the genetics of T2DM. In studies looking at single nucleotide polymorphisms, which have been linked to the development of T2DM, no disease-causing mutations have been discovered (Pinney & Simmons, 2009).

Contemporary genome-wide association studies identified at least 17 genetic loci associated with T2DM (Florez, 2008). Epigenetic modification of gene expression is one mechanism by which genetic susceptibility and environmental insults can lead to T2DM (Pinney & Simmons, 2009). Epigenetic changes are defined as mitotically inheritable alterations in gene expression that are not related to changes in DNA sequence (Pinney & Simmons, 2009).

Much of recent progress in understanding epigenetic phenomena is directly attributable to technologies that allow researchers to pinpoint the genomic location of proteins that package and regulate access to DNA. The advent of DNA microarrays and DNA sequencing allows many of these technologies to be applied to the whole genome (Bernardo et al, 2008, Ozanne et al, 2005, Kim et al, 2005).

There are at least two distinct mechanisms through which epigenetic information can be inherited: histone modifications and DNA methylation (Pinney & Simmons, 2009). The amino termini of histones can be modified by acetylation, methylation, sumoylation, phosphorylation, glycosylation and ADP ribosylation, with acetylation and methylation being the most common modifications. Increased acetylation induces transcription activation whereas transcription repression is usually induced by decreased acetylation. On the other hand methylation of histone is associated with both transcription repression and activation.

The other mechanism of epigenetic regulation is DNA methylation. In which cytosine base is modified, silencing and contributing to X chromosomal inactivation, genomic imprinting, and transcriptional regulation of tissue-specific genes during cellular differentiation. Histone methylation can influence DNA methylation patterns and vice versa (Pinney & Simmons, 2009).

2. T2DM as a thrifty phenotype

Humans represent a thrifty species relative to some other mammals. This indicates that metabolic adaptations had a crucial role in the emergence of present day Homo Sapien lineage, in particular in buffering reproduction from ecological stochasticity (Wells, 2009). In other words, thrifty implies some degree of prosperity deriving from earlier frugality and a careful management of resources. Its use in reference to human metabolism spread after an influential article by James Neel proposed that certain genes relevant to metabolism could have been favored by natural selection in certain environmental conditions (Neel, 1962).

T2DM is considered a thrifty phenotype exceptionally efficient in the intake and utilization of food with basic difference of a quick insulin trigger in response to food-induced hyperglycemia. The survival benefit of this phenotype was to minimize urinary glucose loss when fasting was promptly replaced by feasting, leading to the more efficient utilization of food and tissue-distribution of plasma glucose. A quick insulin trigger that helped primitive man survive famine by storing energy more efficient, now leads eventually to T2DM.

Cahill & Wen (1967) theory postulates that the more insulin resistance an individual, the more efficient will be his ability to decrease proteolysis (and preserve lean body mass) when faced with caloric deprivation. The more efficient one in conserving muscle protein the better changes to withstand prolonged periods of deprivation, to be able to hunt successfully and to escape if preyed upon.

Skeletal muscle takes 80% of insulin-dependent glucose uptake. Hence muscle insulin resistance conserves glucose for utilization by the central nervous system decreasing the amount of muscle protein needed to be converted to glucose (neoglucogenesis).

Summing up the mentioned theories, relative insulin resistance evolved to aid metabolic partitioning between physical activity and other functions during constrained energy supply (Chakravarthy & Booth, 2004) which in turn relate to the selective pressure of a low glycaemic load diet with high meat content (McMichael, 2001) as our gather-hunter ancestors use to eat over ten thousand years ago.

The concept of metabolic programming during early life was prompted nearly 20 years ago in a series of Britain studies by Barker et al, (1989) and Hales et al, (1991) in which the prevalence of T2DM was measured in 64 years old men, whose birth weight records were available. It was shown that those with lower birth weight and lower weight at 1 year of age had a higher prevalence of T2DM and glucose intolerance (Hales et al, 1991) than did those with a normal birthweight.

These findings led to the propositure of the thrifty phenotype hypothesis (Hales & Barker, 2001), which postulates that under conditions of suboptimal in utero nutrition, the fetus must adapt to its environment to ensure survival of the organism, through a "sparing" of vital organs such as the brain at the expense of organs such as pancreas, kidney and skeletal muscle. In addition, it was proposed that metabolic programming occurs to promote nutrient storage to provide a survival advantage in conditions of poor post natal nutrition. However, these adaptations can lead to the post natal development of glucose intolerance, T2DM, CVD and hypertension in conditions of adequate nutrition or overnutrition.

The thrifty phenotype hypothesis is widely used to interpret associations between early nutritional experience and degenerative disease risks (Wells, 2011). Thrifty phenotype represents a short-term adaptive response (preserving vital organs at the expense of less essential traits) to poor energy availability (Wells, 2011).

Many epidemiologic studies in populations worldwide have robustly supported the initial findings that poor fetal growth resulting in low birth weight increases the risk of developing diseases in adulthood, including glucose intolerance, T2DM, CVD and hypertension (Hales & Barker, 2001). The thrifty phenotype hypothesis has served to explain cases such as the high prevalence of T2DM in Pima Indians (Godfrey et al, 2010).

According to the thrifty genes hypothesis (Hales & Baker, 1992) fetal malnutrition as indexed by low-birth weight reduces pancreatic beta cell mass and islet function. These traits then track on into adult life, when they are associated with an increased risk of diabetes, especially if body mass index (BMI) increases (Wells, 2011).

2.1. Alternative hypothesis

T2DM and obesity are not only about energy homeostasis but also about changes in innate immunity, sexual and reproductive function, skin architecture, wound healing and tissue regeneration, memory, cognitive functions, behavior and mechanisms of decision making, social relations and social signaling. Most hypothesis are too glucolipo-centric (e.g. thrifty gene and fetal programming). The only possible exception is the behavioral switch hypothesis by Watve and Yajmik (2007). They argued that insulin resistance is a socioecological adaptation that mediates two phenotypic transitions, reproductive strategy (large number of offspring with little investment in each or smaller number of offspring with more investment in each) and transition from a physically aggressive behavior (soldier) to a socially manipulative one (diplomat). According to this hypothesis, insulin resistance changes the differential budget allocation to tissues, dependent on insulin for nutrient uptake such as skeletal muscle (soldier) to insulin independent tissues such as brain (diplomat). From this hypothesis insulin resistance is likely to have evolved as a switch in reproductive and sustenance strategies rather than an adaptation to feast and famine.

Moalem et al, (2005) hypothesis argued that high plasma glucose lowers the freezing point of blood which prevents formation of ice crystals in cell through super cooling and this has been suggested as an adaptation to the ice age. If high blood glucose is adaptive in cold environment, then ethnic groups who evolved in cold climates should undergo directional selection leading to fixation (Baig et al, 2011).

3. Environment pressures to T2DM

Environmental contributions to the development of T2DM potentially include exposures such as a suboptimal in utero environment, low birth weight, obesity, inactivity and advancing age (Jin & Patti, 2009).

3.1. Suboptimal in utero exposures

Human exposure to an abnormal intrauterine milieu leads to abnormalities in glucose homeostasis and ultimately T2DM (Pinney & Simmons, 2009). Hence pregnant women exposed to the Dutch Hunger Winter, the period in late World War II during which daily caloric intake was limited to 400-800 kcal delivered infants with lower birth weight. By age 50, these offsprings had impaired glucose tolerance compared to offspring who were in utero either the year before or after the famine (Ravelli et al, 1999). Other interactive effects of birth weight and current weight for insulin resistance (Newsome et al, 2003; Fagerberg et al, 2004) and glucose intolerance/diabetes (Forsen et al, 2000; Bhargava et al, 2004) has been demonstrated also.

The epidemiological studies from Hertfordshire (UK) found that men who were the smallest at birth (< 2.5kg) were seven times more likely to have glucose intolerance or T2DM than those who were heaviest at birth (Hales, 1991).

Epigenetic modifications affecting glucose regulation and insulin secretion have been described in the intrauterine growth retardation (IUGR) liver, pancreatic β-cells, and muscle. Studies have demonstrated that genes essential to pancreatic development are susceptible to epigenetic modifications that could ultimately affect gene expression (Pinney & Simmons, 2009).

Pdx-1 is a homeodomain-containing transcription factor that plays a critical role in the early development of both the endocrine and exocrine pancreas and in later differentiation and function of the β-cell. The Pdx-1 is one of 15 genes (of 1749 examined) with cytosines within the promoter that were methylation susceptible (Pinney & Simmons, 2009).

A change in histone acetylation is the first epigenetic modification found in β-cell of IUGR animals. Islets isolated from IUGR fetuses show a significant decrease in histones (H3 and H4) acetylation at the proximal promoter of Pdx-1 leading to a loss of binding of critical activator (USF-1) to the proximal promoter of Pdx-1. This decreased binding markedly decreases Pdx-1 transcription (Park et al, 2008; Qian et al, 1999; Sharma et al, 1996). After birth, histone deacetylation progress is followed by a marked decrease in H3K4 trimethylation and a significant increase in dimethylation of H3K9 in IUGR islets. H3K4 trimethylation is usually associated with active gene transcription, whereas H3K9 dimethylation is usually a repressive chromatin mark. Progressive of these histone modifications parallels the progressive decrease in Pdx-1 expression that manifest as defective glucose homeostasis and increased oxidative stress in aging IUGR (Park et al, 2008).

Oxidative stress plays a significant role in β-cell deterioration (Simmons et al, 2005) that is particularly relevant to T2DM. IUGR induces mitochondrial dysfunction in the β-cell leading to increased production of ROS and oxidative stress (Simmons et al, 2005).

Reduced glucose transport in muscle is a trademark of insulin resistance in IUGR offspring (Thamotharan et al, 2005; Ozanne et al, 2005). Under normal physiological circumstances, glucose transport occurs by facilitated diffusion, a rate-limiting step in glucose utilization (Fueger et al, 2005). This process of glucose transport is mediated by a family of structurally related membrane-spanning glycoproteins, termed facilitative glucose transporters (GLUTs; Slc2 family of transport proteins). Of the isoform cloned GLUT 4 is the major insulin-responsive isoform expressed in insulin-sensitive tissues such as skeletal muscle, adipose tissue and cardiac muscle (Karnieli et al, 2008).

The promoter region of GLUT is the myocyte enhancer factor 2 (MEF2) whereas MyoD is responsible for GLUT 4 expression during myoblast to myocyte differentiation. These two proteins synergistically enhance skeletal muscle GLUT4 transcriptions and gene expression (Moreno et al, 2003).

IUGR is associated with an increase in MEF2D (form that acts as an inhibitor) and a decrease in both MEF2A (that acts as an activator) and MyoD (a coactivator) binding to the GLUT 4 promoter in skeletal muscle. No differential methylation of these three CpG clusters in the GLUT4 promoter was observed but it was found that DNA methyl transferases bindings to the GLUT4 gene were increased and this fact was associated with exposure to increase methyl CpG binding protein 2. Covalent modifications consisted of histone 2 lysine I4 (H3KI4) deacetylation triggering methylase-mediated dimethylation of H3K9 leading to partial inactivation of GLUT4 transcription in post natal and adult IUGR.

Thus, perinatal nutrient restriction resulting in IUGR leads to silencing histone modifications in skeletal muscle which in turn directly decrease GLUT4 gene expression, effectively creating a metabolic knockdown of this important regulator of peripheral glucose transport and insulin resistance and contributing to the adult T2DM phenotype (Raychaudhuri et al, 2008). Studies show that histone modifications can be stably inherited in a caloric-restricted model of IUGR, mimicking the Dutch famine experience (Pinney & Simmons, 2009).

3.2. Low birth weight

Although insulin resistance is considered a hallmark of the thrifty phenotype in later life (Hales & Barker, 1992) studies of small-for-gestational age infants show that the primary initial metabolic adaptations to IUGR comprises greater insulin secretion (Wells, 2011, Mericq et al, 2005, Soto et al, 2003) which seems to promote length gain during the first months of post natal life.

In the Spanish study the body weight differences between small-for-gestational age and normal birth weight infants were 36% at birth, 7% at 2 years and 3% at 4 years of life; however, at 2 years both groups showed similar lean mass and fat mass, from 2 to 4 years the small birth weight gained less lean mass and more abdominal fat than the normal birth weight as well as becoming insulin resistance (Ibanez et al, 2006). Within this pattern of catch-up growth, the onset of insulin resistance appears dependent on a higher level of weight gain (Torre et al, 2008) and is associated with the emergence of central adiposity (Ibanez et al, 2008).

The low birth weight neonates appear to have a higher central fat distribution; however, it would be more appropriated to regard this as a consequence of their reduced peripheral fat (Wells, 2011). In fact, the older English men study (64 to 72 years old) showed that birth size did not directed induce a more central fat distribution. Rather, the primary effect of low-birth weight is to constrain lean mass, muscle mass and peripheral fat. With the post-natal weight gain the fat deficit reduced but the deficit in lean mass remained larger (Kensara et al, 2005). Thus, even though the central fat and insulin resistance emerge post-infancy, they are related to the magnitude on catch-up growth immediately after birth (Wells, 2011). In the Helsinki cohort study T2DM has been associated with rapid weight gain from 7 years (Baker et al, 2009).

3.3. Increased cell fat

Obesity and abdominal fatness courses with insulin resistance as well as myosteatosis named states of glucotoxicity. Serine phosphorylation of the insulin receptor substrate is a critical mechanism of insulin resistance. This process is stimulated by ceramide and cell free-fatty acid and also by C-Jun N-terminal Kinase (JNK), part of a larger mitogen-activated protein kinase (MAPK) family (Exposito et al, 2002). Genetic and diet-induced obesity were shown to markedly increase in JNK activity in liver, muscle and adipose tissue (Hirosumi et al, 2002). Moreover by hyperglycemia/hyperinsulinemia reduces β-oxidation of free-fatty acids by decreasing CPT1 activity due to the increase of MalCoA.

Obesity has been associated with decreased expression of metabolically active genes (e.g. PPAR-α and medium chain acyl-CoA dehydrogenase) in skeletal muscle (Tateishi et al, 2009). Another class of enzymes involved in epigenetic control of metabolism is nicotinamide adenine dinucleotide (NAD+)-dependent sirtuins which target both histone and non-histone proteins (Schwer & Verdin 2008). The most well characterized member, SIRT1, regulates several metabolic pathways including adipogenesis, mitochondrial biogenensis, glucose utilization, fat oxidation and insulin secretion.

3.4. Insulin resistance as muscle mass protector

Insulin resistance emerges post infancy, when weight gain is disproportionate to length and the balance between adipose tissue and muscle mass in high (Ibanez et al, 2006). Such a late emergence of insulin resistance does not strongly support the notion that it represents a metabolic strategy for protecting insulin-insensitive brain (thrifty phenotype hypothesis), whose fuel demands are relatively greatest in the first weeks of life. It does not either represent anticipatory adaptation to poor energy availability in adult life (predictive adaptive response hypothesis). An alternative hypothesis is that insulin resistance in early childhood may supply aid in protecting muscle tissue from high glucose load and corresponding high insulin levels arising from excess weight gain (Lustig 2008), once linear growth is canalized.

Therefore insulin resistance emerges when thrifty growth pattern (low lean mass and reduced metabolic capacity) is subsequently exposure to high metabolic load, and confers protection against it. The lower the skeletal muscle mass the lower tolerance of muscle tissue to a given glucose load (Wells, 2011). Without such metabolic load, growth variability in early life (early growth later disease) appears to have little consequence for metabolic risk (Wells, 2011).

The magnitude of neonate catch-up growth and the muscle mass, fat mass accretion indicates early hormonal adaptations (Martin-Grouet & Ozanne, 2005).

Metabolic capacity comprised by lower pancreatic β-cell mass and the capacity to secret insulin is over passed by the neonate metabolic load of nutrition. Sedentary behavior, which reduces metabolic flexibility, and diet high in refined carbohydrates (Taubes, 2008) challenge the ongoing regulation of blood sugar content and cellular metabolism.

Through many of the components of metabolism considered adaptive for adult life (low metabolic capacity) in the predictive adaptive response hypothesis (insulin resistance and central adiposity) seem to emerge under the "magnifying glass" effect of the modern obesogenic niche (high metabolic load), and may supply represent "protective normalization to preserve homeostasis".

The metabolic costs of body adaptations (e.g. insulin resistance and central adiposity) seem to depend on exposure to an energy-dense diet in childhood, and this is best interpreted as a detrimental effect of the western-industrialized which rather than an adaptive strategy for the long-term future (Wells, 2007).

Moreover while early changes in pancreatic β-cell mass and islet function powerfully determine susceptibility, additional factors such as physical activity, obesity and aging and possibly other process leading to insulin resistance must also play a role in deciding the time of onset and severity of T2DM (Hales & Barker, 1992).

Although obesity, reduced physical activity and aging increase susceptibility to T2DM many people exposed to these risk factors do not develop the disease. Genome-wide association studies have identified a number of genetic variants that explain some of the inter individual variation in diabetes susceptibility (Shahbazian et al, 2007).

In population remaining lean and fit and consuming a traditional diet with low energy density (Prentice & Jobb, 2003), birth weight variability was not associated with adult variability in either the glucose/insulin axis or other risk factors for cardiovascular disease (Moore et al, 2001).

From an evolutionary perspective, those with thrifty or frugal gene who now eat too much and do not get enough exercise are at risk for T2DM.

Ethnic groups, such as the Australian aborigenes, remained hunter gatherers until recently and the recently urbanized individuals of this community developed a high prevalence of diabetes and hypertension (O'Dea 1991).

4. Other exposures

4.1. Oxidative stress

Pancreatic β-cell lost part of their antioxidant defense in association with brain evolution and lost even more in females when placental mammals evolved. Hence pancreatic β-cell and those of females in particular are more susceptible to oxidative damage. Under stress condition the release of stress hormones produces insulin resistance. Reactive oxygen species (ROS) prevent β-cell from secreting insulin at the level required to maintain homeostasis diverts glucose to insulin-independent tissues such as the brain and the fetus (Rashidi et al, 2009).

Excess of deficits in nutrients, hormones or metabolites may trigger changes in DNA or histone gene expression. In addition, changes in small noncoding RNA activity act by modulating gene expression (Godfrey et al, 2010).

Exposure to oxidative stress can directly mediate both DNA methylation and chromatin remodeling in multiple disease models and thus could be a mechanism by which aberrant epigenetic programming leads to T2DM (Yoshida et al, 2006; So et al, 2006; Takahashi et al, 2006; Grady et al, 2008; Feltus et al, 2003; Martin et al, 2008; Cooney et al, 2002; Rauch et al, 2007; Bollati et al, 2009; Franco et al, 2008). Random DNA methylation changes occur during aging in several tissue types and are associated with increased oxidative stress (So et al, 2006; Bollati et al, 2009). Such changes in DNA patterns affect the expression of multiple genes. Replacement of guanine profoundly alters methylation of adjacent cytosines (Franco et al, 2008). Histone sare susceptible to oxidative stress, due to their abundant lysine residues (Ruchko et al, 2009, Tikoo et al, 2008, Drake et al, 2004). It has been discovered that histone demethylases require oxygen as co factor what links epigenetic process to oxygen gradients during development (Hitchler et al, 2007).

Transcriptional PGC 1α coordinates gene expression that stimulates mitochondrial oxidative metabolism in multiple tissues (Puigserver et al, 2003). PGC 1α expression is reduced in diabetic islets and correlates inversely with the degree of DNA methylation (Ling et al, 2008). Importantly, PGC 1α expression correlates positively with glucose-stimulated insulin secretion in human pancreatic islets (Ling et al, 2008).

In β-cells, the insulin gene displays hyperacetylation of H4 and hypermethylation of H3 at lysine 4 typical of active genes.

4.2. Aging

Many of the condition associated with patterns of early growth are traditionally associated with aging. Telomeres are hexameric repeat sequences located at the ends of chromosomes and are considered to be robust biomarkers of cellular aging. In the absence of telomerase, telomeres shorten with every cell division. Progressive telomere shortening causes an alteration in telomeric structure and potently induces the cell cycle inhibitor p53. This can lead to the up-regulation of the cell-cycle inhibitors p21 and p16, which leads to cellular senescence. Accelerated telomere shortening is observed in tissues of the short-lived recuperated maternal low-protein offspring, such as pancreatic islets (Tarry-Adkins et al, 2009). This was accompanied by increased pancreatic islet gene expression of p21 and p16 indicative of accelerated cellular aging. Telomeres are known to shorten in the presence of oxidative stress (Von Zglinicki 2002).

5. Epigenetic of T2DM complications

One major event in the progression of diabetic complications is vascular inflammation with increased expression of inflammatory genes. Enhanced oxidative stress, dyslipidemia and hyperglycemia have also been suggested to influence the development of diabetic complications (Ling & Groop, 2009).

Nuclear factor κB (NFκB) is a transcription factor regulating expression of genes involved in inflammatory diseases, including diabetic complications (Miao et al, 2004).

Poor glycemic control increases NFκB activity through interactions of target genes including the tumoral necrosis factor (TNF) α and cyclooxygenase-2 promoters (Miao et al, 2004). NFκB and interleukin-6 (IL-6) also represent genes with altered histone H3 lysine 9 dimethylation in lymphocytes from patients with diabetes (Miao et al, 2008).

NFκB driven pro inflammatory gene expression seems to play a major role in the pathogenesis of atherosclerosis (Thurberg & Collins et al, 1998, Glass & Witztum et al, 2001). Transient hyperglycemia induces (in vitro) changes in histone methylation at the promoter of NFκB-p65 in vascular epithelial cells, changing NFκB-p65 expression and contributing to vascular complications similar to those seen in T2DM (Brasacchio et al, 2009). Increased NFκB-p65 gene expression was associated with persistently increased H3K4 monomethylation at the NFκB-p65 promoter but not with H3K4 dimethylation or trimethylation. The experiments indicate that increased NFκB-p65 gene expression is associated with persisting epigenetic marks that are maintained when the cell is removed from its hyperglycemic environment, providing evidence that epigenetic modification contribute to altered gene expression and could form the basis for physiologic "hyperglycemic memory".

Interestingly, when genes that reduce mitochondrial superoxide production (e.g. uncoupling protein-1) are over expressed, the changes induced by the transient hyperglycemia are prevented (El-Osta et al, 2008).

An oxidative mechanism seems to mediate the effects of hyperglycemia on inflammatory induction (Exposito et al, 2002). Hyperglycemia-induced oxidative stress occurs along with soluble advanced glycation (AGES) and lipid-peroxidation products which possibly serve as key activation of upstream kinases leading induction of inflammatory gene expression

(Schmidt et al, 1999). Moreover hyperglycemia would induce a higher mitochondrial oxygen reactive species (ROS) production (e.g. muscle cells) that would induce the MAPK with the JNK activation and subsequent transcription of inflammatory mediators (Vallerie et al, 2010).

6. Chromatin remodeling with interventions

6.1. Therapeutic agents

The studies described above clearly showed that environment effects can induce epigenetic alterations. These alterations ultimately affect expression of key genes linked to the development of T2DM including genes critical for pancreatic development and β-cell function, peripheral glucose uptake and insulin resistance. Understanding the role of development of T2DM might unveil a critical window during which epigenetic therapeutic agents could be used as means to prevent the later development of a disease (Pinney & Simmons, 2009).

Experimental treatment of insulinoma cells with incretin hormones such as glucagon-like peptide 1 (GLP-1) and glucose-dependent insulinotropic peptide 1 (GIP) induces β-cell chromatin remodeling which lead to coordinated interactions between specific chromatin-modifying enzymes and transcription factors. The histone modifications (acetylation of lysine and phosphorylation at serine) increase its association with the transcription factor, phosphorylated cAMP-response element-binding protein (phosphor CREB) and with cAMP-response CREB coactivator 2. However it has been noted that changes in histone modifications were not linked to gene expression (Kim et al, 2009).

In addition to incretin hormones, the nuclear receptor proliferator-activated receptor γ (PPARγ) is an important target in diabetes therapy. PPARγ agonist improves glycemic control, increases serum insulin and enhances glucose stimulated insulin release (Finegood et al, 2001; Gerstein et al, 2006; Higa et al, 1999). Whole body glucose homeostasis and insulin secretion improvements were seem in animal with a PPARγ agonist fed either a high fat or normal diet (Evans-Molina et al, 2009).

Cultured islets from animal under oral pioglitazone therapy showed an increase in expression of Ins 1/2 and GLUT2. The specific chromatin remodeling mechanisms described showed increased acetylated H3, increased dimethyl H3K4 association at the proximal promoter of Ins 1/2 and increased mRNA and protein levels (Pinney & Simmons, 2009).

6.2. Physical exercises

Poor physical fitness and a low VO2max predict risk of developing T2DM (Eriksson et al, 1996). Mitochondrial dysfunction, changes in muscle fiber-type composition and insulin resistance are potential mechanisms linking poor physical fitness with an increased risk for disease. All mechanisms of developing insulin resistance can be reversed by physical activity through elevated intracellular PGC-1α (Handschin et al, 2008). Exercise induces the expression of a number of genes that regulate glucose uptake in skeletal muscle, including GLUT isoform 4 (Neufer et al, 1993). GLUT4 expression is further regulated by the transcription factor myocyte enhancer factor 2 (MEF2). Some of the biological changes induced by exercise could be due to histone modifications (Ling & Groop, 2009).

At rest, it has been proposed that MEF2 interacts with histone deacetyltransferase 5 (HDAC 5) in the nucleus (McGee & Hargreaves, 2006). Histone tails at the GLUT4 gene are thereby deacetylated by HDAC 5, resulting in a condense chromatin structure and subsequently reduced GLUT4 expression (McGee & Hargreaves, 2006). After exercise, HDAC 5 is phosphorylated by AMP-activated protein kinase (AMPK), dissociated from MEF2 and exported from the nucleus to the cytosol (McGee & Hargreaves, 2006; McGee et al, 2008; McGee & Hargreaves, 2004). MEF2 may then interact with the co activator protein PPARγ co activatior 1α (PGC 1α) and histone acetyltransferases (HATs) in the nucleus resulting in acetylated histones at the GLUT4 gene, enhanced transcriptional activity, and increased GLUT4 expression (McGee & Hargreaves, 2006; McGee et al, 2006; Vissing et al, 2008). Ca++/Calmodulin dependent protein kinase (CaMK) also seems to modulate MEF activity via histone acetylation in response to acute exercise (Smith et al, 2008). Moreover, there is a positive correlation between a gene expression of HAT with the percentage of Type I fibers and VO2max in human skeletal muscle (Parikh et al, 2008).

6.3. Nutrients and food components

Epigenetic modifications can be altered by external or internal environmental factors. These factors have the ability to change gene expression and are now considered an important mechanism in the unknown etiology of many diseases, including T2DM. Nutrients, food components and specific diets can influence epigenetic phenomena, such as DNA methylation and histone modifications (Choi et al, 2010).

Folate has an effect on DNA methylation for carrying a methyl group in its molecule, which is delivered for the synthesis of AdoMet, the unique methyl donor for DNA methylation reactions. Folate is not the sole determinant of DNA methylation as other methyl donor nutrients (methionine, choline, betaine, and vitamin B-12) as well as other environmental factors can also change DNA methylation status (Choi et al, 2010).

Vitamin B-12 is an essential cofactor of methionine synthase in 1-carbon metabolism and affects genomic DNA methylation (Uekawa et al, 2009). Choline is a methyl donor nutrient and maternal choline availability is essential for fetal neurogenesis such as hippocampal development as well as memory function throughout life. Choline deficiency during the embryonic period could change DNA methylation and thereby alter fetal brain development (Niculescu et al, 2006).

Studies with rats have shown that moderate maternal dietary protein restriction alters phenotypes in the offspring resulting in abnormalities such as hypertension, dyslipidemia, and impaired glucose metabolism, which can be reversed by folate supplementation. The altered phenotype induced by a maternal protein restriction diet during pregnancy involves changes in DNA methylation and histone modifications in specific genes, including the glucocorticoid receptor (GR) and PPARα in the liver of juvenile and adult offspring (Lillycrop et al, 2008; Lillycrop et al, 2007).

Histone acetylation is highly associated with inflammation (Villagra et al, 2008). Calorie restriction reduces the expression of inflammatory genes such as NF-kB, AP1, COX-2, and inducible nitric oxide synthase (iNOS). Histone acetylation activates NF-kB (Villagra et al, 2008) and regulates the expression of COX-2 (Coward et al, 2009).

Individual nutrients and bioactive food components or total diet can modify physiologic and pathologic processes through epigenetic mechanisms that are critical for gene expression. Modulation of these processes through diet or specific nutrients may prevent diseases and maintain health (Choi et al, 2010).

Author details

Katia Cristina Portero McLellan[1], Rodrigo Minoro Manda[1], Lance A. Sloan[2] and Roberto Carlos Burini[1]

1 Sao Paulo State University/ UNESP - School of Medicine, Botucatu/SP, Brazil

2 Texas Institute for Kidney and Endocrine Disorders, Lufkin/TX, USA

References

[1] Baig, U, Belsare, P, Watve, M, & Jog, M. Can Thrifty Gene(s) or Predictive Fetal Programming for Thriftiness Lead to Obesity? J Obesity (2011). ID 861049, 11 pages, doi: 10.1155/2011/861049.

[2] Barker, D. J, Winter, P. D, Osmond, C, Margetts, B, & Simmons, S. J. Weight in infancy and death from ischaemic heart disease. Lancet (1989). , 2, 577-80.

[3] Bernardo, A. S, Hay, C. W, & Docherty, K. Pancreatic transcription factors and their role in the birth, life and survival of the pancreatic beta cell. Mol Cell Endocrinol (2008). , 2008, 294-1.

[4] Bhargava, S. K, Sachdev, H. S, Fall, C. H, Osmond, C, Lakshmy, R, Barker, D. J, Biswas, S. K, Ramji, S, Prabhakaran, D, & Reddy, K. S. Relation of serial changes in childhood body-mass index to impaired glucose tolerance in young adulthood. New Engl J Med (2004). , 350, 865-75.

[5] Bollati, V, Schwartz, J, Wright, R, Litonjua, A, Tarantini, L, Suh, H, et al. Decline in genomic DNA methylation through aging in a cohort of elderly subjects. Mech Ageing Dev (2009). , 130, 234-39.

[6] Brasacchio, D, Okabe, J, Tikellis, C, Balcerczyk, A, George, P, Baker, E. K, et al. Hyperglycemia induces a dynamic cooperativity of histone methylase and demethylase

enzymes associated with gene-activating epigenetic marks that coexist on the lysine tail. Diabetes (2009). , 58, 1229-1236.

[7] Chakravarthy, M. V, & Booth, F. W. Eating, exercise, and 'thrifty' genotypes: connecting the dots toward an evolutionary understanding of modern chronic diseases. J Appl Physiol (2004). , 96, 3-10.

[8] Choi, A. W, & Friso, S. Epigenetics: A New Bridge between Nutrition and Health. Adv Nutr (2010). , 1, 8-16.

[9] Cooney, C. A, Dave, A. A, & Wolff, G. L. Maternal methyl supplements in mice affect epigenetic variation and DNA methylation of offspring. J Nutr (2002). S-2400S.

[10] Coward, W. R, Watts, K, Feghali-bostwick, C. A, Knox, A, & Pang, L. Defective histone acetylation is responsible for the diminished expression of cyclooxygenase 2 in idiopathic pulmonary fibrosis. Mol Cell Biol. (2009). , 29, 4325-39.

[11] Drake, J, Petroze, R, Castegna, A, Ding, Q, Keller, J. N, Markesbery, W. R, et al. Hydroxynonenal oxidatively modifies histones: implications for Alzheimer's disease. Neurosci. Lett (2004). , 356, 155-58.

[12] El-Osta, A, Brasacchio, D, Yao, D, Pocai, A, Jones, P. L, Roeder, R. G, Cooper, M. E, & Brownlee, M. Transient high glucose causes persistent epigenetic changes and altered gene expression during subsequent normoglycemia. J Exp Med (2008). , 205, 2409-2417.

[13] Eriksson, K. F. Lindga°rde F. Poor physical fitness, and impaired early insulin response but late hyperinsulinaemia, as predictors of NIDDM in middle-aged Swedish men. Diabetologia (1996). , 39, 573-579.

[14] Esposito, K, Nappo, F, Marfella, R, Giugliano, G, Giugliano, F, Ciotola, M, et al. Inflammatory Cytokine Concentrations Are Acutely Increased by Hyperglycemia in Humans : Role of Oxidative Stress. Circulation (2002). , 106, 2067-72.

[15] Evans-molina, C, Robbins, R. D, Kono, T, Tersey, S. A, Vestermark, G, Nunemarker, C. S, et al. Peroxisome proliferator-activated receptor g activation restores islet function in diabetic mice through reduction of endoplasmic reticulum stress and maintenance of euchromatin structure. Mol Cell Biol (2009). , 29, 2053-67.

[16] Fagerberg, B, Bondjers, L, & Nilsson, P. Low birth weight in combination with catch-up growth predicts the occurrence of the metabolic syndrome in men at late middle age: the Atherosclerosis and Insulin Resistance study. J Intern Med (2004). , 256, 254-259.

[17] Feltus, F. A, Lee, E. K, Costello, J. K, Plass, C, & Vertino, P. M. Predicting aberrant CpG island methylation. PNAS (2003). , 100, 12253-258.

[18] Finegood DT McArthur MDKojwang D, Thomas MJ, Topp B, Leonard T et al. Beta-cell mass dynamics in Zucker diabetic fatty rats. Rosiglitazone prevents the rise in net cell death. Diabetes (2001). , 1021-29.

[19] Florez, J. The genetics of type 2 diabetes: a realistic appraisal in (2008). J Clin Endocrinol Metab 2008; 93; , 4633-42.

[20] Forsen, T, Eriksson, J, Tuomilehto, J, Reunanen, A, Osmond, C, & Barker, D. The fetal and childhood growth of persons who develop type 2 diabetes. Ann Intern Med (2000). , 133, 176-182.

[21] Franco, R, Schoneveld, O, Georgakilas, A. G, & Panayiotidis, M. I. (2008). Oxidative stress, DNA methylation and carcinogenesis. Cancer Lett 2008; , 266, 6-11.

[22] Fueger, P. T, Shearer, J, Bracy, D. P, Posey, K. A, Pencek, R. R, Mcguinness, O. P, & Wasserman, D. H. Control of muscle glucose uptake: test of the rate-limiting step paradigm in conscious, unrestrained mice. J Physiol (2005). , 562, 925-35.

[23] Mohan, V. Effect of rosiglitazone on the frequency of diabetes in patients with impaired glucose tolerance or impaired fasting glucose: a randomized controlled trial. Lancet (2006). , 368(9541), 1096-105.

[24] Glass, C. K, & Witztum, J. L. Atherosclerosis: the road ahead. Cell (2001). , 104, 503-16.

[25] Godfrey, K. M, Gluckman, P. D, & Hanson, M. A. Developmental origins of metabolic disease: life course and intergenerational perspectives. Trends Endocrinol Metab (2010). , 21, 199-205.

[26] Grady, W. M, & Carethers, J. M. Genomic and epigenetic instability in colorectal cancer pathogenesis. Gastroenterology (2008). , 135, 1079-99.

[27] Hales, C. N, Barker, D. J, Clark, P. M, Cox, L. J, Fall, C, Osmond, C, & Winter, P. D. Fetal and infant growth and impaired glucose tolerance at age 64 years. BMJ (1991). , 303, 1019-22.

[28] Hales, C. N. Barker DJP. The thrifty phenotype hypothesis. Br Med Bull (2001). , 60, 5-20.

[29] Hales, C. N. Barker DJP. Type 2 (non-insulin-dependent) diabetes mellitus: the thrifty phenotype hypothesis. Diabetologia (1992). , 35, 595-601.

[30] Handschin, C, & Spiegelman, B. M. The role of exercise and PGC1α in inflammation and chronic disease. Nature (2008). , 454(7203), 463-69.

[31] Barker, D. J, Osmond, C, Kajantie, E, & Eriksson, J. G. Growth and chronic disease: findings in the Helsinki Birth Cohort. Ann Hum Biol (2009). , 36, 445-458.

[32] Higa, M, Zhou, Y. T, Ravazzola, M, Baetens, D, Orci, L, & Unger, R. H. Troglitazone prevents mitochondrial alterations, beta cell destruction, and diabetes in obese prediabetic rats. PNAC (1999). , 96, 11513-518.

[33] Hirosumi, J, Tuncman, G, Chang, L, Görgün, C. Z, Uysal, K. Y, Maeda, K, Karin, M, & Hotamisligil, G. S. A central role for JNK in obesity and insulin resistance.Nature (2002). , 420, 333-336.

[34] Hitchler, M. J, & Domann, F. E. An epigenetic perspective on the free radical theory of development. Free Radic Biol Med (2007). , 43, 1023-36.

[35] Ibanez, L, Ong, K, & Dunger, D. B. de ZF. Early development of adiposity and insulin resistance after catch-up weight gain in small-for-gestational-age children. J Clin Endocrinol Metab (2006). , 91, 2153-58.

[36] Jin, W, & Patti, M. E. Genetic determinants and molecular pathways in the pathogenesis of type 2 diabetes. Clin Sci (2009). , 116, 99-111.

[37] Karnieli, E, & Armoni, M. Transcriptional regulation of the insulin-responsive glucose transporter GLUT4 gene: from physiology to pathology. Am J Physiol Endocrinol Metab (2008). EE45., 38.

[38] Kensara, O. A, Wootton, S. A, Phillips, D. I, Patel, M, Jackson, A. A, & Elia, M. Fetal programming of body composition: relation between birth weight and body composition measured with dual-energy X-ray absorptiometry and anthropometric methods in older Englishmen. Am J Clin Nutr (2005). , 82, 980-987.

[39] Kim, S. J, & Nian, C. McIntosh CHS. Glucose-dependent insulinotropic polypeptide and glucagon-like peptide-1 modulate b-cell chromatin structure. J Biol Chem (2009). , 284, 12896-904.

[40] Kim TH Barrera LOZheng M, Qu C, Singer MA, Richmond TA. A high-resolution map of active promoters in the human genome. Nature (2005). , 436, 876-80.

[41] Lillycrop, K. A, Phillips, E. S, Torrens, C, Hanson, M. A, Jackson, A. A, & Burdge, G. C. Feeding pregnant rats a protein-restricted diet persistently alters the methylation of specific cytosines in the hepatic PPAR alpha promoter of the offspring. Br J Nutr (2008). , 100, 278-82.

[42] Lillycrop, K. A, Slater-jefferies, J. L, Hanson, M. A, Godfrey, K. M, Jackson, A. A, & Burdge, G. C. Induction of altered epigenetic regulation of the hepatic glucocorticoid receptor in the offspring of rats fed a protein-restricted diet during pregnancy suggests that reduced DNA methyltransferase-1 expression is involved in impaired DNA methylation and changes in histone modifications. Br J Nutr (2007). , 97, 1064-73.

[43] Ling C & Groop LEpigenetics: A Molecular Link Between Environmental Factors and Type 2 Diabetes. Diabetes (2009). , 58, 2718-25.

[44] Ling, C. Del Guerra S, Lupi R, Rönn T, Granhall C, Luthman H, Masiello P, Marchetti P, Groop L, Del Prato S. Epigenetic regulation of PPARGC1A in human type 2 diabetic islets and effect on insulin secretion. Diabetologia (2008). , 51, 615-622.

[45] Lustig, R. H. Which comes first? The obesity or the insulin? The behavior or the biochemistry? J Pediatr (2008). , 152, 601-602.

[46] Martin, D. I, Cropley, J. E, & Suter, C. M. Environmental influence on epigenetic inheritance at the Avy allele. Nutr Rev (2008). Suppl. 1): SS14, 12.

[47] Martin-gronert, M. S, & Ozanne, S. E. Programming of appetite and type 2 diabetes. Early Hum Dev (2005). , 81, 981-88.

[48] Mcgee, S. L, & Hargreaves, M. Exercise and myocyte enhancer factor 2 regulation in human skeletal muscle. Diabetes (2004). , 53, 1208-14.

[49] Mcgee, S. L, & Hargreaves, M. Exercise and skeletal muscle glucose transporter 4 expression: molecular mechanisms. Clin Exp Pharmacol Physiol (2006). , 33, 395-99.

[50] Mcgee, S. L, Sparling, D, Olson, A. L, & Hargreaves, M. Exercise increases MEF2- and GEF DNA-binding activity in human skeletal muscle. Faseb J (2006). , 20, 348-49.

[51] Mcgee, S. L, Van Denderen, B. J, Howlett, K. F, Mollica, J, Schertzer, J. D, Kemp, B. E, & Hargreaves, M. AMP-activated protein kinase regulates GLUT4 transcription by phosphorylating histone deacetylase 5. Diabetes (2008). , 57, 860-67.

[52] Mcmichael, A. J. Diabetes, ancestral diets and dairy foods. In: Macbeth H, Sheety P (eds). Health and Ethnicity. Taylor and Francis: London, (2001). , 133-146.

[53] Mericq, V, Ong, K. K, Bazaes, R, Pena, V, Avila, A, Salazar, T, Soto, N, Iniguez, G, & Dunger, D. B. Longitudinal changes in insulin sensitivity and secretion from birth to age three years in small- and appropriate-for-gestational- age children. Diabetologia (2005). , 48, 2609-14.

[54] Miao, F, Gonzalo, I. G, Lanting, L, & Natarajan, R. In vivo chromatin remodeling events leading to inflammatory gene transcription under diabetic conditions. J Biol Chem (2004). , 279, 18091-97.

[55] Miao, F, Smith, D. D, Zhang, L, Min, A, Feng, W, & Natarajan, R. Lymphocytes from patients with type 1 diabetes display a distinct profile of chromatin histone H3 lysine 9 dimethylation: an epigenetic study in diabetes. Diabetes (2008). , 57, 3189-98.

[56] Moalem, S, Storey, K. B, Percy, M. E, Peros, M. C, & Perl, D. P. The sweet thing about type 1 diabetes: a cryoprotective evolutionary adaptation. Medical Hypotheses (2005). , 65, 8-16.

[57] Moore, S. E, Halsall, I, Howarth, D, Poskitt, E. M, & Prentice, A. M. Glucose, insulin and lipid metabolism in rural Gambians exposed to early malnutrition. Diabet Med (2001). , 18, 646-53.

[58] Moreno, H, Serrano, A. L, Santalucia, T, Guma, A, Canto, C, Brand, N. J, et al. Differential regulation of the muscle-specific GLUT4 enhancer in regenerating and adult skeletal muscle. J Biol Chem (2003). , 278, 40557-564.

[59] Neel, J. V. Diabetes mellitus: a 'thrifty' genotype rendered detrimental by 'progress'? Am J Hum Genet (1962). , 14, 353-362.

[60] Neufer, P. D, & Dohm, G. L. Exercise induces a transient increase in transcription of the GLUT-4 gene in skeletal muscle. Am J Physiol (1993). CC1603, 1597.

[61] Newsome, C. A, Shiell, A. W, Fall, C. H, Phillips, D. I, Shier, R, & Law, C. M. Is birth weight related to later glucose and insulin metabolism?-A systematic review. Diabet Med (2003). , 20, 339-348.

[62] Niculescu, M. D, Craciunescu, C. N, & Zeisel, S. H. Dietary choline deficiency alters global and gene-specific DNA methylation in the developing hippocampus of mouse fetal brains. FASEB J. (2006). , 20, 43-9.

[63] Dea, O, & Westernisation, K. insulin resistance and diabetes in Australian Aborigines. Med J Australia (1991). , 155, 258-64.

[64] Ozanne, S. E, Jensen, C. B, Tingey, K. J, Storgaard, H, Madsbad, S, & Vaag, A. A. Low birthweight is associated with specific changes in muscle insulin-signalling protein expression. Diabetologia (2005). , 48, 547-52.

[65] Parikh, H, Nilsson, E, Ling, C, Poulsen, P, Almgren, P, Nittby, H, Eriksson, K. F, Vaag, A, & Groop, L. C. Molecular correlates for maximal oxygen uptake and type 1 fibers. Am J Physiol Endocrinol Metab (2008). EE1159, 1152.

[66] Park, J. H, Stoffers, D. A, Nicholls, R. D, & Simmons, R. A. Development of type 2 diabetes following intrauterine growth retardation in rats is associated with progressive epigenetic silencing of Pdx1. J Clin Invest (2008). , 118, 2316-24.

[67] Pinney, S. E, & Simmons, R. A. Epigenetic mechanisms in the development of type 2 diabetes. Trends in Endocrinology and Metabolism (2009). , 21(4), 223-229.

[68] Prentice, A. M, & Jobb, S. A. Fast foods, energy density and obesity: a possible mechanistic link. Obesity reviews (2003). , 4, 187-194.

[69] Puigserver, P, & Spiegelman, B. M. Peroxisome proliferator-activated receptor-gamma coactivator 1 alpha (PGC-1 alpha): transcriptional coactivator and metabolic regulator. Endocr Rev (2003). , 24, 78-90.

[70] Qian, J, Kaytor, E. N, Towle, H. C, & Olson, L. K. Upstream stimulatory factor regulates Pdx-1 gene expression in differentiated pancreatic b-cells. Biochem J (1999). , 341, 315-322.

[71] Rashidi, A. Kirkwood TBL, Shanley DP. Metabolic evolution suggests an explanation for the weakness of antioxidant defences in beta-cells. Mechanisms of Ageing and Development (2009). , 130, 216-21.

[72] Rauch, T, Wang, Z, Zhang, X, Zhong, X, Wu, X, Lau, S. K, Kernstine, K. H, Riggs, A. D, & Pfeifer, G. P. Homeobox gene methylation in lung cancer studied by genome-wide analysis with a microarray-based methylated CpG island recovery assay. PNAS (2007). , 104, 5527-32.

[73] Ravelli, A. C, Van Der Meulen, J. H, Osmond, C, Barker, D. J, & Bleker, O. P. Obesity at the age of 50 y in men and women exposed to famine prenatally. Am J Clin Nutr (1999). , 70, 811-816.

[74] Raychaudhuri, N, Raychaudhuri, S, Thamotharan, M, & Devaskar, S. U. Histone code modifications repress glucose transporter 4 expression in the intrauterine growth restricted offspring. J Biol Chem (2008). , 283, 13611-626.

[75] Ruchko, M. V, Gorodnya, O. M, Pastukh, V. M, Swiger, B. M, Middleton, N. S, & Wilson, G. L. Hypoxia-induced oxidative base modifications in the VEGF hypoxia-response element are associated with transcriptionally active nucleosomes. Free Radic Biol Med (2009). , 46, 352-59.

[76] Schmidt, M. I, Duncan, B. B, Sharrett, A. R, Lindberg, G, Savage, P. J, Offenbacher, S, et al. Markers of inflammation and prediction of diabetes mellitus in adults (Atherosclerosis Risk in Communities study): a cohort study. Lancet (1999). , 353, 1649-1652.

[77] Schwer, B, & Verdin, E. Conserved metabolic regulatory functions of sirtuins. Cell Metab (2008). , 7, 104-112.

[78] Shahbazian, M. D, & Grunstein, M. Functions of site-specific histone acetylation and deacetylation. Annu Rev Biochem (2007). , 76, 75-100.

[79] Sharma, S, Leonard, J, Lee, S, Chapman, H. D, Leiter, E. H, & Montminy, M. R. Pancreatic islet expression of the homeobox factor STF-1 (Pdx-1) relies on an E-box motif that binds USF. J Biol Chem (1996). , 271, 2294-99.

[80] Simmons, R. A, Suponitsky-kroyter, I, & Selak, M. A. Progressive accumulation of mitochondrial DNA mutations and decline in mitochondrial function lead to beta-cell failure. J Biol Chem (2005). , 280, 28785-791.

[81] Smith, J. A, Kohn, T. A, Chetty, A. K, & Ojuka, E. O. CaMK activation during exercise is required for histone hyperacetylation and MEF2A binding at the MEF2 site on the Glut4 gene. Am J Physiol Endocrinol Metab (2008). EE704, 698.

[82] So, K, Tamura, G, Honda, T, Homma, N, Waki, T, Togawa, N, Nishizuka, S, & Motoyama, T. Multiple tumor suppressor genes are increasingly methylated with age in non-neoplastic gastric epithelia. Cancer Sci (2006). , 97, 1155-58.

[83] Soto, N, Bazaes, R. A, Pena, V, Salazar, T, Avila, A, Iniguez, G, Ong, K. K, Dunger, D. B, & Mericq, M. V. Insulin sensitivity and secretion are related to catch-up growth in small-for-gestational-age infants at age 1 year: results from a prospective cohort. J Clin Endocrinol Metab (2003). , 88, 3645-3650.

[84] Takahashi, T, Shigematsu, H, Shivapurkar, N, Reddy, J, Zheng, Y, Feng, Z, et al. Aberrant promoter methylation of multiple genes during multistep pathogenesis of colorectal cancers. Int J Cancer (2006). , 118, 924-31.

[85] Tarry-adkins, J. L, Chen, J. H, Smith, N. S, Jones, R. H, Cherif, H, & Ozanne, S. E. Poor maternal nutrition followed by accelerated postnatal growth leads to telomere shortening and increased markers of cell senescence in rat islets. FASEB J (2009). , 23, 1521-8.

[86] Tarry-adkins, J. L, & Ozanne, S. E. Mechanisms of early life programming: current knowledge and future directions. Am J Clin Nutr (2011). suppl):1765S-71S.

[87] Tateishi, K, Okada, Y, Kallin, E. M, & Zhang, Y. Role of Jhdm2a in regulating metabolic gene expression and obesity resistance. Nature (2009). , 458, 757-761.

[88] Taubes, G. The diet delusion. London: Vermillion, 601 , 2008.

[89] Thamotharan, M, Shin, B. C, Suddirikku, D. T, Thamotharan, S, Garg, M, & Devaskar, S. U. GLUT4 expression and subcellular localization in the intrauterine growth-restricted adult rat female offspring. Am J Physiol (2005). EE947, 935.

[90] Thurberg, B. L, & Collins, T. The nuclear factor-kappa B/inhibitor of kappa B autoregulatory system and atherosclerosis. Curr Opin Lipidol (1998). , 9, 387-96.

[91] Tikoo, K, Meena, R. L, Kabra, D. G, & Gaikwad, A. B. Change in post-translational modifications of histone H3, heat-shock protein-27 and MAP kinase expression by curcumin in streptozotocin-induced type I diabetic nephropathy. Br J Pharmacol (2008). , 38.

[92] Torre, P, Ladaki, C, Scire, G, Spadoni, G. L, & Cianfarani, S. Catch-up growth in body mass index is associated neither with reduced insulin sensitivity nor with altered lipid profile in children born small for gestational age. J Endocrinol Invest (2008). , 31, 760-764.

[93] Uauy, R, Kain, J, & Corvalan, C. How can the Developmental Origins of Health and Disease (DOHaD) hypothesis contribute to improving health in developing countries? Am J Clin Nutr (2011). suppl):1759S-64S.

[94] Uekawa, A, Katsushima, K, Ogata, A, Kawata, T, Maeda, N, Kobayashi, K, Maekawa, A, Tadokoro, T, & Yamamoto, Y. Change of epigenetic control of cystathionine beta-synthase gene expression through dietary vitamin B12 is not recovered by methionine supplementation. J Nutrigenet Nutrigenomics. (2009). , 2, 29-36.

[95] Villagra, A, Sotomayor, E. M, & Seto, E. Histone deacetylases and the immunological network: implications in cancer and inflammation. Oncogene (2010). , 29, 157-73.

[96] Vissing, K, Mcgee, S. L, Roepstorff, C, Schjerling, P, Hargreaves, M, & Kiens, B. Effect of sex differences on human MEF2 regulation during endurance exercise. Am J Physiol Endocrinol Metab (2008). EE415, 408.

[97] Von Zglinicki, T. Oxidative stress shortens telomeres. Trends Biochem Sci (2002). , 27, 339-44.

[98] Watve, M. G, & Yajnik, C. S. Evolutionary origins of insulin resistance: a behavioral switch hypothesis. BMC Evolutionary Biology (2007).

[99] Wells JCKEnvironmental quality, developmental plasticity and the thrifty phenotype: a review of evolutionary models. Evol Bioinform Online (2007). , 3, 109-120.

[100] Wells JCKThe Thrifty Phenotype: An Adaptation in Growth or Metabolism? Am J Human Biol (2011). , 23, 65-75.

[101] Wells JCKThrift: a guide to thrifty genes, thrifty phenotypes and thrifty norms. Inter J Obesity (2009). , 33, 1331-38.

[102] Yoshida, H, Broaddus, R, Cheng, W, Xie, S, & Naora, H. Deregulation of the HOXA10 homeobox gene in endometrial carcinoma: role in epithelial-mesenchymal transition. Cancer Res (2006). , 66, 889-897.

Chapter 4

Mitochondrial Metabolism and Insulin Action

Nigel Turner

Additional information is available at the end of the chapter

http://dx.doi.org/10.5772/56449

1. Introduction

The major disease epidemics of modern society are not those of contagion, but are the result of lifestyle imposed upon our genetic pre-disposition. Unrestricted access to calorie-dense food, along with a reduction in physical activity, has resulted in a rapid rise in metabolic disorders. One such condition, type 2 diabetes (T2D), has increased dramatically in recent times, with the International Diabetes Foundation estimating that 371 million people world-wide have T2D, with this number expected to increase to greater than 550 million by 2030 (http://www.idf.org/diabetesatlas/5e/Update2012). T2D is characterized by fasting blood glucose levels higher than 7.0 mM or two-hour blood glucose levels higher than 11.1 mM after a glucose tolerance test. T2D rarely occurs in isolation and is frequently associated with a number of comorbidities, including obesity, dyslipidemia, cardiovascular disease, and inflammation, collectively referred to as the metabolic syndrome.

A central aspect of the disorders comprising the metabolic syndrome is insulin resistance; defined as an impaired ability for insulin to regulate fuel metabolism in target tissues. With respect to glucose homeostasis the main insulin-responsive tissues involved are skeletal muscle, liver and adipose tissue. Under normal physiological conditions, insulin is released into the circulation from the beta cells in the islets of Langerhans in the pancreas in response to the ingestion of a meal. Upon binding to its receptor, insulin stimulates a well-described signaling cascade [1] involving the phosphorylation, docking and translocation of a series of signaling molecules, ultimately leading to alterations in specific endpoints of glucose and lipid metabolism (Figure 1):

- In skeletal muscle, insulin promotes the translocation of the glucose transporter GLUT4 to the plasma membrane to increase glucose uptake and also stimulates glycogen synthesis.
- The major hepatic actions of insulin are the promotion of glycogen and lipid synthesis and the suppression of gluconeogenesis.

• In adipose tissue, insulin stimulates GLUT4-mediated glucose uptake and lipid synthesis, and additionally represses lipolysis, leading to net lipid accumulation.

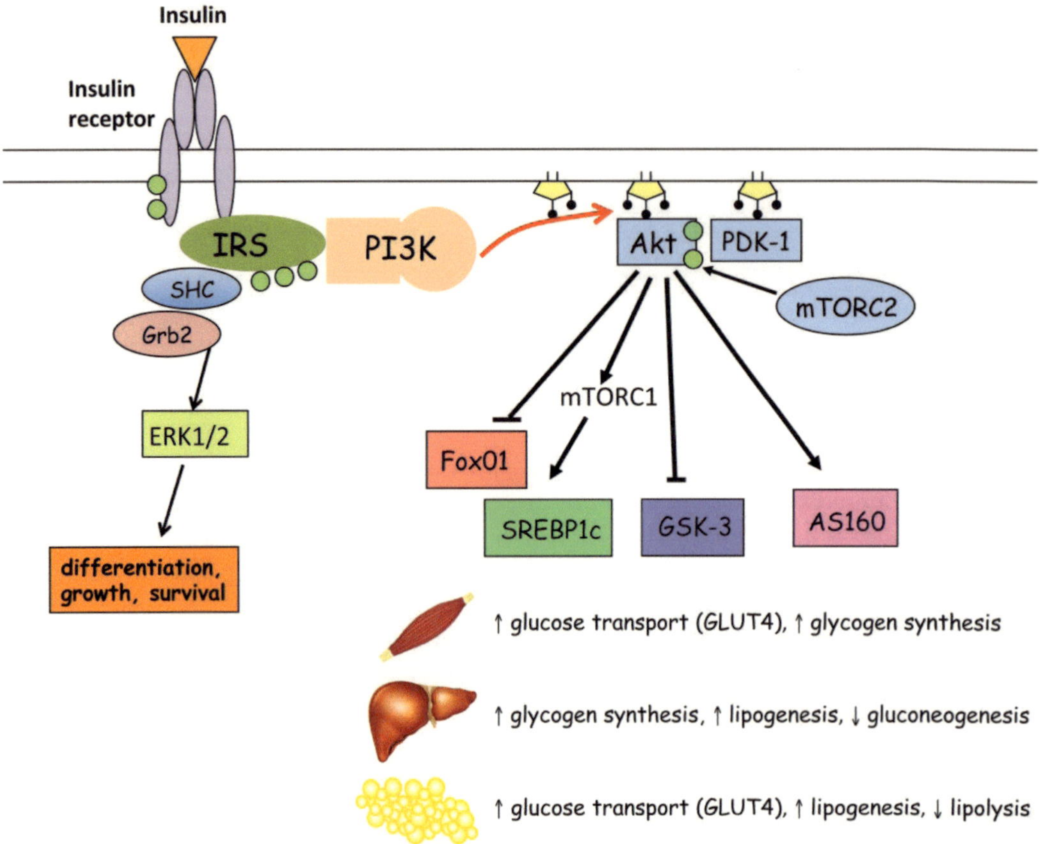

IRS, insulin receptor substrate; SHC, Src Homology 2 domain; GRB2, growth factor receptor-bound protein 2; ERK, extracellular-signal-regulated kinases or classical MAP kinases; PI3K Phosphoinositide 3-kinase; PDK1, phosphoinositide-dependent protein kinase 1; mTORC mammalian target of rapamycin complex; FoxO1 Forkhead box protein O1; SREBP1c sterol regulatory element binding protein 1c; GSK-3, glycogen synthase kinase 3; AS160, 160 kDa Akt substrate.

Figure 1. Insulin signaling pathway. Binding of insulin to the insulin receptor initiates a signaling cascade that involves multiple phosphorylation events (green circles) and leads to alterations in glucose and lipid metabolism.

In the insulin resistant state, the effect of insulin on the above pathways is compromised, leading to insufficient uptake of glucose into tissues and an impaired suppression of hepatic glucose output. To overcome the diminished effectiveness of insulin, the pancreatic beta cells secrete more insulin. The ensuing hyperinsulinemia can adequately compensate for the insulin resistance in most of the population, however in genetically susceptible individuals, the beta cells ultimately fail in the face of the increased workload and this leads to elevated blood glucose levels and T2D. Thus insulin resistance can be considered a very early and important player in the pathogenesis of T2D.

At the molecular level, the precise mechanisms responsible for insulin resistance are not fully elucidated. Studies have reported overactivation of stress-related and inflammatory pathways in tissues of insulin resistant humans and rodents. For example, ER stress was shown by the Hotamisligil lab to be present in the liver of obese mice and subsequent studies using chaperones that reduce ER stress revealed improvements in metabolic homeostatsis [2,3]. Oxidative stress has also been implicated in the development of insulin resistance, with studies showing elevated reactive oxygen species generation in insulin resistant cell models, rodents and humans [4-6]. Finally, inflammation in adipose tissue and liver (and to some extent muscle) has been reported in obese, insulin-resistant humans and rodents [7,8]. While the above factors are often described as causative players in the development of insulin resistance, it still remains unresolved whether they are the primary factors leading to diminished insulin action, or if they arise as a consequence of insulin resistance.

One factor that is one of the earliest defects associated with insulin resistance and T2D is lipid accumulation in non-adipose tissues [9-13]. Under conditions of excess nutrient supply, fatty acids and their metabolites inappropriately spillover into tissues such as skeletal muscle, liver and the heart, precipitating defects in insulin action. More specifically, while elevated triglycerides are frequently reported in tissues of insulin resistant humans and rodents, the accumulation of metabolically active long chain acyl-CoAs (LCACoAs) and other cytosolic lipid metabolites, such as ceramides and diacylglycerol (DAG), are considered to be more directly linked with insulin resistance [9,10]. In support of this, the above lipid metabolites can activate many pathways and factors (e.g. protein kinase C, c-jun N-terminal kinase (JNK), reactive oxygen species, the nuclear factor κB (NFκB) pathway, protein phosphatase A2 (PPA2) and cytokines) that directly antagonize insulin signal transduction and glucose metabolism pathways [9,10].

The extent of lipid accumulation within any given tissue is determined by several factors. Under conditions of elevated lipid availability, enhanced uptake of fat into tissues contributes to greater lipid deposition [14,15]. This increased uptake is associated with greater expression and/or translocation of fatty acid transport proteins (e.g. CD36). Any impairment in the utilization (oxidation) of lipids would also be predicted to increase partitioning of lipids into storage pools. Indeed, over the last decade a popular theory has emerged suggesting that defects in mitochondrial oxidative metabolism, particularly in skeletal muscle, lead to obesity and lipid accumulation and thus may play an important role in the pathogenesis of insulin resistance and T2D [16].

2. Mitochondrial structure and function

The mitochondrion is the key site for energy production in cells, providing a platform for the oxidation of fuel substrates to produce ATP. During the oxidative metabolism of nutrients (primarily glucose and fatty acids under normal circumstances), reducing equivalents (NADH or $FADH_2$) are generated from glycolysis, the TCA cycle and β-oxidation. When NADH and $FADH_2$ are oxidized to NAD^+ or FAD, electrons pass along the mitochondrial electron transport chain coupled to the pumping of protons into the intermembrane space through complex I, III and IV. The electrons are transferred to oxygen at complex IV to produce H_2O. The pumped protons generate an electrochemical gradient across the inner mitochondrial membrane, which is used as the driving force for the ATP synthase (complex V) to produce ATP. The electrochemical gradient may also dissipate through uncoupling proteins (UCP), producing heat in a process referred to as thermogenesis.

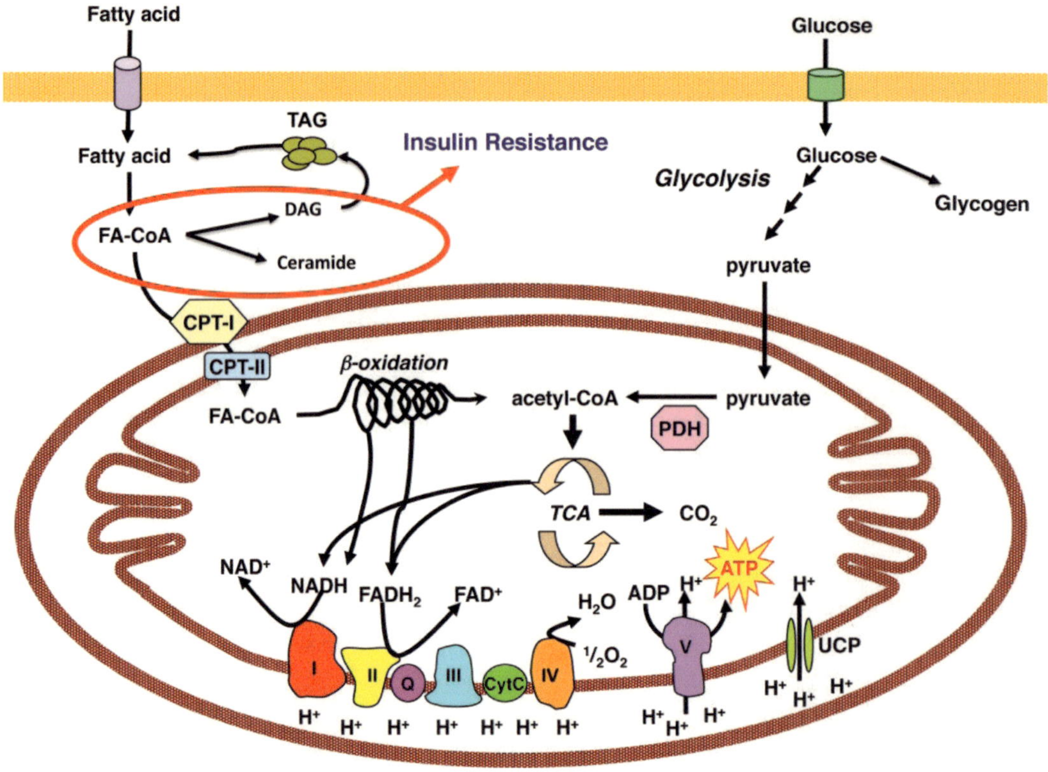

TAG Triacylglycerol; DAG Diacylglycerol; PDH Pyruvate dehydrogenase; CPT Carnitine palmitoyltransferase; UCP Uncoupling Protein

Figure 2. During the oxidative metabolism of glucose and fatty acids, reducing equivalents (NADH or $FADH_2$) are generated from glycolysis, the TCA cycle and β-oxidation. When NADH and $FADH_2$ are oxidized to NAD^+ or FAD, electrons pass along the mitochondrial respiratory chain while protons are pumped into the intermembrane space through complex I, III and IV. The electrons are transferred to oxygen at complex IV to produce H_2O. The pumped protons generate an electrochemical gradient across the inner mitochondrial membrane, which is used as the driving force for ATP synthase (complex V) to produce ATP. Protons can also enter the matrix through uncoupling proteins. Deficiencies in mitochondrial fatty acid oxidation can lead to the buildup of bioactive lipid intermediates (red circle) that can cause insulin resistance.

2.1. Mitochondrial biogenesis

Mitochondrial function within a given tissues is regulated at a number of different levels, including the number or density of mitochondria. The biogenesis of new mitochondria involves a coordinated interaction between the nuclear and mitochondrial genomes [17]. The mitochondrial genome encodes for 13 protein subunits of the mitochondrial respiratory complexes, as well tRNAs and rRNAs necessary for the translation of the mitochondrial-encoded proteins. The nuclear genome therefore encodes the vast majority of mitochondrial proteins and also encodes the transcription factor responsible for controlling mitochondrial transcription, namely TFAM. Proteins encoded by the nucleus are translated in the cytosol and imported into the appropriate mitochondrial compartments via a suite of import complexes [18]. Thus it is obvious that mitochondrial biogenesis is an extremely complex process, reliant upon the exquisite orchestration of separate genomes and multiple cellular processes.

The master regulators of the mitochondrial biogenic program are the peroxisome proliferator-activated receptor gamma (PPARγ) coactivator (PGC-1) family of transcriptional coactivators. The PGC-1 proteins are promiscuous coactivators that interact with and promote transcriptional activity in the key transcription factors (described below) that regulate the expression of genes involved in mitochondrial substrate oxidation, fibre-type determination, mitochondrial biogenesis and mitochondrial function [17,19]. The PGC-1 proteins do not bind directly to DNA, but instead recruit a wide array of chromatin-remodelling cofactors to transcriptional complexes. PGC-1α was the first described member of this family, initially identified in a screen for activators of PPARγ in brown adipocytes [20]. The other members of the family, PGC-1β and PRC were identified based on sequence homology to PGC-1α [21,22]. Overexpression and knockout studies for PGC-1 proteins have provided clear evidence that these coactivator proteins induce increases in mitochondrial oxidative capacity and promote a switch to a more oxidative fibre type in muscle [23-27].

PGC-1α appears to be the most responsive member of this family, with PGC-1β proposed to be important in the regulation of basal mitochondrial content [28]. Environmental stimuli such as exercise, fasting and cold exposure can induce a rapid increase in PGC-1α expression and activity [19]. PGC-1α also promotes its own expression through a feed-forward mechanism [29]. The activity of PGC-1α is regulated by a number of post-translational mechanisms including acetylation and phosphorylation. The relative level of PGC-1α acetylation is determined by the balance between the activity of the acetyltransferase GCN5 and the NAD^+ dependent deacetylase SIRT1 [30,31]. With respect to phosphorylation, the energy sensing kinase AMPK has been shown to directly phosphorylate PGC-1α and alter its transcriptional activity [32]. Thus in responsive to specific stimuli, changes in the concentrations of key molecules within the intracellular milieu (e.g. NAD^+, adenine nucleotides) results in stimulation of upstream regulators of PGC-1α activity and initiaition of the mitochondrial biogenic cascade. While the role of PGC-1α in regulating mitochondrial biogenesis is well established, recent work from the Spiegelman lab has described a novel splice isoform of PGC-1α that also regulates skeletal muscle hypertrophy [33], indicating there is still much to learn about the biology of the PGC-1 transcriptional coactivator proteins.

2.2. Nuclear transcription factors involved in mitochondrial biogenesis

PGC-1 proteins orchestrate the mitochondrial biogenic program by promoting transcriptional activity through a variety of transcription factors. Nuclear transcription factors bind to specific sequences in gene promoter regions to regulate transcription of a subset of specific genes. The key transcription factors that regulate many of the genes involved in the respiratory chain and other mitochondrial pathways are described below.

2.2.1. Nuclear Respiratory Factor 1 (NRF-1)

NRF-1 plays a crucial role in coordinating nuclear and mitochondrial gene expression. It induces the expression of TFAM, as well as other components of the mitochondrial transcriptional machinery (e.g. TFB1M and TFB2M) [34,35]. NRF-1 also promotes the expression of mitochondrial import proteins that are involved in transporting nuclear-encoded proteins into mitochondria. Forced overexpression of NRF-1 in skeletal muscle in mice, results in increased expression of a subset of mitochondrial proteins, but no net increase in mitochondrial oxidative capacity [36]. Deletion of NRF-1 in mice on the other hand has been shown to be embryonic lethal, due to disruption of mitochondrial function [37].

2.2.2. Nuclear Respiratory Factor 2 (NRF-2/GABP)

Nuclear respiratory factor-2 (NRF-2 humans/GABP mice) is a second critical transcription factor that regulates the expression of proteins involved in mitochondrial function and biogenesis. The target genes of NRF-2 include all respiratory complex IV subunits, TFAM and a range of other proteins involved in mitochondrial transcription and replication [38]. Consistent with the findings in NRF-1 knockout animals, NRF-2 deletion also causes a lethal phenotype, underlying the crucial importance of this transcription factor [39].

2.2.3. Estrogen-Related Receptors (ERR)

The estrogen related receptor family contains 3 members, ERRα, ERRβ, ERRγ. ERRs regulate the expression of a wide array of genes involved in substrate uptake, the TCA cycle, fatty acid oxidation (FAO), oxidative phosphorylation and mitochondrial fusion [40,41]. ERRα knockout mice only display a mild phenotype [42], however deletion of the other two isoforms results in a lethal phenotype [43,44].

2.2.4. Peroxisome-Proliferator Activated Receptors (PPAR)

Similar to the ERR family, PPARs nuclear receptors that exist as 3 separate isoforms PPARα, PPARδ, PPARγ. The expression of PPARs varies markedly across different tissues, with PPARα being highly expressed in liver, PPARδ in skeletal muscle and PPARγ in adipose tissue [45]. PPARs are activated by long-chain polyunsaturated fatty acids and a range of lipid derivatives, and several mitochondrial genes, particularly those involved in fatty acid oxidation, are amongst their gene targets [46,47]. Several lipid lowering (e.g. fibrates) and anti-diabetic drugs (e.g. thiazolidinediones) target the PPAR proteins.

2.2.5. Yin Yang 1 (YY1)

A range of mitochondrial genes are also regulated by the transcription factor YY1. Puigserver's group have shown that the regulation of mitochondrial oxidative function by mTOR is regulated through YY1 [48] and recently it has been shown that mitochondrial function and morphology are abnormal in mice with muscle-specific YY1 knockout, highlighting an important role for this transcription factor in regulating mitochondrial function [49].

2.3. Mitophagy

In addition to the biogenesis of new organelles, mitochondrial content is also partly determined by the rate of degradation. Indeed, mitochondrial autophagy (or mitophagy) is now recognized as a key quality control process regulating mitochondrial homeostasis [50]. Autophagy is a conserved cellular event in which damaged organelles and proteins are degraded in a two-step process, that first involves the formation of a double membrane structure called the 'autophagosome', followed by the fusion of the autophagosome with lysosomes and the subsequent degradation of the enveloped contents. Mitophagy can be inititiated by a number of events that signal stress within mitochondria, such as opening of the permeability transition pore or fragmentation of mitochondria [51,52]. The list of proteins that are thought to be involved in the mitophagy process (e.g. PINK1, Parkin, Nix) is increasing rapidly [50]. From a physiological perspective, mitophagy plays important roles in several developmental processes, such as red blood cell maturation and the removal of paternal mitochondria following fertilization of the oocyte [53-55]. However, recent evidence also suggests that abnormal mitophagic activity may contribute to the aging process, as well as a number of different diseases, such as neurodegenerative disorders [56].

2.4. Intrinsic factors regulating mitochondrial function

While the number of mitochondria is obviously an important determinant of the oxidative capacity of different tissues, variations in the intrinsic properties of mitochondria are also critical. Mitochondria from different sites in the body can have different capacities for the same process. For example, mitochondria from red slow-twitch and white fast-twitch muscle display very different rates of fatty acid oxidation [57]. This difference is in line with the functional requirements of these muscles, and is likely related to the differences in protein expression of key enzymes in this pathway [58]. In addition to differential expression of proteins within specific pathways, another emerging factor that may influence mitochondrial oxidative capacity is post-translational modifications of mitochondrial enzymes. Following translation, many different facets of protein function (activity, subcellular localization, protein-protein interactions) can be altered by the addition of functional groups to specific residues in the protein. The most well-described PTM is likely phosphorylation, and proteomics screens have revealed widespread phosphorylation of mitochondrial proteins [59]. The activity of specific mitochondrial proteins, such as uncoupling protein 3, has been shown to be directly regulated by phosphorylation [60]. Other recent work has shown that perhaps the most abundant PTM in mitochondria is lysine acetylation. Acetylation involves the transfer of an acetyl group from acetyl-CoA to a lysine residue in specific proteins. More than 30% of mitochondrial proteins have been shown to be acetylated, and reversible lysine acetylation/deacetylation has been shown to impact on the activity of a large range of mitochondrial enzymes involved in virtually all metabolic pathways within this organelle [61]. In addition to phosphorylation and acetylation, numerous other PTMs (e.g. glutathionylation, nitrosylation, succinylation) have been described as being present in mitochondria [62-64], and their functional importance remains to be determined.

2.5. Mitochondrial dynamics

Mitochondria are not static organelles, but exist largely as a reticular network. Mitochondria are constantly engaged in the process of fusion and fission, providing morphological plasticity to allow adjustments in response to the prevailing cellular stresses and metabolic requirements [65]. Mitochondrial fusion is mediated by the mammalian GTPases mitofusin 1 and mitofusin 2, as well as optic atrophy protein 1 (Opa1). Fusion occurs in a two-step process, which initially involves fusion of the outer membrane (mediated by mitofusins), followed by subsequent fusion of the inner membrane (driven by Opa1) [66,67]. Fission is regulated by another GTPase, dynamin-related protein 1 (Drp1), which resides in the cytosol and is recruited to the mitochondrial surface to engage other key components of the fission machinery (e.g. Fis 1) [68,69]. The fusion process is thought to allow two mitochondria to functionally complement each other through the exchange and repartitioning of their respective components (e.g. copies of the genome, metabolic enzymes and metabolites). Fission on the other hand is important both in the separation of the organelle into daughter cells during cell division and also in isolating and targeting damaged mitochondria for degradation. Collectively the balance of fusion and fission allows mitochondria to form a spectrum of shapes from small individual units to elongated interconnected networks.

In muscle cells, the mitochondrial network is arranged into two discrete, but interconnected pools – the subsarcolemmal (SS) pool near the cell surface, and the intermyofibrillar (IMF) pool in the interior of the cell between myofibres [70-72]. These two pools of mitochondria have been reported to display some differences in their metabolic characteristics, with SS mitochondria appearing to be more responsive to increase their oxidative capacity following an exercise stimuli than IMF mitochondria [57,73]. Despite the differences between mitochondrial pools, it has been proposed that the arrangement of mitochondria may important for efficient mitochondrial function; SS mitochondria have greater access to oxygen and metabolic substrates, and the proton gradient generated through substrate oxidation in the SS pool may potentially contribute fuel ATP synthesis in the IMF pool, where energy demands are highest during contraction [71].

3. Mitochondrial dysfunction in muscle and its association with insulin resistance

As detailed above, mitochondria represent complex organelles and perturbations in any aspect of mitochondrial regulation and function, could impact on metabolic homeostasis. The mitochondrial theory of insulin resistance has developed over the last 10-15 years and is based on the notion that defective mitochondrial metabolism will result in inadequate substrate oxidation, leading to a buildup of lipid metabolites and the subsequent development of insulin resistance. Support for this theory comes from many studies in humans and rodents, which have largely examined skeletal muscle and are reviewed below.

In the late 1990's and early part of last decade, several groups published studies showing that muscle from obese and insulin resistant subjects displayed reduced oxidative enzyme activity [74-76]. Some of these studies also examined lipid oxidation either in muscle homogenates, or by making RQ measurements across the leg, and it was shown that fatty acid oxidation was also decreased in obese, insulin resistant subjects compared to age-matched controls, potentially suggesting that defects in mitochondrial metabolism may be involved in the development of obesity and insulin resistance [74,75]. In 2002, Kelley's group showed that there was lower NADH:O_2 oxidoreductase activity and reduced mitochondrial size, as determined by electron microscopy, in muscle of obese subjects with insulin resistance and/or T2D compared to controls [77]. A year later, two influential microarray studies were published, reporting a coordinated downregulation of genes involved in mitochondrial biogenesis and oxidative phosphorylation in subjects with T2D and non-diabetic individuals with a family history (FH +) of T2D [78,79]. These microarray studies were considered particularly important, as they documented a reduction in the master regulator of mitochondrial biogenesis, PGC-1α, and thus they provided a mechanism for the reduced oxidative gene expression. They were also important, as they showed that abnormal mitochondrial gene expression could be observed in insulin resistant relatives of patients with T2D and thus may be a pathogenic factor in the 'pre-diabetic' state. Overall the conclusion from these studies was that depressed PGC-1α levels, due to genetic predisposition, physical inactivity, or excessive caloric intake, could lead to a reduction in mitochondrial content, predisposing individuals to develop insulin resistance and T2D.

In the ensuing decade since these landmark studies were published, there has been intense research into this field and one issue that has arisen is how to best measure mitochondrial function/dysfunction. Numerous approaches have been employed, including measurements of parameters in frozen muscle samples (e.g. mRNA, protein content, oxidative enzyme activity and mtDNA), functional assessment of substrate oxidation in fresh samples (e.g. radiolabelled fatty acid oxidation, mitochondrial respiration measurements) and non-invasive magnetic resonance spectroscopy (MRS) with ^{31}P or ^{13}C to determine *in vivo* ATP synthesis rates, phosphocreatine resynthesis rates or TCA cycle activity as an index of mitochondrial function. All these assays provide some indication of mitochondrial function, however they may not always correlate with each other and this needs to be considered when interpreting studies in this area. Details of a number of key studies in this area are presented in the following sections.

In line with the microarray studies noted above, mRNA levels for a variety of mitochondrial genes have been shown to be reduced in muscle biopsies obtained from various insulin resistant populations, including lean insulin-resistant offspring of patients with T2D [80], obese subjects [81], patients with polycystic ovarian syndrome [82] and subjects with established T2DM [83,84]. The level of mtDNA was also shown to be lower in both obese, insulin resistant subjects and obese subjects with T2D [85,86]. Heilbronn et al. [81] demonstrated reduced protein expression of respiratory chain subunits in obese insulin-resistant subjects and consistent with these findings, a recent proteomics study comparing lean, obese and T2D subjects, showed patterns of reduced mitochondrial proteins in the insulin-resistant subjects [87]. The activity of specific enzymes involved in oxidative pathways have been reported to be lower in various insulin-resistant populations [81,86,88,89] and additionally electron microscopy studies have reported reduced mitochondrial size and density in insulin-resistant muscle [77,80,86]. Interestingly, in the studies reporting mitochondrial deficiencies, there has been disparate results regarding which population of mitochondria may underlie the functional defects. Ritov et al. [86] reported that the number and functional activity of subsarcolemmal mitochondria was reduced in obesity and T2D, while a more recent study found similar subsarcolemmel mitochondrial content in lean controls, lean insulin-resistant non-diabetic subjects and insulin-resistant T2D subjects, however intermyofibrillar mitochondrial content was reduced in the latter two groups [90]. Differences in mitochondrial function may not only be present within different intramuscular populations, but also between different muscles across the body. Rabol and colleagues used high resolution respirometry to measure mitochondrial function in saponin-permeabilised fibres from m. deltoideus and m. vastus lateralis and observed reduced respiratory capacity only in the leg muscles of type 2 diabetic subjects compared to lean controls [91].

In addition to the above studies, several investigators have also measured *in vivo* mitochondrial function using MRS. Petersen et al. [92] studied lean, healthy elderly subjects using hyperinsulinemic-euglycemic clamps and MRS measurements and observed marked insulin resistance in skeletal muscle of the elderly subjects compared to weight-matched controls. This impairment in insulin action was associated with a 40% reduction in ATP synthesis capacity, and a pronounced accumulation of intramuscular fat. The same group published a paper the following year in which they studied lean insulin-resistant offspring of patients with T2D using the same methods. The insulin-resistant offspring displayed a 60% reduction in insulin-stimulated glucose uptake into muscle and this was again associated with increased intramyocellular lipid and reduced basal mitochondrial ATP synthesis capacity [93]. A subsequent study by Petersen et al. [94] also reported reduced-insulin-stimulated ATP synthesis in first-degree relatives of subjects with T2D and in later work it was shown that family history of T2D was associated with reduced TCA cycle flux [95]. In several other studies, patients with T2D have been shown to have reduced ATP synthesis capacity or phosphocreatine recovery rates, indicative of reduced mitochondrial function in these populations [96-99]. A further interesting case report using MRS showed that a MELAS patient with mtDNA mutations, displayed insulin resistance in muscle association with reduced baseline and insulin-stimulated ATP synthesis capacity [100].

A number of investigations have sought to determine if there is an intrinsic difference in the functional capacity per mitochondrion that may underlie the reductions in mitochondrial function reported with MRS. Some studies examining respiration or fatty acid oxidation in isolated mitochondria or permeabilised muscle fibres, have reported that the functional capacity per mitochondrion in insulin resistant and/or type 2 diabetic subjects is similar or only very mildly reduced [85,88,91,101-103] in insulin-resistant individuals, but when normalized to muscle mass, a substantial reduction is seen in insulin-resistant subjects [85,88,101]. These studies therefore only see marked differences when mitochondrial capacity is expressed per unit mass of skeletal muscle and thus indicate that *in vivo* mitochondrial defects observed with MRS may be more strongly related to reductions in mitochondrial number, than to substantial intrinsic mitochondrial defects. However, an elegant study by Phielix et al. [97] measured both *in vivo* mitochondrial function (with MRS) and *ex vivo* mitochondrial respiration in muscle from the same patients with T2D and they reported that in this population of subjects, the *in vivo* defects in mitochondrial function could be attributed to impairments in intrinsic mitochondrial substrate oxidation. Another study from this group also observed similar differences in intrinsic mitochondrial function in T2D patients compared to BMI-matched controls [96].

One limitation of the aforementioned studies is that they only provide static measurements of different populations at a given time and are unable to delineate whether the observed defects in mitochondrial metabolism are primary drivers of insulin resistance or arise as a consequence of decreases in insulin action. In this regard, intervention studies in rodents and humans have provided some experimental evidence that manipulations which result in declines in insulin action, are also associated with mitochondrial dysfunction. For example, infusion of fatty acids into humans for 6–48h to mimic the effects of chronic lipid overload resulted in a robust induction of whole-body insulin resistance and reduced insulin-stimulated ATP synthesis rates and expression of mRNA encoding PGC1α and other mitochondrial genes in muscle [104-106]. In healthy male subjects, high-fat feeding for 3 days was sufficient to reduce mRNA levels of PGC1α, PGC-1β and several other mitochondrial genes in skeletal muscle [107]. Similarly, genetic, or high-fat diet-induced obesity and insulin resistance in rodents has been reported by several groups to reduce mitochondrial gene expression, protein expression and mitochondrial respiration in skeletal muscle [107-111]. Providing additional evidence of a link between mitochondrial dysfunction and insulin resistance is the fact that antiretroviral therapy used to suppress human immunodeficiency virus infection causes insulin resistance in association with mtDNA copy number [112]. Collectively, the above studies illustrate that there are many instances where defects in mitochondrial metabolism and impairments in insulin action occur in conjunction with each other in skeletal muscle.

4. Mitochondrial dysfunction in tissues other than muscle

4.1. Liver

The liver plays a major role in regulating glucose homeostasis, producing glucose during the fasting state and storing glucose after the ingestion of a meal. Hepatic insulin resistance causes impaired glycogen synthesis and reduced suppression of endogenous glucose and is closely correlated with excess accumulation of lipid in liver. Chronic elevation of liver lipid content is referred to as non-alcoholic liver disease (NAFLD) and this condition progresses to non-alcoholic steatohepatitis (NASH) when inflammatory and fibrotic processes become involved.

A range of different parameters have been studied in rodents and humans with respect to liver mitochondrial metabolism. The collective findings indicate that the liver appears to be able to adapt to an excess of lipid by upregulating fatty acid oxidative capacity and TCA cycle activity, but this is not always coupled to a concomitant increase in electron transport chain activity, and as a consequence reactive oxygen species are produced (see [113] for an excellent review on the topic). There are also some *in vivo* MRS studies that have examined indices of mitochondrial metabolism in individuals with NAFLD and T2D, with the findings generally indicating mild abnormalities in mitochondrial function in these populations [114-116].

4.2. Adipose tissue

4.2.1. White adipose tissue

White adipose tissue (WAT) serves a principal role as the most important energy store in the body. However it has become increasingly clear over the last decade that WAT is also an active endocrine organ, releasing adipokines that influence whole-body energy homeostasis and insulin action. Mitochondrial content in WAT is low compared to other tissues, however the diversity of mitochondrial proteins in WAT has been shown to be greater than in muscle and heart [117]. Intact mitochondrial metabolism is critical for maintaining normal WAT functions, such as the appropriate synthesis and secretion of adipokines and cycling reactions involved in lipid synthesis [118].

WAT mitochondrial content has been reported to be reduced in insulin-resistant humans and rodents. In women with T2D, electron transport chain genes were shown to be downregulated in visceral WAT independently of obesity and perhaps as a consequence of TNFalpha-induced inflammation [119]. In obese humans, mtDNA copy number was reported to be lower than in control subjects and was directly correlated with basal and insulin-stimulated lipogenesis [120]. In rodent models of genetic or dietary-induced obesity and insulin resistance, there are reductions in mtDNA copy number, mitochondrial density and mitochondrial OXPHOS activity [121-123]. Administration of thiazolidinediones promotes mitochondrial biogenesis in WAT in animals and humans, in conjunction with improved whole-body insulin sensitivity [46,123], suggesting that specific changes in WAT mitochondrial metabolism in obesity and T2D, may be imparting whole-body metabolic consequences. Indeed, recent work has shown adipose-restricted alterations in mitochondrial activity can have profound effects on global glucose and lipid homeostasis [124,125].

4.2.2. Brown adipose tissue

Unlike WAT, the principal function of brown adipose tissue (BAT) is energy dissipation, rather than energy storage. BAT has a high mitochondrial density per gram of tissue, and the unique presence of uncoupling protein 1 (UCP1) allows brown adipocytes to couple the oxidation of lipids, not to ATP synthesis, but to heat generation via proton leak across the mitochondrial inner membrane. Interest in brown adipose tissue has recently soared on the back of 3 important papers published in 2009 that unequivocally demonstrated the presence of functional BAT in humans [126-128]. There is an inverse correlation between BAT activity (as assessed by fluorodeoxyglucose PET) and obesity, suggesting that individuals with low BAT mitochondrial activity, may be prone to obesity and other metabolic diseases [126,127,129-131].

4.3. Heart

Like skeletal muscle, translocation of GLUT4 in response to insulin occurs in myocardium. This process is blunted in insulin-resistant humans and animals in association with other abnormalities in fuel metabolism ([132-134]. With respect to mitochondrial metabolism, genetic and diet-induced obesity and type 2 diabetes in rodents is associated impaired mitochondrial function [135-137]. MRS studies in individuals with T1DM, T2DM, obesity and/ or NAFLD have also reported that that there is a decreased ratio of phosphocreatine:ATP in myocardium, potentially indicating derangements in mitochondrial substrate metabolism in these populations [138-142].

5. What factors lead to mitochondrial dysfunction in insulin resistance?

As noted in the previous section, mitochondrial dysfunction is frequently documented in insulin resistant states and there are many possible factors that may underlie this relationship.

5.1. Insulin resistance

Insulin is a potent anabolic hormone and it has been proposed that mitochondrial dysfunction may emerge secondary to insulin resistance. Insulin infusion in humans leads to increases in mitochondrial gene expression, higher oxidative enzyme activity and elevated ATP synthesis in muscle [143,144]. This response is attenuated in insulin-resistant T2D individuals, supporting a direct role for insulin resistance leading to mitochondrial dysfunction [143]. Further evidence for this notion comes from a study by Karakelides et al, who showed that acute insulin removal from subjects with type 1 diabetes, caused reductions in mitochondrial ATP production and in mitochondrial gene expression in skeletal muscle [145]. Additionally a recent study in patients with congenital defects in insulin signal transduction, reported that mitochondrial function (assessed by phosphocreatine recovery rates) in muscle was reduced in this population [146]. Finally a recent study that induced insulin resistance by prolonged fasting, also reported defects in mitochondrial function [147]. Overall these studies indicate that insulin can directly regulate mitochondrial biogenesis and metabolism, and therefore it is plausible that some of the mitochondrial defects observed in insulin-resistant subjects, could be a consequence of the insulin resistance itself.

5.2. Altered mitochondrial dynamics

Any perturbation in the dynamics of the mitochondrial network could potentially contribute to the pathogenesis of insulin resistance in skeletal muscle. The complex process of mitochondrial fission and fusion has been described above and alterations in key proteins mediating these dynamic events have been reported in insulin resistant and obese states. The expression of mitofusin 2 (MFN2), which appears to have additional pleitropic effects in cells beyond the maintenance of the mitochondrial network [148-152], is reduced in the skeletal muscle of obese insulin-resistant humans, type 2 diabetic humans and diabetic Zucker rats [149,153] and correlates with the capacity for glucose oxidation [154]. Repression of MFN2 in L6E9 muscle cells and 10T/2 fibroblasts results in decreased glucose oxidation, cellular respiration, mitochondrial membrane potential, and causes fragmentation of the mitochondrial network [149] and liver-specific deletion of MFN2 results in glucose intolerance and impairments in insulin signaling [155]. Recent work has also shown that mice deficient in the mitochondrial protease OMA1, display obesity and altered metabolic homeostasis, due to altered processing of the inner membrane fusion protein OPA1 and disruptions in mitochondrial morphology and fuel metabolism [156]. It has also been reported that abnormalitieis in mitochondrial fission events may play a role lipid-induced insulin resistance. In C2C12 muscle cells, palmitic acid (but not other long-chain fatty acids) was shown to induce mitochondrial fragmentation in conjunction with insulin resistance and this effect could be blocked by genetic or pharmacological inhibition of Drp1 [157]. Analysis of tissues from *ob/ob* mice and high-fat fed mice in this study revealed increased Drp1 and Fis1 levels and pre-treatment of *ob/ob* mice with the Drp1 inhibitor Mdivi-1 resulted in a mild improvement in insulin action in these animals. Collectively these studies suggest that alterations in the equilibrium of mitochondrial fission and fusions events may play some role in the pathogenesis of insulin resistance.

5.3. Reduced physical activity

Physical inactivity has recently been reported to be as big a risk factor for non-communicable diseases as smoking, stressing the importance of exercise in metabolic health [158]. Exercise is one of the major stimuli for mitochondrial biogenesis and chronic inactivity results in decreases in mitochondrial number in muscle [159]. A number of studies have shown that obesity and other metabolic disorders are characterised by decreased physical activity levels and elevations in sedentary behaviour [160-162]. Interestingly the sedentary behaviours (e.g. sitting time) do not seem to be influenced by changes in weight and have been suggested to be biologically determined [161]. Given these differences, it is likely that some of the mitochondrial defects reported in overweight or obese insulin-resistant subjects may be explained, in part, by low levels of physical activity.

5.4. Genetic and epigenetic factors

There is evidence in the literature that the metabolic phenotype of skeletal muscle may be strongly influenced by genetic programming. For example, despite being cultured under similar conditions for several weeks, studies have shown that primary human skeletal muscle cells in culture display a similar metabolic phenotype (e.g. gene expression and lipid partitioning) to that of the donor subject from which they originated [163,164]. Mutations in nuclear-encoded genes involved in mitochondrial function (e.g. PGC-1α, NDUFB6) have been linked with insulin action and T2D, as have mtDNA deletions [165,166]. An emerging area of research is also the regulation of mitochondrial function by epigenetic factors. Barres et al showed that the promoter of PGC-1a is methylated at non-CpG sites and exposure of primary human myotubes to hyperlipidemia or inflammatory stimuli, promoted PGC-1α hypermethylation. Intriguingly PGC-1α hypermethylation was observed in muscle of T2D patients in conjunction with reduced mitochondrial density [167]. PGC-1α hypermethylation has also been linked with insulin resistance in non-alcoholic fatty liver disease [168]. A number of other studies have also reported that methylation of other mitochondrial genes (e.g. NDUFB6 and ATP50) as well as TFAM, can be regulated by methylation and associated with insulin resistance. [166,168-170]. One recent study has also shown that methylation of mitochondrial DNA is also correlated with severity of NAFLD [171]. In addition to methylation, acetylation can also influence gene transcription and the potential importance of this epigenetic factor is highlighted by a recent study showing that pharmacological inhibition of HDAC1 in cells and obese animals could promote mitochondrial biogenesis and improve metabolic phenotype [172]. Overall the above studies indicate that specific chromatin modifications may influence mitochondrial function in insulin resistance and T2D.

5.5. Oxidative stress

Oxidative stress can be defined as a chronic imbalance between the production of reactive species and the protection against these species by antioxidant defenses, ultimately leading to macromolecular damage. Reactive oxygen species (ROS) are an unavoidable byproduct of metabolic reactions within cells and a major site for ROS production is the mitochondrion [173]. Studies from a number of different groups have shown that in genetic or diet-induced obese rodents, there is increase ROS production [4,5,174,175]. Importantly, most [4,5,175,176], but not all studies [177] show that insulin action is improved by genetic or pharmacological attenuatation of mitochondrial ROS production, indicating an especially important role for generation of reactive species in this organelle. Since mitochondria are particularly susceptible to oxidative attack [178,179], it is possible that overactive ROS generation in response to obesity or high dietary lipid supply, may lead to defects in mitochondrial function. Indeed, Bonnard et al. fed mice a long-term diet rich in fat and sugar and concluded that under their specific experimental conditions, oxidative stress was involved in the induction of mitochondrial dysfunction [108].

5.6. Post-translational regulation of mitochondrial function

As noted above, there is an emerging appreciation for the fact that specific mitochondrial enzymes and pathways may be regulated by post-translational modifications. Several groups have shown that mitochondrial acetylation is increased in tissues of diet-induced obese mice [180,181]. SIRT3 is a key regulator of mitochondrial acetylation and the expression of this deacetylase enzyme is markedly reduced in a number of different experimental models of insulin resistance and diabetes [181-183]. SIRT3 KO mice display insulin resistance in muscle [182] and these mice also exhibit an accelerated development of the metabolic syndrome when challenged with long-term high fat diet, in association with pronounced hyperacetylation of liver mitochondria [181]. Interestingly, in addition to showing that SIRT3 KO mice have a compromised phenotype, Hirschey et al have also shown that a point mutation in SIRT3 that results in reduced activity of this protein, is associated with the development of metabolic syndrome in humans [181]. The above studies suggest that altered acetylation of mitochondrial proteins may associate with insulin resistance and impaired mitochondrial function, and while further study in this field is required, there is some evidence that other mitochondrial PTMs may also be altered in insulin resistance and T2D [184,185].

6. Mitochondrial dysfunction is not always linked with insulin resistance

Despite the frequent association of mitochondrial dysfunction and insulin resistance, evidence of a cause-and-effect relationship between the two is still lacking. In fact, a substantial literature now exists in both humans and rodents directly challenging the notion that deficiencies in mitochondrial oxidative capacity are an obligate part of the link between lipid accumulation (obesity) and insulin resistance.

6.1. Human studies

Trenell and colleagues used MRS to determine basal and maximal ATP turnover in muscle of well-controlled T2D patients compared with physical activity-, age- and weight-matched control subjects and observed no difference between the two groups [186]. A similar finding was reported in a separate population where post-exercise phosphocreatine recovery indicated similar mitochondrial function between obese patients in either the early or advanced stages of T2D and normoglycemic controls matched for age, body composition and habitual physical activity levels [187]. A further study from the same group also recently reported similar *in vivo* mitochondrial function with MRS in prediabetic subjects compared with age, BMI and activity-matched controls, despite the presence of insulin resistance (by HOMA-IR and OGTT) [83]. In young lean men born with low birth-weight, mitochondrial function by MRS and mitochondrial gene expression are intact, despite these subjects displaying several pre-diabetic characteristics [188]. Two groups have also reported measurement of *in vitro* ATP production capacity and respiratory charactersitics in mitochondria isolated from obese subjects and fail to see any difference compared to controls [189,190]. Studies in different ethnic groups have also provided data contrary to the mitochondrial dysfunction theory of insulin resistance. Nair et al. showed that despite being more insulin resistant than age, sex and BMI-matched North American subjects, Asian Indians exhibit higher mtDNA content, elevated expression of genes involved in oxidative phosphorylation, increased oxidative enzyme activity and greater mitochondrial ATP production rates in muscle [191]. In this study the authors also went on to stratify the Asian Indian group into those with T2D and those without, and despite the diabetic individuals displaying impaired insulin sensitivity and increased muscle lipid levels, there was no difference in the various markers of mitochondrial oxidative capacity.

The studies above provide evidence that at least in those populations, mitochondrial dysfunction does not seem to be present in a number of insulin resistant groups. In line with these examples of a discordant relationship between these two variables, several human intervention studies have also shown that changes in insulin sensitivity can occur without concurrent improvements in mitochondrial function. For instance, dietary restriction in overweight and obese subjects enhanced insulin sensitivity, without altering mtDNA, cardiolipin content or NADH-oxidase activity [192]. Improved insulin sensitivity was reported in insulin-resistant subjects with a family history of T2D following 7 days of treatment with the anti-lipolytic agent acipimox, yet mitochondrial gene expression in muscle actually declined in these subjects [193]. Treatment of diabetic patients with rosiglitazone improved insulin sensitivity, without altering *in vivo* mitochondrial function or markers of mitochondrial content [194,195]. Recently Samocha-Bonet also showed that 28 days of high-fat overfeeding was sufficient to induce insulin resistance in health humans, without any detectable defects in various markers of mitochondrial function [6]. Shorter-term overfeeding studies in low birth-weight subjects also revealed a disconnect between the induction of insulin resistance and the response of mitochondrial metabolism [196].

6.2. Rodent studies

To complement the studies in humans, a number of investigators have used gene-manipulated mice to more directly test whether specifically targeting mitochondrial metabolism, can induce changes in insulin sensitivity. Mitochondrial oxidative capacity was shown to be compromised in muscle-specific TFAM knockout mice, however these animals exhibited improved glucose clearance during a glucose tolerance test and maintained insulin-stimulated glucose uptake in muscle [197]. TFAM knockout in adipose tissue was recently shown to protect against diet-induced obesity and insulin resistance, despite causing abnormalities in mitochondrial function [125]. Similar findings were reported in mice with liver or muscle-specific deletion of apoptosis-inducing factor. These animals exhibited a gene expression pattern of mitochondrial oxidative phosphorylation deficiency similar to that observed in human insulin resistance [78,79], however they were lean and insulin-sensitive and did not manifest the usual deleterious effects of a high-fat diet [198]. A number of groups have also targeted other regulators of mitochondrial function in mice. Due to their key role in mitochondrial biogenesis, muscle-specific knockout of PGC-1α or loss-of-function mutation of PGC-1β produced the expected decline in markers of mitochondrial function yet insulin sensitivity in muscle was preserved or in fact slightly enhanced in these animals compared to wild-type counterparts [26,199]. Two separately generated lines of muscle-specific PGC-1α transgenic mice have shown predictable increases in many mitochondrial parameters, but these animals are insulin resistant, potentially due to excessive fatty acid delivery into muscle [200] or decreased GLUT4 expression [201]. In other examples of a dissociation between insulin resistance and mitochondrial dysfunction, it has been shown that Zucker diabetic fatty (ZDF) rats display normal *in vivo* muscle oxidative capacity and improved activity of enzymes involved in lipid oxidation during the progressions to insulin resistance and T2D [202], while *db/db* mice and *ob/ob* mice have been shown to exhibit higher mitochondrial oxidative capacity in liver compared to lean control animals [203,204]. Collectively the above studies clearly demonstrate that targeted manipulation of mitochondrial function, does not produce 'predictable' alterations in insulin action. A caveat to these studies is that in genetically manipulated mice, there is a complete lack or substantial increase in the content/function of a specific protein and thus caution must be exercise when interpreting the findings, as the phenotype (or lack thereof) may be partially related to other compensatory adaptations (e.g. activation of AMP-activated protein kinase or increase in some other lipid metabolism pathway) induced by the alterations in specific genes [197,200].

Dietary studies are another robust approach to test whether mitochondrial defects can be causally linked with changes in insulin action. Feeding rats an iron-deficient diet causes a deficiency in mitochondrial electron transport chain enzymes, however this is not associated with the development of insulin resistance [205]. In 2007, our group showed that high-fat feeding in mice induced insulin resistance and was associated with increased expression of a PGC-1α and a number of mitochondrial proteins, elevated oxidative enzyme activity and higher fatty acid oxidation rates [206]. Furthermore we also demonstrated that similar changes in markers of mitochondrial metabolism were present in muscle from high-fat fed rats, *db/db* mice and *fa/fa* Zucker rats. These findings of enhanced mitochondrial oxidative capacity occurring in parallel with the induction of insulin resistance, suggested that diet-induced insulin resistance does not involve mitochondrial dysfunction. At a similar time Garcia-Roves also showed that high-fat feeding with daily heparin injections in rats resulted in mitochondrial biogenesis in skeletal muscle [207] and subsequent work by the same lab the following year confirmed that oversupply of dietary lipid produced insulin resistance, despite an increase in mitochondria in muscle [208]. Since the time of these publications, a number of other groups have shown that diets rich in fat increase mitochondrial biogenesis in muscle, despite the fact that the same diets robustly induce whole-body and muscle-specific insulin resistance [209-211]. One interpretation of these findings is that skeletal muscle is mounting an appropriate response to the increase in caloric load, by upregulating catabolic pathways, however this response is inadequate or mismatched with the elevation in nutrient intake, thus resulting in ectopic lipid accumulation in muscle and insulin resistance. Interestingly we have shown that the upregulation of mitochondrial oxidative capacity is far greater when medium chain fatty acids are substituted for long chain fatty acids in the diet and this is sufficient to prevent the accumulation of myocellular lipid and the development of insulin resistance in muscle [212]. Enhancing mitochondrial metabolism acutely by genetic means in muscle, also seems to be sufficient to boost mitochondrial fuel oxidation to the point where insulin resistance is ameliorated in muscle in fat-fed animals [25,213].

One interesting observation to come out of the dietary studies in rodents is that from Muoio's group. They reported that the increased mitochondrial fatty acid oxidation that occurs in response to high-fat feeding, results in the generation of acylcarnitines as incomplete oxidation products [214]. This acylcarnitine signature, which is thought to disturb the mitochondrial CoA equilibrium and indicate a state of mitochondrial stress, has also been observed in humans with obesity and T2D [215,216]. Whether the acylcarnitines can directly contribute to the development of insulin resistance is currently unclear, but recent work suggests that these metabolites serve as a marker for the inability of mitochondria to efficiently transition between fuel substrates [217].

In summary, while there are a large number of studies that document an association between mitochondrial dysfunction and insulin resistance in lean and obese subjects, there is now a

http://dx.doi.org/10.5772/56449

significant literature showing that alterations in mitochondrial function in muscle and insulin action are not always correlated. There are a myriad of differences between studies that may explain these discrepancies, including the particular population of individuals studied and their ethnic background and physical fitness level, the muscle group examined, the dietary regime employed in rodent and human studies (e.g. duration of feeding, fat content and composition) and the particular assay/technique used to assess mitochondrial function.

7. Are mitochondria good therapeutic targets for the treatment of insulin resistance and T2D?

While the precise role of mitochondria as pathogenic drivers of insulin resistance and T2D remains controversial, it should be recognized that even if mitochondrial defects arise secondary to the development of insulin resistance or as a consequence of obesity, reductions in oxidative fuel metabolism are likely to accelerate ectopic lipid deposition in non-adipose tissues and thereby exacerbate the insulin-resistant state. Therefore it would appear that stimulating mitochondrial biogenesis and fuel metabolism, could have beneficial effects for treating metabolic diseases. Evidence in this regard is summarised below

7.1. Exercise

Exercise robustly stimulates mitochondrial biogenesis in muscle and has a multitude of health benefits, including improving insulin action. An 8 week cycling regime in sedentary elderly subjects increased muscle fatty acid oxidative capacity and in parallel improved insulin-mediated glucose disposal [218]. A ten week exercise training program produced similar improvements in insulin sensitivity and muscle oxidative enzyme activity in both first degree relatives of T2D patients compared with age-, sex- and BMI-matched controls [219]. Toledo reported that 4 months of exercise training in T2D patients increased skeletal muscle mitochondrial density, cardiolipin content and mitochondrial oxidation enzymes, in conjunction with a 60% improvement in insulin sensitivity [220]. Aerobic cycling training for 10 weeks in obese, T2D male subjects induced an ~20% increase in insulin sensitivity and a 40% increase in mitochondrial content, with these changes of a similar magnitude to that observed in matched control subjects [221]. Twelve weeks of combined progressive training was also sufficient to overcome the *in vivo* mitochondrial impairment observed in a group of T2D patients, with a concomitant improvement in insulin sensitivity also observed [96]

7.2. Caloric restriction and modulation of sirtuin enzymes

Caloric restriction has been shown to improve insulin sensitivity in humans [222,223] and to improve markers of mitochondrial function in muscle of humans and rodents [224,225]. Many of the beneficial effects of calorie restriction have been proposed to be through stimulation of the SIRT1 pathway. Indeed studies have shown that activators of SIRT1 (e.g. resveratrol and more potent specific activators) can enhance mitochondrial metabolism and improve insulin action in rodent models of insulin resistance and T2D [226-229]. Recently it was also shown that 30 days of resveratrol supplementation improved some markers of mitochondrial function in muscle of obese subjects, in parallel with improved HOMA-IR and reduced hepatic lipid levels [230]. These effects seem to be limited to metabolically compromised subjects, as resveratrol did not improve markers of glycaemic control in non-obese women with normal glucose tolerance [231]. An alternative approach to using direct SIRT1 activators to mimic calorie restriction, is to increase the intracellular levels of NAD^+, the obligate co-factor for the sirtuin reaction. Indeed two recent studies using different NAD^+ precursors, nicotinamide mononucleotide or nicotinamide riboside, have both reported beneficial metabolic effects on metabolic homeostasis in animals models of insulin resistance and T2D [232,233].

7.3. Mitochondrial uncoupling

As noted above, energy dissipation or wasting can occur in a process known as mitochondrial uncoupling. While this occurs naturally through uncoupling proteins, there are also a pharmacological agents that can induce mitochondrial uncoupling, such as DNP (2,4-dintirophenol). These uncoupling agents are generally lipophilic weak acids, that cause mitochondrial uncoupling by transporting protons across the mitochondrial inner membrane into the matrix, deprotonating and then exiting as anions before repeating the catalytic cycle. Uncoupling agents have been successfully used in the past as obesity treatments. In the 1930's DNP was shown to be an effective weight-loss drug in humans, providing an important proof-of-concept that the stimulation of energy expenditure by uncoupling is not necessarily compensated for by an increase in caloric intake [234]. Despite its success as an anti-obesity therapy, DNP was withdrawn from the market in 1938 as it (like most uncouplers) has a narrow therapeutic window, with overdoses causing serious complications (even death) by compromising cellular energy homeostasis. Due to the current obesity epidemic, and illicit sales via the internet, it is alarming to see that DNP has made a comeback as a weight loss agent, with predictable lethal results [235,236]. Thus, while mitochondrial uncoupling with DNP does not appears to be a safe weight-loss therapy, other more recently described uncoupling agents may potentially have a safer profile for use in humans [237-239]. An additional approach may to be to upregulate physiological uncoupling in brown adipose tissue, via sympathomimetic agents or agonists for thyroid hormone or bile acid receptors.

7.4. Natural compounds

Natural compounds are another rich source of potential therapeutics for obesity and type diabetes, as there is often a long history of use of these compounds in the treatment of metabolic diseases states. One such compound is berberine, a natural plant alkaloid that has been used as a traditional medicine in many Asian countries. Berberine was shown to improve insulin sensitivity in a range of animal models [240] and there is also evidence of beneficial effects in humans [241]. Although enhancing mitochondrial function appears to be an effective treatment for insulin resistance, we showed that berberine acted through inhibition of Complex 1 of the electron transport chain [242]. This mild mitochondrial inhibition led to the activation of AMPK and subsequent metabolic benefits. Interestingly this pattern of mild inhibition of

http://dx.doi.org/10.5772/56449

mitochondrial metabolism has been reported in other insulin-sensitising medicinal plants [243] and is also a characteristic of metformin and thiazolidinediones, which are frontline anti-diabetic therapies [242,244,245].

8. Concluding remarks

The mitochondrial dysfunction theory of insulin resistance, proposes that defects in mitochondrial metabolism are key events involved in the pathogenesis of insulin resistance. At present, the available literature does not provide strong evidence for this relationship, and there is mounting evidence that mitochondrial defects observed in insulin-resistant individuals are likely acquired (e.g. due to low physical activity or caloric excess), or develop secondary to the insulin resistance itself. Furthermore, with respect to muscle, another important issue that needs to be considered is whether the ~30% reduction in mitochondrial function that has been observed in some insulin-resistant humans would limit the oxidation of fatty acids, leading to lipid accumulation as proposed [16]. At rest the rate of oxygen utilization in muscle is low; and the fact that muscle has enormous capacity to increase substrate oxidation over normal levels, means that there is substantial 'spare' capacity in this system to maintain fatty acid utilization under normal free-living conditions when energy requirements are low. Despite the unanswered questions about the precise role that mitochondria play in insulin resistance and T2D, therapies targeting this important organelle, should be explored for the the treatment of insulin resistance and its associated metabolic disorders.

Acknowledgements

Research on mitochondrial metabolism in the laboratory of NT is funded by the National Health and Medical Research Council of Australia, the Australian Research Council, the Diabetes Australia Research Trust and the Rebecca Cooper Medical Research Foundation.

Author details

Nigel Turner[1,2*]

Address all correspondence to: n.turner@unsw.edu.au

1 Department of Pharmacology, School of Medical Sciences, University of New South Wales, Sydney, Australia

2 Diabetes and Obesity Research Program, Garvan Institute of Medical Research, Darlinghurst, Australia

References

[1] Taniguchi CM, Emanuelli B, Kahn CR. Critical nodes in signalling pathways: insights into insulin action. Nat Rev Mol Cell Biol 2006; 7: 85-96.

[2] Ozcan U, Cao Q, Yilmaz E, Lee AH, Iwakoshi NN, Ozdelen E, Tuncman G, Gorgun C, Glimcher LH, Hotamisligil GS. Endoplasmic reticulum stress links obesity, insulin action, and type 2 diabetes. Science 2004; 306: 457-61.

[3] Ozcan U, Yilmaz E, Ozcan L, Furuhashi M, Vaillancourt E, Smith RO, Gorgun CZ, Hotamisligil GS. Chemical chaperones reduce ER stress and restore glucose homeostasis in a mouse model of type 2 diabetes. Science 2006; 313: 1137-40.

[4] Anderson EJ, Lustig ME, Boyle KE, Woodlief TL, Kane DA, Lin CT, Price JW, 3rd, Kang L, Rabinovitch PS, Szeto HH, Houmard JA, Cortright RN, Wasserman DH, Neufer PD. Mitochondrial H2O2 emission and cellular redox state link excess fat intake to insulin resistance in both rodents and humans. J Clin Invest 2009;

[5] Hoehn KL, Salmon AB, Hohnen-Behrens C, Turner N, Hoy AJ, Maghzal GJ, Stocker R, Van Remmen H, Kraegen EW, Cooney GJ, Richardson AR, James DE. Insulin resistance is a cellular antioxidant defense mechanism. Proc Natl Acad Sci U S A 2009; 106: 17787-92.

[6] Samocha-Bonet D, Campbell LV, Mori TA, Croft KD, Greenfield JR, Turner N, Heilbronn LK. Overfeeding reduces insulin sensitivity and increases oxidative stress, without altering markers of mitochondrial content and function in humans. PLoS One 2012; 7: e36320.

[7] Gregor MF, Hotamisligil GS. Inflammatory mechanisms in obesity. Annu Rev Immunol 2011; 29: 415-45.

[8] Schenk S, Saberi M, Olefsky JM. Insulin sensitivity: modulation by nutrients and inflammation. J Clin Invest 2008; 118: 2992-3002.

[9] Kraegen EW, Cooney GJ. Free fatty acids and skeletal muscle insulin resistance. Curr Opin Lipidol 2008; 19: 235-41.

[10] Samuel VT, Shulman GI. Mechanisms for insulin resistance: common threads and missing links. Cell 2012; 148: 852-71.

[11] Pan DA, Lillioja S, Kriketos AD, Milner MR, Baur LA, Bogardus C, Jenkins AB, Storlien LH. Skeletal muscle triglyceride levels are inversely related to insulin action. Diabetes 1997; 46: 983-8.

[12] Itani SI, Ruderman NB, Schmieder F, Boden G. Lipid-induced insulin resistance in human muscle is associated with changes in diacylglycerol, protein kinase C, and IkappaB-alpha. Diabetes 2002; 51: 2005-11.

[13] Adams JM, 2nd, Pratipanawatr T, Berria R, Wang E, DeFronzo RA, Sullards MC, Mandarino LJ. Ceramide content is increased in skeletal muscle from obese insulin-resistant humans. Diabetes 2004; 53: 25-31.

[14] Hegarty BD, Cooney GJ, Kraegen EW, Furler SM. Increased efficiency of fatty acid uptake contributes to lipid accumulation in skeletal muscle of high fat-fed insulin-resistant rats. Diabetes 2002; 51: 1477-84.

[15] Bonen A, Parolin ML, Steinberg GR, Calles-Escandon J, Tandon NN, Glatz JF, Luiken JJ, Heigenhauser GJ, Dyck DJ. Triacylglycerol accumulation in human obesity and type 2 diabetes is associated with increased rates of skeletal muscle fatty acid transport and increased sarcolemmal FAT/CD36. Faseb J 2004; 18: 1144-6.

[16] Lowell BB, Shulman GI. Mitochondrial dysfunction and type 2 diabetes. Science 2005; 307: 384-7.

[17] Scarpulla RC. Transcriptional paradigms in Mammalian mitochondrial biogenesis and function. Physiol Rev 2008; 88: 611-38.

[18] Mossmann D, Meisinger C, Vogtle FN. Processing of mitochondrial presequences. Biochim Biophys Acta 2012; 1819: 1098-106.

[19] Arany Z. PGC-1 coactivators and skeletal muscle adaptations in health and disease. Curr Opin Genet Dev 2008; 18: 426-34.

[20] Puigserver P, Wu Z, Park CW, Graves R, Wright M, Spiegelman BM. A cold-inducible coactivator of nuclear receptors linked to adaptive thermogenesis. Cell 1998; 92: 829-39.

[21] Lin J, Puigserver P, Donovan J, Tarr P, Spiegelman BM. Peroxisome proliferator-activated receptor gamma coactivator 1beta (PGC-1beta), a novel PGC-1-related transcription coactivator associated with host cell factor. J Biol Chem 2002; 277: 1645-8.

[22] Andersson U, Scarpulla RC. Pgc-1-related coactivator, a novel, serum-inducible coactivator of nuclear respiratory factor 1-dependent transcription in mammalian cells. Mol Cell Biol 2001; 21: 3738-49.

[23] Arany Z, Lebrasseur N, Morris C, Smith E, Yang W, Ma Y, Chin S, Spiegelman BM. The transcriptional coactivator PGC-1beta drives the formation of oxidative type IIX fibers in skeletal muscle. Cell Metab 2007; 5: 35-46.

[24] Lin J, Wu H, Tarr PT, Zhang CY, Wu Z, Boss O, Michael LF, Puigserver P, Isotani E, Olson EN, Lowell BB, Bassel-Duby R, Spiegelman BM. Transcriptional co-activator PGC-1 alpha drives the formation of slow-twitch muscle fibres. Nature 2002; 418: 797-801.

[25] Wright LE, Brandon AE, Hoy AJ, Forsberg GB, Lelliott CJ, Reznick J, Lofgren L, Oscarsson J, Stromstedt M, Cooney GJ, Turner N. Amelioration of lipid-induced insulin

resistance in rat skeletal muscle by overexpression of Pgc-1beta involves reductions in long-chain acyl-CoA levels and oxidative stress. Diabetologia 2011; 54: 1417-26.

[26] Handschin C, Choi CS, Chin S, Kim S, Kawamori D, Kurpad AJ, Neubauer N, Hu J, Mootha VK, Kim YB, Kulkarni RN, Shulman GI, Spiegelman BM. Abnormal glucose homeostasis in skeletal muscle-specific PGC-1alpha knockout mice reveals skeletal muscle-pancreatic beta cell crosstalk. J Clin Invest 2007; 117: 3463-74.

[27] Lelliott CJ, Medina-Gomez G, Petrovic N, Kis A, Feldmann HM, Bjursell M, Parker N, Curtis K, Campbell M, Hu P, Zhang D, Litwin SE, Zaha VG, Fountain KT, Boudina S, Jimenez-Linan M, Blount M, Lopez M, Meirhaeghe A, Bohlooly YM, Storlien L, Stromstedt M, Snaith M, Oresic M, Abel ED, Cannon B, Vidal-Puig A. Ablation of PGC-1beta results in defective mitochondrial activity, thermogenesis, hepatic function, and cardiac performance. PLoS Biol 2006; 4: e369.

[28] Lelliott CJ, Vidal-Puig A. PGC-1beta: a co-activator that sets the tone for both basal and stress-stimulated mitochondrial activity. Adv Exp Med Biol 2009; 646: 133-9.

[29] Handschin C, Rhee J, Lin J, Tarr PT, Spiegelman BM. An autoregulatory loop controls peroxisome proliferator-activated receptor gamma coactivator 1alpha expression in muscle. Proc Natl Acad Sci U S A 2003; 100: 7111-6.

[30] Rodgers JT, Lerin C, Haas W, Gygi SP, Spiegelman BM, Puigserver P. Nutrient control of glucose homeostasis through a complex of PGC-1alpha and SIRT1. Nature 2005; 434: 113-8.

[31] Lerin C, Rodgers JT, Kalume DE, Kim SH, Pandey A, Puigserver P. GCN5 acetyltransferase complex controls glucose metabolism through transcriptional repression of PGC-1alpha. Cell Metab 2006; 3: 429-38.

[32] Jager S, Handschin C, St-Pierre J, Spiegelman BM. AMP-activated protein kinase (AMPK) action in skeletal muscle via direct phosphorylation of PGC-1alpha. Proc Natl Acad Sci U S A 2007; 104: 12017-22.

[33] Ruas JL, White JP, Rao RR, Kleiner S, Brannan KT, Harrison BC, Greene NP, Wu J, Estall JL, Irving BA, Lanza IR, Rasbach KA, Okutsu M, Nair KS, Yan Z, Leinwand LA, Spiegelman BM. A PGC-1alpha Isoform Induced by Resistance Training Regulates Skeletal Muscle Hypertrophy. Cell 2012; 151: 1319-31.

[34] Gleyzer N, Vercauteren K, Scarpulla RC. Control of mitochondrial transcription specificity factors (TFB1M and TFB2M) by nuclear respiratory factors (NRF-1 and NRF-2) and PGC-1 family coactivators. Mol Cell Biol 2005; 25: 1354-66.

[35] Virbasius JV, Scarpulla RC. Activation of the human mitochondrial transcription factor A gene by nuclear respiratory factors: a potential regulatory link between nuclear and mitochondrial gene expression in organelle biogenesis. Proc Natl Acad Sci U S A 1994; 91: 1309-13.

[36] Baar K, Song Z, Semenkovich CF, Jones TE, Han DH, Nolte LA, Ojuka EO, Chen M, Holloszy JO. Skeletal muscle overexpression of nuclear respiratory factor 1 increases glucose transport capacity. FASEB J 2003; 17: 1666-73.

[37] Huo L, Scarpulla RC. Mitochondrial DNA instability and peri-implantation lethality associated with targeted disruption of nuclear respiratory factor 1 in mice. Mol Cell Biol 2001; 21: 644-54.

[38] Bruni F, Polosa PL, Gadaleta MN, Cantatore P, Roberti M. Nuclear respiratory factor 2 induces the expression of many but not all human proteins acting in mitochondrial DNA transcription and replication. J Biol Chem 2010; 285: 3939-48.

[39] Ristevski S, O'Leary DA, Thornell AP, Owen MJ, Kola I, Hertzog PJ. The ETS transcription factor GABPalpha is essential for early embryogenesis. Mol Cell Biol 2004; 24: 5844-9.

[40] Dufour CR, Wilson BJ, Huss JM, Kelly DP, Alaynick WA, Downes M, Evans RM, Blanchette M, Giguere V. Genome-wide orchestration of cardiac functions by the orphan nuclear receptors ERRalpha and gamma. Cell Metab 2007; 5: 345-56.

[41] Liesa M, Borda-d'Agua B, Medina-Gomez G, Lelliott CJ, Paz JC, Rojo M, Palacin M, Vidal-Puig A, Zorzano A. Mitochondrial fusion is increased by the nuclear coactivator PGC-1beta. PLoS ONE 2008; 3: e3613.

[42] Luo J, Sladek R, Carrier J, Bader JA, Richard D, Giguere V. Reduced fat mass in mice lacking orphan nuclear receptor estrogen-related receptor alpha. Mol Cell Biol 2003; 23: 7947-56.

[43] Alaynick WA, Kondo RP, Xie W, He W, Dufour CR, Downes M, Jonker JW, Giles W, Naviaux RK, Giguere V, Evans RM. ERRgamma directs and maintains the transition to oxidative metabolism in the postnatal heart. Cell Metab 2007; 6: 13-24.

[44] Luo J, Sladek R, Bader JA, Matthyssen A, Rossant J, Giguere V. Placental abnormalities in mouse embryos lacking the orphan nuclear receptor ERR-beta. Nature 1997; 388: 778-82.

[45] Michalik L, Auwerx J, Berger JP, Chatterjee VK, Glass CK, Gonzalez FJ, Grimaldi PA, Kadowaki T, Lazar MA, O'Rahilly S, Palmer CN, Plutzky J, Reddy JK, Spiegelman BM, Staels B, Wahli W. International Union of Pharmacology. LXI. Peroxisome proliferator-activated receptors. Pharmacol Rev 2006; 58: 726-41.

[46] Bogacka I, Xie H, Bray GA, Smith SR. Pioglitazone induces mitochondrial biogenesis in human subcutaneous adipose tissue in vivo. Diabetes 2005; 54: 1392-9.

[47] Tanaka T, Yamamoto J, Iwasaki S, Asaba H, Hamura H, Ikeda Y, Watanabe M, Magoori K, Ioka RX, Tachibana K, Watanabe Y, Uchiyama Y, Sumi K, Iguchi H, Ito S, Doi T, Hamakubo T, Naito M, Auwerx J, Yanagisawa M, Kodama T, Sakai J. Activation of peroxisome proliferator-activated receptor delta induces fatty acid beta-oxida-

tion in skeletal muscle and attenuates metabolic syndrome. Proc Natl Acad Sci U S A 2003; 100: 15924-9.

[48] Cunningham JT, Rodgers JT, Arlow DH, Vazquez F, Mootha VK, Puigserver P. mTOR controls mitochondrial oxidative function through a YY1-PGC-1alpha transcriptional complex. Nature 2007; 450: 736-40.

[49] Blattler SM, Cunningham JT, Verdeguer F, Chim H, Haas W, Liu H, Romanino K, Ruegg MA, Gygi SP, Shi Y, Puigserver P. Yin Yang 1 deficiency in skeletal muscle protects against rapamycin-induced diabetic-like symptoms through activation of insulin/IGF signaling. Cell Metab 2012; 15: 505-17.

[50] Ding WX, Yin XM. Mitophagy: mechanisms, pathophysiological roles, and analysis. Biol Chem 2012; 393: 547-64.

[51] Lemasters JJ, Qian T, He L, Kim JS, Elmore SP, Cascio WE, Brenner DA. Role of mitochondrial inner membrane permeabilization in necrotic cell death, apoptosis, and autophagy. Antioxid Redox Signal 2002; 4: 769-81.

[52] Twig G, Elorza A, Molina AJ, Mohamed H, Wikstrom JD, Walzer G, Stiles L, Haigh SE, Katz S, Las G, Alroy J, Wu M, Py BF, Yuan J, Deeney JT, Corkey BE, Shirihai OS. Fission and selective fusion govern mitochondrial segregation and elimination by autophagy. EMBO J 2008; 27: 433-46.

[53] Chen M, Sandoval H, Wang J. Selective mitochondrial autophagy during erythroid maturation. Autophagy 2008; 4: 926-8.

[54] Sandoval H, Thiagarajan P, Dasgupta SK, Schumacher A, Prchal JT, Chen M, Wang J. Essential role for Nix in autophagic maturation of erythroid cells. Nature 2008; 454: 232-5.

[55] Sato M, Sato K. Degradation of paternal mitochondria by fertilization-triggered autophagy in C. elegans embryos. Science 2011; 334: 1141-4.

[56] Santos D, Cardoso SM. Mitochondrial dynamics and neuronal fate in Parkinson's disease. Mitochondrion 2012; 12: 428-37.

[57] Koves TR, Noland RC, Bates AL, Henes ST, Muoio DM, Cortright RN. Subsarcolemmal and intermyofibrillar mitochondria play distinct roles in regulating skeletal muscle fatty acid metabolism. Am J Physiol Cell Physiol 2005; 288: C1074-82.

[58] Glancy B, Balaban RS. Protein composition and function of red and white skeletal muscle mitochondria. Am J Physiol Cell Physiol 2011; 300: C1280-90.

[59] Zhao X, Leon IR, Bak S, Mogensen M, Wrzesinski K, Hojlund K, Jensen ON. Phosphoproteome analysis of functional mitochondria isolated from resting human muscle reveals extensive phosphorylation of inner membrane protein complexes and enzymes. Mol Cell Proteomics 2011; 10: M110 000299.

[60] Kelly OM, McNamara YM, Manzke LH, Meegan MJ, Porter RK. The preservation of in vivo phosphorylated and activated uncoupling protein 3 (UCP3) in isolated skele-

tal muscle mitochondria following administration of 3,4-methylenedioxymethamphetamine (MDMA aka ecstasy) to rats/mice. Mitochondrion 2012; 12: 110-9.

[61] Anderson KA, Hirschey MD. Mitochondrial protein acetylation regulates metabolism. Essays Biochem 2012; 52: 23-35.

[62] Du J, Zhou Y, Su X, Yu JJ, Khan S, Jiang H, Kim J, Woo J, Kim JH, Choi BH, He B, Chen W, Zhang S, Cerione RA, Auwerx J, Hao Q, Lin H. Sirt5 is a NAD-dependent protein lysine demalonylase and desuccinylase. Science 2011; 334: 806-9.

[63] Mailloux RJ, Seifert EL, Bouillaud F, Aguer C, Collins S, Harper ME. Glutathionylation acts as a control switch for uncoupling proteins UCP2 and UCP3. J Biol Chem 2011; 286: 21865-75.

[64] Doulias PT, Tenopoulou M, Greene JL, Raju K, Ischiropoulos H. Nitric oxide regulates mitochondrial Fatty Acid metabolism through reversible protein s-nitrosylation. Sci Signal 2013; 6: rs1.

[65] Ferree A, Shirihai O. Mitochondrial dynamics: the intersection of form and function. Adv Exp Med Biol 2012; 748: 13-40.

[66] Koshiba T, Detmer SA, Kaiser JT, Chen H, McCaffery JM, Chan DC. Structural basis of mitochondrial tethering by mitofusin complexes. Science 2004; 305: 858-62.

[67] Song Z, Ghochani M, McCaffery JM, Frey TG, Chan DC. Mitofusins and OPA1 mediate sequential steps in mitochondrial membrane fusion. Mol Biol Cell 2009; 20: 3525-32.

[68] Yoon Y, Krueger EW, Oswald BJ, McNiven MA. The mitochondrial protein hFis1 regulates mitochondrial fission in mammalian cells through an interaction with the dynamin-like protein DLP1. Mol Cell Biol 2003; 23: 5409-20.

[69] Smirnova E, Griparic L, Shurland DL, van der Bliek AM. Dynamin-related protein Drp1 is required for mitochondrial division in mammalian cells. Mol Biol Cell 2001; 12: 2245-56.

[70] Picard M, White K, Turnbull DM. Mitochondrial morphology, topology, and membrane interactions in skeletal muscle: a quantitative three-dimensional electron microscopy study. J Appl Physiol 2013; 114: 161-71.

[71] Skulachev VP. Mitochondrial filaments and clusters as intracellular power-transmitting cables. Trends Biochem Sci 2001; 26: 23-9.

[72] Westermann B. Molecular machinery of mitochondrial fusion and fission. J Biol Chem 2008; 283: 13501-5.

[73] Krieger DA, Tate CA, McMillin-Wood J, Booth FW. Populations of rat skeletal muscle mitochondria after exercise and immobilization. J Appl Physiol 1980; 48: 23-8.

[74] Kelley DE, Goodpaster B, Wing RR, Simoneau JA. Skeletal muscle fatty acid metabolism in association with insulin resistance, obesity, and weight loss. Am J Physiol 1999; 277: E1130-41.

[75] Kim JY, Hickner RC, Cortright RL, Dohm GL, Houmard JA. Lipid oxidation is reduced in obese human skeletal muscle. Am J Physiol Endocrinol Metab 2000; 279: E1039-44.

[76] Simoneau JA, Veerkamp JH, Turcotte LP, Kelley DE. Markers of capacity to utilize fatty acids in human skeletal muscle: relation to insulin resistance and obesity and effects of weight loss. Faseb J 1999; 13: 2051-60.

[77] Kelley DE, He J, Menshikova EV, Ritov VB. Dysfunction of mitochondria in human skeletal muscle in type 2 diabetes. Diabetes 2002; 51: 2944-50.

[78] Mootha VK, Lindgren CM, Eriksson KF, Subramanian A, Sihag S, Lehar J, Puigserver P, Carlsson E, Ridderstrale M, Laurila E, Houstis N, Daly MJ, Patterson N, Mesirov JP, Golub TR, Tamayo P, Spiegelman B, Lander ES, Hirschhorn JN, Altshuler D, Groop LC. PGC-1alpha-responsive genes involved in oxidative phosphorylation are coordinately downregulated in human diabetes. Nat Genet 2003; 34: 267-73.

[79] Patti ME, Butte AJ, Crunkhorn S, Cusi K, Berria R, Kashyap S, Miyazaki Y, Kohane I, Costello M, Saccone R, Landaker EJ, Goldfine AB, Mun E, DeFronzo R, Finlayson J, Kahn CR, Mandarino LJ. Coordinated reduction of genes of oxidative metabolism in humans with insulin resistance and diabetes: Potential role of PGC1 and NRF1. Proc Natl Acad Sci U S A 2003; 100: 8466-71.

[80] Morino K, Petersen KF, Dufour S, Befroy D, Frattini J, Shatzkes N, Neschen S, White MF, Bilz S, Sono S, Pypaert M, Shulman GI. Reduced mitochondrial density and increased IRS-1 serine phosphorylation in muscle of insulin-resistant offspring of type 2 diabetic parents. J Clin Invest 2005; 115: 3587-93.

[81] Heilbronn LK, Gan SK, Turner N, Campbell LV, Chisholm DJ. Markers of mitochondrial biogenesis and metabolism are lower in overweight and obese insulin-resistant subjects. J Clin Endocrinol Metab 2007; 92: 1467-73.

[82] Skov V, Glintborg D, Knudsen S, Jensen T, Kruse TA, Tan Q, Brusgaard K, Beck-Nielsen H, Hojlund K. Reduced expression of nuclear-encoded genes involved in mitochondrial oxidative metabolism in skeletal muscle of insulin-resistant women with polycystic ovary syndrome. Diabetes 2007; 56: 2349-55.

[83] van Tienen FH, Praet SF, de Feyter HM, van den Broek NM, Lindsey PJ, Schoonderwoerd KG, de Coo IF, Nicolay K, Prompers JJ, Smeets HJ, van Loon LJ. Physical activity is the key determinant of skeletal muscle mitochondrial function in type 2 diabetes. J Clin Endocrinol Metab 2012; 97: 3261-9.

[84] Wang M, Wang XC, Zhang ZY, Mou B, Hu RM. Impaired mitochondrial oxidative phosphorylation in multiple insulin-sensitive tissues of humans with type 2 diabetes mellitus. J Int Med Res 2010; 38: 769-81.

[85] Boushel R, Gnaiger E, Schjerling P, Skovbro M, Kraunsoe R, Dela F. Patients with type 2 diabetes have normal mitochondrial function in skeletal muscle. Diabetologia 2007; 50: 790-6.

[86] Ritov VB, Menshikova EV, He J, Ferrell RE, Goodpaster BH, Kelley DE. Deficiency of subsarcolemmal mitochondria in obesity and type 2 diabetes. Diabetes 2005; 54: 8-14.

[87] Hwang H, Bowen BP, Lefort N, Flynn CR, De Filippis EA, Roberts C, Smoke CC, Meyer C, Hojlund K, Yi Z, Mandarino LJ. Proteomics analysis of human skeletal muscle reveals novel abnormalities in obesity and type 2 diabetes. Diabetes 2010; 59: 33-42.

[88] Holloway GP, Thrush AB, Heigenhauser GJ, Tandon NN, Dyck DJ, Bonen A, Spriet LL. Skeletal muscle mitochondrial FAT/CD36 content and palmitate oxidation are not decreased in obese women. Am J Physiol Endocrinol Metab 2007; 292: E1782-9.

[89] Ritov VB, Menshikova EV, Azuma K, Wood R, Toledo FG, Goodpaster BH, Ruderman NB, Kelley DE. Deficiency of electron transport chain in human skeletal muscle mitochondria in type 2 diabetes mellitus and obesity. Am J Physiol Endocrinol Metab 2010; 298: E49-58.

[90] Chomentowski P, Coen PM, Radikova Z, Goodpaster BH, Toledo FG. Skeletal muscle mitochondria in insulin resistance: differences in intermyofibrillar versus subsarcolemmal subpopulations and relationship to metabolic flexibility. J Clin Endocrinol Metab 2011; 96: 494-503.

[91] Rabol R, Larsen S, Hojberg PM, Almdal T, Boushel R, Haugaard SB, Andersen JL, Madsbad S, Dela F. Regional anatomic differences in skeletal muscle mitochondrial respiration in type 2 diabetes and obesity. J Clin Endocrinol Metab 2010; 95: 857-63.

[92] Petersen KF, Befroy D, Dufour S, Dziura J, Ariyan C, Rothman DL, DiPietro L, Cline GW, Shulman GI. Mitochondrial dysfunction in the elderly: possible role in insulin resistance. Science 2003; 300: 1140-2.

[93] Petersen KF, Dufour S, Befroy D, Garcia R, Shulman GI. Impaired mitochondrial activity in the insulin-resistant offspring of patients with type 2 diabetes. N Engl J Med 2004; 350: 664-71.

[94] Petersen KF, Dufour S, Shulman GI. Decreased insulin-stimulated ATP synthesis and phosphate transport in muscle of insulin-resistant offspring of type 2 diabetic parents. PLoS Med 2005; 2: e233.

[95] Befroy DE, Petersen KF, Dufour S, Mason GF, de Graaf RA, Rothman DL, Shulman GI. Impaired mitochondrial substrate oxidation in muscle of insulin-resistant offspring of type 2 diabetic patients. Diabetes 2007; 56: 1376-81.

[96] Meex RC, Schrauwen-Hinderling VB, Moonen-Kornips E, Schaart G, Mensink M, Phielix E, van de Weijer T, Sels JP, Schrauwen P, Hesselink MK. Restoration of muscle mitochondrial function and metabolic flexibility in type 2 diabetes by exercise training is paralleled by increased myocellular fat storage and improved insulin sensitivity. Diabetes 2010; 59: 572-9.

[97] Phielix E, Schrauwen-Hinderling VB, Mensink M, Lenaers E, Meex R, Hoeks J, Kooi ME, Moonen-Kornips E, Sels JP, Hesselink MK, Schrauwen P. Lower intrinsic ADP-stimulated mitochondrial respiration underlies in vivo mitochondrial dysfunction in muscle of male type 2 diabetic patients. Diabetes 2008; 57: 2943-9.

[98] Schrauwen-Hinderling VB, Kooi ME, Hesselink MK, Jeneson JA, Backes WH, van Echteld CJ, van Engelshoven JM, Mensink M, Schrauwen P. Impaired in vivo mitochondrial function but similar intramyocellular lipid content in patients with type 2 diabetes mellitus and BMI-matched control subjects. Diabetologia 2007; 50: 113-20.

[99] Szendroedi J, Schmid AI, Chmelik M, Toth C, Brehm A, Krssak M, Nowotny P, Wolzt M, Waldhausl W, Roden M. Muscle mitochondrial ATP synthesis and glucose transport/phosphorylation in type 2 diabetes. PLoS Med 2007; 4: e154.

[100] Szendroedi J, Schmid AI, Meyerspeer M, Cervin C, Kacerovsky M, Smekal G, Graser-Lang S, Groop L, Roden M. Impaired mitochondrial function and insulin resistance of skeletal muscle in mitochondrial diabetes. Diabetes Care 2009; 32: 677-9.

[101] Bandyopadhyay GK, Yu JG, Ofrecio J, Olefsky JM. Increased malonyl-CoA levels in muscle from obese and type 2 diabetic subjects lead to decreased fatty acid oxidation and increased lipogenesis; thiazolidinedione treatment reverses these defects. Diabetes 2006; 55: 2277-85.

[102] Larsen S, Stride N, Hey-Mogensen M, Hansen CN, Andersen JL, Madsbad S, Worm D, Helge JW, Dela F. Increased mitochondrial substrate sensitivity in skeletal muscle of patients with type 2 diabetes. Diabetologia 2011; 54: 1427-36.

[103] Mogensen M, Sahlin K, Fernstrom M, Glintborg D, Vind BF, Beck-Nielsen H, Hojlund K. Mitochondrial respiration is decreased in skeletal muscle of patients with type 2 diabetes. Diabetes 2007; 56: 1592-9.

[104] Brehm A, Krssak M, Schmid AI, Nowotny P, Waldhausl W, Roden M. Increased lipid availability impairs insulin-stimulated ATP synthesis in human skeletal muscle. Diabetes 2006; 55: 136-40.

[105] Hoeks J, Hesselink MK, Russell AP, Mensink M, Saris WH, Mensink RP, Schrauwen P. Peroxisome proliferator-activated receptor-gamma coactivator-1 and insulin resistance: acute effect of fatty acids. Diabetologia 2006; 49: 2419-26.

[106] Richardson DK, Kashyap S, Bajaj M, Cusi K, Mandarino SJ, Finlayson J, DeFronzo RA, Jenkinson CP, Mandarino LJ. Lipid infusion decreases the expression of nuclear

encoded mitochondrial genes and increases the expression of extracellular matrix genes in human skeletal muscle. J Biol Chem 2005; 280: 10290-7.

[107] Sparks LM, Xie H, Koza RA, Mynatt R, Hulver MW, Bray GA, Smith SR. A high-fat diet coordinately downregulates genes required for mitochondrial oxidative phosphorylation in skeletal muscle. Diabetes 2005; 54: 1926-33.

[108] Bonnard C, Durand A, Peyrol S, Chanseaume E, Chauvin MA, Morio B, Vidal H, Rieusset J. Mitochondrial dysfunction results from oxidative stress in the skeletal muscle of diet-induced insulin-resistant mice. J Clin Invest 2008; 118: 789-800.

[109] Boudina S, Sena S, Sloan C, Tebbi A, Han YH, O'Neill BT, Cooksey RC, Jones D, Holland WL, McClain DA, Abel ED. Early mitochondrial adaptations in skeletal muscle to diet-induced obesity are strain dependent and determine oxidative stress and energy expenditure but not insulin sensitivity. Endocrinology 2012; 153: 2677-88.

[110] Gomes AP, Duarte FV, Nunes P, Hubbard BP, Teodoro JS, Varela AT, Jones JG, Sinclair DA, Palmeira CM, Rolo AP. Berberine protects against high fat diet-induced dysfunction in muscle mitochondria by inducing SIRT1-dependent mitochondrial biogenesis. Biochim Biophys Acta 2012; 1822: 185-95.

[111] Lionetti L, Mollica MP, Crescenzo R, D'Andrea E, Ferraro M, Bianco F, Liverini G, Iossa S. Skeletal muscle subsarcolemmal mitochondrial dysfunction in high-fat fed rats exhibiting impaired glucose homeostasis. Int J Obes (Lond) 2007; 31: 1596-604.

[112] Fleischman A, Johnsen S, Systrom DM, Hrovat M, Farrar CT, Frontera W, Fitch K, Thomas BJ, Torriani M, Cote HC, Grinspoon SK. Effects of a nucleoside reverse transcriptase inhibitor, stavudine, on glucose disposal and mitochondrial function in muscle of healthy adults. Am J Physiol Endocrinol Metab 2007; 292: E1666-73.

[113] Begriche K, Massart J, Robin MA, Bonnet F, Fromenty B. Mitochondrial adaptations and dysfunctions in nonalcoholic fatty liver disease. Hepatology 2013;

[114] Cortez-Pinto H, Chatham J, Chacko VP, Arnold C, Rashid A, Diehl AM. Alterations in liver ATP homeostasis in human nonalcoholic steatohepatitis: a pilot study. JAMA 1999; 282: 1659-64.

[115] Szendroedi J, Chmelik M, Schmid AI, Nowotny P, Brehm A, Krssak M, Moser E, Roden M. Abnormal hepatic energy homeostasis in type 2 diabetes. Hepatology 2009; 50: 1079-86.

[116] Krssak M, Hofer H, Wrba F, Meyerspeer M, Brehm A, Lohninger A, Steindl-Munda P, Moser E, Ferenci P, Roden M. Non-invasive assessment of hepatic fat accumulation in chronic hepatitis C by 1H magnetic resonance spectroscopy. Eur J Radiol 2010; 74: e60-6.

[117] Pagliarini DJ, Calvo SE, Chang B, Sheth SA, Vafai SB, Ong SE, Walford GA, Sugiana C, Boneh A, Chen WK, Hill DE, Vidal M, Evans JG, Thorburn DR, Carr SA, Mootha

VK. A mitochondrial protein compendium elucidates complex I disease biology. Cell 2008; 134: 112-23.

[118] Kusminski CM, Scherer PE. Mitochondrial dysfunction in white adipose tissue. Trends Endocrinol Metab 2012; 23: 435-43.

[119] Dahlman I, Forsgren M, Sjogren A, Nordstrom EA, Kaaman M, Naslund E, Attersand A, Arner P. Downregulation of electron transport chain genes in visceral adipose tissue in type 2 diabetes independent of obesity and possibly involving tumor necrosis factor-alpha. Diabetes 2006; 55: 1792-9.

[120] Kaaman M, Sparks LM, van Harmelen V, Smith SR, Sjolin E, Dahlman I, Arner P. Strong association between mitochondrial DNA copy number and lipogenesis in human white adipose tissue. Diabetologia 2007; 50: 2526-33.

[121] Choo HJ, Kim JH, Kwon OB, Lee CS, Mun JY, Han SS, Yoon YS, Yoon G, Choi KM, Ko YG. Mitochondria are impaired in the adipocytes of type 2 diabetic mice. Diabetologia 2006; 49: 784-91.

[122] Rong JX, Qiu Y, Hansen MK, Zhu L, Zhang V, Xie M, Okamoto Y, Mattie MD, Higashiyama H, Asano S, Strum JC, Ryan TE. Adipose mitochondrial biogenesis is suppressed in db/db and high-fat diet-fed mice and improved by rosiglitazone. Diabetes 2007; 56: 1751-60.

[123] Wilson-Fritch L, Nicoloro S, Chouinard M, Lazar MA, Chui PC, Leszyk J, Straubhaar J, Czech MP, Corvera S. Mitochondrial remodeling in adipose tissue associated with obesity and treatment with rosiglitazone. J Clin Invest 2004; 114: 1281-9.

[124] Kusminski CM, Holland WL, Sun K, Park J, Spurgin SB, Lin Y, Askew GR, Simcox JA, McClain DA, Li C, Scherer PE. MitoNEET-driven alterations in adipocyte mitochondrial activity reveal a crucial adaptive process that preserves insulin sensitivity in obesity. Nat Med 2012; 18: 1539-49.

[125] Vernochet C, Mourier A, Bezy O, Macotela Y, Boucher J, Rardin MJ, An D, Lee KY, Ilkayeva OR, Zingaretti CM, Emanuelli B, Smyth G, Cinti S, Newgard CB, Gibson BW, Larsson NG, Kahn CR. Adipose-Specific Deletion of TFAM Increases Mitochondrial Oxidation and Protects Mice against Obesity and Insulin Resistance. Cell Metab 2012; 16: 765-76.

[126] Cypess AM, Lehman S, Williams G, Tal I, Rodman D, Goldfine AB, Kuo FC, Palmer EL, Tseng YH, Doria A, Kolodny GM, Kahn CR. Identification and importance of brown adipose tissue in adult humans. N Engl J Med 2009; 360: 1509-17.

[127] van Marken Lichtenbelt WD, Vanhommerig JW, Smulders NM, Drossaerts JM, Kemerink GJ, Bouvy ND, Schrauwen P, Teule GJ. Cold-activated brown adipose tissue in healthy men. N Engl J Med 2009; 360: 1500-8.

[128] Virtanen KA, Lidell ME, Orava J, Heglind M, Westergren R, Niemi T, Taittonen M, Laine J, Savisto NJ, Enerback S, Nuutila P. Functional brown adipose tissue in healthy adults. N Engl J Med 2009; 360: 1518-25.

[129] Ouellet V, Routhier-Labadie A, Bellemare W, Lakhal-Chaieb L, Turcotte E, Carpentier AC, Richard D. Outdoor temperature, age, sex, body mass index, and diabetic status determine the prevalence, mass, and glucose-uptake activity of 18F-FDG-detected BAT in humans. J Clin Endocrinol Metab 2011; 96: 192-9.

[130] Saito M, Okamatsu-Ogura Y, Matsushita M, Watanabe K, Yoneshiro T, Nio-Kobayashi J, Iwanaga T, Miyagawa M, Kameya T, Nakada K, Kawai Y, Tsujisaki M. High incidence of metabolically active brown adipose tissue in healthy adult humans: effects of cold exposure and adiposity. Diabetes 2009; 58: 1526-31.

[131] Pfannenberg C, Werner MK, Ripkens S, Stef I, Deckert A, Schmadl M, Reimold M, Haring HU, Claussen CD, Stefan N. Impact of age on the relationships of brown adipose tissue with sex and adiposity in humans. Diabetes 2010; 59: 1789-93.

[132] Cook SA, Varela-Carver A, Mongillo M, Kleinert C, Khan MT, Leccisotti L, Strickland N, Matsui T, Das S, Rosenzweig A, Punjabi P, Camici PG. Abnormal myocardial insulin signalling in type 2 diabetes and left-ventricular dysfunction. Eur Heart J 2010; 31: 100-11.

[133] Peterson LR, Saeed IM, McGill JB, Herrero P, Schechtman KB, Gunawardena R, Recklein CL, Coggan AR, DeMoss AJ, Dence CS, Gropler RJ. Sex and type 2 diabetes: obesity-independent effects on left ventricular substrate metabolism and relaxation in humans. Obesity (Silver Spring) 2012; 20: 802-10.

[134] Wright JJ, Kim J, Buchanan J, Boudina S, Sena S, Bakirtzi K, Ilkun O, Theobald HA, Cooksey RC, Kandror KV, Abel ED. Mechanisms for increased myocardial fatty acid utilization following short-term high-fat feeding. Cardiovasc Res 2009; 82: 351-60.

[135] Boudina S, Sena S, O'Neill BT, Tathireddy P, Young ME, Abel ED. Reduced mitochondrial oxidative capacity and increased mitochondrial uncoupling impair myocardial energetics in obesity. Circulation 2005; 112: 2686-95.

[136] Boudina S, Sena S, Theobald H, Sheng X, Wright JJ, Hu XX, Aziz S, Johnson JI, Bugger H, Zaha VG, Abel ED. Mitochondrial energetics in the heart in obesity-related diabetes: direct evidence for increased uncoupled respiration and activation of uncoupling proteins. Diabetes 2007; 56: 2457-66.

[137] Zhang Y, Yuan M, Bradley KM, Dong F, Anversa P, Ren J. Insulin-like growth factor 1 alleviates high-fat diet-induced myocardial contractile dysfunction: role of insulin signaling and mitochondrial function. Hypertension 2012; 59: 680-93.

[138] Anderson EJ, Kypson AP, Rodriguez E, Anderson CA, Lehr EJ, Neufer PD. Substrate-specific derangements in mitochondrial metabolism and redox balance in the atrium of the type 2 diabetic human heart. J Am Coll Cardiol 2009; 54: 1891-8.

[139] Perseghin G, Lattuada G, De Cobelli F, Esposito A, Belloni E, Ntali G, Ragogna F, Canu T, Scifo P, Del Maschio A, Luzi L. Increased mediastinal fat and impaired left ventricular energy metabolism in young men with newly found fatty liver. Hepatology 2008; 47: 51-8.

[140] Perseghin G, Ntali G, De Cobelli F, Lattuada G, Esposito A, Belloni E, Canu T, Costantino F, Ragogna F, Scifo P, Del Maschio A, Luzi L. Abnormal left ventricular energy metabolism in obese men with preserved systolic and diastolic functions is associated with insulin resistance. Diabetes Care 2007; 30: 1520-6.

[141] Scheuermann-Freestone M, Madsen PL, Manners D, Blamire AM, Buckingham RE, Styles P, Radda GK, Neubauer S, Clarke K. Abnormal cardiac and skeletal muscle energy metabolism in patients with type 2 diabetes. Circulation 2003; 107: 3040-6.

[142] Metzler B, Schocke MF, Steinboeck P, Wolf C, Judmaier W, Lechleitner M, Lukas P, Pachinger O. Decreased high-energy phosphate ratios in the myocardium of men with diabetes mellitus type I. J Cardiovasc Magn Reson 2002; 4: 493-502.

[143] Asmann YW, Stump CS, Short KR, Coenen-Schimke JM, Guo Z, Bigelow ML, Nair KS. Skeletal muscle mitochondrial functions, mitochondrial DNA copy numbers, and gene transcript profiles in type 2 diabetic and nondiabetic subjects at equal levels of low or high insulin and euglycemia. Diabetes 2006; 55: 3309-19.

[144] Stump CS, Short KR, Bigelow ML, Schimke JM, Nair KS. Effect of insulin on human skeletal muscle mitochondrial ATP production, protein synthesis, and mRNA transcripts. Proc Natl Acad Sci U S A 2003; 100: 7996-8001.

[145] Karakelides H, Asmann YW, Bigelow ML, Short KR, Dhatariya K, Coenen-Schimke J, Kahl J, Mukhopadhyay D, Nair KS. Effect of insulin deprivation on muscle mitochondrial ATP production and gene transcript levels in type 1 diabetic subjects. Diabetes 2007; 56: 2683-9.

[146] Sleigh A, Stears A, Thackray K, Watson L, Gambineri A, Nag S, Campi VI, Schoenmakers N, Brage S, Carpenter TA, Murgatroyd PR, O'Rahilly S, Kemp GJ, Savage DB. Mitochondrial oxidative phosphorylation is impaired in patients with congenital lipodystrophy. J Clin Endocrinol Metab 2012; 97: E438-42.

[147] Hoeks J, van Herpen NA, Mensink M, Moonen-Kornips E, van Beurden D, Hesselink MK, Schrauwen P. Prolonged fasting identifies skeletal muscle mitochondrial dysfunction as consequence rather than cause of human insulin resistance. Diabetes 2010; 59: 2117-25.

[148] de Brito OM, Scorrano L. Mitofusin 2: a mitochondria-shaping protein with signaling roles beyond fusion. Antioxid Redox Signal 2008; 10: 621-33.

[149] Bach D, Pich S, Soriano FX, Vega N, Baumgartner B, Oriola J, Daugaard JR, Lloberas J, Camps M, Zierath JR, Rabasa-Lhoret R, Wallberg-Henriksson H, Laville M, Palacin M, Vidal H, Rivera F, Brand M, Zorzano A. Mitofusin-2 determines mitochondrial

network architecture and mitochondrial metabolism. A novel regulatory mechanism altered in obesity. J Biol Chem 2003; 278: 17190-7.

[150] Pich S, Bach D, Briones P, Liesa M, Camps M, Testar X, Palacin M, Zorzano A. The Charcot-Marie-Tooth type 2A gene product, Mfn2, up-regulates fuel oxidation through expression of OXPHOS system. Hum Mol Genet 2005; 14: 1405-15.

[151] Neuspiel M, Zunino R, Gangaraju S, Rippstein P, McBride H. Activated mitofusin 2 signals mitochondrial fusion, interferes with Bax activation, and reduces susceptibility to radical induced depolarization. J Biol Chem 2005; 280: 25060-70.

[152] Chen KH, Guo X, Ma D, Guo Y, Li Q, Yang D, Li P, Qiu X, Wen S, Xiao RP, Tang J. Dysregulation of HSG triggers vascular proliferative disorders. Nat Cell Biol 2004; 6: 872-83.

[153] Hernandez-Alvarez MI, Thabit H, Burns N, Shah S, Brema I, Hatunic M, Finucane F, Liesa M, Chiellini C, Naon D, Zorzano A, Nolan JJ. Subjects with early-onset type 2 diabetes show defective activation of the skeletal muscle PGC-1{alpha}/Mitofusin-2 regulatory pathway in response to physical activity. Diabetes Care 2010; 33: 645-51.

[154] Mingrone G, Manco M, Calvani M, Castagneto M, Naon D, Zorzano A. Could the low level of expression of the gene encoding skeletal muscle mitofusin-2 account for the metabolic inflexibility of obesity? Diabetologia 2005; 48: 2108-14.

[155] Sebastian D, Hernandez-Alvarez MI, Segales J, Sorianello E, Munoz JP, Sala D, Waget A, Liesa M, Paz JC, Gopalacharyulu P, Oresic M, Pich S, Burcelin R, Palacin M, Zorzano A. Mitofusin 2 (Mfn2) links mitochondrial and endoplasmic reticulum function with insulin signaling and is essential for normal glucose homeostasis. Proc Natl Acad Sci U S A 2012; 109: 5523-8.

[156] Quiros PM, Ramsay AJ, Sala D, Fernandez-Vizarra E, Rodriguez F, Peinado JR, Fernandez-Garcia MS, Vega JA, Enriquez JA, Zorzano A, Lopez-Otin C. Loss of mitochondrial protease OMA1 alters processing of the GTPase OPA1 and causes obesity and defective thermogenesis in mice. EMBO J 2012; 31: 2117-33.

[157] Jheng HF, Tsai PJ, Guo SM, Kuo LH, Chang CS, Su IJ, Chang CR, Tsai YS. Mitochondrial fission contributes to mitochondrial dysfunction and insulin resistance in skeletal muscle. Mol Cell Biol 2012; 32: 309-19.

[158] Lee IM, Shiroma EJ, Lobelo F, Puska P, Blair SN, Katzmarzyk PT, Lancet Physical Activity Series Working G. Effect of physical inactivity on major non-communicable diseases worldwide: an analysis of burden of disease and life expectancy. Lancet 2012; 380: 219-29.

[159] Hoppeler H, Fluck M. Plasticity of skeletal muscle mitochondria: structure and function. Med Sci Sports Exerc 2003; 35: 95-104.

[160] Hamilton MT, Hamilton DG, Zderic TW. Role of low energy expenditure and sitting in obesity, metabolic syndrome, type 2 diabetes, and cardiovascular disease. Diabetes 2007; 56: 2655-67.

[161] Levine JA, Lanningham-Foster LM, McCrady SK, Krizan AC, Olson LR, Kane PH, Jensen MD, Clark MM. Interindividual variation in posture allocation: possible role in human obesity. Science 2005; 307: 584-6.

[162] Levine JA, McCrady SK, Lanningham-Foster LM, Kane PH, Foster RC, Manohar CU. The role of free-living daily walking in human weight gain and obesity. Diabetes 2008; 57: 548-54.

[163] Ukropcova B, McNeil M, Sereda O, de Jonge L, Xie H, Bray GA, Smith SR. Dynamic changes in fat oxidation in human primary myocytes mirror metabolic characteristics of the donor. J Clin Invest 2005; 115: 1934-41.

[164] Hulver MW, Berggren JR, Carper MJ, Miyazaki M, Ntambi JM, Hoffman EP, Thyfault JP, Stevens R, Dohm GL, Houmard JA, Muoio DM. Elevated stearoyl-CoA desaturase-1 expression in skeletal muscle contributes to abnormal fatty acid partitioning in obese humans. Cell Metab 2005; 2: 251-61.

[165] Barroso I, Luan J, Sandhu MS, Franks PW, Crowley V, Schafer AJ, O'Rahilly S, Wareham NJ. Meta-analysis of the Gly482Ser variant in PPARGC1A in type 2 diabetes and related phenotypes. Diabetologia 2006; 49: 501-5.

[166] Ling C, Poulsen P, Simonsson S, Ronn T, Holmkvist J, Almgren P, Hagert P, Nilsson E, Mabey AG, Nilsson P, Vaag A, Groop L. Genetic and epigenetic factors are associated with expression of respiratory chain component NDUFB6 in human skeletal muscle. J Clin Invest 2007; 117: 3427-35.

[167] Barres R, Osler ME, Yan J, Rune A, Fritz T, Caidahl K, Krook A, Zierath JR. Non-CpG methylation of the PGC-1alpha promoter through DNMT3B controls mitochondrial density. Cell Metab 2009; 10: 189-98.

[168] Sookoian S, Rosselli MS, Gemma C, Burgueno AL, Fernandez Gianotti T, Castano GO, Pirola CJ. Epigenetic regulation of insulin resistance in nonalcoholic fatty liver disease: impact of liver methylation of the peroxisome proliferator-activated receptor gamma coactivator 1alpha promoter. Hepatology 2010; 52: 1992-2000.

[169] Gemma C, Sookoian S, Dieuzeide G, Garcia SI, Gianotti TF, Gonzalez CD, Pirola CJ. Methylation of TFAM gene promoter in peripheral white blood cells is associated with insulin resistance in adolescents. Mol Genet Metab 2010; 100: 83-7.

[170] Ronn T, Poulsen P, Tuomi T, Isomaa B, Groop L, Vaag A, Ling C. Genetic variation in ATP5O is associated with skeletal muscle ATP50 mRNA expression and glucose uptake in young twins. PLoS One 2009; 4: e4793.

[171] Pirola CJ, Fernandez Gianotti T, Burgueno AL, Rey-Funes M, Loidl CF, Mallardi P, San Martino J, Castano GO, Sookoian S. Epigenetic modification of liver mitochon-

drial DNA is associated with histological severity of nonalcoholic fatty liver disease. Gut 2012;

[172] Galmozzi A, Mitro N, Ferrari A, Gers E, Gilardi F, Godio C, Cermenati G, Gualerzi A, Donetti E, Rotili D, Valente S, Guerrini U, Caruso D, Mai A, Saez E, De Fabiani E, Crestani M. Inhibition of Class I Histone Deacetylases Unveils a Mitochondrial Signature and Enhances Oxidative Metabolism in Skeletal Muscle and Adipose Tissue. Diabetes 2012;

[173] Andreyev AY, Kushnareva YE, Starkov AA. Mitochondrial metabolism of reactive oxygen species. Biochemistry (Mosc) 2005; 70: 200-14.

[174] Hey-Mogensen M, Jeppesen J, Madsen K, Kiens B, Franch J. Obesity augments the age-induced increase in mitochondrial capacity for H2O2 release in Zucker fatty rats. Acta Physiol (Oxf) 2012; 204: 354-61.

[175] Houstis N, Rosen ED, Lander ES. Reactive oxygen species have a causal role in multiple forms of insulin resistance. Nature 2006; 440: 944-8.

[176] Boden MJ, Brandon AE, Tid-Ang JD, Preston E, Wilks D, Stuart E, Cleasby ME, Turner N, Cooney GJ, Kraegen EW. Overexpression of manganese superoxide dismutase ameliorates high-fat diet-induced insulin resistance in rat skeletal muscle. Am J Physiol Endocrinol Metab 2012; 303: E798-805.

[177] Paglialunga S, van Bree B, Bosma M, Valdecantos MP, Amengual-Cladera E, Jorgensen JA, van Beurden D, den Hartog GJ, Ouwens DM, Briede JJ, Schrauwen P, Hoeks J. Targeting of mitochondrial reactive oxygen species production does not avert lipid-induced insulin resistance in muscle tissue from mice. Diabetologia 2012; 55: 2759-68.

[178] Choksi KB, Boylston WH, Rabek JP, Widger WR, Papaconstantinou J. Oxidatively damaged proteins of heart mitochondrial electron transport complexes. Biochim Biophys Acta 2004; 1688: 95-101.

[179] Lesnefsky EJ, Hoppel CL. Cardiolipin as an oxidative target in cardiac mitochondria in the aged rat. Biochim Biophys Acta 2008; 1777: 1020-7.

[180] Kendrick AA, Choudhury M, Rahman SM, McCurdy CE, Friederich M, Van Hove JL, Watson PA, Birdsey N, Bao J, Gius D, Sack MN, Jing E, Kahn CR, Friedman JE, Jonscher KR. Fatty liver is associated with reduced SIRT3 activity and mitochondrial protein hyperacetylation. Biochem J 2011; 433: 505-14.

[181] Hirschey MD, Shimazu T, Jing E, Grueter CA, Collins AM, Aouizerat B, Stancakova A, Goetzman E, Lam MM, Schwer B, Stevens RD, Muehlbauer MJ, Kakar S, Bass NM, Kuusisto J, Laakso M, Alt FW, Newgard CB, Farese RV, Jr., Kahn CR, Verdin E. SIRT3 deficiency and mitochondrial protein hyperacetylation accelerate the development of the metabolic syndrome. Mol Cell 2011; 44: 177-90.

[182] Jing E, Emanuelli B, Hirschey MD, Boucher J, Lee KY, Lombard D, Verdin EM, Kahn CR. Sirtuin-3 (Sirt3) regulates skeletal muscle metabolism and insulin signaling via

altered mitochondrial oxidation and reactive oxygen species production. Proc Natl Acad Sci U S A 2011; 108: 14608-13.

[183] Yechoor VK, Patti ME, Saccone R, Kahn CR. Coordinated patterns of gene expression for substrate and energy metabolism in skeletal muscle of diabetic mice. Proc Natl Acad Sci U S A 2002; 99: 10587-92.

[184] Hojlund K, Yi Z, Lefort N, Langlais P, Bowen B, Levin K, Beck-Nielsen H, Mandarino LJ. Human ATP synthase beta is phosphorylated at multiple sites and shows abnormal phosphorylation at specific sites in insulin-resistant muscle. Diabetologia 2010; 53: 541-51.

[185] Hojlund K, Wrzesinski K, Larsen PM, Fey SJ, Roepstorff P, Handberg A, Dela F, Vinten J, McCormack JG, Reynet C, Beck-Nielsen H. Proteome analysis reveals phosphorylation of ATP synthase beta -subunit in human skeletal muscle and proteins with potential roles in type 2 diabetes. J Biol Chem 2003; 278: 10436-42.

[186] Trenell MI, Hollingsworth KG, Lim EL, Taylor R. Increased daily walking improves lipid oxidation without changes in mitochondrial function in type 2 diabetes. Diabetes Care 2008; 31: 1644-9.

[187] De Feyter HM, van den Broek NM, Praet SF, Nicolay K, van Loon LJ, Prompers JJ. Early or advanced stage type 2 diabetes is not accompanied by in vivo skeletal muscle mitochondrial dysfunction. Eur J Endocrinol 2008; 158: 643-53.

[188] Brons C, Jensen CB, Storgaard H, Alibegovic A, Jacobsen S, Nilsson E, Astrup A, Quistorff B, Vaag A. Mitochondrial function in skeletal muscle is normal and unrelated to insulin action in young men born with low birth weight. J Clin Endocrinol Metab 2008; 93: 3885-92.

[189] Karakelides H, Irving BA, Short KR, O'Brien P, Nair KS. Age, obesity, and sex effects on insulin sensitivity and skeletal muscle mitochondrial function. Diabetes 2010; 59: 89-97.

[190] Lefort N, Glancy B, Bowen B, Willis WT, Bailowitz Z, De Filippis EA, Brophy C, Meyer C, Hojlund K, Yi Z, Mandarino LJ. Increased reactive oxygen species production and lower abundance of complex I subunits and carnitine palmitoyltransferase 1B protein despite normal mitochondrial respiration in insulin-resistant human skeletal muscle. Diabetes 2010; 59: 2444-52.

[191] Nair KS, Bigelow ML, Asmann YW, Chow LS, Coenen-Schimke JM, Klaus KA, Guo ZK, Sreekumar R, Irving BA. Asian Indians have enhanced skeletal muscle mitochondrial capacity to produce ATP in association with severe insulin resistance. Diabetes 2008; 57: 1166-75.

[192] Toledo FG, Menshikova EV, Azuma K, Radikova Z, Kelley CA, Ritov VB, Kelley DE. Mitochondrial capacity in skeletal muscle is not stimulated by weight loss despite in-

creases in insulin action and decreases in intramyocellular lipid content. Diabetes 2008; 57: 987-94.

[193] Bajaj M, Medina-Navarro R, Suraamornkul S, Meyer C, DeFronzo RA, Mandarino LJ. Paradoxical changes in muscle gene expression in insulin-resistant subjects after sustained reduction in plasma free fatty acid concentration. Diabetes 2007; 56: 743-52.

[194] Pagel-Langenickel I, Schwartz DR, Arena RA, Minerbi DC, Johnson DT, Waclawiw MA, Cannon RO, Balaban RS, Tripodi DJ, Sack MM. A discordance in rosiglitazone mediated insulin sensitization and skeletal muscle mitochondrial content/activity in type 2 diabetes mellitus. Am J Physiol Heart Circ Physiol 2007;

[195] Schrauwen-Hinderling VB, Mensink M, Hesselink MK, Sels JP, Kooi ME, Schrauwen P. The insulin-sensitizing effect of rosiglitazone in type 2 diabetes mellitus patients does not require improved in vivo muscle mitochondrial function. J Clin Endocrinol Metab 2008; 93: 2917-21.

[196] Brons C, Jacobsen S, Hiscock N, White A, Nilsson E, Dunger D, Astrup A, Quistorff B, Vaag A. Effects of high-fat overfeeding on mitochondrial function, glucose and fat metabolism, and adipokine levels in low-birth-weight subjects. Am J Physiol Endocrinol Metab 2012; 302: E43-51.

[197] Wredenberg A, Freyer C, Sandstrom ME, Katz A, Wibom R, Westerblad H, Larsson NG. Respiratory chain dysfunction in skeletal muscle does not cause insulin resistance. Biochem Biophys Res Commun 2006; 350: 202-7.

[198] Pospisilik JA, Knauf C, Joza N, Benit P, Orthofer M, Cani PD, Ebersberger I, Nakashima T, Sarao R, Neely G, Esterbauer H, Kozlov A, Kahn CR, Kroemer G, Rustin P, Burcelin R, Penninger JM. Targeted deletion of AIF decreases mitochondrial oxidative phosphorylation and protects from obesity and diabetes. Cell 2007; 131: 476-91.

[199] Vianna CR, Huntgeburth M, Coppari R, Choi CS, Lin J, Krauss S, Barbatelli G, Tzameli I, Kim YB, Cinti S, Shulman GI, Spiegelman BM, Lowell BB. Hypomorphic mutation of PGC-1beta causes mitochondrial dysfunction and liver insulin resistance. Cell Metab 2006; 4: 453-64.

[200] Choi CS, Befroy DE, Codella R, Kim S, Reznick RM, Hwang YJ, Liu ZX, Lee HY, Distefano A, Samuel VT, Zhang D, Cline GW, Handschin C, Lin J, Petersen KF, Spiegelman BM, Shulman GI. Paradoxical effects of increased expression of PGC-1alpha on muscle mitochondrial function and insulin-stimulated muscle glucose metabolism. Proc Natl Acad Sci U S A 2008; 105: 19926-31.

[201] Miura S, Kai Y, Ono M, Ezaki O. Overexpression of peroxisome proliferator-activated receptor gamma coactivator-1alpha down-regulates GLUT4 mRNA in skeletal muscles. J Biol Chem 2003; 278: 31385-90.

[202] De Feyter HM, Lenaers E, Houten SM, Schrauwen P, Hesselink MK, Wanders RJ, Nicolay K, Prompers JJ. Increased intramyocellular lipid content but normal skeletal

muscle mitochondrial oxidative capacity throughout the pathogenesis of type 2 diabetes. Faseb J 2008; 22: 3947-55.

[203] Holmstrom MH, Iglesias-Gutierrez E, Zierath JR, Garcia-Roves PM. Tissue-specific control of mitochondrial respiration in obesity-related insulin resistance and diabetes. Am J Physiol Endocrinol Metab 2012; 302: E731-9.

[204] Brady LJ, Brady PS, Romsos DR, Hoppel CL. Elevated hepatic mitochondrial and peroxisomal oxidative capacities in fed and starved adult obese (ob/ob) mice. Biochem J 1985; 231: 439-44.

[205] Han DH, Hancock CR, Jung SR, Higashida K, Kim SH, Holloszy JO. Deficiency of the mitochondrial electron transport chain in muscle does not cause insulin resistance. PLoS One 2011; 6: e19739.

[206] Turner N, Bruce CR, Beale SM, Hoehn KL, So T, Rolph MS, Cooney GJ. Excess lipid availability increases mitochondrial fatty acid oxidative capacity in muscle: evidence against a role for reduced fatty acid oxidation in lipid-induced insulin resistance in rodents. Diabetes 2007; 56: 2085-92.

[207] Garcia-Roves P, Huss JM, Han DH, Hancock CR, Iglesias-Gutierrez E, Chen M, Holloszy JO. Raising plasma fatty acid concentration induces increased biogenesis of mitochondria in skeletal muscle. Proc Natl Acad Sci U S A 2007; 104: 10709-13.

[208] Hancock CR, Han DH, Chen M, Terada S, Yasuda T, Wright DC, Holloszy JO. High-fat diets cause insulin resistance despite an increase in muscle mitochondria. Proc Natl Acad Sci U S A 2008;

[209] de Wilde J, Mohren R, van den Berg S, Boekschoten M, Dijk KW, de Groot P, Muller M, Mariman E, Smit E. Short-term high fat-feeding results in morphological and metabolic adaptations in the skeletal muscle of C57BL/6J mice. Physiol Genomics 2008; 32: 360-9.

[210] Sadler NC, Angel TE, Lewis MP, Pederson LM, Chauvigne-Hines LM, Wiedner SD, Zink EM, Smith RD, Wright AT. Activity-based protein profiling reveals mitochondrial oxidative enzyme impairment and restoration in diet-induced obese mice. PLoS One 2012; 7: e47996.

[211] Stephenson EJ, Camera DM, Jenkins TA, Kosari S, Lee JS, Hawley JA, Stepto NK. Skeletal muscle respiratory capacity is enhanced in rats consuming an obesogenic Western diet. Am J Physiol Endocrinol Metab 2012; 302: E1541-9.

[212] Turner N, Hariharan K, TidAng J, Frangioudakis G, Beale SM, Wright LE, Zeng XY, Leslie SJ, Li JY, Kraegen EW, Cooney GJ, Ye JM. Enhancement of muscle mitochondrial oxidative capacity and alterations in insulin action are lipid species dependent: potent tissue-specific effects of medium-chain fatty acids. Diabetes 2009; 58: 2547-54.

[213] Bruce CR, Hoy AJ, Turner N, Watt MJ, Allen TL, Carpenter K, Cooney GJ, Febbraio MA, Kraegen EW. Overexpression of carnitine palmitoyltransferase-1 in skeletal

muscle is sufficient to enhance fatty acid oxidation and improve high fat diet-induced insulin resistance. Diabetes 2009; 58: 550-8.

[214] Koves TR, Ussher JR, Noland RC, Slentz D, Mosedale M, Ilkayeva O, Bain J, Stevens R, Dyck JR, Newgard CB, Lopaschuk GD, Muoio DM. Mitochondrial overload and incomplete fatty acid oxidation contribute to skeletal muscle insulin resistance. Cell Metab 2008; 7: 45-56.

[215] Mihalik SJ, Goodpaster BH, Kelley DE, Chace DH, Vockley J, Toledo FG, DeLany JP. Increased levels of plasma acylcarnitines in obesity and type 2 diabetes and identification of a marker of glucolipotoxicity. Obesity (Silver Spring) 2010; 18: 1695-700.

[216] Adams SH, Hoppel CL, Lok KH, Zhao L, Wong SW, Minkler PE, Hwang DH, Newman JW, Garvey WT. Plasma acylcarnitine profiles suggest incomplete long-chain fatty acid beta-oxidation and altered tricarboxylic acid cycle activity in type 2 diabetic African-American women. J Nutr 2009; 139: 1073-81.

[217] Muoio DM, Noland RC, Kovalik JP, Seiler SE, Davies MN, DeBalsi KL, Ilkayeva OR, Stevens RD, Kheterpal I, Zhang J, Covington JD, Bajpeyi S, Ravussin E, Kraus W, Koves TR, Mynatt RL. Muscle-specific deletion of carnitine acetyltransferase compromises glucose tolerance and metabolic flexibility. Cell Metab 2012; 15: 764-77.

[218] Rimbert V, Boirie Y, Bedu M, Hocquette JF, Ritz P, Morio B. Muscle fat oxidative capacity is not impaired by age but by physical inactivity: association with insulin sensitivity. Faseb J 2004; 18: 737-9.

[219] Ostergard T, Andersen JL, Nyholm B, Lund S, Nair KS, Saltin B, Schmitz O. Impact of exercise training on insulin sensitivity, physical fitness, and muscle oxidative capacity in first-degree relatives of type 2 diabetic patients. Am J Physiol Endocrinol Metab 2006; 290: E998-1005.

[220] Toledo FG, Menshikova EV, Ritov VB, Azuma K, Radikova Z, DeLany J, Kelley DE. Effects of physical activity and weight loss on skeletal muscle mitochondria and relationship with glucose control in type 2 diabetes. Diabetes 2007; 56: 2142-7.

[221] Nielsen J, Mogensen M, Vind BF, Sahlin K, Hojlund K, Schroder HD, Ortenblad N. Increased subsarcolemmal lipids in type 2 diabetes: effect of training on localization of lipids, mitochondria, and glycogen in sedentary human skeletal muscle. Am J Physiol Endocrinol Metab 2010; 298: E706-13.

[222] Larson-Meyer DE, Heilbronn LK, Redman LM, Newcomer BR, Frisard MI, Anton S, Smith SR, Alfonso A, Ravussin E. Effect of calorie restriction with or without exercise on insulin sensitivity, beta-cell function, fat cell size, and ectopic lipid in overweight subjects. Diabetes Care 2006; 29: 1337-44.

[223] Weiss EP, Racette SB, Villareal DT, Fontana L, Steger-May K, Schechtman KB, Klein S, Holloszy JO. Improvements in glucose tolerance and insulin action induced by in-

creasing energy expenditure or decreasing energy intake: a randomized controlled trial. Am J Clin Nutr 2006; 84: 1033-42.

[224] Civitarese AE, Carling S, Heilbronn LK, Hulver MH, Ukropcova B, Deutsch WA, Smith SR, Ravussin E. Calorie restriction increases muscle mitochondrial biogenesis in healthy humans. PLoS Med 2007; 4: e76.

[225] Nisoli E, Tonello C, Cardile A, Cozzi V, Bracale R, Tedesco L, Falcone S, Valerio A, Cantoni O, Clementi E, Moncada S, Carruba MO. Calorie restriction promotes mitochondrial biogenesis by inducing the expression of eNOS. Science 2005; 310: 314-7.

[226] Feige JN, Lagouge M, Canto C, Strehle A, Houten SM, Milne JC, Lambert PD, Mataki C, Elliott PJ, Auwerx J. Specific SIRT1 activation mimics low energy levels and protects against diet-induced metabolic disorders by enhancing fat oxidation. Cell Metab 2008; 8: 347-58.

[227] Lagouge M, Argmann C, Gerhart-Hines Z, Meziane H, Lerin C, Daussin F, Messadeq N, Milne J, Lambert P, Elliott P, Geny B, Laakso M, Puigserver P, Auwerx J. Resveratrol improves mitochondrial function and protects against metabolic disease by activating SIRT1 and PGC-1alpha. Cell 2006; 127: 1109-22.

[228] Milne JC, Lambert PD, Schenk S, Carney DP, Smith JJ, Gagne DJ, Jin L, Boss O, Perni RB, Vu CB, Bemis JE, Xie R, Disch JS, Ng PY, Nunes JJ, Lynch AV, Yang H, Galonek H, Israelian K, Choy W, Iffland A, Lavu S, Medvedik O, Sinclair DA, Olefsky JM, Jirousek MR, Elliott PJ, Westphal CH. Small molecule activators of SIRT1 as therapeutics for the treatment of type 2 diabetes. Nature 2007; 450: 712-6.

[229] Baur JA, Pearson KJ, Price NL, Jamieson HA, Lerin C, Kalra A, Prabhu VV, Allard JS, Lopez-Lluch G, Lewis K, Pistell PJ, Poosala S, Becker KG, Boss O, Gwinn D, Wang M, Ramaswamy S, Fishbein KW, Spencer RG, Lakatta EG, Le Couteur D, Shaw RJ, Navas P, Puigserver P, Ingram DK, de Cabo R, Sinclair DA. Resveratrol improves health and survival of mice on a high-calorie diet. Nature 2006; 444: 337-42.

[230] Timmers S, Konings E, Bilet L, Houtkooper RH, van de Weijer T, Goossens GH, Hoeks J, van der Krieken S, Ryu D, Kersten S, Moonen-Kornips E, Hesselink MK, Kunz I, Schrauwen-Hinderling VB, Blaak EE, Auwerx J, Schrauwen P. Calorie restriction-like effects of 30 days of resveratrol supplementation on energy metabolism and metabolic profile in obese humans. Cell Metab 2011; 14: 612-22.

[231] Yoshino J, Conte C, Fontana L, Mittendorfer B, Imai S, Schechtman KB, Gu C, Kunz I, Rossi Fanelli F, Patterson BW, Klein S. Resveratrol supplementation does not improve metabolic function in nonobese women with normal glucose tolerance. Cell Metab 2012; 16: 658-64.

[232] Canto C, Houtkooper RH, Pirinen E, Youn DY, Oosterveer MH, Cen Y, Fernandez-Marcos PJ, Yamamoto H, Andreux PA, Cettour-Rose P, Gademann K, Rinsch C, Schoonjans K, Sauve AA, Auwerx J. The NAD(+) precursor nicotinamide riboside en-

hances oxidative metabolism and protects against high-fat diet-induced obesity. Cell Metab 2012; 15: 838-47.

[233] Yoshino J, Mills KF, Yoon MJ, Imai S. Nicotinamide mononucleotide, a key NAD(+) intermediate, treats the pathophysiology of diet- and age-induced diabetes in mice. Cell Metab 2011; 14: 528-36.

[234] Tainter ML, Stockton AB, Cutting WC. Use of dinitrophenol in obesity and related conditions. Final report. JAMA 1935; 105: 332-336.

[235] Miranda EJ, McIntyre IM, Parker DR, Gary RD, Logan BK. Two deaths attributed to the use of 2,4-dinitrophenol. J Anal Toxicol 2006; 30: 219-22.

[236] Tewari A, Ali T, O'Donnell J, Butt MS. Weight loss and 2,4-dinitrophenol poisoning. Br J Anaesth 2009; 102: 566-7.

[237] Lou PH, Hansen BS, Olsen PH, Tullin S, Murphy MP, Brand MD. Mitochondrial uncouplers with an extraordinary dynamic range. Biochem J 2007; 407: 129-40.

[238] Severin FF, Severina, II, Antonenko YN, Rokitskaya TI, Cherepanov DA, Mokhova EN, Vyssokikh MY, Pustovidko AV, Markova OV, Yaguzhinsky LS, Korshunova GA, Sumbatyan NV, Skulachev MV, Skulachev VP. Penetrating cation/fatty acid anion pair as a mitochondria-targeted protonophore. Proc Natl Acad Sci U S A 2010; 107: 663-8.

[239] Antonenko YN, Avetisyan AV, Cherepanov DA, Knorre DA, Korshunova GA, Markova OV, Ojovan SM, Perevoshchikova IV, Pustovidko AV, Rokitskaya TI, Severina, II, Simonyan RA, Smirnova EA, Sobko AA, Sumbatyan NV, Severin FF, Skulachev VP. Derivatives of rhodamine 19 as mild mitochondria-targeted cationic uncouplers. J Biol Chem 2011; 286: 17831-40.

[240] Lee YS, Kim WS, Kim KH, Yoon MJ, Cho HJ, Shen Y, Ye JM, Lee CH, Oh WK, Kim CT, Hohnen-Behrens C, Gosby A, Kraegen EW, James DE, Kim JB. Berberine, a natural plant product, activates AMP-activated protein kinase with beneficial metabolic effects in diabetic and insulin-resistant states. Diabetes 2006; 55: 2256-64.

[241] Dong H, Wang N, Zhao L, Lu F. Berberine in the treatment of type 2 diabetes mellitus: a systemic review and meta-analysis. Evid Based Complement Alternat Med 2012; 2012: 591654.

[242] Turner N, Li JY, Gosby A, To SW, Cheng Z, Miyoshi H, Taketo MM, Cooney GJ, Kraegen EW, James DE, Hu LH, Li J, Ye JM. Berberine and its more biologically available derivative, dihydroberberine, inhibit mitochondrial respiratory complex I: a mechanism for the action of berberine to activate AMP-activated protein kinase and improve insulin action. Diabetes 2008; 57: 1414-8.

[243] Eid HM, Martineau LC, Saleem A, Muhammad A, Vallerand D, Benhaddou-Andaloussi A, Nistor L, Afshar A, Arnason JT, Haddad PS. Stimulation of AMP-activated protein kinase and enhancement of basal glucose uptake in muscle cells by quercetin

and quercetin glycosides, active principles of the antidiabetic medicinal plant Vaccinium vitis-idaea. Mol Nutr Food Res 2010; 54: 991-1003.

[244] Brunmair B, Staniek K, Gras F, Scharf N, Althaym A, Clara R, Roden M, Gnaiger E, Nohl H, Waldhausl W, Furnsinn C. Thiazolidinediones, like metformin, inhibit respiratory complex I: a common mechanism contributing to their antidiabetic actions? Diabetes 2004; 53: 1052-9.

[245] Owen MR, Doran E, Halestrap AP. Evidence that metformin exerts its anti-diabetic effects through inhibition of complex 1 of the mitochondrial respiratory chain. Biochem J 2000; 348 Pt 3: 607-14.

Chapter 5

Sympathovagal Imbalance in Type 2 Diabetes — Role of Brainstem Thyrotropin-Releasing Hormone

Hong Yang

Additional information is available at the end of the chapter

http://dx.doi.org/10.5772/56541

1. Introduction

Type 2 diabetes (T2D) is the world's fastest growing disease with high morbidity and mortality rates. The potential to develop effective therapies is severely limited by poor understanding of mechanisms underlying the etiology and progression of T2D.

Increasing evidence suggests that the brain plays a key role in regulating metabolism [1, 2]. In particular, the exquisitely precise adjustments in the sympathetic and parasympathetic outflow by the brain are critical for maintaining metabolic homeostasis. Enhanced sympathetic drive and impaired vagal efferent function contribute to multisystemic pathophysiology of T2D, including reduced insulin secretion, gastroparesis, hypertension, and high cardiovascular mortality [3-6]. The aim of this chapter is to emphasize the importance of the brainstem, which contains sympathovagal regulatory nuclei, in the regulation of metabolism, especially in T2D conditions. I focus on the role of b ainstem thyrotropin-releasing hormone (TRH) in the physiology of autonomic control of metabolism and the pathophysiology of autonomic dysfunction in T2D. TRH is a three amino acid neuropeptide originally discovered in the hypothalamic paraventricular nucleus. Brainstem raphe nuclei are another major locus of TRH neurons, which send TRH-containing projections to innervate brainstem and spinal sympathetic and vagal motor/premotor nuclei. TRH acts at these nuclei to control sympathetic and vagal descending pathways involved in regulating food intake, blood pressure, heart beat, pancreatic insulin secretion, and gastrointestinal secretion/motility. Our studies found an impaired brainstem TRH action on the vagal efferent control in a T2D rat model. Understanding brainstem disorders responsible for the sympathovagal imbalance in T2D is fundamental for revealing the mechanism of T2D development. Targeting on restoring a balanced sympathetic-vagal regulatory function of brainstem TRH could be a new direction for the prevention and therapy of T2D.

2. The autonomic nervous system is a major pathway mediating the brain regulation of metabolism

2.1. Sympathovagal motor and premotor neurons in the brainstem and the spinal cord

The sympathetic and parasympathetic nerves are the two functionally opposite branches innervating visceral organs to mediate and integrate the central control of body metabolism. While numerous studies have well established the metabolic regulatory center of the hypothalamus, more and more recent studies revealed the importance of the brainstem in the neuroanatomically distributed control of energy balance [7]. Studies by Grill et al using the chronically decerebrate rat models demonstrated that the brainstem, also called hindbrain, contains an essential mechanism detecting metabolic need and exhibiting autonomic response to the metabolic challenge [7-9]. The brainstem is sufficient to mediate many aspects of the energetic response to starvation and maintain the normal glucose levels [10]. Indeed, the brainstem contains neural circuits receiving and sensing peripheral neural, nutritional and hormonal signals, and more importantly, including sympathovagal motor neurons and premotor neurons responding to these signals.

2.1.1. The Dorsal Vagal Complex (DVC) and the nucleus Ambiguus (Amb)

The DVC is composed of the dorsal motor nucleus of the vagus (DMV) and the nucleus tractus solitarii (NTS) (Fig.1), which respectively contains somata of parasympathetic efferents projecting to the visceral organs [11-13] and neurons receiving vagal afferent input from the viscera [14]. The nearby area postrema (AP) and portions of the NTS, where the blood-brain barrier is incomplete, can be the portal of entry for circulating hormones entering the brain [15]. The Amb contains vagal motor neurons projecting to the thoracic organs as well as the upper gastrointestinal (GI) tract and the pancreas (Fig. 1).

The DMV receives powerful influence from higher brain levels. Stimulation of the neurons in the paraventricular nucleus of the hypothalamus (PVN) activates DMV neurons projecting to the gut [16,17]. The ventromedial hypothalamic nucleus (VMH), which contains glucose sensitive neurons, also has direct connections with DMV and NTS [18,19]. In addition, the DMV receives descending connections from the locus coeruleus (LC), which is the origin of the noradrenergic innervation of the preganglionic autonomic nuclei in the medulla oblongata [20].

Vagal afferent fibers arise from neurons in the nodose ganglia and their central and peripheral terminals are located respectively in the NTS and visceral organs. A number of NTS neurons directly, or indirectly via interneurons, connect with vagal motor neurons in the DMV, forming vago-vagal reflex, which may result in increased or decreased vagal efferent activity, and thus is an important component in the brainstem circuits controlling the vagal efferent function, independent of the higher brain [21-23].

Acetylcholine is the major transmitter of vagal preganglionic motoneurons in the DMV, which contains intense choline acetyltransferase (ChAT) [24]. By retrograde tracing of subdiaphrag-

http://dx.doi.org/10.5772/56541

matic vagus, the majority (52%) of labeled DMV cells is ChAT positive [25]. Nitric oxide (NO)-synthesizing neurons are identified in the DMV as vagal motoneurons projecting to the GI tract and also in the NTS [26,27]. These neurons are involved in the gastric receptive relaxation reflex [26]. The catecholaminergic NTS neurons are tyrosine hydroxylase (TH) positive that relay the signals received by the NTS to other brain structures [28].

2.1.2. The spinal intermediolateral cell column (IML) and the rostral ventrolateral medulla (RVLM)

The sympathetic preganglionic motor neurons are located in the IML of the spinal cord. A group of brainstem neurons in the RVLM are sympathetic premotor neurons that project monosynaptically to the IML. Brainstem RVLM is the final common point of convergence of most brain pathways regulating sympathetic tone controlling functions of multisystemic visceral organs [29, 30]. The efferent projections of the catecholamine neurons in the C1 area of the RVLM display important central control of the cardiovascular regulation [31]. Trans-neuronal labeling studies also showed that the RVLM is a major brain region involved in sympathetic control of the pancreas [32].

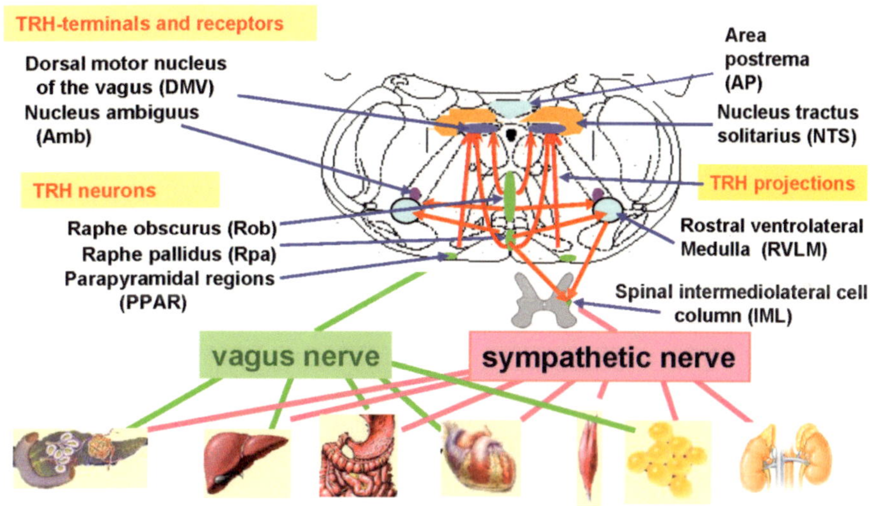

Figure 1. Coronal barainstem section (interaural-4.68 mm) showing the location of THR neurons and THR terminals, and THR regulation of sympathovagal functions.

2.2. sympathovagal-efferent regulation of pancreatic islet hormones secretion and food intake

The autonomic nervous system plays a fundamental role in the brain regulation of metabolism, as this system innervates and tightly controls multisystemic organs involved in food intake and digestion, nutrition absorption, peripheral hormone secretion, blood circulation, and metabolic waste excretion. Here we focus on the pancreatic endocrine secretion and food intake.

2.2.1. Brain regulation of pancreatic endocrine secretion through vagal and sympathetic nerves

The central nervous system requires glucose as an essential source of energy. To maintain blood glucose levels within a narrow range, the brain regulates pancreatic endocrine secretion through rich innervation of vagal and sympathetic nerves in the islets [33]. In rats, three of the five vagal branches, the posterior gastric, anterior gastric, and the hepatic branches, mediate insulin secretion [34]. The direct sympathetic innervation of the pancreas comes from the sympathetic chains and splanchnic and celiac ganglia [35]. Insulin secretion is stimulated by vagal activation and inhibited by sympathetic-adrenal activation [36]. The integrity of vagus-cholinergic component plays an important role in pancreatic islet proliferation and insulin secretion of the cephalic phase and during the early absorption period, and is necessary to maintain normal glucose tolerance [33, 37-40]. Impairment in glucose tolerance is frequently observed in pancreas-transplanted patients due to denervation of the grafted pancreas. These patients have a high basal invariant insulin levels but a reduced insulin secretory capacity in response to glucose challenge; cephalic phase insulin release is absent [41-43]. Decreased β-cell mass was observed in dogs undergone pancreas-transplantation [44]. Acetylcholine is the major neurotransmitter of the vagus nervous and M3 receptor represents the major muscarinic receptor that is functional in pancreatic β-cells [36, 45, 46]. Mutant mice selectively lacking M3 receptor in pancreatic β-cells display impaired glucose tolerance and greatly reduced insulin release. In contrast, mice selectively overexpressing M3 receptors in β-cells show a profound increase in glucose tolerance and insulin release. Moreover, the β-cell M3-overexpressing mice are resistant to diet-induced glucose intolerance and hyperglycemia [47]. These findings indicate that autonomic nerves play a key role in maintaining proper insulin release and glucose homeostasis.

2.2.2. The importance of the vagus nerve in food intake regulation

Food intake provides body energy. Autonomic innervation, especially cholinergic processes of the vagus control hunger, meal initiation, and food digestion. Vagal-cholinergic (muscarinic) activation regulates gastric ghrelin biosynthesis and secretion [48, 49]. Elevation of plasma ghrelin induced by food deprivation can be blocked by subdiaphragmatic vagotomy and atropine treatment [50]. Circulating ghrelin levels in humans are increased or reduced by cholinergic agonists or antagonists, respectively [51].

2.3. Brainstem sympathovagal-controlling circuits respond to metabolic alterations

Hypoglycemia is a well established central stimulus that enhances autonomic activities [52-55]. The neuronal activations in the PVN, DVC and other autonomic-regulatory nuclei are initiated when blood glucose levels are immediately below the normal range; the extent of neuronal activation negatively correlates with glucose levels [55]. Microinjection of glucose into the DVC prevents hypoglycemia-induced gastric motility response, indicating a direct influence of glucose concentration on the DVC neurons [56, 57]. Acute glucose deprivation by 2-deoxy-glucose induces Fos expression in NADPH-positive neurons in the NTS and DMV [58] and in catecholamine neurons in the RVLM [59]. Electrophysiological data suggest that some DMV neurons have an enteroceptor function detecting changes in glucose concentration in their environment [60]; however, another study found that glucose had no direct effect on DMV neurons, which appear to be affected by glucose action on NTS neurons [61]. The NTS neurons transmit information of local glucose availability and peripheral glucose metabolic signals received from the vagal afferents toward other brain areas, such as the nearby DMV, via circuits mediating vagal-vagal reflex, and the hypothalamus, including the PVN, via the ascending adrenergic and noradrenergic pathways [61-64]. The response of medullary vagal-regulatory circuits to altered blood glucose levels seems independent of the higher brain structures. In dogs, decerebration and mid-brain or pontine section did not prevent insulin-hypoglycemia-induced gastric acid secretion, which was drastically reduced after destruction of the DMV [65]. Beside the enhanced vagal efferent outflow, which mediates hypoglycemia induced food intake, neuronal activation in the RVLM by glucose deprivation increases sympathetic efferent activity [59], which is important for the liver to produce and release more glucose. These findings indicate that activating brainstem autonomic regulatory circuits is an important counterregulatory response for changed metabolic status.

3. Brainstem Thyrotropin-Releasing Hormone (TRH)-containing circuits regulate sympathovagal outflow to visceral organs

3.1. Brainstem TRH synthesizing neurons and their projections to the autonomic motor/premotor nuclei

TRH is a three amino acid neuropeptide originally discovered in the hypothalamic PVN, where it regulates pituitary thyrotropin release. Brainstem raphe nuclei, including the raphe pallidus (Rpa), raphe obscurus (Rob) and the parapyramidal regions (PPR) are among other major loci capable of TRH synthesis in the brain (Fig.1). Raphe nuclei project TRH-containing fibers to sympathetic and vagal motor neurons located respectively in the brainstem DVC, the RVLM, and the spinal IML, areas densely clustered with TRH-immunoreactive nerve terminals and TRH receptor 1 [66-69] (Figs.1,2). Electron microscopic studies revealed that TRH terminals make direct synaptic contacts with dendrites of neurons in medial NTS and vagal motoneurons throughout the DMV [68]. The direct effects of TRH are to excite DMV neurons and inhibit NTS neurons [70]. TRH-containing fibers also innervate sympathetic premotor loci, particularly the RVLM [69, 71, 72]. These TRH-containing brainstem-spinal circuits are important central components of autonomic regulation of visceral organ functions and in particular, the baroreflex pathways [73].

3.2. Brainstem TRH regulation of gastric, pancreatic, and cardiovascular functions

Studies in the 1980s by Amir S et al and others found that intracerebroventricular (icv) injection of TRH induces hyperglycemia through pathways involving the adrenal gland in rats, but prevents central and peripheral stimuli-induced hyperglycemia in mice through stimulating insulin release [74-78].

Our studies demonstrated that injection of TRH or its stable analog RX77368 into brain ventricles activates both sympathetic and vagal descending pathways, inducing sympatheti-

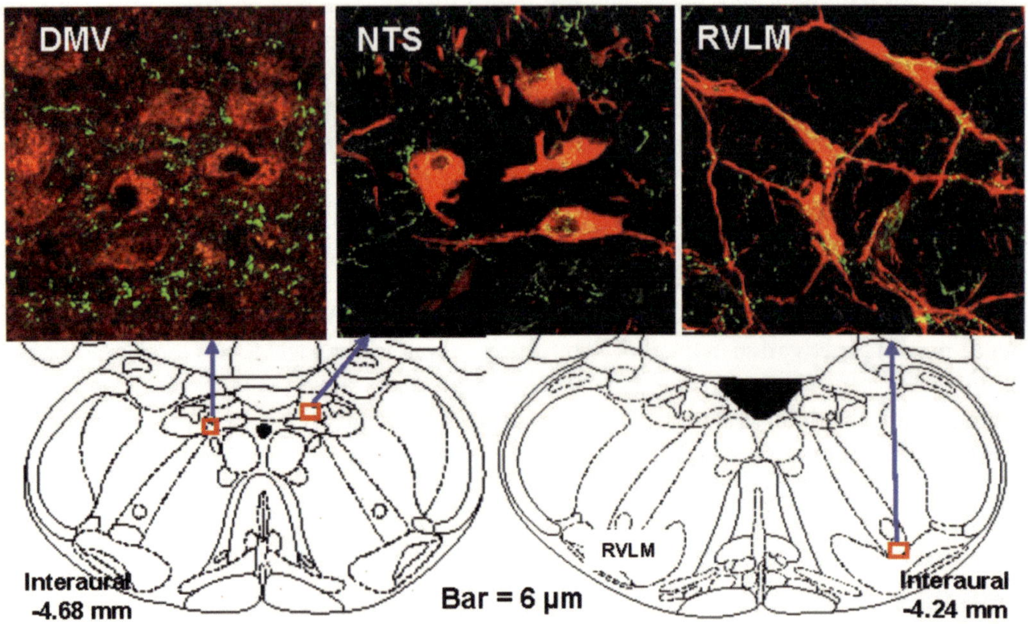

Figure 2. PreproTHR-containing fibres (green) and ChAT neurons (red) in the DMV and TH neurons (red) in the RLVM and NTS.

cally driven hyperglycemia, hypertension and tachycardia, and vagally mediated stimulation of gastric secretion/contractility, pancreatic insulin secretion, and ghrelin release [49, 69, 79-82]. The gastric myenteric plexus innervates smooth muscle and mucosal layers and receives dense and intricate network of vagal efferent axons [83-86]. Electrical stimulation of the rat cervical vagus nerve induces widespread Fos expression in the gastric myenteric plexus in rats [87, 88]. Similarly, intracisternal injection of TRH analog, known to activate vagal preganglionic neurons in the DMV and increase gastric vagal efferent discharges [80, 89,90], activates gastric myenteric neurons in rats [91]. Brainstem microinjection and intrathecal (it) injection studies revealed that pontine locus coeruleus, brainstem RVLM and spinal IML are TRH action sites for activating sympathetic efferent pathways [69, 79, 92, 93], whereas the DMV, the Amb, and the dorsal portion of the RVLM are among those responsible for the resulting stimulation of vagal efferent outflow [69, 94-96]. Substantial evidence shows that TRH is the only brain peptide fulfilling all of the criteria as a neurotransmitter and/or neuromodulator activating vagal motor neurons in the DMV [49, 69, 80, 82, 97]. TRH knockout mice are significantly hyperglycemic with impaired insulin secretion in response to glucose [98].

3.3. Physiological and pathophysiological regulation of brainstem TRH gene expression

Autonomic response to external and internal environmental changes is associated with activation of brainstem TRH containing pathways. Brainstem TRH gene expression is upregulated by energy deficiency or increased energy demand, such as starvation, hypothermia, and hypothyroidism [49, 99, 100].

The physiological role of brainstem TRH in regulating sympathovagal efferent activities responding to metabolic challenge was first evidenced in the animal model of cold exposure, which is wildly used to induce sympathetic-vagally mediated gastric ulceration [99, 101, 102]. Cold exposure activates not only TRH system in the hypothalamus but also TRH-containing Rpa/Rob/PPR-DVC pathways in the brainstem [99, 103]. The hypothermia resulting from cold exposure induces Fos expression in the Rpa, Rob, PPR and DVC neurons and enhances brainstem TRH gene expression, especially in the Rpa and Rob [99, 104, 105]. These brainstem changes are with strongly concomitant activation of gastric myenteric neurons through the excitement of vagal-nicotinic pathways and therefore responsible for the vagal-mediated increases of gastric acid secretion/motility and sympathetic-mediated decrease of mucosal blood flow, leading to gastric ulcer formation [102, 106-108]. Cold exposure induced gastric ulceration and increased gastric emptying were prevented by icv injection of TRH antiserum or antisense oligodeoxynucleotides of TRH receptor, respectively [109, 110].

Brainstem TRH gene expression is influenced by thyroid hormone levels in a feedback regulatory manner. Thyroidectomy increases TRH mRNA levels in the raphe nuclei and the effect is reversed by thyroid hormone replacement [100]. This finding indicates that abnormal brainstem TRH gene expression and altered TRH regulation of sympathovagal efferent outflow may be involved in the autonomic disorders observed in hypo- or hyperthyroidism.

Our recent studies demonstrated that brainstem TRH is involved in food intake regulation. Intracisternal injection of the stable TRH analog RX77368 (7.5-25 ng) dose-dependently stimulated solid food intake by 2.4- to 3-fold in freely fed rats, an effect that lasted for 3 hours. By contrast, RX77368 at 25 ng injected into the lateral ventricle induced a delayed and insignificant orexigenic effect only in the first hour. In pentobarbital-anesthetized rats, intracisternal injection of TRH analog (50 ng) induced a significant bi-peak increase in serum total ghrelin levels from the basal of 8.7 ± 1.7 ng/ml to 13.4 ± 2.4 ng/ml at 30 min and 14.5 ± 2.0 ng/ml at 90 min, which was prevented by either bilateral vagotomy (-60 min) or atropine pretreatment (2 mg/kg, -30 min) but magnified by bilateral adrenalectomy (-60 min). TRH analog induced food intake in freely fed rats was abolished by either peripheral atropine or ghrelin receptor antagonist (D-Lys-3)-GHRP-6 (10 μmol/kg), or intracisternal Y1 receptor antagonist 122PU91 (10 nmol/5 μl). Brainstem TRH mRNA and TRH receptor1 mRNA increased by 57-58% and 33-35% in 24-48 h fasted rats and returned to the fed levels after a 3 hour re-feeding. Natural food intake in overnight fasted rats was significantly reduced by intracisternal TRH antibody, Y1 antagonist, and peripheral atropine. These data establish a physiological role of brainstem TRH in vagal-ghrelin-mediated stimulation of food intake, which involves interaction with brainstem Y1 receptors [49].

3.4. Interaction of TRH with other neurotransmitters and neuropeptides in the DVC

The TRH-synthesizing neurons in brainstem raphe nuclei contain other neuropeptides and neurotransmitters, such as substance P (SP) and serotonin (5-HT). These transmitters/peptides co-release with TRH in the raphe projections innervating the target autonomic-regulatory neurons. In the DVC, 5-HT potentiates and SP suppresses the vagal-activating action of TRH [111, 112].

3.5. Upper GI afferent signals influence TRH regulation of vagal efferent activity

The upper gut mechano-/chemo- signals and their impact on ascending sympathetic-vagal afferents are crucial information for the brain to adjust sympathetic-vagal efferent functions involved in controlling glucose and energy homeostasis [113, 114]. GI peptides, such as cholecystokinin (CCK) and secretin, released from the proximal small intestine, and peptide YY (PYY) and glucagon-like peptide-1 (GLP-1), released from the hindgut, all appear to accomplish their gastric/pancreatic regulatory functions through both the humoral route and the vagus nerve [113]. These peptides modulate, mostly inhibit, efferent vagal outflow at least partly through brainstem vago-vagal reflexive neurocircuits that initiated with stimulating vagal afferent pathways, acting on either vagal afferent terminals in the GI enteric plexuses, vagal afferent neurons in the nodose ganglions that express all the relevant receptors for these gut hormones, or brainstem AP/NTS neurons, where receptors of these peptides are localized [113, 114]. Glucose itself is an activator of vagal afferents [114]. In addition, information of glucose metabolism in the liver is sent to the brainstem via the afferent fibers in the hepatic vagal branch. Sensors localized in the portal vein pass nutrition signals to the brain through sympathetic-spinal pathways [113, 114]. Of particular noticeable, the vagal-efferent activation by brainstem TRH is inhibited by these signals from proximal gut. We have found that intraduodenal infusion of lipid or intravenous infusion of glucose, CCK, secretin, or PYY inhibits intracisternal TRH-induced gastric acid secretion that is mediated by vagal efferent activation [115-117].

Collectively, research findings show that the TRH containing raphe-DVC pathways and raphe-IML pathways play important physiological roles in maintaining metabolic homeostasis, through balancing sympathovagal outflow that controls multisystemic visceral organs.

4. Sympathovagal imbalance is the linchpin of T2D pathophysiology

Relative to healthy peers, diabetic patients have increased sympathetic and decreased parasympathetic activity that appears to be present at early stages of metabolic impairment, regardless of the presence or absence of autonomic neuropathy [118-121]. T2D patients have higher resting muscle sympathetic nerve activity burst incidence and arterial norepinephrine levels, lower plasma norepinephrine clearance and reduced neuronal reuptake, compared with obese metabolic syndrome patients [122]. The progression from obesity to T2D is associated with increased central sympathetic drive, blunted sympathetic responsiveness, and altered norepinephrine disposition [122]. Unbalanced autonomic function leads to the development of diabetes and its complications, including hypertension [123], increased risk of cardiovascular events such as arrhythmia [4, 124, 125], enhanced activity of hypothalamus-pituitary-adrenal axis [126], potentiated hepatic glucose output [127], suppression of insulin release [128], insulin resistance [6], lipemia and increased visceral fat [129], chronic renal failure [130], reduced gastric secretion/motility and altered gut hormone secretion [131, 132]. Moreover, sympathetic overactivity may be a contributing factor to the development of T2D in non-obese men [133]. Vagal impairment contributes significantly to the predominance of sympathetic activity in T2D [4].

http://dx.doi.org/10.5772/56541

4.1. The vagal regulation of visceral function is altered by abnormal blood glucose levels in T2D

Converging evidence suggests that hyper- or hypoglycemia affects GI functions by influencing vagal-cholinergic outflow to the viscera. GI functions stimulated by vagal efferent activation, such as sham feeding-induced pancreatic polypeptide (PP) release and gastric acid secretion, were remarkably reduced in humans during hyperglycemia [134]. In the rat, experimental diabetes lowered gastric acid secretion, which did not decrease further after vagotomy [135]. Hyperglycemia induced by intravenous glucose infusion completely prevented the gastric acid secretion stimulated by intracisternal TRH analog [115]. In contrast to hyperglycemia, insulin-hypoglycemia induces central-vagal stimulus of upper GI functions and has been widely used to test vagus nerve integrity [136-139]. These findings establish the mediating role of the vagus nerve in GI functional alternations induced by altered glucose metabolism.

Gastroparesis is a common complication of diabetes [140]. Gastric acid secretion is markedly lower and gastric emptying abnormalities occur in about 30-50% of diabetic patients [141-144]. Although morphological changes in the vagus nerve were identified in diabetic patients [145], many observations indicate that hyperglycemia itself may play a major role in the abnormal GI motility of T2D patients, in addition to the traditionally-attributed irreversible autonomic neuropathy [143, 146]. Acute hyperglycemia causes reversible motility impairment in the GI tract in both healthy subjects and in diabetic patients and animals [147-151]. Delay in gastric emptying is observed within one week after streptozotocin treatment in rats, when there is no autonomic neuropathy developed [152]. Even changes in blood glucose levels within the normal postprandial range significantly impact gastric emptying in both normal subjects and diabetic patients [153]. These observations show that hyperglycemia in diabetes can influence vagal-mediated visceral functions through functional alteration, in addition to morphological damage, of the vagus nerve.

4.2. Sympathovagal imbalance in T2D suppresses insulin secretory response to glucose

T2D Patients frequently lose the first phase insulin release that is mainly triggered by vagal activation [154]. The vagal-mediated acute insulin response to glucose is absent in those with glucose levels above 115 mg/dL [155]. In fact, after intravenous glucose infusion, both the first and second phases of insulin secretion are impaired in T2D patients [156]. The impaired second phase insulin secretion may result from reduced incretin secretory response and the reduction of absolute incretin effect in T2D [156-158], both can be attributed to impaired vagal efferent activity [159]. The impaired vagal function reduces the proliferation of pancreatic islet β-cells, resulting in an approximately 60% reduction in β-cell mass in T2D patients [38, 160]. With increasing duration of T2D, the decrease of postprandial insulin secretion becomes more prominent [161]. The contribution of sympathetic overactivity to the inhibition of insulin secretion in T2D was evidenced in a patient, who underwent a spinal-sympathetic blockage for treating a disorder that was not directly related to diabetes but resulted in a dramatic 50% decrease in her insulin need [162]. Adrenalectomy increases basal insulin secretion in rats [82].

4.3. Sympathetic hyperactivity contributes to cardiovascular diseases in T2D

Cardiovascular disease is the leading cause of mortality in patients with T2D. T2D patients have a high incidence of hypertension and nonischemic heart failure, and worse outcomes in acute cardiovascular events compared to non-diabetic controls [163, 164]. A key mechanism underlying cardiovascular disorders is an increase in sympathetic nerve activity [73, 165], in addition to pathological cardiovascular changes due to inflammation and over-activity of the renin-angiotensin system [164, 166-168], which are associated with altered sympathovagal function as well. The cardiac vagal and sympathetic nerve functions are both abnormal in T2D patients, but particularly shown as decreased cardiac vagal baroreflex sensitivity [169]. These autonomic dysregulation contribute to increased blood pressure (BP), cardiac arrhythmias and atrial fibrillation, and the resulting progression to heart failure [4, 118, 170-173]. The attenuated sympathetic response to hypotension may contribute directly to mortality in diabetes and cardiovascular disease [174]. Autonomic dysfunction has become one of the most powerful predictor of risk for cardiac mortality in T2D patients [169, 175].

5. Brainstem TRH dysfunction is involved in the sympathovagal imbalance in T2D: Studies with T2D Goto-Kakizaki (GK) rats

Our lab in the last 10 years used a T2D rat model and combined systemic T2D pathophysiology and autonomic neuroscience to assess the role of brainstem TRH in the central mechanism responsible for the sympathovagal imbalance in T2D.

5.1. GK rat is a suitable animal model for studying sympathovagal imbalance in T2D

The GK rat is an extensively studied polygenic model of non-obese T2D that was obtained by selective breeding of individuals with glucose intolerance from a non-diabetic Wistar rat colony [176,177]. GK rats are used to dissect genetic etiology of T2D [178,179], and exhibit well-characterized features typical of human T2D, such as fasting hyperglycemia, impaired insulin-secretory response to glucose, reduced β-cell mass, chronic inflammation, disruption of hepatic lipid metabolism, hypertension, and insulin resistance [97, 176, 178, 180, 181]. GK rats and human T2D share similar late complications, such as neuropathy, nephropathy, and cardio-vascular disorders including heart failure [180, 182-184]. Glucose-stimulated insulin release was reduced by 90% in the first phase and by 75% in the second phase in GK rats [185]. Vagal-dependent increase of islet blood flow, which is required for glucose-induced insulin secretion, is diminished in GK rats [186]. Carbachol, an agonist for muscarinic acetylcholine receptors, fully normalizes insulin secretion in GK rats responding to 16.7 mmol/L glucose through an effect abolished by atropine [187].

http://dx.doi.org/10.5772/56541

5.2. Impaired brainstem TRH action on activating vagal efferents in T2D GK rats

5.2.1. Increased fat content and elevated serum leptin levels in T2D GK rats

Higher amounts of visceral fat is a sign of a high ratio of sympathetic vs parasympathetic reactivity [129]. We measured the lean and fat body mass quantities in awake rats by non-invasive magnetic resonance imaging. Compared to Wistar rats with same body weight, GK rats have doubled fat mass and significantly less lean mass. During rat growth from 285 g to 320 g, the increase in Wistar rats is mainly lean weight while that in GK rats is mainly fat weight. Coinciding with this finding, serum leptin levels elevated in GK rats in normally feed, fast, and refeed status. Hyperleptinemia is associated with increased sympathetic activity as leptin increases sympathetic nerve activity to influence cardiovascular, renal, muscle, endocrine, and adrenal gland functions [188, 189].

5.2.2. Absence of vagally mediated gastric acid response to intracisternal TRH analog in T2D GK rats

TRH is a physiological stimulator on DMV neurons to induce a vagally mediated excitation of gastric secretory/motility functions [80]. The well-known gastric acid-stimulatory effect of intracisternal injection of TRH analog was totally absent in T2D GK rats, indicating that TRH action in the DMV to activate vagal efferent outflow is severely damaged in GK rats.

5.2.3. Potentiated hyperglycemic and suppressed insulin early-phase responses to TRH analog injected intracisternally, intrathecally into the subarachnoid space at the thoracic 8-11 level, or microinjected into the RVLM in T2D GK rats

TRH analog RX77368 (50 ng) injected intracisternally induced markedly greater hyperglycemic and weaker insulin responses in GK rats than in Wistar rats. Bilateral vagotomy blocked RX77368-induced insulin secretion while adrenalectomy abolished its hyperglycemic effect. In adrenalectomized GK but not Wistar rats, RX77368 dramatically increased serum insulin levels by 6.5-fold and decreased blood glucose levels from 154 to 98 mg%; these changes were prevented by simultaneous vagotomy. These results indicate that central-vagal activation-induced insulin secretion is susceptible in T2D GK rats and the dominant sympathetic-adrenal response to brainstem TRH plays a suppressing role on vagal-mediated insulin secretion. This unbalanced sympathovagal activation by medullary TRH may contribute to the impaired insulin secretion in T2D [82].

TRH analog RX77368 injected intrathecally or microinjected into the RVLM, the TRH action sites for activating the sympathetic efferent function, induced a significantly potentiated hyperglycemic response and an impaired first hour insulin response in T2D GK rats, compared to Wistar rats, indicating a sympathetic overactivation together with an impaired vagal counterregulatory response to hyperglycemia in GK rats [69, 82].

5.2.4. Brainstem TRH-triggered cardioacceleration results in death from congestive heart failure in T2D GK rats, showing diminished vagal efferent function in baroreceptor reflex

In comparison with Wistar rats, GK rats exhibited basal systolic hypertension (152 ± 2 mmHg) and a significantly potentiated, dose-related hypertensive response to intracisternal injection of TRH analog RX77368 (10-60 ng). In GK rats only, intracisternal RX77368 (30-60 ng) markedly increased heart rate (+88 bpm) and induced acute cardiac mortality (100%) resulting from congestive heart failure, concurrent with extreme hyperglycemia (>480 mg%), increased plasma H_2O_2 and 8-isoprostane, and increased heart mRNA levels of NADPH oxidase 4 and vascular cell adhesion molecule-1, which are the oxidative stress and inflammation markers. GK rats also had elevated basal levels of plasma epinephrine, higher adrenal gene expression of epinephrine-synthesizing enzymes tyrosine hydroxylase and dopamine β-hydroxylase, and greater responses of plasma catecholamines and the adrenal enzymes to intracisternal TRH analog, compared to Wistar rats. Pretreatment with the nicotine receptor blocker hexamethonium prevented intracisternal TRH analog induced hypertensive and tachycardic responses, and cardiac mortality in GK rats. The α-receptor blockage with phentolamine abolished the hypertensive response but enhanced tachycardia (+160 bpm), and reduced mortality by 50%. The angiotensin II type 1 receptor antagonist irbesartan prevented intracisternal RX77368-induced increases in blood pressure, heart rate, and mortality. These findings indicate that sympathetic overactivation triggered by brainstem TRH and the lack of effective vagal counterregulation contribute to the cardiovascular morbidity and mortality in T2D, which involves heightened cardiac inflammation and peripheral oxidative stress responses to the sympathetic drive and a mediating role of renin-angiotensin system [97]. The cardiovascular autonomic imbalance in GK rats further confirms a diminished vagal-activating function of brainstem TRH, which is responsible for the damaged vagal arm function in the baroreceptor reflex.

6. Summary and perspectives

Using the T2D GK rat model, we found a damaged brainstem TRH action on activating the vagal efferent functions, which contributes to reveal the central mechanism of the sympatho-vagal imbalance in T2D. Further studies are warranted to investigate in the cellular and molecular levels of the abnormal vagal motor neuronal functions in T2D, such as insulin and TRH signaling in the DVC neurons.

Author details

Hong Yang*

Address all correspondence to: hoyang@ucla.edu.

Research & Development, Department of Veterans Affairs, Greater Los Angeles Health Care System and Department of Medicine, David Geffen School of Medicine, University of California at Los Angeles and Los Angeles, California, USA

http://dx.doi.org/10.5772/56541

References

[1] Seeley RJ and Tschop M. How diabetes went to our heads. Nat Med 2006; 12: 47-49.

[2] Schwartz MW and Porte DJ. Diabetes, obesity, and the brain. Science 2005; 307: 375-379.

[3] Oida E, Kannagi T, Moritani T and Yamori Y. Diabetic alteration of cardiac vago-sympathetic modulation assessed with tone-entropy analysis. Acta Physiol Scand 1999; 165: 129-134.

[4] Perin PC, Maule S and Quadri R. Sympathetic nervous system, diabetes, and hypertension. Clin Exp Hypertens 2001; 23: 45-55.

[5] Huggett RJ, Scott EM, Gilbey SG, Stoker JB, Mackintosh AF and Mary DA. Impact of type 2 diabetes mellitus on sympathetic neural mechanisms in hypertension. Circulation 2003; 108: 3097-3101.

[6] Lindmark S, Wiklund U, Bjerle P and Eriksson JW. Does the autonomic nervous system play a role in the development of insulin resistance? A study on heart rate variability in first-degree relatives of Type 2 diabetes patients and control subjects. Diabet Med 2003; 20: 399-405.

[7] Grill HJ and Hayes MR. Hindbrain neurons as an essential hub in the neuroanatomically distributed control of energy balance. Cell Metab 2012; 16: 296-309.

[8] Grill HJ and Norgren R. Chronically decerebrate rats demonstrate satiation but not bait shyness. Science 1978: 201: 267-269.

[9] Grill HJ and Kaplan JM. Sham feeding in intact and chronic decerebrate rats. Am J Physiol 1992; 262: R1070-R1074.

[10] Harris RB, Kelso EW, Flatt WP, Bartness TJ and Grill HJ. Energy Expenditure and Body Composition of Chronically Maintained Decerebrate Rats in the Fed and Fasted Condition. Endocrinology 2006; 147: 1365-1376.

[11] Shapiro RE and Miselis RR. The central organization of the vagus nerve innervating the stomach of the rat. J Comp Neurol 1985; 238: 473-488.

[12] Pagani FD, Norman WP, Kasbekar DK and Gillis RA. Localization of sites within dorsal motor nucleus of vagus that affect gastric motility. Am J Physiol 1985; 249: G73-G84.

[13] Berthoud HR, Carlson NR and Powley TL. Topography of efferent vagal innervation of the rat gastrointestinal tract. Am J Physiol 1991; 260: R200-R207.

[14] Kalia M and Sullivan JM. Brainstem projections of sensory and motor components of the vagus nerve in the rat. J Comp Neurol 1982; 211: 248-265.

[15] Gross PM, Wall KM, Pang JJ, Shaver SW and Wainman DS. Microvascular specializations promoting rapid interstitial solute dispersion in nucleus tractus solitarius. Am J Physiol 1990; 259: R1131-R1138.

[16] Kannan H and Yamashita H. Electrophysiological study of paraventricular nucleus neurons projecting to the dorsomedial medulla and their response to baroreceptor stimulation in rats. Brain Res 1983; 279: 31-40.

[17] Zhang X, Fogel R and Renehan WE. Stimulation of the paraventricular nucleus modulates the activity of gut-sensitive neurons in the vagal complex. Am J Physiol 1999; 277: G79-G90.

[18] Nishimura H and Oomura Y. Effects of hypothalamic stimulation on activity of dorsomedial medulla neurons that respond to subdiaphragmatic vagal stimulation. J Neurophysiol 1987; 58: 655-675.

[19] Ashford ML, Boden PR and Treherne JM. Tolbutamide excites rat glucoreceptive ventromedial hypothalamic neurones by indirect inhibition of ATP-K+ channels. Br J Pharmacol 1990; 101: 531-540.

[20] Ter Horst GJ, Toes GJ and Van WJD. Locus coeruleus projections to the dorsal motor vagus nucleus in the rat. Neuroscience 1991; 45: 153-160.

[21] Tougas G and Wang L. Pseudoaffective cardioautonomic responses to gastric distension in rats. Am J Physiol 1999; 277: R272-R278.

[22] Li Y, Hao Y, Zhu J and Owyang C. Serotonin released from intestinal enterochromaffin cells mediates luminal non-cholecystokinin-stimulated pancreatic secretion in rats. Gastroenterology 2000; 118: 1197-1207.

[23] McCann MJ and Rogers RC. Functional and Chemical Anatomy of a Gastric Vago-Vagal Reflex. In: Innervation of the Gut: Pathophysiological Implications, edited by Taché Y, Wingate D. and Burks TF. London: CRC Press, 1993.

[24] Oh JD, Woolf NJ, Roghani A, Edwards RH and Butcher LL. Cholinergic neurons in the rat central nervous system demonstrated by in situ hybridization of choline acetyltransferase mRNA. Neuroscience 1992; 47: 807-822.

[25] Sang Q and Young HM. The origin and development of the vagal and spinal innervation of the external muscle of the mouse esophagus. Brain Res 1998; 809: 253-268.

[26] Zheng ZL, Rogers RC and Travagli RA. Selective gastric projections of nitric oxide synthase-containing vagal brainstem neurons. Neuroscience 1999; 90: 685-694.

[27] Lin LH, Sahai AK, Rockland KS and Talman WT. The distribution of neuronal nitric oxide synthase in the nucleus tractus solitarii of the squirrel monkey. Brain Res 2000; 856: 84-92.

[28] Dong YX, Xiong KH and Rao ZR. Medullary catecholaminergic neurons projecting to lateral hypothalamic area and expressing Fos after chemical stimulation of the stomach in the rat. J Hirnforsch 1997; 38: 3-7.

[29] Allen AM, O'Callaghan EL, Chen D and Bassi JK. Central Neural Regulation of Cardiovascular Function by Angiotensin: A Focus on the Rostral Ventrolateral Medulla. Neuroendocrinology 2009; 89:361-369.

[30] Oshima N, Kumagai H, Kawai A, Sakata K, Matsuura T and Saruta T. Three types of putative presympathetic neurons in the rostral ventrolateral medulla studied with rat brainstem-spinal cord preparation. Auton Neurosci 2000; 84: 40-49.

[31] Card JP, Sved JC, Craig B, Raizada M, Vazquez J and Sved AF. Efferent projections of rat rostroventrolateral medulla C1 catecholamine neurons: Implications for the central control of cardiovascular regulation. J Comp Neurol 2006; 499: 840-859.

[32] Jansen AS, Hoffman JL and Loewy AD. CNS sites involved in sympathetic and parasympathetic control of the pancreas: a viral tracing study. Brain Res 1997; 766: 29-38.

[33] Berthoud HR and Jeanrenaud B. Acute hyperinsulinemia and its reversal by vagotomy after lesions of the ventromedial hypothalamus in anesthetized rats. Endocrinology 1979; 105: 146-151.

[34] Berthoud HR, Fox EA and Powley TL. Localization of vagal preganglionics that stimulate insulin and glucagon secretion. Am J Physiol 1990; 258: R160-R168.

[35] Quinson N, Robbins HL, Clark MJ and Furness JB. Locations and innervation of cell bodies of sympathetic neurons projecting to the gastrointestinal tract in the rat. Arch Histol Cytol 2001; 64: 281-294.

[36] Ahren B. Autonomic regulation of islet hormone secretion--implications for health and disease. Diabetologia 2000; 43: 393-410.

[37] Trimble ER, Berthoud HR, Siegel EG, Jeanrenaud B and Renold AE. Importance of cholinergic innervation of the pancreas for glucose tolerance in the rat. Am J Physiol 1981; 241: E337-E341.

[38] Kiba T, Tanaka K, Numata K, Hoshino M, Misugi K and Inoue S. Ventromedial hypothalamic lesion-induced vagal hyperactivity stimulates rat pancreatic cell proliferation. Gastroenterology 1996; 110: 885-893.

[39] Kiba T. Relationships Between the Autonomic Nervous System and the Pancreas Including Regulation of Regeneration and Apoptosis: Recent Developments. Pancreas 2004; 29: E51-E58.

[40] Benthem L, Mundinger TO and Taborsky GJJ. Meal-induced insulin secretion in dogs is mediated by both branches of the autonomic nervous system. Am J Physiol Endocrinol Metab 2000; 278: E603-E610.

[41] Secchi A, Caldara R, Caumo A, Monti LD, Bonfatti D, Di CV and Pozza G. Cephalic-phase insulin and glucagon release in normal subjects and in patients receiving pancreas transplantation. Metabolism 1995; 44: 1153-1158.

[42] Smets YF, van der Pijl JW, Frolich M, Ringers J, de FJ and Lemkes HH. Insulin secretion and sensitivity after simultaneous pancreas-kidney transplantation estimated by continuous infusion of glucose with model assessment. Transplantation 2000; 69: 1322-1327.

[43] Christiansen E, Tibell A, Volund AA, Holst JJ, Rasmussen K, Schaffer L and Madsbad S. Metabolism of oral glucose in pancreas transplant recipients with normal and impaired glucose tolerance. J Clin Endocrinol Metab 1997; 82: 2299-2307.

[44] Earnhardt RC, Veldhuis JD, Cornett G and Hanks JB. Pathophysiology of hyperinsulinemia following pancreas transplantation: altered pulsatile versus Basal insulin secretion and the role of specific transplant anatomy in dogs. Ann Surg 2002; 236: 480-490.

[45] Henquin JC and Nenquin M. The muscarinic receptor subtype in mouse pancreatic B-cells. FEBS Lett 1988; 236: 89-92.

[46] Duttaroy A, Zimliki CL, Gautam D, Cui Y, Mears D and Wess J. Muscarinic stimulation of pancreatic insulin and glucagon release is abolished in m3 muscarinic acetylcholine receptor-deficient mice. Diabetes 2004; 53: 1714-1720.

[47] Gautam D, Han SJ, Hamdan FF, Jeon J, Li B, Li JH, Cui Y, Mears D, Lu H, Deng C, Heard T and Wess J. A critical role for beta cell M(3) muscarinic acetylcholine receptors in regulating insulin release and blood glucose homeostasis in vivo. Cell Metab 2006; 3: 449-461.

[48] Toshinai K, Mondal MS, Nakazato M, Date Y, Murakami N, Kojima M, Kangawa K and Matsukura S. Upregulation of Ghrelin expression in the stomach upon fasting, insulin-induced hypoglycemia, and leptin administration. Biochem Biophys Res Commun 2001; 281: 1220-1225.

[49] Ao Y, Go VL, Toy N, Li T, Wang Y, Song MK, Reeve JRJ, Liu Y and Yang H. Brainstem Thyrotropin-Releasing Hormone Regulates Food Intake through Vagal-Dependent Cholinergic Stimulation of Ghrelin Secretion. Endocrinology 2006; 147: 6004-6010.

[50] Williams DL, Grill HJ, Cummings DE and Kaplan JM. Vagotomy dissociates short- and long-term controls of circulating ghrelin. Endocrinology 2003; 144: 5184-5187.

[51] Broglio F, Gottero C, Van KP, Prodam F, Destefanis S, Benso A, Gauna C, Hofland L, Arvat E, Van Der Lely AJ and Ghigo E. Acetylcholine regulates ghrelin secretion in humans. J Clin Endocrinol Metab 2004; 89: 2429-2433.

[52] Niimi M, Sato M, Tamaki M, Wada Y, Takahara J and Kawanishi K. Induction of Fos protein in the rat hypothalamus elicited by insulin- induced hypoglycemia. Neurosci Res 1995; 23: 361-364.

[53] Horn CC, Addis A and Friedman MI. Neural substrate for an integrated metabolic control of feeding behavior. Am J Physiol 1999; 276: R113-R119.

[54] Cai XJ, Evans ML, Lister CA, Leslie RA, Arch JR, Wilson S and Williams G. Hypoglycemia activates orexin neurons and selectively increases hypothalamic orexin-B levels: responses inhibited by feeding and possibly mediated by the nucleus of the solitary tract. Diabetes 2001; 50: 105-112.

[55] Yuan PQ and Yang H. Neuronal activation of brain vagal-regulatory pathways and upper gut enteric plexuses by insulin hypoglycemia. Am J Physiol Endocrinol Metab 2002; 283: E436-E448.

[56] Sakaguchi T, Aono T, Ohtake M and Sandoh N. Interaction of glucose signals between the nucleus of the vagus nerve and the portal vein area in the regulation of gastric motility in rats. Brain Res Bull 1994; 33: 469-471.

[57] Sakaguchi T and Nakadaira K. Interaction of glucose signals between the nucleus of the tractus solitarius and the portal vein area in the control of gastric acid secretion in rats. Brain Res 1991; 568: 299-302.

[58] Briski KP. Induction of Fos immunoreactivity by acute glucose deprivation in the rat caudal brainstem: relation to NADPH diaphorase localization [In Process Citation]. Histochem Cell Biol 1999; 111: 229-233.

[59] Ritter S, Llewellyn-Smith I and Dinh TT. Subgroups of hindbrain catecholamine neurons are selectively activated by 2-deoxy-D-glucose induced metabolic challenge. Brain Res 1998; 805: 41-54.

[60] Kobashi M and Adachi A. Effect of topical administration of glucose on neurons innervating abdominal viscera in dorsal motor nucleus of vagus in rats. Jpn J Physiol 1994; 44: 729-734.

[61] Ferreira MJ, Browning KN, Sahibzada N, Verbalis JG, Gillis RA and Travagli RA. Glucose effects on gastric motility and tone evoked from the rat dorsal vagal complex. J Physiol 2001; 536: 141-152.

[62] Niijima A. Glucose-sensitive afferent nerve fibres in the hepatic branch of the vagus nerve in the guinea-pig. J Physiol 1982; 332: 315-323.

[63] Yettefti K, Orsini JC and Perrin J. Characteristics of glycemia-sensitive neurons in the nucleus tractus solitarii: possible involvement in nutritional regulation. Physiol Behav 1997; 61: 93-100.

[64] Cunningham ETJ, Bohn MC and Sawchenko PE. Organization of adrenergic inputs to the paraventricular and supraoptic nuclei of the hypothalamus in the rat. J Comp Neurol 1990; 292: 651-667.

[65] Kerr FW and Preshaw RM. Secretomotor function of the dorsal motor nucleus of the vagus. J Physiol 1969; 205: 405-415.

[66] Lynn RB, Kreider MS and Miselis RR. Thyrotropin-releasing hormone-immunoreactive projections to the dorsal motor nucleus and the nucleus of the solitary tract of the rat. J Comp Neurol 1991; 311: 271-288.

[67] Sasek CA, Wessendorf MW and Helke CJ. Evidence for co-existence of thyrotropin-releasing hormone, substance P and serotonin in ventral medullary neurons that project to the intermediolateral cell column in the rat. Neuroscience 1990; 35: 105-119.

[68] Rinaman L, Miselis RR and Kreider MS. Ultrastructural localization of thyrotropin-releasing hormone immunoreactivity in the dorsal vagal complex in rat. Neurosci Lett 1989; 104: 7-12.

[69] Ao Y, Ko M, Chen A, Marvizon JC, Adelson D, Song MK, Go VL, Liu YY and Yang H. Potent hyperglycemic and hyperinsulinemic effects of thyrotropin-releasing hormone microinjected into the rostroventrolateral medulla and abnormal responses in type 2 diabetic rats. Neuroscience 2010; 169: 706-719.

[70] McCann MJ, Hermann GE and Rogers RC. Thyrotropin-releasing hormone: effects on identified neurons of the dorsal vagal complex. J Auton Nerv Syst 1989; 26: 107-112.

[71] Underwood MD, Iadecola C and Reis DJ. Lesions of the rostral ventrolateral medulla reduce the cerebrovascular response to hypoxia. Brain Res 1994; 635: 217-223.

[72] Ross CA, Ruggiero DA, Park DH, Joh TH, Sved AF, Fernandez-Pardal J, Saavedra JM and Reis DJ. Tonic vasomotor control by the rostral ventrolateral medulla: effect of electrical or chemical stimulation of the area containing C1 adrenaline neurons on arterial pressure, heart rate, and plasma catecholamines and vasopressin. J Neurosci 1984; 4: 474-494.

[73] Malpas SC. Sympathetic nervous system overactivity and its role in the development of cardiovascular disease. Physiol Rev 2010; 90: 513-557.

[74] Marubashi S, Kunii Y, Tominaga M and Sasaki H. Modulation of plasma glucose levels by thyrotropin-releasing hormone administered intracerebroventricularly in the rat. Neuroendocrinology 48: 640-644, 1988.

[75] Amir S and Rivkind AI. Prevention of clonidine-stimulated hyperglycemia by thyrotropin-releasing hormone. Peptides 1988; 9: 527-531.

[76] Amir S, Harel M and Rivkind AI. Thyrotropin-releasing hormone potently reverses epinephrine-stimulated hyperglycemia in mice. Brain Res 1987; 435: 112-122.

[77] Amir S and Jackson IM. Immunological blockade of endogenous thyrotropin-releasing hormone impairs recovery from hyperglycemia in mice. Brain Res 1988; 462: 160-162.

[78] Amir S and Butler PD. Thyrotropin-releasing hormone blocks neurally-mediated hyperglycemia through central action. Peptides 1988; 9: 31-35.

[79] Paakkari I, Siren AL, Nurminen ML and Svartstrom-Fraser M. Injection of thyrotropin releasing hormone into the locus coeruleus increases blood pressure. Eur Heart J 1987; 8 Suppl B: 147-151.

[80] Taché Y and Yang H. Role of medullary TRH in the vagal regulation of gastric function. In: Innervation of the Gut: Pathophysiological Implications, edited by Wingate DL and Butkd TF. Boca Raton: CRC, 1994.

[81] Yang H, Tache Y, Ohning G and Go VL. Activation of raphe pallidus neurons increases insulin through medullary thyrotropin-releasing hormone (TRH)-vagal pathways. Pancreas 2002; 25: 301-307.

[82] Ao Y, Toy N, Song MK, Go VL and Yang H. Altered glucose and insulin responses to brain medullary thyrotropin-releasing hormone (TRH)-induced autonomic activation in type 2 diabetic Goto-Kakizaki rats. Endocrinology 2005; 146: 5425-5432.

[83] Furness JB, Lloyd KC, Sternini C and Walsh JH. Evidence that myenteric neurons of the gastric corpus project to both the mucosa and the external muscle: myectomy operations on the canine stomach. Cell Tissue Res 1991; 266: 475-481.

[84] Pfannkuche H, Reiche D, Sann H and Schemann M. Different subpopulations of cholinergic and nitrergic myenteric neurones project to mucosa and circular muscle of the guinea-pig gastric fundus. Cell Tissue Res 1998; 292: 463-475.

[85] Holst MC, Kelly JB and Powley TL. Vagal preganglionic projections to the enteric nervous system characterized with Phaseolus vulgaris-leucoagglutinin. J Comp Neurol 1997; 381: 81-100.

[86] Berthoud HR. Anatomical demonstration of vagal input to nicotinamide acetamide dinucleotide phosphate diaphorase-positive (nitrergic) neurons in rat fundic stomach. J Comp Neurol 1995; 358: 428-439.

[87] Zheng H and Berthoud HR. Functional vagal input to gastric myenteric plexus as assessed by vagal stimulation-induced Fos expression. Am J Physiol Gastrointest Liver Physiol 2000; 279: G73-G81.

[88] Zheng H, Lauve A, Patterson LM and Berthoud HR. Limited excitatory local effector function of gastric vagal afferent intraganglionic terminals in rats. Am J Physiol 1997; 273: G661-G669.

[89] Berthoud HR, Patterson LM and Zheng H. Vagal-enteric interface: Vagal activation-induced expression of c-Fos and p-CREB in neurons of the upper gastrointestinal tract and pancreas. Anat Rec 2001; 262: 29-40.

[90] O-Lee TJ, Wei JY and Taché Y. Intracisternal TRH and RX 77368 potently activate gastric vagal efferent discharge in rats. Peptides 1997; 18: 213-219.

[91] Miampamba M, Yang H, Sharkey KA and Tache Y. Intracisternal TRH analog induces Fos expression in gastric myenteric neurons and glia in conscious rats. Am J Physiol Gastrointest Liver Physiol 2001; 280: G979-G991.

[92] Assadian H, Ishikawa Y, Shimatsu A, Tanoh T and Imura H. Serotoninergic denervation suppresses the sympathetic outflow induced by thyrotropin-releasing hormone in conscious rats. J Auton Nerv Syst 1991; 35: 193-198.

[93] Ishikawa Y, Shimatsu A, Kato Y, Murakami Y and Imura H. Effects of intrathecal administration of thyrotropin releasing hormone and its analogue, DN1417, on plasma glucose and catecholamine levels in conscious rats. Brain Res 1990; 514: 1-4.

[94] Ishikawa T, Yang H and Taché Y. Medullary sites of action of the TRH analogue, RX 77368, for stimulation of gastric acid secretion in the rat. Gastroenterology 1988; 95: 1470-1476.

[95] Stephens RL, Ishikawa T, Weiner H, Novin D and Taché Y. TRH analogue, RX 77368, injected into dorsal vagal complex stimulates gastric secretion in rats. Am J Physiol 1988 254: G639-G643.

[96] Yoneda S, Kadowaki M, Kuramoto H, Fukui H and Takaki M. Enhanced colonic peristalsis by impairment of nitrergic enteric neurons in spontaneously diabetic rats. Auton Neurosci 2001; 92: 65-71.

[97] Yang H, Nyby MD, Ao Y, Chen A, Adelson DW, Smutko V, Wijesuriya J, Go VL and Tuck ML. Role of brainstem thyrotropin-releasing hormone-triggered sympathetic overactivation in cardiovascular mortality in type 2 diabetic Goto-Kakizaki rats. Hypertens Res 2012; 35: 157-165.

[98] Yamada M, Saga Y, Shibusawa N, Hirato J, Murakami M, Iwasaki T, Hashimoto K, Satoh T, Wakabayashi K, Taketo MM and Mori M. Tertiary hypothyroidism and hyperglycemia in mice with targeted disruption of the thyrotropin-releasing hormone gene. Proc Natl Acad Sci U S A 1997; 94: 10862-10867.

[99] Yang H, Wu SV, Ishikawa T and Taché Y. Cold exposure elevates thyrotropin-releasing hormone gene expression in medullary raphe nuclei: relationship with vagally mediated gastric erosions. Neuroscience 1994; 61: 655-663.

[100] Yang H, Yuan P, Wu V and Tache Y. Feedback regulation of thyrotropin-releasing hormone gene expression by thyroid hormone in the caudal raphe nuclei in rats. Endocrinology 1999; 140: 43-49.

[101] Arai I, Muramatsu M and Aihara H. Body temperature dependent decrease of gastric blood flow in restraint and water-immersion stressed rats. J Pharmacobiodyn 1986; 9: 678-682.

[102] Arai I, Muramatsu M and Aihara H. Body temperature dependency of gastric regional blood flow, acid secretion and ulcer formation in restraint and water-immersion stressed rats. Jpn J Pharmacol 1986; 40: 501-504.

[103] Zoeller RT, Kabeer N and Albers HE. Cold exposure elevates cellular levels of messenger ribonucleic acid encoding thyrotropin-releasing hormone in paraventricular nucleus despite elevated levels of thyroid hormones. Endocrinology 1990; 127: 2955-2962.

[104] Bonaz B and Taché Y. Induction of Fos immunoreactivity in the rat brain after cold-restraint induced gastric lesions and fecal excretion. Brain Res 1994; 652: 56-64.

[105] Yang H, Yuan PQ, Wang L and Taché Y. Activation of the parapyramidal region in the ventral medulla stimulates gastric acid secretion through vagal pathways in rats. Neuroscience 95: 773-779, 2000.

[106] Yuan PQ, Tache Y, Miampamba M and Yang H. Acute cold exposure induces vagally mediated Fos expression in gastric myenteric neurons in conscious rats. Am J Physiol Gastrointest Liver Physiol 2001; 281: G560-G568.

[107] Hayase M and Takeuchi K. Gastric acid secretion and lesion formation in rats under water- immersion stress. Dig Dis Sci 1986; 31: 166-171.

[108] Witty RT and Long JF. Effect of ambient temperature on gastric secretion and food intake in the rat. Am J Physiol 1970; 219: 1359-1362.

[109] Basso N, Bagarani M, Pekary AE, Genco A and Materia A. Role of thyrotropin-releasing hormone in stress ulcer formation in the rat. Dig Dis Sci 1988; 33: 819-823.

[110] Martinez V, Wang L and Tache Y. Central TRH receptor 1 antisense blocks cold-induced gastric emptying but not brain c-Fos induction. Peptides 2001; 22: 81-90.

[111] Yang H and Taché Y. Substance P in the dorsal vagal complex inhibits medullary TRH-induced gastric acid secretion in rats. Am J Physiol 1997; 272: G987-G993.

[112] Yoneda M and Taché Y. Serotonin enhances gastric acid response to TRH analogue in dorsal vagal complex through 5-HT2 receptors in rats. Am J Physiol 1995; 269: R1-R6.

[113] Berthoud HR. Vagal and hormonal gut-brain communication: from satiation to satisfaction. Neurogastroenterol Motil 2008; 20 Suppl 1: 64-72.

[114] Thorens B and Larsen PJ. Gut-derived signaling molecules and vagal afferents in the control of glucose and energy homeostasis. Curr Opin Clin Nutr Metab Care 2004; 7: 471-478.

[115] Doong ML and Yang H. Intravenous glucose infusion decreases intracisternal thyrotropin-releasing hormone induced vagal stimulation of gastric acid secretion in anesthetized rats. Neurosci Lett 2003; 340: 49-52.

[116] Yang H. Central and peripheral regulation of gastric acid secretion by peptide YY. Peptides 2002; 23: 349-358.

[117] Yang H, Kawakubo K, Wong H, Ohning G, Walsh J and Tache Y. Peripheral PYY inhibits intracisternal TRH-induced gastric acid secretion by acting in the brain. Am J Physiol Gastrointest Liver Physiol 2000; 279: G575-G581.

[118] Urbancic-Rovan V, Meglic B, Stefanovska A, Bernjak A, Azman-Juvan K and Kocijancic A. Incipient cardiovascular autonomic imbalance revealed by wavelet analysis of heart rate variability in Type 2 diabetic patients. Diabet Med 2007; 24: 18-26.

[119] Carnethon MR, Jacobs DRJ, Sidney S and Liu K. Influence of autonomic nervous system dysfunction on the development of type 2 diabetes: the CARDIA study. Diabetes Care 2003; 26: 3035-3041.

[120] Frontoni S. Comment on: Straznicky et al. neuroadrenergic dysfunction along the diabetes continuum: a comparative study in obese metabolic syndrome subjects. Diabetes 2012;61:2506-2516. Diabetes 2013; 62: e1.

[121] Straznicky NE, Lambert EA and Lambert GW. Response to Comment on: Straznicky et al. neuroadrenergic dysfunction along the diabetes continuum: a comparative study in obese metabolic syndrome subjects. Diabetes 2012;61:2506-2516. Diabetes 2013; 62: e2.

[122] Straznicky NE, Grima MT, Sari CI, Eikelis N, Lambert EA, Nestel PJ, Esler MD, Dixon JB, Chopra R, Tilbrook AJ, Schlaich MP and Lambert GW. Neuroadrenergic dysfunction along the diabetes continuum: a comparative study in obese metabolic syndrome subjects. Diabetes 2012; 61: 2506-2516.

[123] Frontoni S, Bracaglia D and Gigli F. Relationship between autonomic dysfunction, insulin resistance and hypertension, in diabetes. Nutr Metab Cardiovasc Dis 2005; 15: 441-449.

[124] Mori A, Maruyama T, Ohashi N, Shibuya T, Sakai K, Tatebe H, Inoue H, Kato T and Okuno M. Impaired autonomic function in type 2 diabetic patients during upper gastrointestinal endoscopy. J Gastroenterol 2008; 43: 603-608.

[125] Manzella D and Paolisso G. Cardiac autonomic activity and Type II diabetes mellitus. Clin Sci (Lond) 2005; 108: 93-99.

[126] Chiodini I, Di LS, Morelli V, Epaminonda P, Coletti F, Masserini B, Scillitani A, Arosio M and Adda G. Hypothalamic-pituitary-adrenal activity in type 2 diabetes mellitus: role of autonomic imbalance. Metabolism 2006; 55: 1135-1140.

[127] Dicostanzo CA, Dardevet DP, Neal DW, Lautz M, Allen E, Snead W and Cherrington AD. Role of the hepatic sympathetic nerves in the regulation of net hepatic glucose

uptake and the mediation of the portal glucose signal. Am J Physiol Endocrinol Metab 2006; 290: E9-E16.

[128] Hu X, Friedman D, Hill S, Caprioli R, Nicholson W, Powers AC, Hunter L and Limbird LE. Proteomic exploration of pancreatic islets in mice null for the alpha2A adrenergic receptor. J Mol Endocrinol 2005; 35: 73-88.

[129] Lindmark S, Lonn L, Wiklund U, Tufvesson M, Olsson T and Eriksson JW. Dysregulation of the autonomic nervous system can be a link between visceral adiposity and insulin resistance. Obes Res 2005; 13: 717-728.

[130] Schlaich MP, Socratous F, Hennebry S, Eikelis N, Lambert EA, Straznicky N, Esler MD and Lambert GW. Sympathetic Activation in Chronic Renal Failure. J Am Soc Nephrol 2009; 20:933-939.

[131] el-Salhy M. Neuroendocrine peptides of the gastrointestinal tract of an animal model of human type 2 diabetes mellitus. Acta Diabetol 1998; 35: 194-198.

[132] Kashyap P and Farrugia G. Diabetic gastroparesis: what we have learned and had to unlearn in the past 5 years. Gut 2010; 59: 1716-1726.

[133] Grantham NM, Magliano DJ, Tanamas SK, Soderberg S, Schlaich MP and Shaw JE. Higher heart rate increases risk of diabetes among men: The Australian Diabetes Obesity and Lifestyle (AusDiab) Study. Diabet Med 2013; 30:421-427.

[134] Lam WF, Masclee AA, De Boer SY and Lamers CB. Hyperglycemia reduces gastric secretory and plasma pancreatic polypeptide responses to modified sham feeding in humans. Digestion 1993; 54: 48-53.

[135] Mehta N, Veliath S and Thombre DP. The effect of bilateral gastric vagotomy and histamine stimulation on parietal cell activity in streptozotocin induced diabetic rat model. Indian J Physiol Pharmacol 1993; 37: 30-34.

[136] Vu MK, Straathof JW, Schaar PJ, Arndt JW, Ringers J, Lamers CB and Masclee AA. Motor and sensory function of the proximal stomach in reflux disease and after laparoscopic Nissen fundoplication. Am J Gastroenterol 1999; 94: 1481-1489.

[137] Nilsell K and Ewerth S. The acid secretory response to betazole and insulin hypoglycemia after selective proximal vagotomy for duodenal ulcer. Acta Chir Scand 1981; 147: 431-434.

[138] Stenquist B. Studies on vagal activation of gastric acid secretion in man. Acta Physiol Scand Suppl 1979; 465: 1-31.

[139] Smith RB, Edwards JP and Johnston D. Effect of vagotomy on exocrine pancreatic and biliary secretion in man. Am J Surg 1981; 141: 40-47.

[140] Quigley EM. The pathophysiology of diabetic gastroenteropathy: more vague than vagal [editorial; comment]. Gastroenterology 1997; 113: 1790-1794.

[141] Horowitz M, Harding PE, Maddox A and et al. Gastric and oesophageal emptying in insulin-dependent diabetes mellitus. J Gastroenterol Hepatol 1986; 1: 97.

[142] Horowitz M, Harding PE, Maddox AF, Wishart JM, Akkermans LM, Chatterton BE and Shearman DJ. Gastric and oesophageal emptying in patients with type 2 (non-insulin- dependent) diabetes mellitus. Diabetologia 32: 151-159, 1989.

[143] Kong MF and Horowitz M. Gastric emptying in diabetes mellitus: relationship to blood-glucose control. Clin Geriatr Med 1999; 15: 321-338.

[144] Nakamura T, Takebe K, Imamura K, Miyazawa T, Ishii M, Kudoh K, Terada A, Machida K, Kikuchi H and Kasai F. Decreased gastric secretory functions in diabetic patients with autonomic neuropathy. Tohoku J Exp Med 1994; 173: 199-208.

[145] Britland ST, Young RJ, Sharma AK, Lee D, Ah-See AK and Clarke BF. Vagus nerve morphology in diabetic gastropathy. Diabet Med 1990; 7: 780-787.

[146] Fraser R, Horowitz M and Dent J. Hyperglycaemia stimulates pyloric motility in normal subjects. Gut 1991; 32: 475-478.

[147] Fraser RJ, Horowitz M, Maddox AF, Harding PE, Chatterton BE and Dent J. Hyperglycaemia slows gastric emptying in type 1 (insulin-dependent) diabetes mellitus. Diabetologia 1990; 33: 675-680.

[148] Bjornsson ES, Urbanavicius V, Eliasson B, Attvall S, Smith U and Abrahamsson H. Effects of hyperglycemia on interdigestive gastrointestinal motility in humans. Scand J Gastroenterol 1994; 29: 1096-1104.

[149] Morgan LM, Tredger JA, Hampton SM, French AP, Peake JC and Marks V. The effect of dietary modification and hyperglycaemia on gastric emptying and gastric inhibitory polypeptide (GIP) secretion. Br J Nutr 1988; 60: 29-37.

[150] Barnett JL and Owyang C. Serum glucose concentration as a modulator of interdigestive gastric motility. Gastroenterology 1988; 94: 739-744.

[151] Chang FY, Lee SD, Yeh GH and Wang PS. Influence of blood glucose levels on rat liquid gastric emptying. Dig Dis Sci 1996; 41: 528-532.

[152] Yamano M, Kamato T, Nagakura Y and Miyata K. Effects of gastroprokinetic agents on gastroparesis in streptozotocin-induced diabetic rats. Naunyn Schmiedebergs Arch Pharmacol 1997; 356: 145-150.

[153] Schvarcz E, Palmer M, Aman J, Horowitz M, Stridsberg M and Berne C. Physiological hyperglycemia slows gastric emptying in normal subjects and patients with insulin-dependent diabetes mellitus. Gastroenterology 1997; 113: 60-66.

[154] Gallwitz B, Kazda C, Kraus P, Nicolay C and Schernthaner G. Contribution of insulin deficiency and insulin resistance to the development of type 2 diabetes: nature of early stage diabetes. Acta Diabetol 2013; 50: 39-45.

[155] Brunzell JD, Robertson RP, Lerner RL, Hazzard WR, Ensinck JW, Bierman EL and Porte DJ. Relationships between fasting plasma glucose levels and insulin secretion during intravenous glucose tolerance tests. J Clin Endocrinol Metab 1976; 42: 222-229.

[156] Woerle HJ, Carneiro L, Derani A, Goke B and Schirra J. The role of endogenous incretin secretion as amplifier of glucose-stimulated insulin secretion in healthy subjects and patients with type 2 diabetes. Diabetes 2012; 61: 2349-2358.

[157] Vollmer K, Gardiwal H, Menge BA, Goetze O, Deacon CF, Schmidt WE, Holst JJ and Meier JJ. Hyperglycemia acutely lowers the postprandial excursions of glucagon-like Peptide-1 and gastric inhibitory polypeptide in humans. J Clin Endocrinol Metab 2009; 94: 1379-1385.

[158] Knop FK, Aaboe K, Vilsboll T, Volund A, Holst JJ, Krarup T and Madsbad S. Impaired incretin effect and fasting hyperglucagonaemia characterizing type 2 diabetic subjects are early signs of dysmetabolism in obesity. Diabetes Obes Metab 2012; 14: 500-510.

[159] Rocca AS and Brubaker PL. Role of the vagus nerve in mediating proximal nutrient-induced glucagon-like peptide-1 secretion. Endocrinology 1999; 140: 1687-1694.

[160] Butler AE, Campbell-Thompson M, Gurlo T, Dawson DW, Atkinson M and Butler PC. Marked Expansion of Exocrine and Endocrine Pancreas with Incretin Therapy in Humans with increased Exocrine Pancreas Dysplasia and the potential for Glucagon-producing Neuroendocrine Tumors. Diabetes 2013.

[161] Shim WS, Kim SK, Kim HJ, Kang ES, Ahn CW, Lim SK, Lee HC and Cha BS. Decrement of postprandial insulin secretion determines the progressive nature of type-2 diabetes. Eur J Endocrinol 2006; 155: 615-622.

[162] Kapural L, Hayek SM, Stanton-Hicks M and Mekhail N. Decreased insulin requirements with spinal cord stimulation in a patient with diabetes. Anesth Analg 2004; 98: 745-746.

[163] Kannel WB and McGee DL. Diabetes and cardiovascular disease. The Framingham study. JAMA 1979; 241: 2035-2038.

[164] Lockhart CJ, Hamilton PK, McVeigh KA and McVeigh GE. A cardiologist view of vascular disease in diabetes. Diabetes Obes Metab 2008; 10: 279-292.

[165] Palatini P and Julius S. The role of cardiac autonomic function in hypertension and cardiovascular disease. Curr Hypertens Rep 2009; 11: 199-205.

[166] Taegtmeyer H, Golfman L, Sharma S, Razeghi P and van AM. Linking gene expression to function: metabolic flexibility in the normal and diseased heart. Ann N Y Acad Sci 2004; 1015: 202-213.

[167] Boudina S and Abel ED. Diabetic cardiomyopathy revisited. Circulation 2007; 115: 3213-3223.

[168] Guha A, Harmancey R and Taegtmeyer H. Nonischemic heart failure in diabetes mellitus. Curr Opin Cardiol 2008; 23: 241-248.

[169] Paolillo S, Rengo G, Pagano G, Pellegrino T, Savarese G, Femminella GD, Tuccillo M, Boemio A, Attena E, Formisano R, Petraglia L, Scopacasa F, Galasso G, Leosco D, Trimarco B, Cuocolo A and Perrone-Filardi P. Impact of Diabetes Mellitus on Cardiac Sympathetic Innervation in Patients With Heart Failure: A 123I meta-iodobenzylguanidine (123IMIBG) scintigraphic study. Diabetes Care 2013.

[170] Aso Y, Wakabayashi S, Nakano T, Yamamoto R, Takebayashi K and Inukai T. High serum high-sensitivity C-reactive protein concentrations are associated with relative cardiac sympathetic overactivity during the early morning period in type 2 diabetic patients with metabolic syndrome. Metabolism 2006; 55: 1014-1021.

[171] Dublin S, Glazer NL, Smith NL, Psaty BM, Lumley T, Wiggins KL, Page RL and Heckbert SR. Diabetes mellitus, glycemic control, and risk of atrial fibrillation. J Gen Intern Med 2010; 25: 853-858.

[172] Esler M. Sympathetic nervous activation in essential hypertension: commonly neglected as a therapeutic target, usually ignored as a drug side effect. Hypertension 2010; 55: 1090-1091.

[173] Voulgari C, Papadogiannis D and Tentolouris N. Diabetic cardiomyopathy: from the pathophysiology of the cardiac myocytes to current diagnosis and management strategies. Vasc Health Risk Manag 2010; 6: 883-903.

[174] Adler GK, Bonyhay I, Failing H, Waring E, Dotson S and Freeman R. Antecedent hypoglycemia impairs autonomic cardiovascular function: implications for rigorous glycemic control. Diabetes 58: 360-366, 2009.

[175] Vinik AI and Erbas T. Cardiovascular autonomic neuropathy: diagnosis and management. Curr Diab Rep 2006; 6: 424-430.

[176] Goto Y, Suzuki K, Sasaki M, Ono T and Abe S. GK rat as a model of nonobese, noninsulin-dependent diabetes. Selective breeding over 35 generations. In: Frontiers in Diabetes Research. Lessons from Animal Diabetes II, edited by Renold AE and Renold. London, UK: John Libbey, 1988.

[177] Galli J, Li LS, Glaser A, Ostenson CG, Jiao H, Fakhrai-Rad H, Jacob HJ, Lander ES and Luthman H. Genetic analysis of non-insulin dependent diabetes mellitus in the GK rat. Nat Genet 12: 31-37, 1996.

[178] Almon RR, DuBois DC, Lai W, Xue B, Nie J and Jusko WJ. Gene expression analysis of hepatic roles in cause and development of diabetes in Goto-Kakizaki rats. J Endocrinol 200: 331-346, 2009.

[179] Galli J, Fakhrai-Rad H, Kamel A, Marcus C, Norgren S and Luthman H. Pathophysiological and genetic characterization of the major diabetes locus in GK rats. Diabetes 48: 2463-2470, 1999.

[180] Porte DJ and Kahn SE. beta-cell dysfunction and failure in type 2 diabetes: potential mechanisms. Diabetes 50 Suppl 1: S160-S163, 2001.

[181] Xue B, Sukumaran S, Nie J, Jusko WJ, DuBois DC and Almon RR. Adipose tissue deficiency and chronic inflammation in diabetic goto-kakizaki rats. PLoS One 6: e17386, 2011.

[182] Chandler MP, Morgan EE, McElfresh TA, Kung TA, Rennison JH, Hoit BD and Young ME. Heart failure progression is accelerated following myocardial infarction in type 2 diabetic rats. Am J Physiol Heart Circ Physiol 293: H1609-H1616, 2007.

[183] Goto Y, Kakizaki M and Masaki N. Production of spontaneous diabetic rats by repetition of selective breeding. Tohoku J Exp Med 119: 85-90, 1976.

[184] Portha B. Programmed disorders of beta-cell development and function as one cause for type 2 diabetes? The GK rat paradigm. Diabetes Metab Res Rev 21: 495-504, 2005.

[185] Hughes SJ, Suzuki K and Goto Y. The role of islet secretory function in the development of diabetes in the GK Wistar rat. Diabetologia 37: 863-870, 1994.

[186] Svensson AM, Ostenson CG and Jansson L. Age-induced changes in pancreatic islet blood flow: evidence for an impaired regulation in diabetic GK rats. Am J Physiol Endocrinol Metab 279: E1139-E1144, 2000.

[187] Guenifi A, Simonsson E, Karlsson S, Ahren B and Abdel-Halim SM. Carbachol restores insulin release in diabetic GK rat islets by mechanisms largely involving hydrolysis of diacylglycerol and direct interaction with the exocytotic machinery. Pancreas 22: 164-171, 2001.

[188] Haynes WG, Sivitz WI, Morgan DA, Walsh SA and Mark AL. Sympathetic and cardiorenal actions of leptin. Hypertension 30: 619-623, 1997.

[189] Haynes WG, Morgan DA, Walsh SA, Sivitz WI and Mark AL. Cardiovascular consequences of obesity: role of leptin. Clin Exp Pharmacol Physiol 25: 65-69, 1998.

Chapter 6

Arterial Stiffness: A Review in Type 2 Diabetes

Mariella Catalano, Giovanni Scandale and
Gabriel Dimitrov

Additional information is available at the end of the chapter

http://dx.doi.org/10.5772/56582

1. Introduction

Diabetes is a growing health problem worldwide in [1]. In a prospective study the risk of cardiovascular death in patients with diabetes, without previous coronary heart disease (CHD) is equal to that of patients with CHD without diabetes, with a higher risk factor in women in [2]. This excessive risk is not explained by classic risk factors for cardiovascular disease such as smoking, LDL-cholesterol, hypertension in [3]. This has led to a search for early markers of vascular dysfunction (arterial stiffness) in diabetic patients that may pre-date the development of overt clinical disease, offer a target for early intervention and delay the progress of cardiovascular disease complications. Arterial walls stiffen with age. Once, the aging-associated changes in arterial structural and functional changes were thought to be part of natural aging, but this concept changed when data emerged showing that these changes are accelerated with coexistent cardiovascular disease. For example, patients with diabetes exhibit increased stiffness even after adjusting for age in [4] and this 'accelerated' arterial aging is well confirmed to be a risk. Several non-invasive methods are currently used to assess vascular stiffness. An extensive theoretical review of models underlying the definitions and assessment methods of arterial stiffness estimates have been recently published in [5].

Pulse wave velocity is a recognized marker of large artery stiffness. Increased arterial stiffness may be an important pathway linking diabetes to increased cardiovascular risk in [6]. Indeed, increased arterial stiffness predicts the development of cardiovascular disease and mortality in several groups of patients in [7] and has been shown to be elevated and predict premature mortality in patients with type 2 diabetes (T2DM) in [8]. Abnormalities in rigidity markers have been reported in patients with T2DM in [9,10] although not in all the arteries in [11], and also without T2DM though predisposed to diabetes suggesting that genetic influences operate through a mechanism different from structural alterations where body mass index (BMI), and glucose metabolism may be involved in [12,13,14]. Diabetic patients are subject to a myriad of abnormalities (poor glycaemic control, dyslipidaemia etc) and it is difficult to determine which abnormality accounts for arterial stiffening in [15]. We present the results of an analysis that examined the independent association of PWV c-f with cardiovascular risk factors. This may be useful to interpret its variations and is of clinical relevance, as arterial stiffening is an independent predictor of an increase in cardiovascular risk in [16]. For this reason we used PubMed for bibliographic research from 1990 to 2012 using the key words : diabetes non-insulin dependent, T2DM, "PWVc-f," "aortic pulse wave velocity," and "aortic stiffness," which were combined with the terms determining and predictive. Articles with multiple regression analysis were included to evaluate factors independently associated with PWV c-f without any restriction on sample size or type. Variables not included in the regression analysis model were considered not independently associated with PWV c-f. Pathogenetic mechanisms, pathophysiological implications and strategies to reduce arterial stiffening will be discussed.

2. Pulse wave velocity carotid-femoral measurement

Pulse wave velocity carotid-femoral (PWVc-f) is currently considered the "gold standard" in [5] of aortic distensibility, a biophysical property of the arterial wall that allows the pressure waves generated by the left ventricle (buffering function) to be absorbed. PWVc-f, the velocity of arterial wave propagation between two arterial sites, can be measured non-invasively, is simple to determine, precise and reproducible in [17,18]. PWVc-f is calculated by dividing the distance between the carotid and the femoral artery by the time delay of the arterial pulse between these two arterial sites. The speed at which the pulse wave travels through an arterial segment increases with increasing stiffness in [19].

3. Factors associated with Pulse wave velocity carotid-femoral

Age is a powerful determinant of PWVc.f in [20,21]. The results of this review confirm that this is also the case for patients with T2DM. In particular, age is the main determinant of PWV c-f in the multiple regression analysis in 89% of nineteen studies (Table 1). Age exposes the aortic wall to degenerative phenomena such as collagen accumulation, fragmentation of elastic fibers and calcification of the media responsible for the increase in aortic rigidity in [22,23,24]. This interpretation gives a possible explanation of the relationship with arterial blood pressure that is another major determinant of PWVc-f in 95% of the included studies. Longstanding arterial pulsation in the central artery has a direct effect on the structural matrix proteins, collagen and elastin in the arterial wall, disrupting muscular attachments and causing elastin fibers to fatigue and fracture in [25]. This would explain why age and blood pressure are major determinants of PWV c-f in [26]. It should be stressed that aortic stiffening is not only a consequence of hypertension but is also in itself a pathogenetic mechanism of the disease. Several studies report an independent association between heart rate (HR) and PWVc-f. The underlying mechanism is unknown, however several observations indicate that the rate of elastin fatigue fracture depends on the number of stress cycles that is, the number of heartbeats experienced which may explain the relationship between HR and PWVc-f in [27,28]. The relationship between HR and PWV c-f suggests that HR may be a confounding factor that should be incorporated into any analysis relating to PWVc-f. T2DM was associated with an increase in PWVc-f in some studies in [29,30,31,32,33] but not in others in [34,35,36,37]. One explanation for the variable association of PWVcf with diabetes mellitus is that it is gender dependent, with a stronger association in women than in men in [38]. A relation between duration of diabetes and PWV c-f has also been described in [39,40] although other authors have failed to show this in [41]. Glycaemia and glycate hemoglobin (HbA1c) were associated with an increase in PWV c-f in [42] that persisted in the multivariate analysis. In the study by Smith et al [43] there was a weak association between PWV c-f and fasting plasma glucose that persisted in the multivariate analysis. PWV c-f was unrelated to elements of the metabolic syndrome (waist circumference, BMI, and triglycerides) and smoking. Only in [44] BMI was associated to PWVc-f and waist-hip ratio in Strain et al [45]. More importantly, fasting glucose concentration, 2 h post-challenge glucose and homeostasis model assessment for insulin resistance (HOMA-IR) were independently related to PWV c-f after adjustment for age, gender, mean arterial pressure, HR, BMI, renal function and antihypertensive medication in [46]. Implying hyperglycaemic excursion and insulin resistance play important roles in the pathogenesis of atherosclerosis. Possible contributors to increased arterial stiffening in T2DM include impaired glycaemic control and the formation of advanced glycation. The aforementioned are end products which lead to structural changes in the vessel walls. Kimoto et al 2006 showed that gender is a determinant of PWV c-f. In the study by Smith et al women have greater age-related aorta stiffening than men, a finding consistent with the enhanced vascular risk in women with diabetes. In the study by Taniwaki et al aortic stiffness while increased in females, was not a risk factor of PWV c-f in the multiple regression analysis. None of the selected studies report smoking as a determining factor in patients with T2DM. Dyslipidaemia did not play an important role in atherosclerosis therefore it is plausible that hyperlipidaemia and foam-cell-driven plaque formation may affect vascular wall integrity at a later stage in the pathogenic process in [47]. Increased aortic stiffness was associated with retinopathy and peripheral neuropathy after adjusting for possible confounding variables. Other variables associated with increased aortic stiffness were old age, HR, diabetes duration, 24 h pulse pressure, dyslipidaemia and physical inactivity in [48].

4. Coefficient of determination (R^2) values

Thirteen studies (68%) reported R^2 values, representing the amount of variability in PWVc-f. Furthermore, regression models could predict a part of the variability of PWVc-f (22–73%) indicating that other factors (e.g. insulin resistance, advanced glycation end-products, genetic factors) may play a more important role in arterial stiffness in T2DM.

5. Pathogenetic mechanism of arterial stiffening

Arterial stiffness depends on the structure and function of the vessel wall. Alterations in the extracellular matrix of the media and adventitia have long been implicated in the pathogenesis of age and blood pressure-related increase in arterial stiffness in [49,50]. Data suggest that such alterations may be caused not only by short-term hyperglycemia, but also by carbonyl and oxidative stress and endothelial dysfunction in [51,52]. Impaired glucose tolerance also enhances nonenzymatic glycation of proteins with covalent cross-linking of collagen (AGEs) and alters the mechanical properties of interstitial tissue of the arterial wall in [53,54]. Chronic hyperglycemia and hyperinsulinemia increases the local activity of renin-angiotensin-aldosterone system (RAAS) and expression of angiotensin type I receptor in vascular tissue in [55] promoting development of wall hypertrophy and fibrosis in [56,57]. In recent years there has been growing evidence of the important role played by inflammation which can influence, by different mechanisms, the increase in arterial stiffness (endothelial dysfunction, smooth muscle proliferation and activation, changes in composition of extracellular matrix) in [58].

6. Pathophysiological implications

The principal function of the arterial system is to deliver an adequate supply of blood to tissues and organs. In performing this primary conduit function, the arteries transform the pulsatile flow generated by ventricular contraction into a continuous flow of blood in the periphery. This latter cushioning function is dependent on the mechanical properties of the arterial walls. Increased aortic stiffness has several detrimental effects on cardiovascular performance. A less distensible aorta cannot efficiently accommodate the blood volume ejected by the left ventricle, which results in high systolic pressure. In addition, diastolic pressure is decreased and pulse pressure (PP) is thus increased. These haemodynamic modification influence ventricular afterload and impair coronary perfusion in [59]. Indeed, PP is more closely predictive of mortality in individuals with T2DM than systolic (SBP) and diastolic blood pressure (DBP) in [60]. PWVc-f seems closely related to PP. Excessive pressure pulsatility enhances regional stress and flow abnormalities in the central aorta and proximal large arteries and may contribute to the propensity for focally severe atherosclerosis in these regions. Thus, excessive aortic stiffness and increased pressure pulsatility contribute to damage the arterial wall and may represent both a cause and a consequence of atherogenesis in [61]. Increased local pulsatile pressure and strain increase the likelihood of plaque rupture and thereby contribute to the increased risk of overt clinical events in individuals with atherosclerotic disease. In addition, high pulsatility may be transferred down to arterioles, resulting in disruption of microcirculation leading to stroke, dementia, and to renal failure in [62,63]. A positive relationship between PP and proteinuria has been observed in [64,65]. Such microvascular disease is accentuated in patients with T2DM.

7. Strategies to reduce arterial stiffening in type 2 diabetes

In patients at high risk of developing CVD, such as diabetic patients, it is important to improve arterial stiffness. There are many studies reporting changes in arterial stiffness after various interventions, either non-pharmacological or pharmacological. Non-pharmacological treatment able to reduce arterial stiffness include exercise training, weight loss, and various dietary modifications, including low-salt diet, moderate alcohol consumption, α-linoleic acid, dark chocolate, and fish oil in [66]. It is still debated whether the reduction in arterial stiffness after antihypertensive treatment is only attributable to blood pressure (BP) lowering, or if additional BP-independent effects are involved. However, renin–angiotensin–aldosterone system (RAAS) inhibitors, such as ACE inhibitors and angiotensin II receptor blockers (ARBs), have been widely suggested to have a BP-independent effect on arterial stiffness in [66,68]. Currently, ARBs are recommended as first-line drugs for hypertension treatment in T2DM patients. Several studies have reported that angiotensin receptor blockers (ARBs) also reduce arterial stiffness in patients with hypertension and T2DM in [69,70]. Fish oil ingestion improved vascular compliance in patients with T2DM by increasing nitric oxide (NO) production or release in [71]. Aerobic exercise has been reported to restore the loss of central arterial compliance and would likely improve arterial stiffening in patients with T2DM in [72]. A combined nutrition and walking program in [73] as well as a pure walking intervention in [74] have also demonstrated prospectively a decrease in arterial stiffness in the middle-aged diabetic population. In T2DM, 3 months of pioglitazone treatment reduced PWVc-f while increasing adiponectin in [75] and lowering C-reactive protein. Interestingly, the decrease of PWVc-f and C-reactive protein levels occurred irrespective of improved diabetic control, suggesting that vascular and antidiabetic effects of glitazones may be partially independent. Studies have shown reduction of arterial stiffness using compounds that affect or break the structure of advanced glycation end-product crosslinks (AGEs) in [76].

8. Conclusions

Arteries stiffen with advancing age, even in the absence of clinically detectable atherosclerotic disease. Diabetes has been shown to accelerate this age associated stiffening in [77] mainly through nonenzymatic glycation, the reaction between glucose and the extracellular matrix proteins in the arterial wall. Nonenzymatic glycation leads to the formation of increased collagen crosslinks that result in increased arterial stiffness in [78]. The results of this review show that in T2DM, the increase in aortic stiffness is independent from other common atherosclerotic risk factors. The principal determinants of PWV c-f are age and arterial blood pressure suggesting that an increase in aortic stiffness could be explained in terms of age and blood pressure. This review has certain limits: First, the studies were cross-sectional, and could not reveal causal relationships. Future studies should include prospective studies to elucidate the contribution of environmental-genetic factors over time to arterial stiffening. Secondly, only studies reporting PWV c-f as a measure of arterial stiffness were included. There is considerable variability in agreement between measures of stiffness and PWVc-f is clinically

References	Sample (n°)	Men %	Age	M	PWVc-f m/s	R2 (%)	Variables associated with PWVc-f	Other variables
Tanokuchi et al 1995 [34]	107 T2DM	54	59	H	9,4	-	Age, SBP,DBP	-
Taniwaki et al 1999 [39]	271 T2DM 285 C	44 51	51 50	U	9 7	33	Age-Diabetes duration	-
Amar et al 2001[4]	247 T2DM,HC	52	54	C	8,8	34	Age.SBP,HR	Apolipoprotein
Aoun et al 2001[41]	122 T2DM 122 Ccontrol	66 66	58 58	C	13 12	-	Age,MBP	-
Kimoto et al 2003 [30]	161 T2DM, 129 Control	53 43	60 59	N	- -	47	Age-SBP-T2DM	-
Lacy et al 2004 [29]	66 T2DM 66 Control	68 68	55 55	S	9,3 7,7	73	Age. SBP,DBP,HR,T2DM	Previous history of cardiovascular disease
Tedesco et al 2004 [42]	50 T2DM 85 T2DM -HT	60 39	53 55	C	11 13,8	22	MBP	FPG
Silva et al 2004 [37]	102 T2DM	37	55	C	12,6	-	Age.24-h SBP	-
Smith et al 2005 [43]	134 T2DM	66	61	S	10,2	55	Age,,PP, Diabetes duration	HT drugs, ACEI/ARB use
Paini et al 2006 [44]	126 T2DM	58	63	C	18,3	33	Age,SBP,	BMI
Kimoto et al 2006 [31]	434 T2DM with and without CKD	56	62 59	H	12,5	55	Age,SBP, T2DM,	Sex male, GFR, non cholesterol HDL
Strain et al 2006 [45]	51 European T2DM 66 African Caribbean T2DM	49 36	57 57	C C	14 15	-	Age,SBP,MBP,HR Age,MBP	Waist:hip ratio
Lee et al 2007 [33]	18 T2DM 20 Control		66 63	MR	8,8 6,2	70	Age,SBP,T2DM	-
Matsumae et al 2008 [40]	94 Hemodialysis with T2DM 148 Hemodialysis without T2DM	59	65	H	11	32	SBP, Diabetes duration Age,SBP,HR,	HbA1c Duration HD, HbA1c
Saez et al 2008 [32]	318 Renal transplant with and without T2DM	49	52	S	9	-	Age,SBP,T2DM	-
Rahman et al 2008 [36]	T2DM 30 IGT 30 NG 30		47 47 47	S	10,4 9,5 8,7	29	Age,SBP	2hPPG
Cardoso et al 2009 [48]	482 T2DM 334 148	38 37	59 67	C	<12 >12	-	Age,24-hPP,HR,Diabetes duration	Dyslipidemia,retinopathy, physical inactivity, peripheral neuropathy
Webb et al 2010 [46]	176 NGM 219 IGR 175 T2DM	58 59 59	55 53 57	U	8,9 9,7 10	51	Age, MBP,HR Sex Female	FPG,2HPG,HOMA-IR
Naka et al 2012 [35]	165 T2DM	30	66	S	10,2	25	Age, SBP	-

Table 1. Characteristic of studies on PWVc-f included in the review

the most relevant. PWV c-f is easy to measure with specifically designed devices. High aortic stiffness doubles the risk of cardiovascular events or mortality compared to low aortic stiffness, and the predictive value of high PWV c-f is greater in high-risk patients, such as patients with T2DM. PWVc-f expresses the cumulative effect of various factors on the arterial system and their interplay with genetic predisposition. In contrast to cardiovascular risk factors, such as blood pressure or cholesterol, that may fluctuate over time, PWVc-f is relatively stable, since it is mostly influenced by alterations of arterial wall structure. The 2007 European Society of Hypertension & European Society of Cardiology guidelines for the management of hypertension rightfully included increased PWVc-f as subclinical target-organ damage, and recommended aggressive management of patients with high PWVc-f in [79]. The World Health Organization estimates that by the year 2025 more than 300 million people worldwide will have diabetes [80]. Measurement of aortic PWV c-f should be integrated in the examination and risk stratification of patients with T2DM.

M, method, C, compilor; S, SphygmoCor; U, ultrasound; H, Hasegawa method MR, magnetic resonance, N, indicates noninvasivepressure recordings. R2,coefficient of determination, SBP, systolic blood pressure, DBP, diastolic blood pressure, PP, pulse pressure, MBP, mean blood pressure, HR, heart rate, FPG, fasting plasma glucose, T2DM, type 2 diabetes; BMI, body mass index, ACE angiotensin-converting enzyme ARB, angiotensin receptor blocker, GFR glomerular filtration rate, HbA1c, glycate hemoglobin, 2HPG, 2 h post-challenge glucose HOMA-IR, homeostasis model assessment for insulin resistance, IGT impaired glucose tolerance IR insulin resistance, IGR, impaired glucose regulation, HT, hypertensive HC, hypercholesterolemia.

Acknowledgements

We would like to thank Mrs Rotolo MR, (Prof. A. Malliani Library, University of Milan) for her help with the bibliographic research.

Author details

Mariella Catalano, Giovanni Scandale and Gabriel Dimitrov

Research Center on Vascular Diseases and Angiology Unit, University of Milan L.Sacco Hospital Milan, Italy

References

[1] Wild, S, Roglic, G, Green, A, Sicree, R, & King, H. Global prevalence of diabetes: estimates for the year 2000 and projection for 2030. Diabetes Care (2004). , 27, 1047-1053.

[2] Whiteley, L, Padmanabhan, S, & Hole, D. Isles C: Should diabetes be considered a coronary heart disease risk equivalent ? Results from 25 years of follow-up in the Renfrew and paisley Survey. Diabetes Care (2005). , 28, 1588-1593.

[3] Pyörälä, K. Relationship of glucose tolerance and plasma insulin in the incidence of coronary heart disease.Results from two population studies in Finland. Diabetes Care (1979). , 2, 131-141.

[4] Amar, J, Ruidavets, J. B, Chamontin, B, & Drouet, L. Ferrieres J: Arterial stiffness and cardiovascular risk factors in a population- based study. J Hypertens (2001). , 19, 381-387.

[5] Laurent, S, & Cockcroft, J. Van Bortel L Butourye P, Giannattasio C et al. Expert consensus document on arterial stiffness: methodological issues and clinical applications. Eur Heart J (2006). , 27, 2588-2605.

[6] Stehouwer, C. D, Henry, R. M, & Ferreira, I. Arterial stiffness in diabetes and the metabolic syndrome: a pathway to cardiovascular disease. Diabetologia (2008). , 51, 527-39.

[7] Vlachopoulos, C, Aznaouridis, K, & Stefanadis, C. Prediction of cardiovascular events and all-cause mortality with arterial stiffness. A systematic review and meta-analysis. J Am Coll Cardiol; (2010). , 55, 1318-27.

[8] Cruickshank, K, Riste, L, Anderson, S. G, Wright, J. S, & Dunn, G. Gosling RG: Aortic pulse-wave velocity and its relationship to mortality in diabetes and glucose intolerance: An integrated index of vascular function? Circulation (2002). , 106, 2085-2090.

[9] Lehmann, E. D, Gosling, R. G, & Sonksen, P. H. Arterial wall compliance in diabetes. Diabet Med (1992). , 9, 114-119.

[10] Schram, M. T, Henry, R. M, Van Dijk, R. A, Kostense, P. J, Dekker, J. M, et al. Increased central artery stiffness in impaired glucose metabolism and type 2 diabetes: the Hoorn Study. Hypertension (2004). , 43, 176-181.

[11] Catalano, M, Scandale, G, Minola, M, Carzaniga, G, Carotta, M, et al. Elastic properties and structure of the radial artery in patients with type 2 diabetes. Diabetes & Vascular Disease Research (2009). , 6, 244-248.

[12] Henry, R. M, Kostense, P. J, Spijkerman, A. M, Dekker, J. M, Nijpels, G, et al. Arterial stiffness increases with deteriorating glucose tolerance status: the Hoorn Study. Circulation. (2003). , 107, 2089-2095.

[13] Mceleavy, O. D, Mccallum, R. W, & Petrie, J. R. Higher carotid-radial pulse wave velocity in healthy offspring of patients with type 2 diabetes. Diabetic Med. (2004). , 21, 262-266.

[14] Giannattasio, C, Failla, M, Capra, A, Scanziani, E, Amigoni, M, Boffi, L, Whistock, C, Gamba, P, Paleari, F, & Mancia, G. Increased arterial stiffness in normoglycemic normotensive offspring of type 2 Diabetic parents. Hypertension. (2008). , 51, 182-187.

[15] Salomaa, V, Riley, W, Kark, J. D, Nardo, C, & Folsom, A. R. Non-insulin-dependent diabetes mellitus and fasting glucose and insulin concentrations are associated with arterial stiffness indexes. The ARIC Study. Atherosclerosis Risk in Communities Study. Circulation (1995). , 91, 1432-1443.

[16] Blacher, J, Safar, M. E, Guerin, A. P, Pannier, B, Marchais, S. J, & London, G. M. Aortic pulse wave velocity index and mortality in end-stage renal disease. Kidney Int. (2003). , 63, 1852-1860.

[17] Asmar, R, Benetos, A, Topouchian, J, Laurent, P, Pannier, B, Brisac, A. M, Target, R, & Levy, B. Assessment of arterial distensibility by automatic pulse wave velocity measurement. Validation and clinical application studies. Hypertension (1995). , 26, 485-90.

[18] Wilkinson, I. B, Fuchs, S. A, Jansen, I. M, Spratt, J. C, Murray, G. D, & Cockcroft, J. R. Webb DJ: Reproducibility of pulse wave velocity and augmentation index measured by pulse wave analysis. J Hypertens (1998). , 16, 2079-2084.

[19] Oliver, J. J. Webb DJ: Noninvasive assessment of arterial stiffness and risk of atherosclerotic events. Arterioscler Thromb Vasc Biol (2003). , 23, 554-566.

[20] Avolio, A. P, Chen, S. G, Wang, R. P, Zhang, C. L, Li, M. F, & Rourke, O. MF. Effects of aging on changing arterial compliance and left ventricular load in a northern Chinese urban community. Circulation.(1983). , 68, 50-58.

[21] Smulyan, H, Csermely, T. J, & Mookherjee, S. Warner RA: Effect of age on arterial distensibility in asymptomatic humans. Arteriosclerosis (1983). , 3, 199-205.

[22] Zieman, S. J, Melenovsky, V, & Kass, D. A. Mechanisms, pathophysiology, and therapy of arterial stiffness. Arterioscler Thromb Vasc Biol ;(2005).

[23] Atkinson, J. Age-related medial elastocalcinosis in arteries: Mechanisms, animal models, and physiological consequences. J Appl Physiol (2008). , 105, 1643-1651.

[24] Jacob, M. P. Extracellular matrix remodeling and matrix metalloproteinases in the vascular wall during aging and in pathological conditions. Biomed Pharmacother (2003). , 57, 195-202.

[25] Greenwald, S. E. Ageing of the conduit arteries. J Pathol. (2007). , 211, 157-172.

[26] Mceniery, C. M. Yasmin, Hall IR, Qasem A, Wilkinson IB, Cockcroft JR.Normal vascular ageing: differential effects on wave reflection and aortic pulse wave velocity-the Anglo-Cardiff Collaborative Trial (ACCT 1). J Am Coll Cardiol. (2005). , 46, 1753-1760.

[27] Sa Cunha RPannier B, Benetos A, Siche J-P, London GM, Mallion JM, Safar ME. Association between high heart rate and high arterial rigidity in normotensive and hypertensive subjects. J Hypertens. (1997). , 15, 1423-1430.

[28] Lantelme, P, Mestre, C, Lievre, M, Gressard, A, & Milon, H. Heart rate: an important confounder of pulse wave velocity assessment. Hypertension. (2002). , 39, 1083-1087.

[29] Lacy, P. S, Brien, O, Stanley, D. G, & Dewar, A. G. MM, Swales PPR, Williams B. Increased pulse wave velocity is not associated with elevated augmentation index in patients with diabetes. J Hypertens. (2004). , 22, 1937-1944.

[30] Kimoto, E, Shoji, T, Shinohara, K, Inaba, M, Okuno, Y, et al. Preferential stiffening of central over peripheral arteries in type 2 diabetes. Diabetes (2003). , 52, 448-452.

[31] Kimoto, E, Shoji, T, Shinohara, K, Hatsuda, S, Mori, K, et al. Regional arterial stiffness in patients with type 2 diabetes and chronic kidney disease. J Am Soc Nephrol (2006). , 17, 2245-52.

[32] Saez, A. O, Kos, M, Witzke, O, Kribben, A, & Nürnberger, J. Effect of new-onset diabetes mellitus on arterial stiffness in renal transplantation. Transpl Int. (2008). , 21, 930-935.

[33] Lee JMSShirodaria C, Jackson CE, Robson MD, Antoniades C et al. Multi-modal magnetic resonance imaging quantifies atherosclerosis and vascular dysfunction in patients with type 2 diabetes mellitus. Diab Vasc Dis Res. (2007). , 4, 44-48.

[34] Tanokuchi, S, Okada, S, & Ota, Z. Factors related to aortic pulse wave velocity in patients with non-insulindependent diabetes mellitus. J Int Med Res (1995). , 23, 423-430.

[35] Naka, K. K, Papathanassiou, K, Bechlioulis, A, Kazakos, N, Pappas, K, et al. Determinants of vascular function in patients with type 2 diabetes.Cardiovascular Diabetology (2012). , 11, 127-134.

[36] Raham, S, Ismail, A. A, Ismail, S. B, & Naing, N. N. Rahman AR Early manifestation of macrovasculopathy in newly diagnosed never treated type II diabetic patients with no traditional CVD risk factors. Diabetes Res Clin Pract (2008). , 80, 253-258.

[37] Silva, J. A, Barbosa, L, Bertoquini, S, Maldonado, J, & Polónia, J. Relationship between aortic stiffness and cardiovascular risk factors in a population of normotensive, white coat normotensive, white-coat hypertensive, sustained hypertensive and diabetic patients. Rev Port Cardiol. (2004). , 23, 1533-1547.

[38] De Angelis, L, Millasseau, S. C, Smith, A, Viberti, G, Jones, R. H, Ritter, J. M, & Chowienczyk, P. J. Sex differences in age-related stiffening of the aorta in subjects with type 2 diabetes. Hypertension (2004). , 44, 67-71.

[39] Taniwaki, H, Kawagishi, T, Emoto, M, Shoji, T, Kanda, H, Maekawa, K, & Nishizawa, Y. Morii H: Correlation between the intima-media thickness ofthe carotid artery

and aortic pulse-wave velocity in patients with type 2diabetes. Vessel wall properties in type 2 diabetes. Diabetes Care (1999). , 22, 1851-1857.

[40] Matsumae, T, Abe, Y, Murakami, G, Ueda, K, & Saito, T. Effects of glucose metabolism on aortic pulse wave velocity in hemodialysis patients with and without diabetes. Hypertens Res. (2008). , 31, 1365-1372.

[41] Aoun, S, Blacher, J, Safar, M. E, & Mourad, J. J. Diabetes mellitus and renal failure: effects on large artery stiffness. J Hum Hypertens (2001). , 15, 693-700.

[42] Tedesco, M. A, & Natale, F. Di Salvo G, Caputo S, Capasso M, Calabro R. Effects of coexisting hypertension and type II diabetes mellitus on arterial stiffness. J Hum Hypertens (2004). , 18, 469-473.

[43] Smith, A, Karalliedde, J, De Angelis, L, & Goldsmith, D. Viberti G: Aortic pulse wave velocity and albuminuria in patients with type 2 diabetes. J Am Soc Nephrol (2005). , 16, 1069-1075.

[44] Paini, A, Boutouyrie, P, Calvet, D, Tropeano, A. I, Laloux, B, & Laurent, S. Carotid and aortic stiffness: determinants of discrepancies. Hypertension. (2006). , 47, 371-376.

[45] Strain, W. D, Chaturvedi, N, Dockery, F, Shiff, R, Shore, A. C, Bulpitt, C. J, et al. Increased arterial stiffness in Europeans and African Caribbeans with type 2 diabetes cannot be accounted for by conventional cardiovascular risk factors. Am J Hypertens (2006). , 19, 889-96.

[46] Webb, D. R, Khunti, K, Silverman, R, Gray, L. J, Srinivasan, B, Lacy, P. S, & Williams, B. Davies MJ Impact of metabolic indices on central artery stiffness: independent association of insulin resistance and glucose with aortic pulse wave velocity. Diabetologia (2010). , 53, 1190-1198.

[47] Zureik, M, Bureau, J. M, Temmar, M, Adamopoulos, C, Courbon, D, Bean, K, Touboul, P. J, & Benetos, A. Ducimetie`re P. Echogenic carotid plaques are associated with aortic arterial stiffness in subjects with subclinical carotid atherosclerosis. Hypertension. (2003). , 41, 519-527.

[48] Cardoso CRLFerreira MT, Leite NC, Barros PN, Conte PH, Salles GF. Microvascular degenerative complications are associated with increased aortic stiffness in type 2 diabetic patients. Atherosclerosis (2009). , 205, 472-476.

[49] Glagov, S, Vito, R, Giddens, D. P, & Zarins, C. K. Microarchitecture and composition of artery walls: relationships to location, diameter and the distribution of mechanical stress. J Hypertens (1992). Suppl 6): SS104., 101.

[50] Tayebjee, M. H. MacFadyen RJ, Lip GY. Extracellular matrix biology: a new frontier in linking the pathology and therapy of hypertension? J Hypertens (2003). , 21(12), 2211-2218.

[51] Eckel, R. H, Wassef, M, Chait, A, Sobel, B, Barret, E, King, G, et al. Prevention conference VI: diabetes and cardiovascular diseases writing group II: pathogenesis of atherosclerosis in diabetes. Circulation (2002). , 105, 138-43.

[52] Bruno, R. M, Penno, G, Daniele, G, Lucchesi, D, Stea, F, Landini, L, Cartoni, G, Taddei, S, & Ghiadoni, L. Del Prato S. Type 2 diabetes mellitus worsens arterial stiffness in hypertensive patients through endothelial dysfunction. Diabetologia (2012). , 55, 1847-55.

[53] Brownlee, M, Cerami, A, & Vlassara, H. Advanced glycosylation end products in tissue and the biochemical basis of diabetic complications. N Engl J Med. (1988). , 318, 1315-1321.

[54] Airaksinen, K. E, Salela, P. I, Linnaluoto, M. K, Ikaheimo, M. J, Anola, K, & Rynanen, L. J. Diminished arterial elasticity in diabetes: association with fluorescent advanced glycosylation end products in collagen. Cardiovasc Res (1993). , 27, 942-945.

[55] Nickenig, G, Roling, J, Strehlow, K, Schnabel, P, & Bohm, M. Insulin induces upregulation of vascular AT1 receptor gene expression by posttranscriptional mechanisms. Circulation (1998). , 98, 2453-2460.

[56] Jesmin, S, Sakuma, I, Hattori, Y, & Kitabatake, A. Role of angiotensin II in altered expression of molecules responsible for coronary matrix remodeling in insulin-resistant diabetic rats. Arterioscler Thromb Vasc Biol. (2003). , 23, 2021-2026.

[57] Rizzoni, D, Porteri, E, Guelfi, D, Muiesan, M. L, Valentini, U, Cimino, A, Girelli, A, Rodella, L, Bianchi, R, Sleiman, I, & Rosei, E. A. Structural alterations in subcutaneous small arteries of normotensive and hypertensive patients with non-insulin-dependent diabetes mellitus. Circulation. (2001). , 103, 1238-1244.

[58] Maki-petaja, K. M. Wilkinson IB Inflammation and large arteries: Potential mechanisms for inflammation-induced arterial stiffness. Artery Research (2012). , 6, 59-64.

[59] Nichols, W. W, Rourke, O, & Mcdonald, M. F. s blood flow in arteries: theoretical, experimental and clinical principles. 5th ed. London: Hodder Arnold; (2005).

[60] Schram, M. T, & Kostense, P. J. van Dijk RAJM, Dekker JM, Nijpels G, Bouter LM, Heine RJ, Stehouwer CDA. Diabetes, pulse pressure and cardiovascular mortality: the Hoorn study. J Hypertens. (2002). , 20, 1743-1751.

[61] Sako, H, Miura, S, Kumagai, K, & Saku, K. Associations between augmentation index and severity of atheroma or aortic stiffness of the descending thoracic aorta by transesophageal echocardiography. Circ J (2009). , 73, 1151-1156.

[62] Mitchell, G. F, Vita, J. A, Larson, M. G, Parise, H, Keyes, M. J, et al. Cross-sectional relations of peripheral microvascular function, cardiovascular disease risk factors, and aortic stiffness: the Framingham Heart Study. Circulation (2005). , 112, 3722-28.

[63] Rourke, O, & Safar, M. F. ME. Relationship between aortic stiffening and microvascular disease in brain and kidney. Cause and Logic of therapy. Hypertension. (2005)., 46, 200-204.

[64] Pedrinelli, R. Dell'Omo G, Penno G, Bandinelli S, Bertini A, Di BV, Mariani M: Microalbuminuria and pulse pressure in hypertensive and atherosclerotic men. Hypertension (2000)., 35, 48-54.

[65] Ishimura, E, Taniwaki, H, Tsuchida, T, Obatake, N, Emoto, M, et al. Urinary albumin excretion associated with arterial stiffness rather than thickness in type 2 diabetes. J Nephrol (2007)., 20, 204-11.

[66] Laurent, S, & Boutouyrie, P. Recent advances in arterial stiffness and wave reflection in human hypertension. Hypertension (2007)., 49, 1202-1206.

[67] Mitchell, G. F, Dunlap, M. E, Warnica, W, Ducharme, A, Arnold, J. M, Tardif, J. C, et al. Long-term trandolapril treatment is associated with reduced aortic stiffness: The prevention of events with angiotensin converting enzyme inhibition hemodynamic substudy. Hypertension (2007)., 49, 1271-1277.

[68] Tropeano, A. I, Boutouyrie, P, Pannier, B, Joannides, R, Balkestein, E, et al. Brachial pressure-independent reduction in carotid stiffness after long-term angiotensin-converting enzyme inhibition in diabetic hypertensives. Hypertension. (2006)., 48, 80-86.

[69] Asmar, R, Gosse, P, Topouchian, J, Tela, N, Dudley, G, & Shepherd, A. GL. Effects of telmisartan on arterial stiffness in type 2 diabetes patients with essential hypertension. J Renin Angiotensin Aldosterone Syst (2002)., 3, 176-80.

[70] Karalliedde, J, Smith, A, De Angelis, L, Mirenda, V, Kandra, A, Botha, J, Ferber, P, & Viberti, G. Valsartan improves arterial stiffness in type 2 diabetes independently of blood pressure lowering. Hypertension (2008)., 51, 1617-23.

[71] Mcveigh, G. E, Brennan, G. M, Johnston, G. D, Mc Dermott, B. J, Mc Grath, L. T, et al. Dietary fish oil augments nitric oxide production or release in patients with type 2 (non-insulin-dependent) diabetes mellitus. Diabetologia (1993)., 36, 33-8.

[72] Madden, K. M, Lockart, C, Cuff, D, & Potter, T. F. Meneilly G Short-term aerobic exercise reduces arterial stiffness in older adults with Type 2 diabetes, hypertension and hypercholesterolemia. Diabetes Care (2009)., 32, 1531-1535.

[73] Yamamoto, A, Katayama, Y, Tomiyama, K, Hosoai, H, Hirata, F, & Yasuda, H. A short-term admission improved brachial-ankle pulse wave velocity in type 2 diabetic patients. Diabetes Res Clin Pract (2005)., 70, 248-252.

[74] Yokoyama, H, Emoto, M, Fujiwara, S, Motoyama, K, Morioka, T, et al. Short-term aerobic exercise improves arterial stiffness in type 2 diabetes. Diabetes Res Clin Pract (2004)., 65, 85-93.

[75] Satoh, N, Ogawa, Y, Usui, T, Tagami, T, Kono, S, Uesugi, H, et al. Antiatherogenic effect of pioglitazone in type 2 diabetic patients irrespective of the responsiveness to its antidiabetic effect. Diabetes Care. (2003). , 26, 2493-2499.

[76] Kass, D. A, Shapiro, E. P, Kawaguchi, M, et al. Improved arterial compliance by a novel advanced glycation end-product crosslink breaker. Circulation (2001). , 104, 1464-1470.

[77] Cameron, J. D, Bulpitt, C. J, Pinto, E. S, & Rajkumar, C. The aging of elastic and muscular arteries: a comparison of diabetic and nondiabetic subjects. Diabetes Care (2003). , 26, 2133-2138.

[78] Lakatta, E. G. Arterial and cardiac aging: major shareholders in cardiovascular disease enterprises. Part III: cellular and molecular clues to heart and arterial aging. Circulation (2003). , 107, 490-497.

[79] Mancia, G, De Backer, G, Dominiczak, A, Cifkovar, R, Fagard, R, et al. ESH-ESC Task force on the management of arterial hypertension. J Hypertens (2007). , 25, 1105-87.

[80] Zimmet, P, Alberti, K. G, & Shaw, J. Global and societal implications of the diabetes epidemic. Nature (2001). , 414, 782-787.

Chapter 7

Association Between Creatinine Clearance and Insulin-Resistance in Healthy Adolescent Boys

Valeria Hirschler

Additional information is available at the end of the chapter

http://dx.doi.org/10.5772/56483

1. Introduction

Prevalence of high levels of BMI in both adults and children has been observed in USA [1,2]. Argentina as well, has experienced marked increases in the prevalence of childhood overweight/obesity (OW/OB) over the last few decades [3]. Studies in adults have shown that excess weight is an independent risk factor for end-stage renal disease [4, 5]. Chronic kidney disease is a significant public health problem in the United States, affecting 11% of the U.S. adult population and it has been associated with increased cardiovascular morbidity and mortality [6].

Given the high prevalence and the low awareness of chronic kidney disease, it becomes inevitable to formulate appropriate strategies for the prevention of the chronic kidney disease to control the escalating healthcare cost [7]. A screening program in communities would detect previously unidentified persons at high risk for chronic kidney disease in the general population [8]. OB has been shown to be a strong predictor of chronic kidney disease [4,9,10]. Additionally, studies have suggested an association between insulin resistance and chronic kidney disease [11,12]. A large study performed in a community population in Shanghai, China, showed that OB, hypertension, and anemia, were positively correlated with the development of chronic kidney disease [7].

Few studies have examined the significance of BMI, insulin-resistance and hemoglobin, as risk factors for the development of chronic kidney disease in normal adolescents. The aim of this study was to determine the association between calculated creatinine clearance (CrC) and risk factors for chronic kidney disease such as, BMI, insulin resistance (HOMA-IR), and hemoglobin in healthy adolescents.

2. Methods

2.1. Study design and participants

Data were collected cross-sectionally from 195 adolescent boys aged 16.7 ± 1.8 years, age ranged 15-21 years, in an amateur rugby club in the west side of the Buenos Aires suburbs in April 2009. Exclusion criteria included: missing BMI, blood pressure information, known diabetes or other chronic disease, the use of medication that could alter blood pressure, glucose or lipid metabolism, and the informed consent not being signed. Of the 207 adolescents recruited, 4 were missing the BMI information and 8 declined to participate. The remaining 195 children were included. All subjects were examined by the same physician. The study was approved by the Human Rights Committee of Durand Hospital in Buenos Aires. Each subject and parent gave written informed consent after an explanation of the study and before the initiation of the research studies.

Although Argentina is a Spanish-speaking country, the population differs greatly from what is usually referred to as Hispanic in the U.S. About 85% of the population is of European descent (largely Spanish and Italian), with the remainder of mixed European and American Indian (12%) or American Indian (3%) descent [13]. Socio-demographic characteristics included age, level of education and the presence or absence of a refrigerator and/or a dirt floor. Questionnaires for socio economic status have been described in detail elsewhere [14].

2.2. Anthropometric measures, stage of puberty and blood pressure

Height and weight were measured with subjects wearing light clothing and without shoes. Weight was measured to the nearest 0.1 kg on a medical balance scale. Height was measured to the nearest 0.1 cm. with a wall-mounted stadiometer. Adolescents were classified as normal weight (BMI< 85%), OW (BMI 85% to < 95%), or OB (BMI > or = 95%) according to CDC norms [15]. When participants were older than 18 years they were classified as normal weight (BMI < 25 kg/m^2), OW (25 kg/m^2 ≤ BMI < 30 kg/m^2), or OB (≥30 kg/m^2) according to the adult definition [16]

Waist circumference measurement was taken at the level of the umbilicus and recorded to 0.1cm. A non-elastic flexible tape measure was employed with the subject standing without clothing covering the waist area. Central OB was defined as waist circumference ≥ 94cm per international diabetes federation criteria (IDF) [17].

Three separate blood pressure measurements were recorded by a trained technician using a random-zero sphygmomanometer after the participant was seated at rest for 5 minutes. The averages of the last 3 measurements of systolic and diastolic blood pressures were used [18]. Hypertension was defined according to IDF criteria [17].

Metabolic syndrome was defined according to IDF criteria [17]. Metabolic syndrome is a constellation of metabolic abnormalities that predicts premature coronary artery disease. Recently the IDF [17] developed a simple unified definition for children over 10 years of age. The IDF definition for adolescents included the presence of ≥3 of the following 5 conditions:

[1] central OB (waist circumference >94cm), [2] fasting triglycerides ≥150 mg/dL, [3] HDL-C <40 mg/dL, [4] hypertension with systolic blood pressure ≥ 130 and/or diastolic blood pressure ≥85 mm Hg percentile [5] fasting glucose >100 mg/dL.

The physical examination also included determination of the stage of puberty according to the criteria of Tanner [19].

2.3. Biochemistry

Baseline blood samples were obtained from subjects while they were fasting for 12 hours, for measurement of complete blood count (CBC), levels of glucose, insulin, lipid profile and creatinine. Plasma glucose was obtained by the glucose oxidase technique and serum lipids were measured with a Hitachi Modular P analyser (Hitachi High Technologies Corp., Tokyo, Japan). Serum insulin levels were determined by radioimmunoassay (Diagnostic Products, Los Angeles, CA, USA) and did not cross-react with proinsulin or C-peptide (%CV 5.2-6.8%). Serum creatinine was obtained by the enzymatic method (Bayer, ID-MS, HPLC).

The following equation for HOMA-IR index was used: fasting insulin (uU/l) x fasting glucose (mmol/l)/22.5) [20].

2.4. Estimated glomerular filtration rate

Kidney Disease Improving Global Outcome organization [21] recommended the estimation of glomerular filtration rate, using the simplified equation. Several formulas are widely used in clinical practice: The Schwartz equation is used and validated for adolescents [22]. The abbreviated Modification of Diet in Renal Disease and quadratic equation (MDRD) is used for individuals older than 18 years old [23].The Cockcroft–Gault equation [24] was not used for analysis because it introduces a major methodological problem. Since weight is already included in the numerator of the equation, the association between BMI and CrC would be obvious.

2.5. Data analysis

Chi squared test was used to compare proportions. When more than 20% of the cells had expected frequencies <5, Fisher's exact test was used. The fit to normal distribution of continuous variables was assessed using the Shapiro-Wilks test. When comparing two groups with normally distributed data, a student t test was performed. When comparing more than three groups and with data that were normally distributed, one-way Analysis of Variance was used (Student-Newman-Keuls post hoc test). When the homogeneity of the variances could not be proven, we used the non-parametric Kruskal Wallis instead of Analysis of Variance, with Dunn post hoc test. We evaluated the correlation of plasma CrC with components of the metabolic syndrome using Spearman correlation coefficients. The primary focus of the analysis was to determine the association between calculated CrC and risk factors for chronic kidney disease. Multiple linear regression analysis using CrC as the dependent variable was used. In order to obtain an r squared in each step, a stepwise method was used. P values <0.05 were considered significant in the two-tailed situation. Data are presented as mean ± SD unless otherwise stated.

Analyses were done using the SPSS (Chicago, IL) statistical software package SPSS version 10.0 ®.

3. Results

3.1. Physical and metabolic characteristics:

Participants came from a middle-low socioeconomic class, reflected in their parents' educational background, with 51.8% of mothers and 53.3% of fathers having completed an elementary school education or less. All of the families had a refrigerator and none had a dirt floor. All participants were at pubertal or post pubertal stage. Accordingly, clinical and metabolic characteristics are presented in Table 1.

	Mean	**±Std. Deviation**
Age (years)	16.73	±1.78
BMI(Kg/m^2)	25.20	±4.99
Waist Circumference (cm)	83.58	±12.95
Systolic BP(mmHg)	115.90	±11.59
Diastolic BP(mmHg)	71.16	±8.56
Hemoglobin (g/dL)	14.76	±0.911
Creatinine (mg/dl)	0.93	±0.17
Cholesterol(mg/dl)	157.13	±33.93
HDL-C(mg/dl)	44.09	±11.77
Insulin(mU/l)	7.69	±5.81
LDL-C(mg/dl)	99.89	±33.06
HOMA-IR	1.61	±1.32
Cr C(ml/min)	128.44	±28.16
OB%	24.1%	(47/195)
OW %	21.0%	(41/195)
Central OB	23.6%	(45/191)
Tanner 3	11.3%	(20/195)
Tanner 4	32.1%	(57/195)
Tanner 5	55.4%	(95/195)

BP, blood pressure. Data are mean ±S.D. or percentage.

Table 1. Clinical and metabolic characteristics

3.2. Physical and metabolic characteristics according to the presence of OW/OB

Adolescents were divided by the presence of OW/OB. The prevalence of OB adolescents was 47 (24.1%), and of OW 41 (21.0%). There was no significant difference in age between the groups. Clinical and metabolic characteristics according to the presence of OW/ OB are presented in Table 2. Mean values of BMI, triglycerides, systolic blood pressure, diastolic blood pressure, insulin, and HOMA-IR were significantly higher while HDL-C was significantly lower in the group of children with OW or OB (Table 2). Mean values of CrC were not significantly different among normal weight and OW or OB adolescents.

	Normal Weight			OW			OB		
	N=107			N=41			N=47		
Age (c) (years)	16.52	+	1.73	16.45	+	1.81	16.52	+	1.80
BMI(a) (Kg/m^2)	21.74	+	2.33	26.14	+	1.41	32.27	+	3.36
WC(a) (cm)	75.05	+	6.88	85.80	+	6.72	101.12	+	8.43
S BP(b) (mm Hg)	113.43	+	9.98	113.59	+	10.63	123.55	+	12.64
D BP(b) (mm Hg)	69.78	+	8.22	68.44	+	6.35	76.70	+	8.70
Hemoglobin (g/dL) (c)	14.76	+	0.98	14.83	+	0.90	14.74	+	0.74
TG (b) (mg/dl)	75.42	+	33.92	95.44	+	60.67	125.98	+	71.51
Cholesterol (b)	153.65	+	34.93	149.85	+	25.59	171.38	+	34.56
HDL-C(b) (mg/dl)	47.36	+	13.22	42.00	+	9.14	38.47	+	6.92
LDL-C(b) (mg/dl)	94.63	+	34.39	93.24	+	24.36	117.68	+	30.69
Ccr(c)(ml/min)	131.85	+	27.21	122.24	+	28.88	126.09	+	29.14
HOMA-IR(b)	1.25	+	0.71	1.30	+	0.59	2.68	+	2.07

SBP, systolic blood pressure, DBP diastolic blood pressure, HDL-C, high density lipoprotein; LDL-C, low density lipoprotein; Data are mean ± standard deviation

(a) Significance found between each group

(b) Significance found in comparison of obese to normal weight and OW

(c) No significant differences found between any of the groups

Table 2. Clinical and Metabolic Characteristics according to the presence of OW/OB.

The prevalence of metabolic syndrome was 6.7% (13/195) overall, 0% in normal weight; 4.9% in OW and 23.4% in OB (p<0.001]. None had all 5 risk factors. None had diabetes. There was not a significant difference in the mean values of CrC between children with and without metabolic syndrome.

3.3. Hemoglobin quartiles

Subjects were divided for comparison of mean values of CrC, into four groups according to hemoglobin quartiles: 1st (12.2–14.1g/dL), 2nd (14.2–14.7 g/dL), 3rd (14.8-15.3 g/dL), and 4th (15.4–17.6 g/dL). None of the adolescents had anemia (Hb<12g/dL). Mean CrC was significantly higher in quartile 1 than in quartiles 2, 3 and 4 (Figure 1).

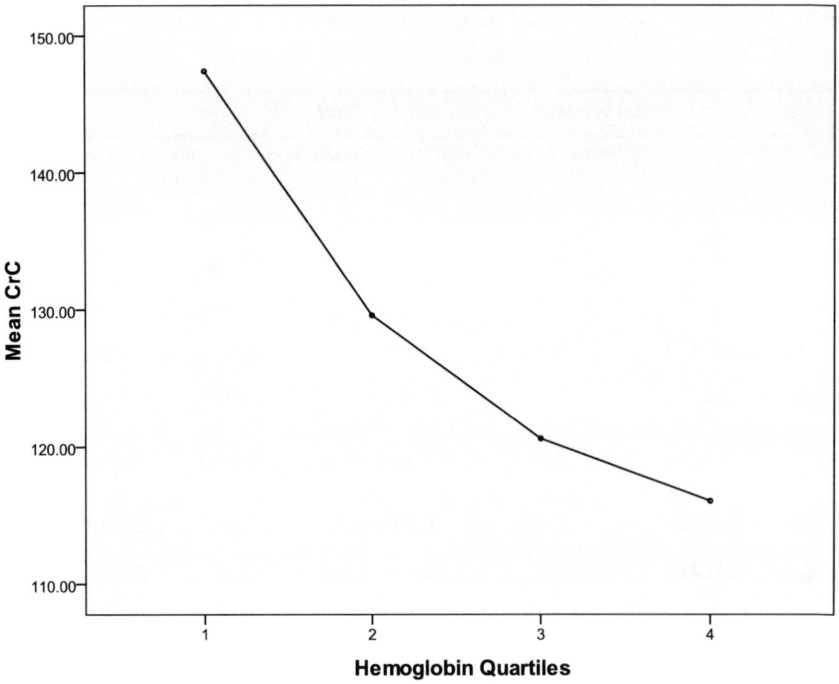

Figure 1. Mean Values of CrC according to Hemoglobin Quartiles

3.4. Insulin resistance quartiles

Subjects were divided into four groups by HOMA-IR quartiles for comparison of their means. As insulin resistance increased, BMI, waist circumference, systolic blood pressure, triglycerides and CrC increased significantly from the lowest to the highest quartiles of HOMA-IR levels (Table 3). There was not a significant difference in age, LDL-C, HDL-C, and total cholesterol between HOMA-IR quartiles.

3.5. Univariate and multivariate analysis

There was a univariate association ($p<0.01$) between CrC and age (r=--0.60), Tanner (r=-0.51), BMI (r = -0.29), waist circumference (r = -0.22), systolic blood pressure (r = -0.18), diastolic blood pressure (r =- 0.22), hemoglobin (r = -0.39), triglycerides (r = -0.15), insulin (r = 0.25), and HOMA-

	Quartile I (0.14-0.87)			Quartile II (0.88-1.30)			Quartile III (1.31-1.85)			Quartile VI (1.9-9.80)		
	N=47			N=48			N=48			N=48		
Age (years) (e)	16.32	+	1.75	16.92	+	1.73	16.62	+	1.96	16.10	+	1.45
BMI[(a)] (Kg/m^2)	22.77	+	3.36	25.35	+	4.50	24.86	+	4.56	28.12	+	5.87
WC[(a)] (cm)	76.63	+	8.93	83.69	+	11.85	82.38	+	11.40	92.00	+	14.48
Systolic BP[(b)] (mmHg)	111.45	+	9.09	114.85	+	9.80	117.69	+	13.52	119.77	+	12.31
Triglycerides[(c)] (mg/dl)	67.17	+	28.89	84.71	+	46.94	91.42	+	46.68	125.46	+	73.76
Cholesterol(e) (mg/dl)	155.77	+	36.82	150.08	+	32.88	157.04	+	34.28	166.98	+	31.33
HDL-C(e) (mg/dl)	45.87	+	9.16	43.92	+	9.96	44.38	+	17.19	41.92	+	8.98
LDL-C(e) (mg/dl)	99.64	+	35.80	93.06	+	31.88	101.48	+	33.93	107.65	+	30.19
Ccr[(c)](ml/min)	122.33	+	19.78	119.16	+	28.22	133.83	+	31.93	137.28	+	27.30
Insulin(mU/l) (a)	3.21	+	1.05	5.46	+	1.03	7.65	+	1.07	14.34	+	7.93
HOMA-IR(a)	0.60	+	0.20	1.08	+	0.14	1.58	+	0.16	3.18	+	1.78

[(a)] Significance found in comparison of quartile I to II, and quartile IV to I,II &III

[(b)] Significance found in comparison of quartile I to III & IV

[(c)] Significance found in comparison of quartile IV to I,II &III

[(d)] Significance found in comparison of quartile I to III and quartile IV to I,II &III

[(e)] No significance found between any of the groups

Table 3. Clinical and metabolic patient characteristics according to HOMA-IR quartiles. Analysis by analysis of variance: mean (± SD)

IR (r = 0.24). There was neither a significant correlation between CrC and white leukocytes count, nor with HDL-C.

When significant factors chosen by univariate analysis were entered in the multiple linear regression analysis, it showed that age, BMI, hemoglobin and HOMA-IR were significantly associated with CrC adjusted for Tanner stage, waist circumference, systolic, diastolic blood pressure, and triglycerides (r^2=0.52) (Table 4). In order to obtain an r^2 in each step, a stepwise method was used. The first step, which incorporated only age, explained 37% of the total variance. The second step, which included hemoglobin, produced an increase of 6% and the third step which included BMI, produced an increase of 3%. The fourth step, which included HOMA-IR, produced an increase of 6% of the variance, reaching 52%.

	Unstandardized Coefficients		T	Significance	R^2
	B	Std. Error			
Age	-5.84	1.06	-5.50	<0.001	0.52
BMI	-1.86	0.41	-4.49	<0.001	
Hb	-6.93	1.91	-3.64	<0.001	
HOMA-IR	6.40	1.47	4.36	<0.001	

Table 4. Multiple Regression Analysis (stepwise method)

Dependent variable: CrC. Adjusted for waist circumference, Tanner stage. systolic blood pressure, diastolic BP, triglycerides.

4. Discussion

The most important findings in this report were that age, insulin-resistance, BMI, and hemoglobin were associated with CrC in normal adolescents. These findings were supported by the results of the univariate correlations and the multiple regression analysis with the use of lipid profile, blood pressure, and waist circumference as independent factors. Adolescents with insulin-resistance had a higher CrC compared to adolescents without insulin-resistance of a similar age and pubertal development. We also found that mean CrC was significantly higher in adolescents in the lower hemoglobin quartile than in the other quartiles.

The rise in the prevalence of OW/OB in adolescents is one of the most alarming public health issues facing the world today. The 2003-2004 US National Health and Nutrition Examination Survey of adolescents aged 12 to 19 years found that 35% of children were OW/OB [25]. The prevalence of OW/OB in this cohort of Argentinean adolescents (45.1%) was higher than the high rate of OW/OB among adolescents in the United States. This could be due to the fact that OW/OB adolescents are especially encouraged to practice a sport. Furthermore, bigger adolescents are specially selected for certain positions on the rugby field due to their size. Therefore, the prevalence of OW/OB in this group of rugby amateurs could be overrepresented.

Clinical and pathologic characteristics of a distinct nephropathy have emerged independent of that of diabetic or hypertensive glomerulosclerosis including a silent presentation in OB individuals [26-28]. Tomaszewski et al. [29] was the first to demonstrate that OB could explain the relationship between hyperfiltration and BMI. However, as Cockcroft–Gault equation was used to estimate glomerular filtration rate, it introduced a major methodological problem since weight was included in the formula [29]. Consistent with this study, several papers showed that OB was associated with elevated glomerular filtration rate [30-,33]. In contrast several studies [34,35] noted that glomerular filtration rate in OB patients was lower. The mechanism could be due to increased fat in the renal helium that may compress renal vessels and parenchyma, decreasing renal blood flow and tubular flow rates [34,35]. Consistent with these studies this paper shows a significant inverse association between BMI and glomerular filtration rate in healthy adolescents. Therefore, increased renal blood flow and hyperfiltration may not be universal findings in OB individuals. The potential mechanisms involving OB and CrC are perhaps unknown [10].

A recent retrospective cohort study showed that BMI was an independent predictor of chronic kidney disease progression on multivariate analysis but no significant difference was observed between normal weight and OW/OB individuals [36]. Another methodological issue is the categorization of individuals as OW or OB. Consistent with this fact, though we found that mean CrC was higher in the normal weight than in OW/ OB adolescents the difference did not reach a significant level. However, we found a significant inverse association between BMI and glomerular filtration rate in the univariate and in the multivariate analysis.

Insulin resistance has been implicated as a predictor of renal function [11,37,38]. The National Health and Nutrition Examination Study (NHANES) III population [11] showed that after adjustment for multiple confounders, the odds ratios of prevalent kidney disease significantly increased from the lowest to the highest quartiles of HOMA-IR. Consistent with these studies we found that CrC increased as HOMA-IR quartiles increased. Our findings are also in accordance with previous community-based studies in adults [11, 38] which have investigated the association of insulin resistance and CrC. Impaired insulin sensitivity and hyperinsulinemia have been suggested to contribute to the development of renal injury via a number of different pathophysiologic pathways. Insulin per se stimulates the expression and activation of IGF-1, and components of the renin-angiotensin-aldosterone system [39]. These factors have been shown to promote mitogenic and fibrotic processes in the kidney, such as proliferation of mesangial cells and extracellular matrix expansion [39]. Moreover, insulin resistance and hyperinsulinemia are closely associated with oxidative stress [40], which could promote renal injury via decreased production and availability of nitric oxide [41]

Our study shows that hemoglobin was inversely associated with CrC. Different studies performed to investigate the risk factors of chronic kidney disease in communities showed that OB, and anemia, were positively correlated with the development of the disease [7,8]. This research found that adolescents in the lower quartile of hemoglobin had significantly higher mean CrC than adolescents in the other quartiles, even if none of the adolescents had anemia. Consistent with these previous studies we found in the regression analysis that there was a significant inverse association between CrC and hemoglobin, adjusted by several confounding factors.

Several limitations of this study should be acknowledged. First, it was a cross-sectional analysis, and thus, the directionality of the associations could not be established. However, appropriate analysis of cross-sectional data represent a useful initial step in identifying relationships between OB and CrC. Secondly, CrC was estimated with serum creatinine and not with the gold standard measure of renal function [21] Therefore, an incorrect conclusion may derive from our results. Thirdly, as the sample included only adolescent boys, girls were not represented. However, the strengths of our study included our amateur rugby club sample, which was more likely to represent the healthy population, the good response rate of the adolescents, the measurement of creatinine concentration for all participants by the same laboratory and method, and the use of regression models and simultaneous adjustments of confounding variables.

5. Conclusions

In summary, we have identified BMI, hemoglobin and insulin-resistance as strong and potentially modifiable risk factors for the development of chronic kidney disease in adolescents. Therefore, efforts to prevent and treat OB and insulin resistance in the general population could possibly have a beneficial impact on the incidence, progression and related co-morbidities and costs of chronic kidney disease. However, further longitudinal studies are needed in order to shed further light on this issue.

Acknowledgements

Claudia Molinari for her help in statistics. Claudio Aranda and Gustavo Maccallini for their help in lab analyses.

Author details

Valeria Hirschler*

Address all correspondence to: vhirschler@intramed.net

Hospital Durand, Maipu, Capital Federal, Argentina

References

[1] Flegal KM, Carroll MD, Ogden CL, Curtin LR.Prevalence and trends in obesity among US adults, 1999-2008. JAMA. 2010 Jan 20;303(3):235-41.

[2] Ogden CL, Carroll MD, Curtin LR, Lamb MM, Flegal KM. Prevalence of high body mass index in US children and adolescents, 2007-2008. JAMA. 2010 Jan 20;303(3): 242-9.

[3] Hirschler V, Oestreicher K, Maccallini G, Aranda C. Relationship between obesity and metabolic syndrome among Argentinean elementary school children. Clin Biochem. 2010 Mar;43(4-5):435-441.

[4] Iseki K, Ikemiya Y, Kinjo K, Inoue T, Iseki C, Takishita S: Body mass index and the risk of development of end-stage renal disease in a screened cohort. Kidney Int 2004: 65 :1870 –1876.

[5] Hsu CY, McCulloch CE, Iribarren C, et al. Body mass index and risk for end-stage renal disease. Ann Intern Med 2006: 144:21–28.

[6] Levey AS, Coresh J, Balk E, Kausz AT, LevinA, Steffes MW, Hogg RJ, Perrone RD, Lau J, Eknoyan G: National Kidney Foundation practice guidelines for chronic kidney disease: evaluation, classification, and stratification. Ann Intern Med 2003:139: 137-147.

[7] Chen N, Wang W, Huang Y, Shen P, Pei D, Yu H, Shi H, Zhang Q, Xu J, Lv Y, Fan Q. Community-based study on CKD subjects and the associated risk factors. Nephrol Dial Transplant. 2009;24(7):2117-23.

[8] Brown WW, Peters RM, Ohmit SE, Keane WF, Collins A, Chen SC, King K, Klag MJ, Molony DA, Flack JMEarly detection of kidney disease in community settings: the Kidney Early Evaluation Program (KEEP). Am J Kidney Dis. 2003;42(1):22-35.

[9] Kramer H, Luke A, Bidani A, Cao G, Cooper R, McGee D: Obesity and prevalent and incident CKD: the Hypertension Detection and Follow-Up Program. 2005 Am J Kidney Dis 46. 587-594.

[10] Hall JE, Henegar JR, Dwyer TM, Liu J, Da Silva AA, Kuo JJ, Tallam L: Is obesity a major cause of chronic kidney disease? Adv Ren Replace Ther 2004 11. 41-54.

[11] J, Muntner P, Hamm LL, Fonseca V, Batuman V, Whelton PK, He J: Insulin resistance and risk of chronic kidney disease in nondiabetic US adults. J Am Soc Nephrol 200314. 469-477.

[12] Singleton JR, Smith AG, Russell JW, Feldman EL: Microvascular complications of impaired glucose tolerance. Diabetes 2003 52. 2867-2873.

[13] Composición étnica de Argentina; http:// es.wikipedia.org/wiki/Composición_étnica_de_Argentina.

[14] Hirschler V, Roque M, Calcagno ML, Gonzalez C, Aranda C. Maternal waist circumference and the prediction of children's metabolic syndrome Arch Pediatr Adolesc Med. 2007: 161(12):1205-10.

[15] Kuczmarski R, Ogden C, Guo SS, Grummer-Strawn LM, Flegal KM, Mei Z, Wei R, Curtin LR, Roche AF, Johnson CL .: 2000 CDC growth charts for the United States: methods and development. Vital Health Stat 2002:11:1–190.

[16] Clinical Guidelines on the Identification, Evaluation and Treatment of Overweight and Obesity in Adults: The Evidence Report. NIH publication no. 98-4083. Bethesda, MD: National Institutes of Health; 1998.

[17] Zimmet P, Alberti KG, Kaufman F, Tajima N, Silink M, Arslanian S, Wong G, Bennett P, Shaw J, Caprio S; IDF Consensus Group. The metabolic syndrome in children and adolescents - an IDF consensus report. Pediatr Diabetes. 2007: 8 :299-306.

[18] National High Blood Pressure Education Working Group on High Blood Pressure in Children and Adolescents. The Fourth Report on the Diagnosis, evaluation and treatment on High Blood Pressure in Children and Adolescents. Pediatrics 2004:114: 555-76.

[19] Tanner JM: Growth at Adolescence: With a General Consideration of the Effects of Hereditary and Environmental Factors upon Growth and Maturation from Birth to maturity, 2nd ed. Oxford, UK: Blackwell Scientific, 1962

[20] Mc Auley K, Williams S, Mann J, Walker R,Lewis Barned N, Temple L Duncan A. Diagnosing Insulin Resistance in the General Population. Diabetes Care 2001:24:460-464.

[21] Levey AS,. Eckardt K.U and Tsukamoto Y. Levin A, Coresh J, Rossert J, De Zeeuw D, Hostetter TH,Lameire N, Eknoyan G, Definition and classification of chronic kidney disease: a position statement from kidney disease: Improving Global Outcomes (KDIGO), Kidney Int. 2005: 67: 2089–2100.

[22] Schwartz G.J, Haycock G.B, Edelmann C.M and Spitzer A., A simple estimate of glomerular filtration rate in children derived from body length and plasma creatinine, Pediatrics 1976: 58: 259–263.

[23] Rosenthal SH, Bökenkamp A, Hofmann W. How to estimate GFR-serum creatinine, serum cystatin C or equations? Clinical Biochemistry 40 (2007) 153–161.

[24] Cockcroft D.W. and Gault M.H., Prediction of creatinine clearance from serum creatinine, Nephron 1976:16: 31–41.

[25] Ogden CL, Carroll MD, Flegal KM High Body Mass Index for Age Among US Children and Adolescents, 2003-2006. JAMA. 2008: 299(20):2401-2405.

[26] Abitbol CL.; Rodrigez MM..Obesity-Related Nephropathy in Children Pediatr Health. 2009;3(2):141-153.

[27] Fox CS, Larson MG, Leip EP, et al. Predictors of new-onset kidney disease in a community-based population. JAMA 2004: 291:844–850.

[28] Wang Y, Chen X, Song Y, et al. Association between obesity and kidney disease: a systematic review and meta-analysis. Kidney Int 2008; 73:19–33.

[29] Tomaszewski M, Charchar FJ, Maric C et al Glomerular hyperfiltration: a new marker of metabolic risk. Kidney Int 2007 71:816–821.

[30] Chagnac A, Weinstein T, Korzets A, Ramadan E, Hirsch J, Gafter U: Glomerular hemodynamics in severe obesity. Am J Physiol 2000 278 :F817 –F822,

[31] Henegar JR, Bigler SA, Henegar LK, Tyagi SC, Hall JE: Functional and structural changes in the kidney in the early stages of obesity. J Am Soc Nephrol 2001 12 :1211 – 1217.

[32] Kambham N, Markowitz GS, Valeri AM, Lin J, D'Agati VD: Obesity-related glomerulopathy: An emerging epidemic. Kidney Int 2001 59:1498 –1509.

[33] Praga M, Hernandez E, Morales E, Campos AP, Valero MA, Martinez MA, Leon M: Clinical features and long-term outcome of obesity-associated focal segmental glomerulosclerosis. Nephrol Dial Transplant 2001 16:1790 –1798.

[34] Anastasio P, Spitali L, Frangiosa A, Molino D, Stellato D, Cirillo E, Pollastro RM, Capodicasa L, Sepe J, Federico P, Gaspare De Santo N: Glomerular filtration rate in severely overweight normotensive humans. Am J Kidney Dis 2000 35:1144 –1148.

[35] Hall JE: Mechanisms of abnormal renal sodium handling in obesity hypertension Am J Hypertens. 1997;10(5 Pt 2):49S-55S

[36] Othman M, Kawar B, El Nahas AM. Influence of obesity on progression of non-diabetic chronic kidney disease: a retrospective cohort study. Nephron Clin Pract. 2009; 113(1):c16-23.

[37] Chen J, Muntner P, Hamm LL, Jones DW, Batuman V, Fonseca V, Whelton PK, He J: The metabolic syndrome and chronic kidney disease in U.S. adults. Ann Intern Med 2004; 140. 167-174.

[38] Kubo M, Kiyohara Y, Kato I, Iwamoto H, Nakayama K, Hirakata H, Fujishima M: Effect of hyperinsulinemia on renal function in a general Japanese population: the Hisayama study. Kidney Int 1999; 55:2450–2456.

[39] Sarafidis PA, Ruilope LM: Insulin resistance, hyperinsulinemia, and renal injury: mechanisms and implications. Am J Nephrol 2006; 26:232–244.

[40] Riserus U, Basu S, Jovinge S, Fredrikson GN, Arnlov J, Vessby B: Supplementation with conjugated linoleic acid causes isomer-dependent oxidative stress and elevated C-reactive protein: a potential link to fatty acid-induced insulin resistance. Circulation 2002; 106:1925–1929.

[41] Prabhakar SS: Role of nitric oxide in diabetic nephropathy. Semin Nephrol 2004: 24:333–344.

Chapter 8

HDL, apo B/apo A1 ratio, Diabetes Mellitus and Cardiovascular Disease

Dhastagir Sultan Sheriff, Sachu P. and Elshaari F.A.

Additional information is available at the end of the chapter

http://dx.doi.org/10.5772/56476

1. Introduction

In India, diabetes is not an epidemic anymore but has turned into a pandemic. According to the International Journal of Diabetes in developing Countries India is labelled as the diabetic capital of the world. The International Diabetes Federation estimates that the number of diabetic patients in India more than doubled from 19 million in 1995 to 40.9 million in 2007. It is projected to increase to 69.9 million by 2025.Type II diabetes and its complications constitute a major worldwide public health problem. Patients with type II diabetes have 2 - 4 times higher risk of experiencing cardiovascular disease(CVD) than adults without diabetes (Fox et al. 2004; Laakso,2001) and their relative risk for CVD is about twice as high(Liu et al. 2005), much of which may be preventable with appropriate treatment of dyslipidemia.

The elevated CVD risk affecting patients with Type II diabetes may be attributed to a combined dyslipidemia characterized by elevated triglycerides, elevated triglyceride rich remnant lipoproteins(TGRLP), elevated apolipoprotein (apo) B and low levels of HDL cholesterol, with a predominance of small, dense low density lipoprotein(LDL) particles amid relatively normal LDL Cholesterol levels (Chih-yuan wang et al. 2004).

The association of low plasma levels of high-density lipoprotein (HDL) with states of impaired glucose metabolism and type 2 diabetes mellitus is well established, but the mechanistic links remain to be fully elucidated. Recent data suggests that HDL directly influences glucose metabolism through multiple mechanisms. (Drew et al., 2012).

The association of low plasma levels HDL with states of impaired glucose metabolism and type 2 diabetes mellitus is well established, but the mechanistic links remain to be fully elucidated. Recent data suggests that HDL directly influences glucose metabolism through multiple mechanisms. (Drew et al., 2009)

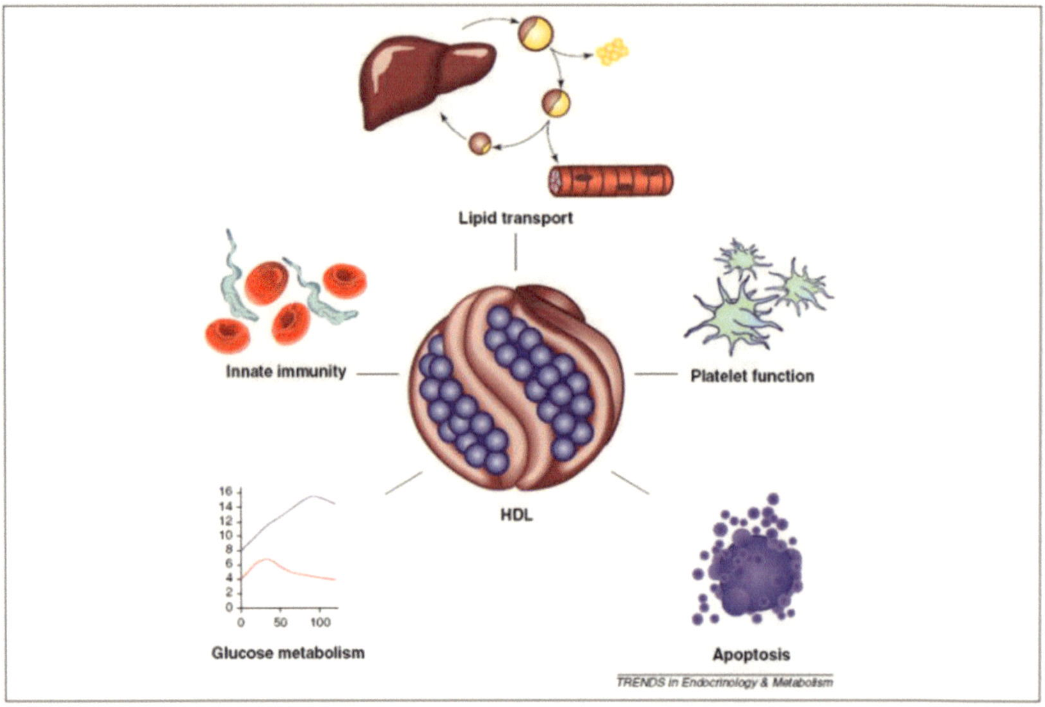

Figure 1. High density Lipoprotein- Main Functions

2. Materials and methods

Study was done on 109 subjects aged 40-75 years from HIGH-Tech Hospital, Cardiology Unit, Vinayaka Missions, Salem, India. Subjects were selected by simple random technique from the group of patients who were referred to the department of cardiology for coronary angiography and who met the inclusion criteria set out above. From all patients a written informed consent was obtained All data collected during a regular visit to the hospital included, anthropometric parameters including weight, height and waist circumference were measured using standard protocols Also a completed questionnaire regarding their medical history, coronary artery disease(CAD) and its complications, hypertension, age of onset of diabetes mellitus, chronic diseases other than CAD and diabetes mellitus, medications, socio-economic factors, dietary habits as well as the family medical history.

3. Grouping of patients

The patients were sub divided into two groups

1. Group I comprised of 52 coronary artery disease patients without type 2 diabetes(T2D) mellitus.(CAD WDM)

http://dx.doi.org/10.5772/56476

2. Group II comprised 57 coronary artery disease patients with type 2 diabetes mellitus(T2D).(CAD WNDM).
3. Control Subjects comprised of 71 age-matched healthy subjects.

PARAMETERS	CONTROL (N=71)	CAD WNDM(N=52)	CAD WDM (N=57)
Age(Years)	52.42 ±6.7	55.4 ± 5.657	52 ±9.5
BMI (kg/m2)	20.05±0.95	27.82 ± 3.359[a]	32.05 ± 0.33[a,b]
SBP (mmHg)	116.14±10.25	140.9 ± 16.97[a]	147.5 ± 28.28[a,b]
DBP (mmHg)	77.14±7.8	88.92± 14.14[a]	95.78 ± 21.21[a,b]

BMI: Body mass index,, SBP: Systolic blood pressure, DBP: diastolic blood pressure. Data are expressed as (mean ± S.D).All comparisons by t- test. Statistical analysis was done by Anova (post hoc test : Bonferroni.[a]: Statistically significant from control group at $p<0.05$; [b]:Statistically significant from CAD patients without type 2 DM at $p<0.05$..

Table 1. Demographic details of study subjects.

4. Coronary angiography and grading of CAD patients

The coronary angiogram was assessed by two cardiologists who were unaware of the current study. Selective coronary angiography was performed with Judkins technique in all patients. The severity of coronary atherosclerosis was estimated by calculating the coronary atherosclerotic score (CAS). Jenkins et al.,1978., based on the number of stenotic coronary artery segments, the degree of their lumen stenosis. The extend and severity of the CAD was assessed by assigning points to each lesion as follows: less than 50% stenosis of the luminal diameter 1;50-74% stenosis,2;75-100%, 3.The point for each lesion in coronary arteries including proximal,medial and distal segments were summed and a cumulative CAS obtained. The severity of CAD was further classified as one, two, three vessel disease according to the number of stenotic coronary artery in the three major vessels.Significant CAD was defined as more than 50% stenosis in at least one coronary artery segment.(Fievet. et al.,1991).(Table.2-given below)

GRADE I	<50% stenosis with single vessel disease .(mild)
GRADE II	50-74% stenosis with double vessel disease.(moderate)
GRADE III	75-100% stenosis with triple vessel disease.(severe).

Table 2. Add caption

Anthropometric measurements like Body Mass Index (BMI), Waist Circumference (WC) and Blood Pressure(BP) were done by standard procedures.

5. Measurement of Mean Arterial Pressure (MAP)

MAP = [(2 x diastolic) +systolic] / 3 Diastole counts twice as much as systole because 2/3 of the cardiac cycle is spent in diastole (Zheng et al 2008)

5.1. Biochemical estimations

Routine biochemical investigations were done using serum and plasma. Serum was used for the determination of insulin and blood glucose on the same day of sample collection. Remaining serum and plasma were stored at -20^0C for analyzing other parameters.

5.2. Determination of Homeostasis Model Assessment (HOMA) — IR

The Homeostasis Model Assessment (HOMA) estimates steady state beta cell function (%B) and insulin sensitivity (%S), as percentages of a normal reference population. (HOMA-IR) is used in clinical diabetes research to measure insulin sensitivity. The calculation helps correct for the effects of fasting hyperglycemia (high blood sugar). (Levy JC *et al.*,1998.)

HOMA IR = (FBS mmol/L)X(Fasting Insulin μU/ml.)/22.5

5.3. Biochemical studies

Serum samples taken were subjected to estimations of glucose, Glycated hemoglobin, insulin, lipid profile including apo A 1 and apo B. by standard automated methods

5.4. Result

Study was done on 109 subjects who were selected by simple random technique from the group of patients referred to the department of cardiology for coronary angiography and who met the inclusion criteria. Study subjects were 39% control subjects(n=71), 29% coronary artery disease patients without type 2 DM (CAD WNDM, n=52) and 32 % were coronary artery disease patients with type 2 DM (CAD WDM, n=57). Among the control subjects 65% were males and 35% were female. Among the CAD WNDM patients 88% were males and 12% were female and in CAD WDM 82% were male and 18% were female.The base line characteristics of study subjects are shown in Table 1. Age of the study subjects were from 40 to 75 years. The mean age of onset of CAD in the group with type 2 DM was 52 ± 4.5 when compared to 59± 6.4 in CAD WNDM. 79% of CAD WDM subjects and 48% of CAD WNDM subjects were of the age group 51-60 years. The mean duration of diabetes in CAD WDM was 6.2±2.5. Statistically no significant difference in SBP and DBP was observed in CAD WDM when compared to CAD WNDM. Significant difference in BMI was observed in the CAD WDM subjects when compared to CAD WNDM and control (with $p<0.001$).The mean BMI level was 32.05 ± 0.33 in CAD WDM, 27.82 ± 3.359 in CAD WNDM and 20.05±0.95 in the control group respectively.

The occurrence of CAD was computed in relation to age, BMI, and hypertension. (Table. 3.below)

Variables		CAD WNDM N(%)	CAD WDM N(%)	P value
Age (years)	40-50	15 (29 %)	1 (2%)	0.0001
	51-60	25 (48 %)	45(79%)	
	61-70	12 (23%)	11(19 %)	
BMI (kg/m^2)	18.5-24.9	1(2 %)	6(11 %)	0.0004
	25. - 30	28(54 %)	12(21 %)	
	>30	23(44 %)	39(68%)	
Smoking	Yes	13(25%)	9(16 %)	0.6807
	No	39(75 %)	48(84 %)	
Alcoholism	Yes	5(10 %)	11(19 %)	0.2445
	No	47(90 %)	46(81 %)	
SBP	<140mmofHg	2(4 %)	4 (7 %)	0.6807
	>140m of Hg	50(96 %)	53 (93 %)	

BMI: Body mass index, SBP: Systolic blood pressure Statistical analysis was done by Chi square test. Statistically significant from CAD patients without type 2 DM at $p<0.001$.

Table 3. Relation of Coronary Artery Disease (CAD) to different variables.

Among the study subjects 2% of CAD WNDM had BMI in the range of 18.5-24.9 kg/m^2 compared to 11% in CAD WDM. 54% of CAD WNDM had BMI in the range of 25-30 kg/m^2,when compared to 21% in CAD WDM. Also 44% of CAD WNDM had BMI value >30 kg/m^{2}when compared to 68% in CAD WDM.

CADsubjects		Severity of CAD	
Grade I	Grade II	Grade III	
CAD WNDM	24(46%)	15(29%)	13(25%)
CAD WDM	9(16%)	12(21%)	36(63%)

CAD WDM: coronary artery disease with diabetes. CAD WNDM coronary artery disease without diabetes.. Statistical analysis was done by Chi square test.

Table 4. Severity of CAD among the study subjects.

According to the percentage of stenosis and involvement of coronary vessels, severity of CAD was assessed and classified as Grade I(mild), Grade II(Moderate) and Grade III(Severe). Analysis on frequency of distribution has revealed that severity was significantly high in CAD WDM. (Table : 4) The percentage of patients with severe coronary artery disease-Grade III was 63% in CAD WDM Vs 25 % in CAD WN DM($p<0.001$). 21% of CAD WDM patients had Grade

II (moderate) compared to 29% in CAD WNDM.16% of CAD WDM had Grade I (mild) disease compared to 46% in CAD WNDM. A significantly high percentage of multivessel atherosclerosis was observed in CAD WDM when compared to CAD WNDM.

PARAMETERS	CONTROL(N=71)	CAD WNDM (N=52)	CAD WDM (N=57)
FBS (mg/dL)	85.04±6.20	85.65 ± 5.66	147.05 ± 30.40[a,b]
PPBS (mg/dL)	101.81±5.10	109.4± 7.07	403.00 ± 53.70[a,b]
Insulin (µIU/ml)	8.41±0.33	8.76 ± 5.37	22.93 ± 3.25[a,b]
HOMA - IR	1.77±0.33	1.80± 0.45	9.70 ± 1.10[a,b]

Table 5. Serum Fasting Blood glucose, Insulin and HOMA-IR of study subjects

Data are expressed as (mean ± S.D). Statistical analysis was done by Anova (post hoc test : Bonferroni) [a]: Statistically significant from control group at $p<0.05$; [b]:Statistically significant from CAD patients without type 2 DM ($p<0.05$.).

The mean fasting blood glucose of the normal controls, CAD WNDM and CAD WDM subjects were 85.04±6.2, 85.65 ± 5.657 and 147.05 ± 30.4 respectively. There was significant ($p < 0.05$) increase in mean Fasting blood glucose in CAD WDM when compared to CAD WNDM and control. The mean Post prandial blood glucose of the normal controls, CAD WNDM and CAD WDM were 101.81±5.1, 109.4± 7.071and 403 ± 53.7 respectively. The mean Post Prandial blood glucose in CAD WDM was significantly high ($p<0.05$) when compared to CAD WNDM and control. The mean insulin level among the three groups were 8.41±0.334, 8.76 ± 5.37 and 22.93 ± 3.25 respectively. The CAD WDM patients had significantly high insulin level ($p<0.05$) when compared to CAD WNDM and control. The mean HOMA IR of controls, CAD WNDM and CAD WDM were 1.77±0.33, 1.8± 0.445 and 9.7 ± 1.1 respectively. The CAD WDM patients had significantly high IR level ($p<0.05$) when compared to CAD WNDM and control.(Table.5.)

One of the basic factor which was found to be significantly elevated in CAD WDM group when compared to other two groups was Insulin resistance – which is the underlying defect in >90% of patients with type 2 diabetes mellitus.

IR		SEVERITY OF CAD	
Grade I	Grade II	Grade III	
<1.6	30(58%)	18(35%)	4(8%)
>1.6	9(16%)	12(21%)	36(69%)

Table 6. IR and Severity of CAD among the CAD subjects

The median value 1.6 was considered as Cut off values in our study.IR: Insulin resistance. Statistical analysis was done by Analysis was done by Chi square test. (Gary *et al.*, 1997)

http://dx.doi.org/10.5772/56476

Analysis on frequency of distribution has revealed that severity was significantly high in CAD subjects with IR >1.6. (Table 6) The percentage of patients with IR >1.6 and Grade III-coronary artery disease - was 69%, Grade II coronary artery disease - was 21% and Grade I -coronary artery disease- was 16% respectively. The percentage of subjects with IR <1.6 and Grade III - severity- was 8%, Grade II coronary artery disease - was 35% and Grade I -coronary artery disease- was 30% respectively.

6. Body Mass Index (BMI)

Body mass index (BMI) is a simple index of weight-for-height that is commonly used to classify overweight and obesity in adults. The WHO defines a BMI greater than or equal to 25 is overweight and a BMI greater than or equal to 30 is obesity(World Health Organization,2007).

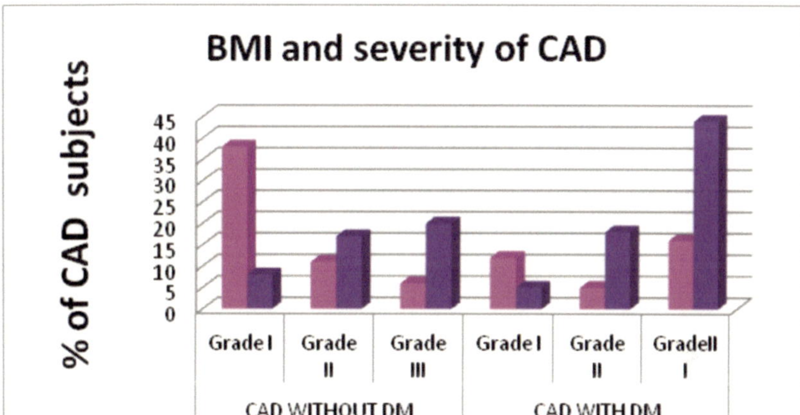

	CAD WITHOUT DM			CAD WITH DM		
	Grade I	Grade II	Grade III	Grade I	Grade II	GradeII I
<30 kg/m2	38	11	6	12	5	16
>30 kg/m2	8	17	20	5	18	44

BMI: Body mass index. The subjects were graded into I,II,III based on severity Statistical analysis was done by Chi square test.

Table 7. BMI and severity of CAD among CAD subjects.

Analysis on frequency of distribution has revealed that severity was significantly high in CAD subjects with BMI >30kg/m^2.The percentage of CAD WDM patients with BMI>30 kg/m^2 and Grade III-coronary artery disease - was 44%, Grade II coronary artery disease - was 18% and Grade I -coronary artery disease- was 5% respectively. The percentage of CAD WDM subjects with BMI<30 kg/m^2 and Grade III -severity- was 16%, Grade II coronary artery disease - was 5% and Grade I -coronary artery disease- was 12% respectively.(Table.7.)

The percentage of CAD WNDM patients with BMI>30 kg/m^2 and Grade III-coronary artery disease - was 20%, Grade II coronary artery disease - was 17% and Grade I -coronary artery disease- was 8% respectively. The percentage of CAD WDM subjects with BMI<30 kg/m^2 and Grade III -severity- was 6%, Grade II coronary artery disease - was 11% and Grade I -coronary artery disease- was 38% respectively.

7. Lipid parameters

7.1. Total cholesterol, triglycerides, HDL-C, LDL-C and VLDL

CAD WDM subjects were 169±3.0, 182.2 ± 8.485 and 197.49 ± 7.77 respectively. The level of total cholesterol was significantly high in CAD WDM and CAD WNDM) when compared to control. But no difference was observed between the CAD WDM and CAD WNDM. The triglyceride level was I21.35±11.28, 131.6 ± 6.4 and 157.5 ± 8.5 in normal controls, CAD WNDM and CAD WDM subjects respectively.The triglyceride level in CAD WDM was significantly high ($p<0.05$) when compared to CAD WNDM. The mean HDL cholesterol level of the normal controls, CAD WNDM and CAD WDM subjects were 41.48±5.59, 38.4 ± 2.07 and 35.05 ±1.44 respectively.Also the HDL level in CAD WDM was found to be low when compared to normal controls but was not significant in CAD WDM Vs CAD WNDM. The LDL-cholesterol level was 104.48±33.5, 129.50 ± 8.8 and 144.25 ± 8.2 respectively in normal controls, CAD WNDM and CAD WDM subjects. LDL level was significantly($p<0.05$) high in CAD WDM when compared to CAD WNDM and control subjects. The mean VLDL level of the normal controls, CAD WNDM and CAD WDM subjects were 24.27±2.26, 26.3±13.01 and 31.5 ± 9.617 respectively.(Table.8.)

PARAMETERS	CONTROL(N=71)	CAD WDM(N= 52)	CAD WNDM(N=57)
Total cholesterol (mg/dL)	169.00±8.00	182.20 ± 8.49^{a}	197.49 ± 7.77^{a,}
Serum Triglycerides (mg/dL)	I21.35±11.28	131.60 ± 6.40	157.50 ± 8.50^{a,b}
HDL cholesterol (mg/dL)	41.48±5.59	38.40 ± 2.07^{a}	35.05 ± 1.44^{a,b}
LDL cholesterol (mg/dL)	104.48±33.50	129.50 ± 8.80^{a}	144.25 ± 8.20^{a,b}
VLDL (mg/dL)	24.27±2.26	26.3± 13.01	31.5 ± 9.62^{a}
ApoA1(g/L)	1.39±0.31	1.187 ± 0.21	0.873 ± 0.07^{a,b}
ApoB (g/L)	0.79±0.12	1.64±0.62^{a}	1.66±1.10^{a,b}
ApoB/A1 ratio	0.59±0.17	2.04±0.84	2.069±1.23^{a}

Table 8. Lipid profile and Apolipoproteins of study subjects.

Data are expressed as (mean ± S.D). Statistical analysis was done by Anova analysis (post hoc test : Bonferroni).a: Statistically significant from Control group at $p<0.05$; b: Statistically significant from CAD WNDM at $p<0.05$. HDL-high density lipoprotein; LDL-low density lipoprotein; VLDL-very low density lipoprotein

http://dx.doi.org/10.5772/56476

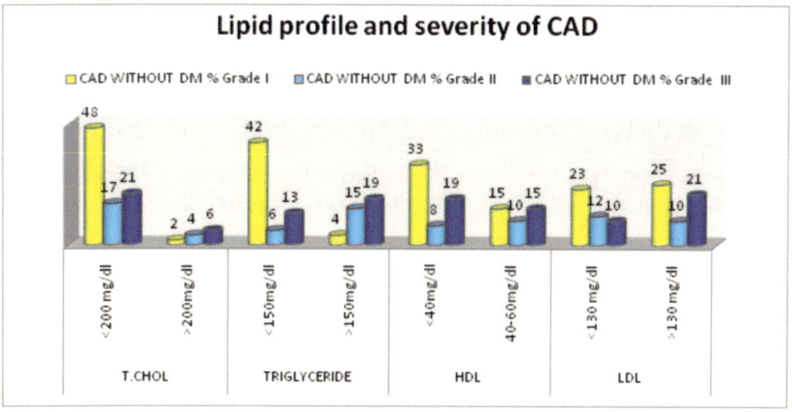

Statistical Analysis was done by Chi Square Test

Figure 2. Lipid profile and severity of CAD in non diabetic subjects.

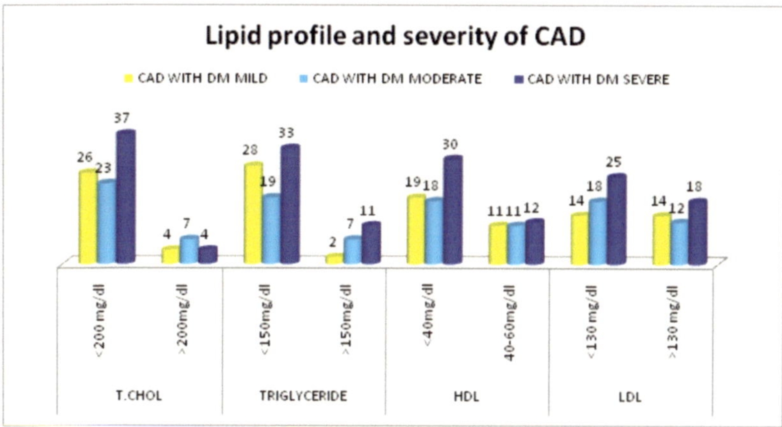

Figure 3. Lipid profile and severity of CAD in Diabetic subjects.

The CAD patients without diabetes and with total cholesterol level <200 mg/dl were 21% with grade III stenosis, 18% with grade II and 48% with grade I stenosis. The CAD subjects without diabetes and Total cholesterol level >200 mg/dl had 6% with grade III stenosis, 4% with grade II and 2% with grade I stenosis. Among the CAD without diabetes subjects with total triglyceride level <150 mg/dl 13% subjects had grade III stenosis, 6% had grade II and 42% had grade I stenosis. Compared to 19% subjects with grade III stenosis, 15% with grade II and 4% with grade I stenosis and triglyceride level >150 mg/dl. The CAD subjects without diabetes and HDL level <40 mg/dl had 19% with grade III stenosis, 8% with grade II and 33% with grade I stenosis. The CAD subjects without diabetes and HDL >40 mg/dl had 15% with grade III stenosis, 10% with grade II and 15% with grade I stenosis. Among the CAD without diabetes subjects with LDL level <130 mg/dl 10% subjects had grade III stenosis, 12% had grade II and 23% had grade I stenosis,compared to 21% subjects with grade III stenosis, 10% with grade II and 23% with grade I stenosis with LDL level >130 mg/dl.

Among the CAD with diabetes subjects with total cholesterol level <200 mg/dl 37% subjects had grade III stenosis, 7% had grade II and 4% had grade I stenosis. Among the CAD subjects with >200 mg/dl cholesterol level,4% of subjects had Grade III,7% had grade II and 4% had grade I stenosis.Among CAD with diabetes and triglyceride level <150 mg/dl 33% had grade III stenosis, 19% had grade II and 28% had grade I stenosis. Among CAD subjects with triglyceride level >150 mg/dl were found to have 11% of subjects with grade III,7% with grade II and 2% with grade I stenosis. Among the CAD with diabetes subjects with total HDL level <40 mg/dl 30% subjects had grade III stenosis, 18% had grade II and 19% had grade I stenosis. Among the CAD subjects with 40-60 mg/dl HDL level 12% of subjects had Grade III,11% had grade II and 11% had grade I stenosis.

The CAD subjects with diabetes and LDL level <130 mg/dl had 25% with grade III stenosis, 18% with grade II and 14% with grade I stenosis. The CAD subjects with diabetes and LDL level >130 mg/dl had 18% with grade III stenosis, 12% with grade II and 14% with grade I stenosis.

Lipid parameters	**IR IN CAD WITH DM**	
r value	**p value**	
T.Cholesterol (mg/dl)	-0.211	0.115
Triglyceride (mg/dl)	0.343	0.009**
HDL-C (mg/dl)	0.026	0.847
LDL-C (mg/dl)	-0.109	0.12
VLDL (mg/dl)	-0.357	0.006**

** significant at p<0.01 and * denoted significant at p<0.001. statistical analysis was done by Pearson correlation.

Table 9. Correlation analysis of Lipid profile with Insulin Resistance

Table.9.depicts the results of the Pearson correlation analysis between different variables in CAD patients. In CAD with type 2 diabetes population triglyceride showed significant association with IR (r=..343, p<0.01) and VLDL showed significant correlation with IR.(r=. 357,p<0.01).

In CAD WDM subjects 77% had HDL-C level less than 40 mg/dl when compared to 56% in CAD WNDM. In CAD WDM 23% had HDL-C level >40mg/dl when compared to 44% in CAD WNDM.The HDL-C level was found to be not significant between the CAD WDM and CAD WNDM.

http://dx.doi.org/10.5772/56476

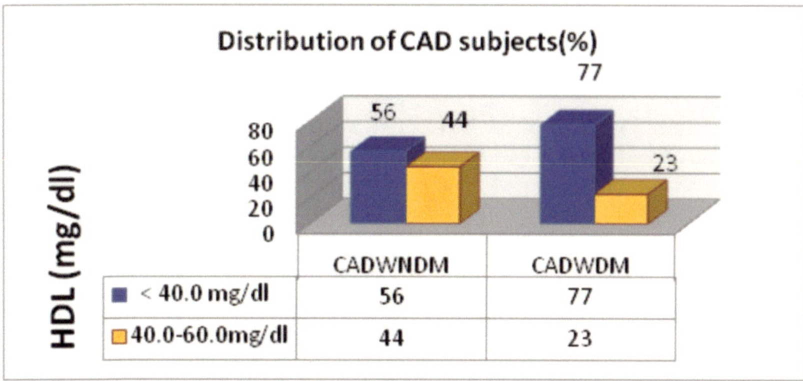

CADWDN: Coronary artery disease patients with DM and CAD WNDM : Coronary artery disease patients without type 2 diabetes.. Statistical analysis was done by Anova(post hoc test : Bonferroni).

Table 10. HDL C level in CAD subjects

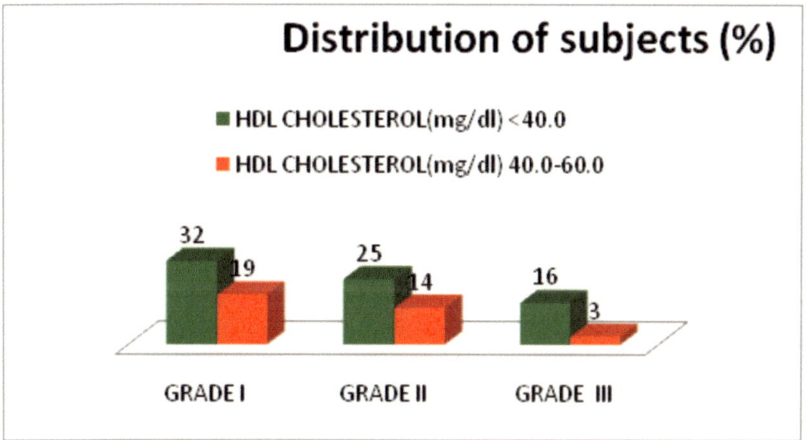

Figure 4. HDL –C among the CAD subjects based on severity of CAD.

The CAD subjects were graded into I,II,III based on severity. Statistical analysis was done by Chi square test.

The distribution of subjects based on HDL cholesterol level <40 mg/dl had shown that 32% had Grade I stenosis,25% had Grade II stenosis and 16% had Grade III stenosis.. Among the CAD subjects with HDL level 40-60 mg/dl 19% had grade I stenosis,14% had Grade II stenosis and 3% had Grade III stenosis.(Fig.4)

The mean ApoA1 level was 1.39±0.31, 1.187 ± 0.205 and 0.873 ± 0.007 in normal controls, CAD WNDM and CAD WDM subjects.ApoA1was found to be significant with p<0.05 in CAD WDM

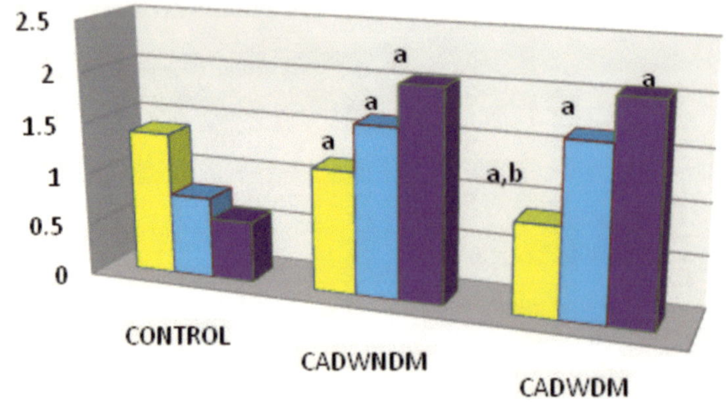

	CONTROL	CADWNDM	CADWDM
ApoA1(g/L)	1.39	1.187	0.873
ApoB (g/L)	0.79	1.64	1.66

Figure 5. ApoA1,ApoB,and ApoB/A ratio in study subjects

compared to normal control. ApoB level was 0.79±0.12, 1.64± 0.621and for 1.66 ± 1.10 respectively in normal controls,

CAD WNDM and CAD WDM subjects. ApoB/A1 ratio in normal subjects in CAD WNDM and in CAD WDM was 0.59±0.173, 2.04 ± 0.84712 and 2.06 ± 0.84712 respectively. ApoB/A ratio was found to be significant at $p<0.05$ in CAD with diabetic subjects when compared to CAD with no diabetes and normal controls. (Fig.5)

Data are expressed as (mean ± S.D). a: significantly different from control group at $p<0.05$; b: significantly different from CAD patients without DM at $p<0.05$.. Statistical analysis was done by Anova analysis (post hoc test : Bonferroni)

Cut off values: ApoB/A1 ratio above 1.0 was considered to be at risk. (Benton *et al.,* 2005). Statistical analysis was done by chi square test.

In CAD WNDM 8% had grade I CAD and ApoB/A ratio less than 1.0 g/L when compared to 4% with grade I CAD in CAD WDM,4% of CAD WNDM had grade II CAD and ApoB/A ratio less than 1.0 g/L when compared to an equal 4% in CAD WDM. 4%of subjects had CAD WNDM and grade III when compared to5% in CAD WDM and grade III severity with an ApoB/A1 ratio < 1.0. In CAD WNDM 48%had ApoB/A ratio >1.0 and grade I CAD when compared to 14%in CAD WDM.15% of CAD WNDM had ApoB/A ratio >1.0and grade II CAD when compared to 28% in CAD WDM.21% of CAD WNDM subjects had ApoB/A ratio >1.0 and grade III CAD when compared to 49%in CAD WDM. (Fig.6)

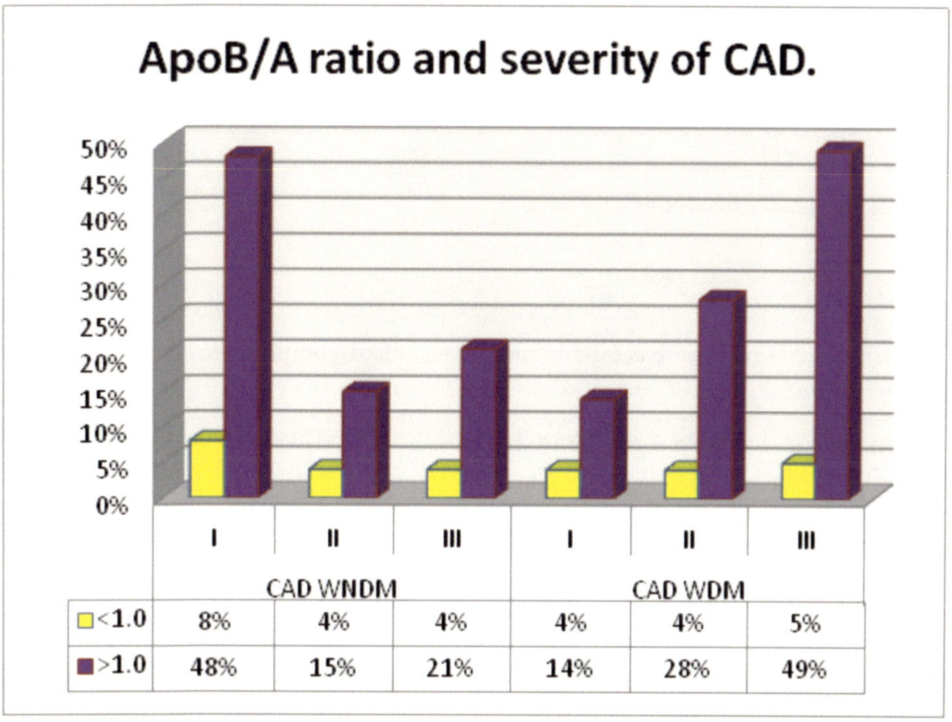

Figure 6. ApoB/Apo A1 ratio and Severity of CAD.

Apolipoproteins	IR IN CAD WDM	
	r value	p value
ApoA1**(g/L)**	.098	-.073
ApoB **(g/L)**	.467	.591
ApoB/A1 ratio	**-.413**	**.001****
Statistical Analysis was done by Pearson correlation		

Table 11. Correlation studies of Apoproteins with Insulin resistance in CAD subjects

Table 11 depicts the results of the Pearson correlation analysis between different variables in CAD patients.. In CAD with type 2 diabetes population,ApoB/A1 ratio showed negative correlation with IR (r,-..413, p,0.001).

Statistical analysis was done by Anova analysis (post hoc test : Bonferroni)

The level of Apo A1 was found to be significantly low ($p < 0.001$) in CAD WDM compared to CAD WNDM.18% of CAD WDM patients had ApoA1 level >1g/L compared to 38% in CAD

CAD subjects	**Apo A1(g/L)**	
<1.0	>1.0	
CAD WN DM	**32(62%)**	**20(38%)**
CAD W DM	**47(82%)**	**10(18%)**
ApoA1 level of 1.0 g/L. was considered as cut off value		

Table 12. Level of ApoA1 in CAD patients

WNDM. 82%of CAD WDM subjects had ApoA1 level <1g/L compared to 62 % in CAD WNDM. (Table.11)

Correlation analysis between ApoA1 and lipid profile in CAD WDM had shown a significant positive association with HDL-C (r,.755, p=.000).ApoA1 also showed significant positive association with HDL-C (r,.415, p=.002) in CAD WNDM.(Table.12)

7.2. Discussion

Age has not been considered to be a modifiable risk factor but, it out-ranks all other factors like lipids, blood pressure, and smoking—as a predictor of clinical events(Lloyd-Jones *et al.*, 2004). Conventional analyses do not distinguish between the biological changes of ageing within arteries—the non-modifiable effects of disintegration of tissues over time—and those produced by exposure over time to risk factors such as atherogenic dyslipoproteinaemia. (Lloyd-Jones *et al.*, 2004). The incidence of CAD was high among the patients of the age group 51-60 (77%) in CAD with type 2 DM patients when compared to CAD without DM (46%).

Smoking has been considered as a predictor of the transition from normoglycaemia to impaired fasting glucose and was found to increase the risk of type 2 diabetes, independent from possible confounders. Smoking and diabetes are two important hazards to the health of many individuals and contribute substantially to the global burden of disease in various ways. Smoking can not only aggravate the diabetes complications such as macro- or microvascular disease, but has also been shown to deteriorate glucose metabolism in normal subjects and thereby may provoke the onset of type 2 diabetes (Robert, Fagard, Nilsson, 2009)

Pathophysiological mechanisms by which smoking causes glucose intolerance and worsens clinical outcomes in established diabetes include greater insulin resistance, impaired beta-cell function and insulin secretion, chronic low grade inflammation, endothelial dysfunction, as well as interacting indirectly with other factors known to aggravate diabetes and lifestyle factors. (Robert *et al.*, 2009) Table 1. had shown that there was no significant difference between two groups with respect to smoking, alcoholism and SBP.

According to the percentage of stenosis and involvement of coronary vessels, severity of CAD was assessed and classified as Grade I(mild), Grade II(Moderate) and Grade III(Severe). Analysis on frequency of distribution has revealed that severity was significantly high in CAD WDM. (Table : 4) The percentage of patients with severe coronary artery disease-Grade III was

63% in CAD WDM Vs 25 % in CAD WN DM(p<0.001). 21% of CAD WDM patients had Grade II (moderate) compared to 29% in CAD WNDM.16% of CAD WDM had Grade I (mild) disease compared to 46% in CAD WNDM. A significantly high percentage of multivessel atherosclerosis was observed in CAD WDM when compared to CAD WNDM. These findings showed a delayed recognition of CAD in type 2 DM. The typical symptoms of cardiac ischemia are often masked in diabetic patients. Hence the pathological events are not identified at the preliminary stages (Hanif *et al.*, 2009). This might be the reason for the observed high frequency of grade III severity in CAD WDM and high percentage of CAD related mortality in diabetic patients as observed in various epidemiological studies. (Goraya *et al.*, 2002)

8. Insulin resistance

Insulin resistance has been defined as a condition of low insulin sensitivity, in which the ability of insulin to lower circulating glucose levels is impaired (DeFronzo 2009). The gold standard for assessing insulin resistance and insulin sensitivity is the hyperinsulinemic euglycemic clamp technique; however, this test was found to be too labor intensive, time consuming, and costly for routine clinical practice. The Homeostasis Model Assessment (HOMA) may be used alternatively as it is minimally invasive, easy to apply in a standard office setting and provide reasonable indices of insulin action in pre diabetes and diseases of recent onset(Matthews *et al.*, 1985; Katz A *et al.*, 2000). The biochemical defects that provoke insulin resistance involve impaired insulin signaling as well as reductions in glucose transport within insulin-sensitive tissues. (Lewis *et al.*, 2002).So subjects with insulin resistance require more insulin to promote glucose uptake by peripheral tissues, and genetically predisposed individuals may lack the necessary beta-cell secretory capacity. Insulin resistance mainly influence the metabolism related to Liver, Muscle and fat cells. Thus resulting relative insulin insufficiency disrupts the regulation of glucose production in the liver, glucose uptake in muscle, and the release of fatty acid from adipose tissue, the outcome being postprandial, and later fasting hyperglycemia. (Hajer GR *et al.*, 2007)

Analysis on frequency of distribution has revealed that severity was significantly high in CAD subjects with IR >1.6. (Table 6)The percentage of patients with IR >1.6 and Grade III-coronary artery disease - was 69%, Grade II coronary artery disease - was 21% and Grade I -coronary artery disease- was 16% respectively. The percentage of subjects with IR <1.6 and Grade III - severity- was 8%, Grade II coronary artery disease - was 35% and Grade I -coronary artery disease- was 30% respectively. Our results have shown that severity was significantly high in patients with an elevated IR level.(p<0.0001) and coincide with the findings of Bodlaj. (Bodlaj et al. 2006).

Insulin resistance not only contributes to the pathogenesis of type 2 diabetes but also linked to cardiovascular risk factors and premature cardiovascular disease. It has been reported that insulin resistance predisposes individuals to the development of obesity and dyslipidemia which are considered as the traditional risk factors.

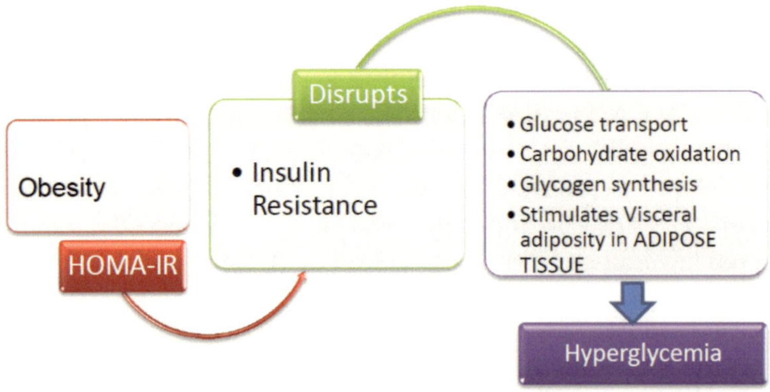

Figure 7. Obesity and IR related to hyperglycemia

As insulin stimulates the production of NO which has both antiatherogenic and anti inflammatory effects, IR is considered as an endothelial dysfunction risk equivalent (Zeng G *et al.*, 2000;. Kuboki K *et al.*, 2000) IR results in the down regulation of the antiatherogenic phosphatidylinositol-3-kinase–mediated insulin receptor signaling pathway, and maintained activity of the proatherogenic mitogenic activated protein kinase pathway(Bansilal S *et al.*, 2007). It also results in a state of low-grade, chronic, systemic inflammation, which in turn links the metabolic and the vascular pathologies (Romano *et al.*, 2003; Hsueh and Law,2003; Haffner SM.,2003) All these might have lead to accelerated atherosclerosis and increased severity of CAD in patients with type 2 DM.

9. Body Mass Index (BMI)

Body mass index (BMI) is a simple index of weight-for-height that is commonly used to classify overweight and obesity in adults. The WHO defines a BMI greater than or equal to 25 is overweight and a BMI greater than or equal to 30 is obesity(World Health Organization, 2007).BMI provides the most useful population-level measure of overweight and obesity as it is the same for both sexes and for all ages of adults. Raised BMI is a major risk factor for non-communicable diseases such as CAD (Niraj et al.2007) In our study significantly high level of BMI was observed in the CAD WDM subjects when compared to CAD WNDM and control (with $p<0.001$).The mean BMI level was 32.05 ± 0.33 in CAD WDM, 27.82 ± 3.359 in CAD WNDM and 20.05±0.95 in the control group respectively (Table.7.). Abbasi *et al* had shown similar results in their studies. (Abbasi *et al.*, 2002).

This increase in BMI might be due to the Insulin resistance, the major causative factor for type 2 DM. (Goossens, 2008) IR greatly reduces the sensitivity of cell walls to insulin. So the vital process whereby glucose passes through the cell wall via insulin to be converted into energy gets greatly impaired.

As a result, excess glucose remains in the blood stream, causing elevated levels of blood sugar, which are sent to the liver. (Niraj et al/ 2007) Once it reaches there, the sugar gets converted into fat and carried via the blood stream throughout the body. This process can lead to weight gain and obesity.

Evidences have revealed that normal function of Adipose issue is disturbed during obesity and adipose tissue dysfunction plays a prominent role in the development and/or progression of insulin resistance (Goossens.,2008). Boden and Chen et al had identified that Insulin-resistant fat cells of obesity can confer insulin resistance to muscle through the excessive release of free fatty acids into the general circulation and/or through the accumulation of intra myocellular triglyceride (Boden, 1997 and Chen *et al.*, 1988). Since obesity has been recognized as a significant contributor to hypertension, dyslipidemia and Insulin resistance, it has been recognized as a major modifiable risk factor for cardiovascular disease (Sharma,2003). This might be the reason for the observed significantly high percentage of incidence of CAD and severity in CAD patients with BMI >30 kg/m^2.

The athero-thrombotic process that underlies CVD implies a central role for cholesterol metabolism. The average concentration of blood cholesterol within a population has been found to be an important determinant of the risk of CHD in the population (Corti Salive *et al.*, 1997). Girard, had found that high cholesterol levels augments the risk of several diseases, most notably cardiovascular diseases(Girard-Mauduit,2010). In the present study cholesterol level was found to be significantly high in CAD patients when compared to control subjects. As its concentration increases, Cholesterol-rich apoproteins B containing lipoproteins may infiltrate the subendothelial space and initiate an inflammatory process that leads to atherosclerotic lesions. This progresses to fibrous plaques, with necrotic scores. (Paik.and Blair.,1995). Abnormal concentration of cholesterol also increase platelet aggregation, which exacerbates the severity of athero-thrombotic process. Hence cholesterol metabolism occupies a central role in the pathophysiology of CVD and found to be high in CAD patients (Enas,yousuf, Mehta, 1992).

In the present study total cholesterol level in CAD patients does not show any significant change with severity of CAD which underlines the fact that blood cholesterol alone may be a relatively poor predictor for CHD. (Table 9) This might be due to the fact that the other major risk factors might have exerted a component of their adverse effects via their effects on the above mentioned aspects of cholesterol metabolism. (David.,2001)

In the study, plasma triglyceride and VLDL were found to be significantly high in CAD WDM when compared to control and CAD WNDM.(Table 9) Hypertriglyceridemia has been found to be one of the most consistent finding in type 2 diabetes patients (Saxena et al., 2005).

Evidence from both animal and human studies implied that insulin resistance which causes increased synthesis and/or decreased clearance of VLDL – has been an important underlying cause of hypertriglyceridemia in subjects with type 2DM (Hopkinns et al.2009).

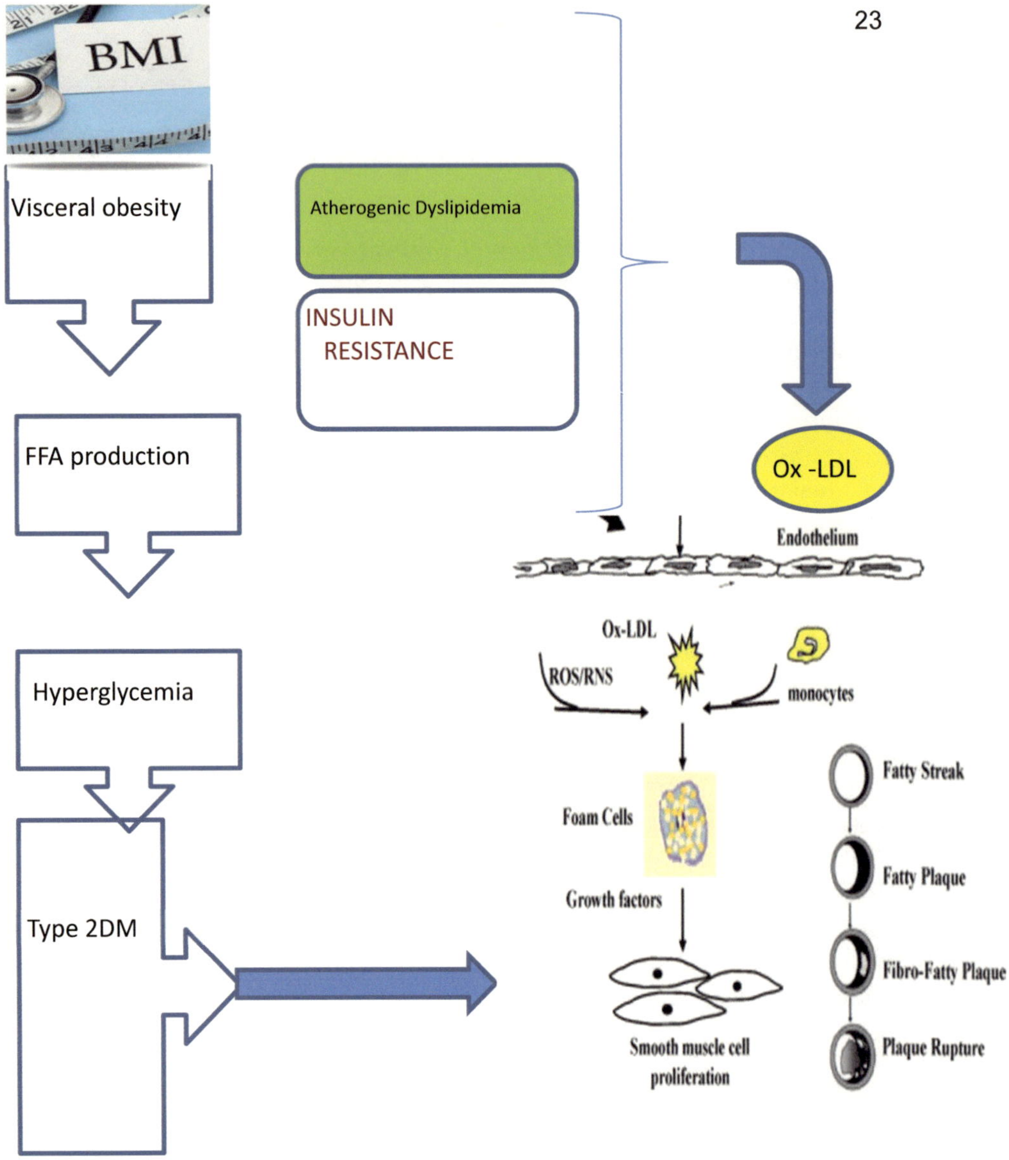

Figure 8. Possible Link Between Body Mass Index (BMI),Type 2 Diabetes Mellitus T2DM) And Coronary Artery Disease(CAD).FFA-Free fatty acid

Insulin an anabolic hormone was found to play a central role in the lipid synthesis and inhibition of lipolysis. Insulin inhibit VLDL production from the liver indirectly by decreasing FFA flux from adipose tissue to the liver and directly by its inhibitory effect on the rate of ApoB 100 synthesis and degradation in hepatocytes It has also been identified that Insulin can inhibit the assembly and secretion of VLDL by increasing posttranslational degradation of ApoB and reducing the expression of MTP (microsomal triglyceride transfer protein) in the liver(Meshkani and Adeli 2009).

One of the major abnormalities in insulin resistance was found to be hepatic overproduction of VLDL(Meyer *et al.,* 1996). It influences hepatic VLDL production by increasing the free fatty acid flux to liver and by affecting the rate of ApoB synthesis. It also reduces VLDL and intermediate density lipoprotein(IDL) catabolism by reducing the activity of lipoprotein lipase and decrease the hepatic uptake of VLDL and IDL. (Miller M;1999) These could have been the reason behind the significantly high level of TG and VLDL in CAD with diabetes subjects. (Figure 2 and 3)

Triglyceride was widely accepted as a CAD risk factor synergistic with other lipid risk factors. Helsinki Heart Study and 6-year follow-up of the observational Prospective Cardiovascular Muenster (PROCAM) study, revealed the importance of triglyceride as major risk factor. (Antonio Jr, 1998) Gianturco *et al.,* had shown that macrophages may take up triglyceride-rich lipoproteins by a mechanism that was independent of the ApoB/E receptor, there by facilitating the formation of atherogenic foam cells. (Gianturco *et al.,* 1994) Hypertriglyceridemia was found to have some adverse effect on endothelial dysfunction and activation on coagulation.These involvement of hyper triglyceridemia in atherogenesis at various level could have resulted in positive correlation of TG level with severity of CAD. (Table 9).

10. Low density lipoprotein — C

The concentration of serum LDL was found to be directly related to the development of atherosclerosis. One current theory which relates the role of LDL in the institution of atherosclerosis propose that oxidized LDL plays a major role in the development of foam cell-laden fatty streaks in the arterial wall. Elevated low-density lipoprotein cholesterol (LDL-C) has been a well-established independent risk factor for coronary artery disease (CAD). A number of primary and secondary trials have demonstrated that lowering of LDL-C decreases the incidence of CAD.

The present study has shown that LDL level was significantly elevated in CAD with diabetes subjects when compared to the CAD without diabetic group and normal controls. Reports have revealed that T2D patients show decreased hepatic uptake of VLDL, IDL and LDL that lead to increased plasma levels of these lipoproteins particularly in the postprandial state. This condition is observed particularly when there is marked insulin deficiency or poor glycemic control in type T2D (Lewis *et al.,* 2002). It has also been reported that clearance of LDL was limited due to the decreased availability of LDL receptors. So the high insulin resistance reported in CAD WDM might be the etiology behind the observed high level of LDL.

Patients with type 2 diabetes frequently have normal or only slightly elevated LDL-cholesterol concentrations but increased numbers of atherogenic LDL particles owing to the predominance of small, dense LDL particles. The basis for formation of sdLDL in insulin resistant states relates to the action of two proteins; cholesteryl ester transfer protein (CETP) and hepatic lipase. CETP mediates the exchange of VLDL triglyceride for LDL cholesteryl ester, creating a triglyceride-enriched, cholesterol depleted LDL particle. This LDL particle is a substrate for hepatic lipase leading to hydrolysis of triglyceride and formation of the sdLDL (Olofsson *et al.*, 2005) Increased CETP and hepatic lipase activity, observed in insulin resistant and type 2diabetes subjects, favor the formation of sdLDL (Bagdade *et al.*, 1993 and Riemens *et al.*, 1998)A predominance of small, dense LDL particles is associated with increased risk of CHD (Austin *et al.*, 1988, Gardner *et al.*, 1996).These particles are more powerful than larger LDL particles to penetrate the vessel intimal wall and are more exposed to oxidation; oxidized LDL are then taken up by macrophages as part of atherosclerotic plaque formation. Small, dense LDL is also associated with early vascular dysfunction in the form of impaired endothelial response in patients with diabetes independent of other risk factor variables, including lipid levels, body mass index (BMI), blood pressure and severity. (Tan *et al.*, 1999).

Hence the absolute LDL-cholesterol concentration could be misleading, since it does not directly reflect the increased number of atherogenic particles. This might have led to the lack of positive correlation between LDL cholesterol with Insulin resistance and severity of CAD. (Tan *et al.*, 1999).

The CAD patients without diabetes and with total cholesterol level <200 mg/dl were 21% with grade III stenosis, 18% with grade II and 48% with grade I stenosis. The CAD subjects without diabetes and Total cholesterol level >200 mg/dl had 6% with grade III stenosis, 4% with grade II and 2% with grade I stenosis. Among the CAD without diabetes subjects with total triglyceride level <150 mg/dl 13% subjects had grade III stenosis, 6% had grade II and 42% had grade I stenosis. Compared to 19% subjects with grade III stenosis, 15% with grade II and 4% with grade I stenosis and triglyceride level >150 mg/dl. The CAD subjects without diabetes and HDL level <40 mg/dl had 19% with grade III stenosis, 8% with grade II and 33% with grade I stenosis.

The CAD subjects without diabetes and HDL >40 mg/dl had 15% with grade III stenosis, 10% with grade II and 15% with grade I stenosis. Among the CAD without diabetes subjects with LDL level <130 mg/dl 10% subjects had grade III stenosis, 12% had grade II and 23% had grade I stenosis,compared to 21% subjects with grade III stenosis, 10% with grade II and 23% with grade I stenosis with LDL level >130 mg/dl.

Among the CAD with diabetes subjects with total cholesterol level <200 mg/dl 37% subjects had grade III stenosis, 7% had grade II and 4% had grade I stenosis. Among the CAD subjects with >200 mg/dl cholesterol level,4% of subjects had Grade III,7% had grade II and 4% had grade I stenosis.Among CAD with diabetes and triglyceride level <150 mg/dl 33% had grade III stenosis, 19% had grade II and 28% had grade I stenosis. Among CAD subjects with triglyceride level >150 mg/dl were found to have 11% of subjects with grade III,7% with grade II and 2% with grade I stenosis. Among the CAD with diabetes subjects with total HDL level <40 mg/dl 30% subjects had grade III stenosis, 18% had grade II and 19% had grade I stenosis. Among the CAD subjects with 40-60 mg/dl HDL level 12% of subjects had Grade III,11% had grade II and 11% had grade I stenosis.

The CAD subjects with diabetes and LDL level <130 mg/dl had 25% with grade III stenosis, 18% with grade II and 14% with grade I stenosis. The CAD subjects with diabetes and LDL level >130 mg/dl had 18% with grade III stenosis, 12% with grade II and 14% with grade I stenosis.

The distribution of subjects based on HDL cholesterol level <40 mg/dl had shown that 32% had Grade I stenosis,25% had Grade II stenosis and 16% had Grade III stenosis.. Among the CAD subjects with HDL level 40-60 mg/dl 19% had grade I stenosis,14% had Grade II stenosis and 3% had Grade III stenosis.

HDL-C has been considered as an antiatherogenic lipid factor as it helps in reverse cholesterol transport (Hersberger et.al.,2005). Furthermore HDL particles have been shown to have cardioprotective nature due to its - antioxidant properties, protective effect on endothelial cells, inhibitory effect on endothelial adhesion and activation of leukocytes, inhibitory action on platelet activation (Nofer *et al.,* 2002). In our study, HDL-C level has been found to be significantly lowered in CAD patients when compared to normal. These results draw a parallel with the existing reports (Grundy,et.al., 2004). Reduced HDL levels have been commonly observed in metabolic syndrome and type 2 diabetes subjects. The reduced HDL cholesterol levels found in CAD WDM may be due to the high Apo E-containing triglyceride-rich lipoproteins found in these patients. Apo E is involved in HDL catabolism and can transfer from triglyceride-rich lipoproteins to HDL. Furthermore, when present on HDL particles, apo E is predominantly associated with LpAI/AII (Lipoprotein lipase AI/AII) particles. Therefore, the elevation of circulating apo E-containing triglyceride- rich lipoproteins could lead to increased transfer of apo E to LpAI/AII (Lipoprotein AI/AII) and enhanced catabolism of this fraction. (Juying Ji *et al.,* 2006)

Functions and properties of HDL particle vary according to its particle size and apoproteins content. It exists as particles of different sizes, with HDL- 2 being the largest and containing the most lipid in its core. HDL-3 particles are smaller and pre-b-HDL is the smallest, and these may be the most active particles in taking up peripheral cholesterol (Benton *et al.,* 2005). Apolipoprotein composition can be used to separate HDL into subpopulations: HDL containing apo A-I and apo A-II (HDL A-I : A-II), and HDL containing apo A-I but not apo A-II (HDL A-I)(Kuller *et al.,* 2002). HDL A-I is more effective than HDL A-I : A-II in promoting cholesterol efflux (Kuller *et al.,* 2002), which is consistent with the atheroprotective effect of apo A-I on LCAT (Walldius *et al.,* 2001 and Sharet *et al.,* 1994). The Prospective Epidemiological Study of Myocardial Infarction (PRIME) study examined the association between the incidence of CHD and several HDL related parameters, including HDL-C itself, apo A-I, HDL A-I, and HDL A-I : A-II (Ensign *et al.,* 2006). All four parameters were related to CHD risk, however, HDL apo A-I, and apo A-I were the strongest predictor. This might be the reason why HDL had no positive correlation with severity of CAD in the present study.

10.1. Apolipoprotein A1

An inverse relationship between the concentration of high-density lipoprotein (HDL) cholesterol and the risk of developing cardiovascular is well established. There are several documented functions of HDLs that may contribute to a protective role of the lipoproteins. These include the ability of HDLs to promote the efflux of cholesterol from macrophages and foam cells in the artery wall and to anti inflammatory/antioxidant properties of these lipoproteins. (Gotto AM J *et al.,* 1983) The fact that the main apolipoprotein of HDLs, ApoA-I, plays a prominent role in each of these functions adds support to the view that ApoA-I should be measured as a component of the assessment of cardiovascular risk in humans (Robinson D *et al.,* 1987). Moreover there is mounting evidence that HDL subpopulations vary in terms of their ability to protect against CHD. Case-control studies have suggested that the inverse relationship between HDL cholesterol concentration and CHD is a function of the concentration of the HDL subfractions (Miller *et al.,* 1987). In another study relating HDL subpopulations to CHD, it was found that both the severity and the rate of progression of coronary lesions correlate significantly and inversely with the concentration of types of HDL(Stamper *et al.,* 1991).

Level of Apolipoproteins overwhelms the lipids because ApoA1are under more genetic control than lipid components and hence depicts the number of lipoprotein particles more accurately (Walldius G and I Jungner I, 2006) The present study has shown that the level of Apo A1 was significantly low in CAD with diabetic subjects when compared to CAD without diabetes. This might be due to the presence of high level of Apo E which cause the catabolism of Apo A1 and HDL.

APO-A1 is the major structural protein of HDL(70%)and it has major role is centripetal movement of cholesterol from peripheral tissues including the arterial wall to the liver for eventual elimination of through the biliary system in to the gut.(Sniderman A D *et al.,* 2003)The transport of cholesterol and formation of HDL are the basic roles of APO-A1.,low levels of this proteins have been identified as the risk factor in the development and progression of coronary damage. (Sniderman A D et *al.,* 1997). Apo A1 not only initiates the reverse cholesterol transport by activating the LCAT but also manifests antioxidant and antiinflammatory effects (Walldius G and Jungner I.,2004) It also removes oxidative seeding molecules from endothelium, Scavenges toxic products from arterial wall, 'Reduces smooth muscle cell, apoptosis/ necrosis', Reduces plaque lipid content, Reduces plaque macrophage content and Improves endothelial dysfunction. Furthermore, apo A-I is the ligand for the ATP-binding cassette (ABC) protein, ABCA1,and hence is involved in the docking procedure by which excess cholesterol in peripheral cells is externalized to HDL (Oram et al., 2000 and Wang N et al., 2001) for further reverse cholesterol transport either directly or indirectly via LDL back to the liver Hence it can be considered as a better marker than HDL-C (Oram et al., 2000).

10.2. Apolipoprotein B(apoB)

For over three decades it has been recognized that a high level of total blood cholesterol, particularly in the form of LDL cholesterol (LDL-C), is a major risk factor for developing coronary heart disease (CHD) (Walldius G and Jungner I.,2001)However, recent research has shown that LDL-C is not the only lipoprotein species involved in atherogenesis. Elevated levels of intermediate- density lipoprotein (IDL) and very low density lipoprotein (VLDL) are also associated with increased cardiovascular risk. All these potentially atherogenic lipoprotein contain one Apo B molecule.and therefore the total apo B value indicates the total number of potentially atherogenic lipoproteins (Scharnagl H et al., 2001 and Nissen et al. 2003)

In our study Apo B was found to be significantly high in CAD with type 2 DM when compared to CAD without DM and control subjects. This observation coincide with the findings several studies related to coronary heart disease

Apo B is essential for the binding of LDL particles to the LDL receptor, allowing cells to internalize LDL and thus absorb cholesterol (Alfonso Troisia,, Alberto D'Argeniob,2006). The concentration of plasma apo B particles is highly correlated with the level of non-HDL cholesterol (non-HDL-C), defined as TC minus HDL-C (Chapman and Caslek, 2004) As HDL is known to be protective against cardiovascular risk, non-HDL-C reflects the fraction of blood cholesterol that is not contained in atheroprotective lipoproteins. Thus apo B has been found to be a better predictor of risk than LDL-c, VLDL and chylomicrons. In most conditions, more than 90% of all ApoB in blood is found in LDL. In some cases where LDL C is in the normal/low range, high ApoB levels were observed which indicate an increased number of sd-LDL particles, - most atherogenic particles as they are easily oxidized and promote an inflammatory response and the growth of plaques. Furthermore Apo B has been found to be an independent predictor of endothelial vasodilatory function, increased carotid IMT and arterial stiffness. These properties and the observation from the present study that Apo B is positively correlated to the severity of the CAD underline the simple fact that an excess of apo B- particles always denote proatherogenic condition.

10.3. ApoB/A ratio

An early detection of the people at high risk for CAD can reverse or reduce the worsening of condition by modification of lifestyle of patient, an establishment of robust and precise risk indicator for lipid imbalance and atherogenesis will be of great practical advantage for patients and physicians. (Nam BH, 2006).

LDL-C had been considered as the major atherogenic lipoprotein particles for many years and the prime predictor for CAD (Vogel RA, 1998).Now it has been identified that Apolipoprotein B represent total atherogenic particles and is better predictor than other lipoproteins. (Walldius G, Jungner I.,2004). ApoA-I the major apolipoprotein in HDL particles has a central role in the 'reverse cholesterol transport'and manifests anti-inflammatory and antioxidant effects. It has been identified that Apo A1 can be risk factor than HDL cholesterol and can be considered as for antiatherogenic marker. (Walldius G and Jungner I. 2004).

So to get a precise picture of both atherogenic and antiatherogenic lipid related risk, ratio of ApoB/ApoA1 was considered. The ratio between the concentrations of ApoB and ApoAI (henceforth ApoB/A) reflect the balance between the opposing processes of arterial internalization of cholesterol and the reverse transport of cholesterol back to the liver (Walldius G and Jungner I.,2005). The reason for improved predictive effect of ApoB/A ratio might be due to the fact that the ratio reflects and integrates the " cholesterol balance " between potentially atherogenic lipoprotein particles (ApoB) in relation to all antiatherogenic particles.(ApoA1). It has been found to be better than one single lipid fraction or the LDL-C/HDL-C ratio. Another contributing explanation is that the methodological errors of the apolipoprteins are smaller than those for lipids. (Walldius G and Jungner I, 2005).

In the present study the ApoB/A ratio was found to be markedly elevated ($p \leq 0.001$)in CAD patients irrespective of their Diabetes status. The ApoB/A ratio and severity of CAD was not found to be significant in CAD WNDM (r=1.000,p =.809) whereas the ratio and severity was significant(p<.05) in CAD WDM with(r=.547 p =.034.The risk relationship between ApoB and ApoA1 was expressed as Odds ratio. The Odds ratio for CAD WNDM was 0.48 while Odds ratio for CAD WDM was found to be 4.5 (95% CI: 1.122 - 18.31).(Table.8-10)

The ratio reflects the balance of cholesterol transport and can be expressed as one number which integrates the risk associated with an imbalance between atherogenic and antiatherogenic lipoproteins. The strongest single variable in AMORIS, related to increased risk of fatal MI, was the ApoB/ApoA-I ratio. AMORIS study showed that the ratio of ApoB /A1 can indicate the risk of MI irrespective of lipid phenotype and even if lipid levels are normal/low.(van Lennep *el al.*, 2008) This ratio had a stronger relationship with CV risk than any other lipid ratio such as total cholesterol (TC)/HDL-C, LDL-C/HDL-C, or non-HDL-C/HDL-C. Talmud et al have confirmed the results from the AMORIS study and found that the ratio was a better predictor of cardiac risk than LDL-C, and that both apo B with TG and found to have the strongest associations with CHD. (Talmud PJ *et al.*, 2002)

Epidemiologic studies indicated that the ratio of ApoB to ApoA-I was the strongest predictor of CAD (Barter etal.,2006). Similarly, van Lennep et al. (van Lennep *et al.*, 2000) reported in patients with CAD on statin therapy that only ApoB and the ApoB/ApoA-I ratio predicted myocardial infarction and all-cause mortality, whereas LDL-C and TG did not. In both men and women from the AMORIS (Apolipoprotein-Related Mortality Risk) study, the superiority of the ratio of ApoB to ApoA-I, compared with the TC/HDL-C ratio, became more obvious as risk of CAD increased.

Our study had shown that instead of still remaining with the old paradigm:'LDL cholesterol-the lower the better, a new paradigm ApoB/A1 ratio indicating the cholesterol balance –the lower the better 'might be more appropriate.

11. Conclusion

Type 2 diabetes mellitus is associated with a three to fourfold increase in risk for coronary artery disease (CHD). (Diabetes mellitus is associated with sharp increased risk of CVD and mortality). People with type 2 DM develop CVD at a younger age, have a high rate of multi-vessel disease. The typical symptoms of cardiac ischemia are often masked in diabetic patients Hence the pathological events are not identified at the preliminary stages. Despite advances in our knowledge, the established risk factors could not fully explain its occurrence: and cannot be explained by conventional risk factors which lead to delayed recognition of CAD in type 2 DM. Mechanism underlying the accelerated atherosclerosis in DM patients are not fully understood. Insulin resistance which is the major etiological factor of T2DM influence (affect)

http://dx.doi.org/10.5772/56476

HDL,LDL and TG level- which can increase the risk of CAD. ApoB/ApoA1 ratio which reflects both atherogenic and antiatherogenic lipid related risk, can be used as a better predictor than traditional lipid markers like LDL and HDL to analyze the atherogenicity.

12. Future implications

It is now reported that HDL can influence glucose metabolism directly and possibly improve insulin resistance by altering plasma membrane composition through enhanced cholesterol efflux. Balancing cholesterol efflux and influx HDL can promote insulin sensitivity enhancing or activating insulin receptor function, its tyrosine kinase activity and downstream regulation of cellular function. It is reported that glycation of certain residues of apo A1 could inhibit its anti-oxidant activity converting HDL into a dysfunctional molecule which may affect its protective properties including its newly emerging role in insulin action and glucose metabolism.

Author details

Dhastagir Sultan Sheriff[1*], Sachu P.[1] and Elshaari F.A.[1]

1 Department of Biochemistry, Faculty of Medicine, Benghazi, Libya

2 VMKV Medical College, Salem, India

References

[1] Abbasi F; Brown BW JrLamendola C, et al. Relationship between obesity, insulin resistance,and coronary heart disease risk. J Am Coil Cardiol. (2002). , 40, 937-943.

[2] Alfonso Troisia and Alberto D'Argeniob Apolipoprotein A-I/apolipoprotein B ratio and aggression in violent and nonviolent young adult males Journal of Psychiatric Research 2006;40 : 466-472

[3] Antonio, M. Gotto, Jr, TG-The Forgotten Risk Factor. Circulation (1998).

[4] Austin, M. A, Breslow, J. L, Hennekens, C. H, Buring, J. E, Willett, W. C, & Krauss, R. M. Low-density lipoprotein subclasspatterns and risk of myocardial infarction, J. Am.Med. Assoc. (1988).

[5] Bagdade, J. D, Lane, J. T, Subbaiah, P. V, Otto, M. E, & Ritter, M. C. Accelerated cholesteryl ester transfer in non insulin-dependent diabetes mellitus. Atherosclerosis (1993). , 104, 69-77.

[6] BansilalSameer; Farkouh, Michael E.; Fuster, Valentin. Role of Insulin Resistance and Hyperglycemia in the Development of Atherosclerosis. 2007; The American Journal of Cardiology (2007)., 99, 6-14.

[7] Barter, P. J, Ballantyne, C. M, Carmena, R, et al. Apo B versus cholesterol in estimating cardiovascular risk and in guiding therapy: report of the Thirty-Person/Ten-Country Panel J Intern Med (2006)., 259, 247-258.

[8] Boden, G. Role of fatty acids in the pathogenesis of insulin resistance and NIDDM. Diabetes. (1997)., 46, 3-10.

[9] Bodlaj, G, Berg, J, Pichler, R, & Biesenbach, G. Prevalence, severity and predictors of HOMA-estimated insulin resistance in diabetic and nondiabetic patients with end-stage renal disease.J Nephrol. (2006)., 19(5), 607-12.

[10] Chapman, M. J. and M Caslake Non-high-density lipoprotein cholesterol as a risk factor: addressing risk associated with apolipoprotein B-containing lipoproteins Eur Heart J Suppl (2004).

[11] Chen, H, Wertheimer, S. J, & Lin, C. H. et al.Protein-tyrosine phosphatases PTP1B and syp are modulators of insulin-stimulated translocation of GLUT4 in transfected rat adipose cells.J Biol Chem, (1997)., 272, 8026-8031.

[12] Chih-yuan wang and Tien-Chun ChangNon-HDL cholesterol level is reliable to be an early predictor for vascular inflammation in type 2 diabetes mellitus. J of Clin. Endocrinol. Met. (2004)., 89(9), 4762-4767.

[13] Corti, M. C, Guralnik, J. M, Salive, M. E, et al. HDL cholesterol predicts coronary heart disease mortality in older persons. JAMA(1995)., 274, 539-44.

[14] Defronzo, R. A. Banting Lecture. From the triumvirate to the ominous octet:a new paradigm for the treatment of type 2 diabetes mellitus.Diabetes (2009)., 58, 773-95.

[15] Drew, B. G, Rye, K, Duffy, A, Barter, S. J, & Kingwell, P. B. A. ((2012). The emerging role of HDL in glucose metabolism. NATURE REVIEWS | ENDOCRINOLOGY, doi: 10.1038/nrendo.2011.235, 1-9.

[16] Enas, E. A, Yusuf, S, & Mehta, J. Prevalence of coronary artery disease in Asian Indians. Am J Cardiol (1992)., 70, 945-949.

[17] Ensign, W, et al. Clin Chem (2006)., 52, 1722-27.

[18] Fox, C. S, Coady, S, Sorlie, P. D, Levy, D, Meigs, J. B, Agostino, D, & Sr, R. B. Wilson PWF, Savage PJ. Trends in cardiovascular complications of diabetes. JAMA, (2004)., 292, 2495-2499.

[19] Gardner, C. D, Fortmann, S. P, & Krauss, R. M. Associationof small low-density lipoprotein particles with the incidenceof coronary artery disease in men and women, J.Am. Med. Assoc. (1996).

[20] Gianturco, S. H, Ramprasad, M. P, Lin, A. H, Song, R, & Bradley, W. A. Cellular binding site and membrane binding proteins for triglyceride-rich lipoproteins in human monocyte-macrophages and THP-1 monocytic cells.J Lipid Res. 994;, 35(9), 1674-87.

[21] Girard-MauduitS "The lipid triad, or how to reduce residual cardiovascular risk?". Ann Endocrinol (Paris) :(2010)., 71(2), 89-94.

[22] Goossens, G. H. The role of adipose tissue dysfunction in the pathogenesis of obesity-related insulin resistance. Physiol Behav. (2008).

[23] Goraya, T. Y, Leibson, C. L, & Palumbo, P. J. et al.Coronary aterosclerosis in diabetes mellitus: a population based autopsy study J Am Coll Cardiol, (2002)., 40, 946-953.

[24] Gotto AM JrPownall HJ, Havel RJ. Introduction to the plasma lipoproteins. Methods Enzymol (1986)., 128, 3-41.

[25] Gotto AM JrTriglyceride as a risk factor for coronary artery disease. Am J Cardiol. (1998). A):22Q-25Q

[26] Grundy, S. M, Cleeman, J. I, & Merz, C. N. Brewer HB Jr, Clark LT, Hunninghake DB, Pasternak RC, Smith SC Jr, Stone NJ.Implications of recent clinical trials for the National Cholesterol Education Program Adult Treatment Panel III guidelines. Circulation. (2004). Jul 13;, 110(2), 227-39.

[27] Haffner, S. M, Stern, M, Hazuda, H. P, Mitchell, B. D, & Patterson, J. K. Cardiovascular risk factors in confirmed prediabetic individuals.Does the clock for coronary heart disease start ticking before theonset of clinical diabetes.JAMA(1990)., 263, 2893-2898.

[28] Hajer, G. R, Van Der Graaf, Y, Olijhoek, J. K, & Edlinger, M. Visseren FLJ. Low plasma levels of adiponectin are associated with low risk for future cardiovascular events in patients with clinical evident vascular disease. Am Heart J (2007).

[29] Hanif, W, & Muhammad, A. K. Cultural aspects, in: K. Khunti,S. Kumar (Eds.), Diabetes UK and South Asian Health Foundation Recommendations on Diabetes Research Priorities for British South Asians, first ed., Diabetes UK,London, UK, (2009)., 27-35.

[30] Hopkins, P. N, Wu, L. L, Hunt, S. C, & Brinton, E. A. Plasma triglycerides and type III hyperlipidemia are independently associated withpremature familial coronary artery disease. J Am Coll Cardiol. (2005)., 45(7), 1003-12.

[31] Hsueh, W. A, & Law, R. E. Cardiovascular risk continuum: implicationsof insulin resistance and diabetes.Am J Med (1998). S-14S.

[32] Juying JiGerald F. Watts, Anthony G. Johnson, Dick C. Chan, Esther M. M. Ooi Kerry-Anne Rye Adrian P. Serone and P. Hugh R. BarrettThe Journal of Clinical Endocrinology & Metabolism(2006).

[33] Katz, A. Nambi 55, Mather K, et al. Quantitative insulin sensitivity check index: A simple,accurate method for assessing insulin sensitivity in humans. J Chin EndocrinolMetab. (2000). , 85, 2402-2410.

[34] Kuboki, K, Jiang, Z. Y, Takahara, N, Ha, S. W, Igarashi, M, et al. Regulation of endothelial constitutive nitric oxide synthase gene expression in endothelial cells and in vivo : a specific vascular action of insulin. Circulation (2011). , 101, 676-681.

[35] Kuller, . . Nuclear magnetic resonance spectroscopy of lipoproteins and risk of coronary heart disease in the cardiovascular health study. Arterioscler Thromb Vasc Biol. 2002;22:1175-1180.

[36] Laakso, M. Cardiovascular disease in type 2 diabetes:challenge for treatment and prevention. J Intern Med,(2001). , 249, 225-235.

[37] Levy, J. C, & Matthews, D. R. Hermans MP: Correct homeostasis model assessment (HOMA) evaluation uses the computer program (Letter).Diabetes Care (1998).

[38] Lewis, G. F, Carpentier, A, Adeli, K, & Giacca, A. Disordered fat storage and mobilization in the pathogenesis of insulin resistance and type 2 diabetes. Endocr Rev (2002). , 23, 201-29.

[39] Lewis, G. F, Carpentier, A, Adeli, K, & Giacca, A. Disordered fat storage and mobilization in the pathogenesis of insulin resistance and type 2 diabetes. Endocr Rev (2002). , 23, 201-29.

[40] Liu, J, Sempos, C, Donahue, R. P, Dorn, J, Trevisan, M, & Grundy, S. M. Joint distribution of Non-HDL and LDL cholesterol and coronary heart disease risk prediction among individuals with and without diabetes. Diabetes care, (2005). , 28, 1916-1921.

[41] Lloyd-jones, D. M, Leip, E. P, Larson, M. G, et al. Prediction of lifetime risk for cardiovascular disease by risk factor burden at 50 years of age. Circulation. (2006). , 113, 791-798.

[42] Ma°kimattila SM.-L. Liu, J. Vakkilainen, et al., Impairedendothelium-dependent vasodilatation in type 2 diabetes. Relation to LDL size, oxidized LDL, and antioxidants,Diabetes Care 22; (1999).

[43] Matthews, D. R. Hosker Je Rudenski AS, et al. Homeostasis model assessment: Insulin resistance and beta-cell function from fasting plasma glucose and insulin concentrationsin man. Diabetologia. (1985). , 28, 412-419.

[44] Mayer, E. L, Jacobsen, D. W, & Robinson, K. Homocysteine and coronary atherosclerosis.J Am Coll Cardiol (1996). , 27, 517-27.

[45] Meshkani, R, & Adeli, K. Hepatic insulin resistance, metabolic syndrome and cardiovascular disease., Clin Biochem. (2009).

[46] Miller, N. E. Associations of high-density lipoprotein sub- classes and apolipoproteins with ischemic heart disease and coronary atherosclerosis, Am Heart J (1987).

[47] Nam, B. H, Kannel, W. B, & Agostino, D. RB. Search for an optimal atherogenic lipid risk profile: from the Framingham Study. Am J Cardiol. (2006). , 97, 372-375.

[48] Niraj, A, Pradahan, J, Fakhry, H, Veeranna, V, & Afonso, L. Severity of coronary artery disease in obese patients undergoing coronary angiography: "obesity paradox" revisited. Clin Cardiol (2007). , 30, 391-6.

[49] Nissen, S. E, Tsunoda, T, Tuzcu, E. M, et al. Effect of recombinant ApoA-I Milano on coronary atherosclerosis in patients with acute coronary syndromes: a randomized controlled trial. JAMA (2003). , 290, 2292-2300.

[50] Nofer, J. R, Van Der Giet, M, Tolle, M, & Wolinska, I. von Wnuck Lipinski K, Baba HA, Tietge UJ, Godecke A, Ishii I, Kleuser B, et al HDL induces NO-dependent vasorelaxation via the lysophospholipid receptor S1J Clin Investig. (2004). , 3.

[51] Olofsson, S. O, Boren, J, & Apolipoprotein, B. a clinically important apolipoprotein which assembles atherogenic lipoproteins and promotes the development of atherosclerosis. J Intern Med (2005). , 258, 395-410.

[52] Oram, J. F. (2001). Novel approaches to treating cardiovascular disease: lessons from Tangier disease. Expert Opin. Investig. Drugs, , 10, 427-38.

[53] Paik, I. K, & Blair, R. Atherosclerosis,cholesterol and ECG Review, AJAS (1995).

[54] Riemens, S, Vantoll, A, & Sluiter, . . Elevated plasma cholesteryl ester transfer in NIDDM relationships with apo B-containing lipoproteins and phospholipid transfer protein. Atherosclerosis 1998;140:71-9

[55] Robert, H. Fagard, Peter M. Nilsson, Smoking and diabetes-The double health hazard!, Primary Care Diabetes,, (2009).

[56] Robert VogelListening to endothelium A Story of Signal and Noise J Am Coll Cardiol, (2008). , 51, 1965-1966.

[57] Saxena, R, Madhu, S. V, Shukla, R, Prabhu, K. M, & Gambhir, J. K. Postprandial hypertriglyceridemia and oxidative stress in patients of type 2diabetes mellitus with macrovascular complications. Clin Chim Acta. (2005).

[58] Schaefer, E. J, Gregg, R. E, Ghiselli, G, Forte, T. M, Ordovas, J. M, & Zech, L. A. Brewer Schwenke DC, Carew TE: Determination of LDL degradation rate, content, and residence time in lesioned and nonlesioned aorta. Circulation (1987). IV- 313

[59] Scharnagl, H, Nauck, M, Wieland, H, & März, W. The Friedewald formula underestimates LDL cholesterol at low concentrations. Clin Chem Lab Med(2001). , 39, 426-431.

[60] Sharett, A. R, Patsch, W, Sorlie, P. D, Heiss, G, Bond, M. G, & Davis, C. E. Associations of lipoprotein cholesterols, apolipoproteins A-Iand B, and triglycerides with carotid atherosclerosis andcoronary heart disease. The Atherosclerosis Risk in Communities (ARIC) Study. Arterioscler Thromb (1994). , 14, 1098-104.

[61] Sharma, A. M. Obesity and cardiovascular risk; Growth Hormone & IGF Research : (2003).

[62] Stampfer, M. J, Sacks, F. M, Salvini, S, Willett, W. C, & Hennekens, C. H. A prospective study of cholesterol, apolipoproteins and the risk of myocardial infarction. N Engl J Med (1991). , 325, 373-81.

[63] Talmud, P. J, Hawe, E, Miller, G. J, & Humphries, S. E. Nonfasting apolipoprotein B and triglyceride levels as a useful predictor of coronary heart disease risk in middle-aged UK men. Arterioscler Thromb Vasc Biol (2002). , 22, 1918-23.

[64] Tan, K. C. B, Ai, V. H. G, Chow, W. S, Chau, M. T, Leong, L, & Lam, K. S. L. Influence of low density lipoprotein(LDL) subfraction profile and LDL oxidation on endothelium-dependent and independent vasodilatation in patientswith type 2 diabetes, J. Clin. Endocrinol. Metab. (1999).

[65] Van Lennep, J. E, & Westerveld, H. T. van Roeters Lennep HWO, et al. Apolipoprotein concentrations during treatment and recurrent coronary artery disease events Arterioscler Thromb Vasc Biol (2000). , 20, 2408-2413.

[66] Walldius, G, Jungner, I, Holme, I, Aastveit, A, Kolar, W, & Steiner, E. High apolipoprotein B, low apolipoprotein A-I, and improvement in the prediction of fatal myocardial infarction (AMORIS study): a prospective study. Lancet (2001). , 358, 2026-33.

[67] Walldius, G, Jungner, I, Holme, I, Aastveit, A, Kolar, W, & Steiner, E. High apolipoprotein B, low apolipoprotein A-I, and improvement in the prediction of fatal myocardial infarction (AMORIS study): a prospective study. Lancet (2001). , 358, 2026-33.

[68] Walldius, G, & Jungner, I. Rationale for using apolipoprotein Ba nd apolipoprotein A-I as indicators of cardiac risk and as targets for lipid-lowering therapy. Eur Heart J (2005). , 26, 210-2.

[69] Walldius, G, Jungner, I, & Apolipoprotein, B. and apolipoprotein A-I: risk indicators of coronary heart disease and targets for lipid-modifying therapy. J Intern Med. (2004). , 255(2), 188-205.

[70] Walldius, G, & Jungner, I. The apoB/apoA-I ratio: a strong, new risk factor for cardiovascular disease and a target for lipid-lowering therapy- a review of the evidence, Journal of Internal Medicine (2006). , 259, 493-519.

[71] Wang, C. H, Li, S. H, Weisel, R. D, et al. C-reactive protein upregulates angiotensin type 1 receptors in vascular smooth muscle. Circulation (2003). , 107, 1783-90.

[72] Wang, N, Silver, D. L, Thiele, C, & Tall, A. R. ATP-binding cassette transporter A1 (ABCA1) functions as a cholesterol efflux regulatory protein. J Biol Chem (2001). , 276, 23742-7.

[73] Wang, T. J, Gona, P, Larson, M. G, Tofler, G. H, Levy, D, Newton-cheh, C, et al. Multiple biomarkers for the prediction of first major cardiovascular events and death. N Engl J Med. (2006). , 355(25), 2631-9.

[74] Wang, X. L, Badenhop, R, Humphrey, K. E, Wilcken, D. E, & To, T. and/or G to A transitions are responsible for loss of a MspI restriction site at the 50-end of the human apolipoprotein AI gene;Hum Genet (1995). , 95, 473-474.

[75] WHO expert consultationAppropriate body-mass index for Asian populations and its implications for policy and intervention strategies. The Lancet, (2004). , 157-163.

[76] Zeng, G, Nystrom, F. H, Ravichandran, L. V, et al. Roles for insulin receptor, PI3-kinase, and Akt in insulin-signaling pathways related to production of nitric oxide in human vascular endothelial cells. Circulation (2000). , 101, 1539-45.

[77] Zouki, C, Haas, B, et al. Loss of pentameric symmetry of endothelial cell adhesion. J Immunol (2001). , 167, 5355-61.

Section 2

Complications

Chapter 9

Diabetes Mellitus Type 2 and Proteinuria

Relu Cernes and Reuven Zimlichman

Additional information is available at the end of the chapter

http://dx.doi.org/10.5772/56434

1. Introduction

Worldwide the prevalence of diabetes was estimated to be 2.8% in 2000 and 4.4% in 2030. The total number of people with diabetes is projected to rise from 171 million in 2000 to 366 million in 2030 [1]. The spread will be higher in developing countries (69%) compared to developed countries (20%). Most of diabetic patients will have type 2 diabetes [2].

Chronic kidney disease (CKD) is prevalent in people with diabetes; a recent analysis of NHANES data found that 39.6% of people with diagnosed diabetes, 41.7% of those with undiagnosed diabetes and 17.7% of those with prediabetes had CKD [3]. Increased urinary protein excretion may be an early clinical manifestation of diabetic nephropathy. However, when assessing protein excretion, the urine dipstick is a relatively insensitive marker for initial increases in protein excretion, not becoming positive until protein excretion exceeds 300 to 500 mg/day (upper limit of normal less than 150 mg/day, with most individuals excreting less than 100 mg/day) [4]. Microalbuminuria is delimited as an albumin excretion rate of 30-300 mg/24 h or a spot urine albumin to creatinine Ratio (ACR) of 30-300 mg/g (3.5-35 mg/mmol) in males and 20-200 mg/g (2.5-25 mg/mmol) in females. Overt diabetic nephropathy (DN) is settled by proteinuria >500 mg/24 h or albuminuria >300 mg/24 h. Also DN can be defined by an estimated glomerular filtration rate (eGFR) less than 60 ml/min/1.73 m^2 [5]. 5097 subjects with type 2 diabetes were followed from 1977 to 1997 to determine the rate of progression of kidney disease. From diagnosis of diabetes, progression to microalbuminuria occurred at 2.0% per year, from microalbuminuria to macroalbuminuria at 2.8% per year, and from macroalbuminuria to elevated plasma creatinine (>or=175 micromol/L) or renal replacement therapy (RRT) at 2.3% per year. Ten years following diagnosis of diabetes, the prevalence of microalbuminuria was 24.9%, of macroalbuminuria was 5.3%, and of elevated plasma creatinine or RRT was 0.8% [6]. Renal dysfunction, including proteinuria and microalbuminuria, is predictive of cardiovascular events, and cardiovascular and all-cause mortality [7-11]. Although these cut-offs defining normoalbuminuria, microalbuminuria, and macroalbuminuria facilitate determining the risk for progression of nephropathy, the risk of developing overt diabetic nephropathy is probably directly related to albumin excretion rates at all levels. A recent collaborative meta-analysis of general population cohorts involving more than 1 million participants has provided strong evidence of the direct relationship between renal dysfunction and cardiovascular risk [12]. eGFR < 60 ml/min/1.73 m 2 and (ACR) 1.1 mg/mmol (10 mg/g) were both independent predictors of mortality risk in the general population. The two parameters increased mortality in a multiplicative fashion, without evidence of interaction [12]. The clinical significance, screening, prevention and management of proteinuria in patients with type 2 diabetes will be reviewed here.

Mortality rates for those with nephropathy are high, increasing from 1.4% per year in normoalbuminuria to 4.6% per year (clinical grade proteinuria), and to 19.2% per year those with renal impairment. More intensive blood glucose control resulted in both a 33% reduction in relative risk of development of microalbuminuria or clinical grade proteinuria at 12 years, and a significant reduction in the proportion doubling their plasma creatinine (0.91 vs. 3.52%, P = 0.0028). These data underline the importance of glycaemic and blood pressure control in type 2 diabetes in order to prevent diabetic nephropathy [13]. Asian and hispanic patients with type 2 diabetes had a high prevalence of proteinuria and reduced kidney function [14,15]. In Caucasian non-insulin dependent diabetic baseline microalbuminuria, male gender, presence of retinopathy, S-cholesterol, HbA1c, and age was found to predict the development of incipient/overt diabetic nephropathy [16]. To estimate the frequency of remission/regression of microalbuminuria and to identify factors affecting such outcomes 216 Japanese patients with type 2 diabetes and microalbuminuria were enrolled and observed during an initial 2-year evaluation period. Remission was defined as shift to normoalbuminuria and regression as a 50% reduction in urinary albumin excretion rate (UAER)from one 2-year period to the next. Reduction of urinary UAER was frequent, with a 6-year cumulative incidence of 51% (95% CI 42-60) for remission and 54% for regression, whereas the frequency of progression to overt proteinuria was 28%. Microalbuminuria of short duration, the use of renin-angiotensin system-blocking drugs, and lower tertiles for HbA(1c) (<6.95%) and systolic blood pressure (<129 mmHg) were independently associated with remission or regression in the pooled logistic regression analysis. Early detection of microalbuminuria and a multifactorial control may result in improved outcomes for diabetic nephropathy and cardiovascular events [17].

2. Pathogenesis

Microalbuminuria and macroalbuminuria are not only markers of nephropathy but also causes of disease progression. Proteinuria may accelerate kidney disease progression to end-stage renal failure through multiple pathways, including induction of tubular chemokine expression and complement activation that lead to inflammatory cell infiltration in the interstitium and sustained fibrogenesis [18]. The precise mechanisms by which albumin leaves the bloodstream, crosses the endothelial suface layer, glomerural endothelial fenestrae, the glomerural basement membrane, the sleet pores between the foot processes of the podocytes and the subpodocyte space and by which albumin passes through Bowman's space and the tubuli and at the end enters into the urine remain an area of research and debate [19].

Glomerular hemodynamics and renin-angiotensin system (RAS). Proteinuria may be detected in healthy people after sustained exercise. Unbalance between afferent artery and efferent artery may appear during vigorous physical effort. Renal blood flow decreases and GFR is maintained by increment in intraglomerural pressure. Intraglomerural hypertension induces albuminuria. Also in DN, albuminuria is induced by a reduction in renal mass. Preserved glomeruli compensate the sclerotic ones by dilatation of afferent arterioles, constriction of efferent arterioles, increment of intraglomerural hydrostatic pressure. When this process continues, the glomerular barrier is compromised and albumin enters into the urine [20]. Leak of albumin into the urine is partly blocked by RAS inhibition also in healthy subjects [21]. RAS plays a central role as a mediator of glomerural hemodynamic and injury. Therapeutic blockade of RAS slows the disease progression not only by hemodynamic action but also by induction of profibrotic agents. Angiotensin II (Ang II) also plays an important role in glomerulosclerosis through induction of transforming growth factor –β (TGF- β) expression in mesangial cell [22]. Angiotensin-converting enzyme (ACE) inhibitors and angiotensin receptor blockers (ARBs) can attenuate progressive glomerulosclerosis without altering glomerular pressures. Because agents that interfere with Ang II action may decrease glomerular injury, it has been suggested that Ang II has direct effects on glomerular cells to induce sclerosis independent of its hemodynamic actions.Antagonizing the profibrotic effects of angiotensin II may also be a significant factor in benefits observed with ACE inhibitors and ARBS [22].

3. Endothelial barrier and glomerural basement membrane

The endothelium of glomerural capillaries is fenestrated. The diameter of endothelial pores is 60-100 nm. Although the albumin diameter is smaller than the pore diameter (8nm) the endothelium is not working like a sieve [24]. A glycoprotein coat covers capillary endothelium like a gel-like diaphragm. Damage of diaphragm in diabetic patients is associated with proteinuria [25].

The glomerural basement membrane was considered a mechanical and electrostatic barrier. The loss negatively charged proteoglycans is associated with albumin cross. Today,the mechanical role of glomerural basement membrane is less important [14,26]. Although the glomerural basement membrane is thick in diabetic patients, the leakage of albumin is increased [26].

4. Podocytes

Podocytes are highly specialized cells of the kidney glomerulus that help to prevent proteinuria through regulation of the actin cytoskeleton in their foot processes. Podocytopenia correlates with disease progression and is related inversely to the control of hypertension and diabetes. Diabetes mellitus induces podocytopenia through several mechanisms.

Podocyte morphological changes in DN are flattening and retraction. Podocyte dysfunction reduces ultrafiltration and induces intraglomerural hypertension and proteinuria. Podocytes are detected in the urine of diabetic patients and proves that this type of cells are in a proliferation apoptosis cycle [27].

Defects in podocyte-specific insulin signaling may contribute to diabetic nephropathy. Two mouse models have been engineered in which the gene encoding the insulin receptor from the podocyte is deleted [28]. In the absence of hyperglycemia, affected mice develop albuminuria, effacement of foot processes, apoptosis, glomerular basement membrane thickening, accumulation of mesangial matrix and glomerulosclerosis. Activation of the insulin receptor appears to trigger remodeling of the actin cytoskeleton through the mitogen-activated protein kinase 42/44 (MAPK) and phosphatidylinositol 3 (PI3) kinase signaling pathways, suggesting a possible mechanism of proteinuria. The podocyte insulin receptor is an attractive target for agents that prevent proteinuria and development and progression of diabetic nephropathy [29].

Podocytes are linked by a porous diaphragm with pores diameter of 12 nm. The integrity of the diaphragm has a great importance in prevention of proteinuria, Several diaphragm protein mutations like nephrin and podocin are associated with nephritic syndrome. When compared with nondiabetic patients with minimal change nephropathy and controls, patients with diabetic nephropathy had a downregulation of nephrin expression and fewer electron dense slit diaphragms [30].

5. Bowman 's space and proximal tubule

Bowman's space is situated between the parietal layer of Bowman's capsule and podocytes. Bowman's space is important in ultrafiltration and hydraulic resistance. The hydrostatic pressure is reduced in diabetic patients and appears to be associates with albuminuria [31]. Tubules suffer a number of structural and functional changes in DN. Tubules are hypertrophic and tubular basement membrane is thickened before proteinuria appearance. Tubular filtration is impaired through several mechanisms: lysosomal dysfunction; albumin transporters' reduction like megalin and cubilin; apical brush border changes and cathepsin-mediated proteolytic activity decrease [32,33].

Advanced Glycation End Products (AGEs) AGEs are the product of nonenzymatic reaction between the aldehyde group of sugars and carbonyls of proteins, lipids and nucleic acids. The first stable product is Amadori complex like HBA1c [34]. AGEs induce mesangial expansion and injury, through activation of AGE receptors (RAGE) perhaps in part via increased matrix production or glycation of matrix proteins [34]. The potential significance of RAGE in diabetic kidney is demonstrated by prevention of indices of mesangial expansion, thickening of the glomerural basement membrane and reduced albuminuria in RAGE knockout (KO) mice and following intervention with RAGE antibodies; on the other hand RAGE activation may produce renal damage [35,36]. The net effect is tissue accumulation of AGEs, in part by crosslinking with collagen, which can contribute to the associated renal and microvascular complications [37].

Prorenin — Renin is an aspartyl-protease that exists in two forms, the proenzyme prorenin and mature renin. Prorenin is transformed into mature renin by cleavage of the 43 amino acids of the pro-segment. Prorenin, although synthesized by a restricted number of tissues, represents up to 90% of total plasma renin in normal subjects. Experimental data on transgenic rats confirm a link between the overexpression of the receptor and cardiovascular and renal dysfunctions possibly involving direct activation of the receptor by (pro)renin [38]. Prorenin receptor blockade with a short peptide of prorenin practically abolished the increased mitogen-activated protein kinase (MAPK) activation and nephropathy despite unaltered increase in AngII in diabetic kidney. These results indicate that the MAPK activation signal leads to the diabetic nephropathy but not other renin-angiotensin system-activated mechanisms in the glomeruli. It is not only AngII but also intraglomerular activation of MAPK by the receptor-associated prorenin that plays a pivotal role in diabetic nephropathy [39].

Cytokines — Angiogenetic factors may explain pathologic changes in DN. Vascular endothelial growth factor (VEGF) is one of the main angiogenetic factors. Its expression and signaling in the kidney are amplified early on in the diabetic state. Moreover, counteracting its effects reverses the albuminuria and other hemodynamic and structural features of experimental DN. Finally, experimental overexpression of VEGF in adult mice replicates several aspects of diabetic kidney disease [41]. Under the influence of a variety of diabetic mediators, the podocyte becomes the main source of increased expression of VEGF in the kidney. The cytokine then exerts its multitude of effects in an autocrine fashion on the podocyte itself, on the endothelial cell in a paracrine manner, and finally contributes to macrophage recruitment acting as a chemokine [41,42]. The angiopoietins consist primarily of two main factors acting in contrast to each other: Ang I--an antiangiogenic ligand, and Ang II--its competitive inhibitor. Both, however, seem to have important roles in the maintenance of glomerular homeostasis [43]. Diabetes disrupts the tight balance that controls angiopoietin expression and function and decreases theAngI/AngII ratio. The end physiologic result seems to be dependent on the concomitant VEGF changes in the kidney. Because of the intricacy of their control, angiogenic factors are difficult to manipulate therapeutically [41,43].

TGF- β is a key factor in the development of diabetic complications by activating downstream mediators called Smad2 and Smad3. Hyperglycemia can induce TGF- β and Smads stimulation and renal fibrosis through MAPK and NF-kB pathways [44]

6. Detection and screening

Establishing the diagnosis of microalbuminuria requires the demonstration of an elevation in albumin excretion (30 to 300 mg/day). An elevated ratio should be confirmed with at least two additional tests performed over the subsequent three to six months, with confirmation of the diagnosis requiring at least two of three positive samples [45]. Patients with diabetes mellitus type 2 must be screened annually, starting at diagnosis. Fever, exercise, heart failure, and poor glycemic control are among the factors that can cause transient microalbuminuria [46]. There are many methods to screen for abnormal amounts of proteinuria to identify patients at risk for progression of renal disease. 701 patients with type 2 diabetes and nephropathy participating in the Reduction of Endpoints in Non Insulin Dependent Diabetes Mellitus with the Angiotensin II Antagonist Losartan (RENAAL) trial were enrolled to compare the ability of urinary protein excretion (UPE) and urinary albumin excretion (UAE) from a 24-hour urine collection and urinary albumin concentration (UAC) and the albumin:creatinine ratio (ACR) from a first-morning void in predicting renal events. The primary outcome measure was the time to a doubling of serum creatinine or end-stage renal disease. During follow-up, 202 events occurred. The hazard ratios for the risk of a renal outcome (95% CIs) associated with 1-SD increment in the log-transformed measures were 3.16 (2.60 to 3.86) for UAE, 3.02 (2.53 to 3.62) for UPE, 3.23 (2.67 to 3.91) for UAC, and 4.36 (3.50 to 5.45) for ACR. The area under the ROC curve was significantly higher for ACR compared with the other measures. In conclusion, measurement of the albumin:creatinine ratio in a first-morning void is the superior method to predict renal events in patients with type 2 diabetes and nephropathy,but the difference compared to spot urine samples at other times was not significant [46,47]. The recommended albumin (microg)/creatinine (mg) ratio (ACR) (30 microg/mg) to detect microalbuminuria does not account for sex or racial differences in creatinine excretion. Mean urine albumin concentration were not significantly different between men and women, but urine creatinine concentrations is significantly higher. No significant difference in the prevalence of microalbuminuria between men and women was noted when sex-specific ACR cutpoints are used (> or =17 microg/mg in men and > or =25 microg/mg in women). The use of one ACR value to define microalbuminuria may underestimate microalbuminuria in subjects with higher muscle mass (men) and possibly members of certain racial/ethnic groups [48]. The most pronounced benefits of glycaemic control are on retinal and renal complications in both normoalbuminuric and microalbuminuric patients considered together, with little or no evidence of any greater benefit in those with microalbuminuria. Hence, microalbuminuric status may be a false boundary when considering the benefits of glycaemic control. Classification of a person as normoalbuminuric must not serve to suggest that they will derive less benefit from optimal glycaemic control than a person who is microalbuminuric. All hypertensive patients benefit from blood pressure lowering [49].

7. Treatment and prevention

Glycemic and blood pressure control, particularly with angiotensin converting enzyme (ACE) inhibitors or angiotensin II receptor blockers (ARBs), have shown to reduce proteinuria, preserve renal function in diabetic patients and reduce cardiovascular events [50].

Lifestyle improvement is the first step in the treatment of DN. This includes a number of measures: avoidance or cessation of smoking, weight reduction and maintaining body mass index (BMI) between 18.5 and 24.9; physical activity, especially regular aerobic physical activity such as brisk walking for more than 30 minutes per day, most days of the week; low protein diet and reducing protein intake to 0.8-1.0 g/kg body weight per day, most days of the week; low sodium intake to less than 100 mmol /d (2.4 g of sodium or 6 g of sodium chloride) consuming a diet rich in fruits, vegetables, and low fat diary products (DASH diet); low alcohol intake, not more than two drinks for men and one drink for women). For patients with diabetes, clinical practice guidelines recommend treating to a low-density lipoprotein cholesterol (LDL-C) goal of < 100 mg/dL and <70 mg/dl for very high risk patients, using statins as first line treatment [46,51].

8. Blood pressure control and renin-angiotensin blockade

All current guidelines recommend a blood pressure goal in patients with diabetes <130/80 mm Hg. The proportion of diabetic individuals taking lipid- and BP-lowering agents has increased significantly in recent years. However, while there has been a significant improvement in LDL-C goal attainment, nearly one-half of all U.S. adults with diabetes are not at recommended LDL-C or BP treatment goals [52]. Patients with HTN and diabetes have a 7-fold greater risk for progressing to end-stage renal disease (ESRD) and 2 to 4-fold greater risk of developing cardiovascular disease. The first lone treatment are ACEI and ARBS due to renoprotective effect [53,54]. If the baseline BP is >150/90 mm Hg, a second agent should be added, preferably a thiazide diuretic, because they can add cardiovascular protection [54,55]. However, recent evidence suggests that calcium channel blockers, especially amlodipine can comparatively reduce cardiovascular events [56].

Several clinical trials have proved evidence that the conventional treatments for renoprotection including blood pressure regulation, tight glucose control, renin-angiotensin system inhibition, lifestyle modifications and medical team improvement reduce the morbidity and mortality associated with proteinuria. The benefit of ACEI and ARBS in reducing proteinuria and renal preservation in DN has been confirmed in several large randomized trials. Some of them are summarized in Table 1 and detailed in this paragraph.

9. ACEI

In a randomized, double-blind, placebo-controlled trial 94 patients with normal blood pressure and microalbuminuria were assigned to receive enalapril, 10 mg per day, or placebo. After 5 years albuminuria decreased from 143 +/- 64 (mg/24 h to 122 +/- 67 mg/24 h during the first year. In the placebo group microalbuminuria slowly increased to 140 +/- 134 mg/24 [P<0.05]). Kidney function (expressed as mean reciprocal creatinine) declined by 13% in the placebo group and remained stable (-1%) in the enalapril group (P<0.05) [57]. Later this study was done on diabetic patients with normal blood pressure and normoalbuminuria. In a randomized, double-blind, placebo-controlled trial, 156 patients were assigned to receive enalapril, 10 mg/d, or placebo for a period of 6 years. Enalapril therapy decreased albumin excretion from 11.6 +/- 7 mg/24 h to 9.7 +/- 6 mg/24 h at 2 years. This was followed by a gradual increase to 15.8 +/- 8 mg/24 h at 6 years. In the placebo group, albumin excretion increased from 10.8 +/- 8 mg/24 h to 26.5 +/- 10 mg/24 h at 6 years (P = 0.001 for enalapril compared with placebo). Transition to microalbuminuria occurred in 15 of 79 (19%) placebo recipients and 5 of 77 (6.5%) enalapril recipients. Enalapril treatment resulted in an absolute risk reduction of 12.5% (95% CI, 2% to 23%; P = 0.042) for development of microalbuminuria. After 6 years, creatinine clearance decreased from 1.78 +/- 0.13 mL/s to 1.63 +/- 0.12 mL/s (mean decrease, 0.025 mL/s per year) in enalapril recipients and from 1.81 +/- 0.15 mL/s to 1.57 +/- 0.17 mL/s (mean decrease, 0.04 mL/s per year) in placebo recipients (P = 0.040) [58].

10. ARBS

In IRMA-2 (Irbesartan Microalbuminuria in Hypertensive Patients with Type 2 Diabetes),the renoprotective effect of the angiotensin-II-receptor antagonist irbesartan independently of its blood-pressure-lowering effect was evaluated in hypertensive patients with type 2 diabetes and microalbuminuria. 590 patients were enrolled in a randomized, double-blind, placebo-controlled study of irbesartan, at a dose of either 150 mg daily or 300 mg daily, and were followed for two years. The primary outcome was the time to the onset of diabetic nephropathy, defined by persistent albuminuria in overnight specimens, with a urinary albumin excretion rate that was greater than 200 ucg per minute and at least 30 percent higher than the base-line level. Ten of the 194 patients in the 300-mg group (5.2 percent) and 19 of the 195 patients in the 150-mg group (9.7 percent) reached the primary end point, as compared with 30 of the 201 patients in the placebo group (14.9 percent) (hazard ratios, 0.30 [95 percent confidence interval, 0.14 to 0.61; P<0.001]and 0.61 [95 percent confidence interval, 0.34 to 1.08; P=0.081 for the two irbesartan groups, respectively) [59]. The Angiotensin II Antagonist Losartan (RENAAL) study investigated renoprotective role of albuminuria reduction in 1428 patients with hypertension and diabetic nephropathy from the placebo-controlled Reduction of Endpoints in NIDDM with the Angiotensin II Antagonist Losartan (RENAAL) study. Among patients with a reduced blood pressure during treatment, a lack of albuminuria reduction was observed in 37, 26, and 51% (total, losartan, and placebo, respectively) at month 6. Blood pressure or albuminuria reduction was associated with a lower risk for end stage renal failure, whereas combined blood pressure and albuminuria reduction was associated with the lowest risk for events [60]. The MicroAlbuminuria Reduction With VALsartan (MARVAL) study investigated the BP-independent effect of valsartan to reduce microalbuminuria in type 2 diabetic patients. Three hundred thirty-two patients with type 2 diabetes and microalbuminuria, with or without hypertension, were randomly assigned to 80 mg/d valsartan or 5 mg/d amlodipine for 24 weeks. The primary end point was the percent change in UAER from baseline to 24 weeks. The UAER at 24 weeks was 56% (95% CI, 49.6 to 63.0) of baseline with valsartan and 92% (95% CI, 81.7 to 103.7) of baseline with amlodipine, a highly significant between-group effect (P<0.001). Valsartan lowered UAER similarly in both the hypertensive and normotensive subgroups. More patients reversed to normoalbuminuria with valsartan (29.9% versus 14.5%; P=0.001)., valsartan lowered UAER more effectively than amlodipine in patients with type 2 diabetes and microalbuminuria, including the subgroup with baseline normotension [61]. In ROADMAP trial olmesartan was associated with a delayed onset of microalbuminuria, even though blood-pressure control in both groups was excellent according to current standards [62]. Although in other studies ARBS were effective in reducing cardiovascular morbidity and mortality as well as mortality from all causes in patients with hypertension, diabetes, and left ventricular hypertrophy, in ROADMAP study the higher rate of fatal cardiovascular events with olmesartan among patients with preexisting coronary heart disease is of concern [62,63]. Several trials do not permit a conclusion about the efficacy of angiotensin inhibition for the prevention of new onset microalbuminuria in normotensive patients with type 2 diabetes. The DIRECT (Diabetic Retinopathy Candesartan Trials) Program are three randomized studies. 3326 and 1905 patients with type 1 and type 2 diabetes, respectively, most were normotensive, and all had normoalbuminuria (median urinary albumin excretion rate, 5.0 microg/min) were assigned to receive candesartan, 16 mg/d increasing to 32 mg/d, versus placebo, for a period of 4.7 years. The primary end point was new microalbuminuria (3 or 4 collections of urinary albumin excretion rate>or=20 microg/min). Individual and pooled results of the 3 trials showed that candesartan had little effect on risk for microalbuminuria (pooled hazard ratio, 0.95 [95% CI, 0.78 to 1.16]; P = 0.60). Pooled results showed that the annual rate of change in albuminuria was 5.53% lower (CI, 0.73% to 10.14%; P = 0.024) with candesartan than with placebo. Candesartan, 32 mg/d, for 4.7 years did not prevent microalbuminuria in mainly normotensive patients with type 1 or type 2 diabetes [64]. The normotensive Appropriate Blood pressure Control in Diabetes (ABCD) trial study investigated the effect of intensive versus moderate diastolic blood pressure (DBP) control on diabetic vascular complications in 480 normotensive type 2 diabetic patients. 480 patients randomized to intensive (10 mm Hg below the baseline DBP) versus moderate (80 to 89 mm Hg) DBP control. Patients in the moderate therapy group were given placebo, while the patients randomized to intensive therapy received either nisoldipine or enalapril in a blinded manner for 5.3 years. The primary end point evaluated was the change in creatinine clearance with the secondary endpoints consisting of change in urinary albumin excretion, progression of retinopathy and neuropathy and the incidence of cardiovascular disease. Mean BP in the intensive group was 128 +/- 0.8/75 +/- 0.3 mm Hg versus 137 +/- 0.7/81 +/- 0.3 mm Hg in the moderate group, P<0.0001. Although no difference was demonstrated in creatinine clearance (P = 0.43), a lower percentage of patients in the intensive group progressed from normoalbuminuria to microalbuminuria (P = 0.012) and microalbuminuria to overt albuminuria (P = 0.028). The intensive BP control group also demonstrated less progression of diabetic retinopathy (P = 0.019) and a lower incidence of strokes (P = 0.03). The results were the same whether enalapril or nisoldipine was used as the initial antihypertensive agent [65].

11. ACEI and ARBS

A number of trials were designed to address the lack of comparative data on the long-term effects of ARBS versus ACEI on renoprotection. The Diabetics Exposed to Telmisartan And enalaprIL (DETAIL) trial is a randomized comparative of these agents. 250 patients with type 2 diabetes and early nephropathy as defined by albuminuria (82 percent microalbuminuria and 18 percent macroalbuminuria to a maximum of 1.4 g/day) and a baseline GFR (measured isotopically) of approximately 93 mL/min per 1.73 m2 patients were assigned to receive an ACEI, enalapril to an ARB,telmisartan. A greater fall in GFR of at least 10.0 mL/min per 1.73 m2 at five years was predefined as suggesting a clinically significant difference between the two treatment groups.At five years, there was a smaller decline in GFR with enalapril that was not significant (14.9 versus 17.9 mL/min per 1.73 m2 with telnmisartan). Both groups had similar rates or findings for the secondary end points, which included annual changes in the GFR, blood pressure, serum creatinine concentration, urinary albumin excretion, end-stage kidney disease, cardiovascular events, and mortality [66]. In the candesartan and lisinopril microalbuminuria (CALM) study was assessed and compared the effects of candesartan or lisinopril, or both, on blood pressure and urinary albumin excretion in patients with microalbuminuria, hypertension, and type 2 diabetes. Candesartan 16 mg once daily, lisinopril 20 mg once daily were administered to 199 patients in a prospective, randomised, parallel group, double blind study.It run in period and 12 weeks' monotherapy with candesartan or lisinopril followed by 12 weeks' monotherapy or combination treatment. the reduction in urinary albumin:creatinine ratio with combination treatment (50%, 36% to 61%, P<0.001) was greater than with candesartan (24%, 0% to 43%, P=0.05) and lisinopril (39%, 20% to 54%, P<0.001) [67]. In other trials the benefit of combination therapy of ACEI along with ARB reduce proteinuria to a greater extent than monotherapy, overall it worsens major renal outcomes [68]. The ONTARGET study investigated the renal effects of ramipril (an ACE inhibitor), telmisartan (an ARB), and their combination in patients aged 55 years or older with established atherosclerotic vascular disease or with diabetes with end-organ damage. The trial ran for six years. After a 3-week run-in period, 25 620 participants were randomly assigned to ramipril 10 mg a day (n=8576), telmisartan 80 mg a day (n=8542), or to a combination of both drugs (n=8502; median follow-up was 56 months), and renal function and proteinuria were measured. The primary renal outcome was a composite of dialysis, doubling of serum creatinine, and death. The number of events for the composite primary outcome was similar for telmisartan (n=1147 [13.4%]) and ramipril (1150 [13.5%]; hazard ratio [HR] 1.00, 95% CI 0.92-1.09), but was increased with combination therapy (1233 [14.5%]; HR 1.09, 1.01-1.18, p=0.037). The secondary renal outcome, dialysis or doubling of serum creatinine, was similar with telmisartan (189 [2.21%]) and ramipril (174 [2.03%]; HR 1.09, 0.89-1.34) and more frequent with combination therapy (212 [2.49%]: HR 1.24, 1.01-1.51, p=0.038). Estimated glomerular filtration rate (eGFR) declined least with ramipril compared with telmisartan (-2.82 [SD 17.2] mL/min/1.73 m(2)vs -4.12 [17.4], p<0.0001) or combination therapy (-6.11 [17.9], p<0.0001). The increase in urinary albumin excretion was less with telmisartan (p=0.004) or with combination therapy (p=0.001) than with ramipril [68]. The ORIENT study examined the effects of olmesartan, an ARB, on primary composite outcome of doubling of serum creatinine, endstage renal disease and death in type 2 diabetic patients with overt nephropathy [69]. Secondary outcome included composite cardiovascular outcomes, changes in renal function and proteinuria. Five hundred and seventy-seven (377 Japanese, 200 Chinese) patients treated with antihypertensive therapy (73.5%) received concomitant ACEI), were given either once-daily olmesartan (10-40 mg) or placebo over 3.2 years (In the olmesartan group, 116 developed the primary outcome (41.1%) compared with 129 (45.4%) in the placebo group (HR 0.97, 95% CI 0.75, 1.24; p=0.791). Olmesartan significantly decreased blood pressure, proteinuria and rate of change of reciprocal serum creatinine. Cardiovascular death was higher in the olmesartan group than the placebo group (ten vs three cases), whereas major adverse cardiovascular events (cardiovascular death plus non-fatal stroke and myocardial infarction) and all-cause death were similar between the two groups (major adverse cardiovascular events 18 vs 21 cases, all-cause deaths; 19 vs 20 cases). Hyperkalaemia was more frequent in the olmesartan group than the placebo group (9.2% vs 5.3%) [69]. The benefit of the combined use of a renin-angiotensin system inhibitor with other antihypertensive drugs such as diuretics or nondihydropyridine calcium channel blockers was studied.

12. Aliskiren, spironolactone and others

The ADVANCE trial investigated if controlling the blood pressure with a fixed combination of perindopril and indapamide or matching placebo, in addition to current therapy reduces the risks of major macrovascular and microvascular events, defined as death from cardiovascular disease, non-fatal stroke or non-fatal myocardial infarction, and new or worsening renal or diabetic eye disease.

Study	Patient population and duration	Treatment	Primary endpoint	Benefit and outcomes
Ravid (1993) [57]	Normotensive+microalbuminuria (5 years)	Enalapril vs placebo	Microalbuminuria reduction	Confirmed
Ravid (1998) [58]	Normotensive+normoalbuminuria (6 years)	Enalapril vs placebo	Albuminuria prevention	Confirmed
IRMA-2 [59]	Hypertension+microalbuminuria (2 years)	Irbesartan vs placebo	Albuminuria reduction	Confirmed, independently of BP
RENAAL [60]	Hypertension+microalbuminuria (6 months)	Losartan vs placebo	Albuminuria reduction	Confirmed, independently of BP
MARVAL [61]	Hypertension(or normotensive) +microalbuminuria (24 weeks)	Valsartan vs placebo	Albuminuria reduction	Confirmed, independently of BP
ROADMAP [62]	Hypertension +normoalbuminuria (3.2 years)	Olmesartan vs. placebo	Albuminuria prevention	Confirmed Higher fatal CV events
ABCD [65]	Hyper or normotension without overt DN (5 years)	Intensive / standard BP treatment	Overt DN prevention and reduction	Overt DN can not be reversed
DIRECT [64]	Normotensive+normoalbuminuria (4.7 years)	Candesartan vs placebo	Albuminuria prevention	Did not prevent microalbuminuria

Study	Patient population and duration	Treatment	Primary endpoint	Benefit and outcomes
DETAIL [66]	Hypertension+microalbuminuria (5 years)	Telmisartan vs enalapril	Noniferiority renoprotection	Confirmed
CALM [67]	Hypertension+microalbuminuria (24 weeks)	Candesartan+lisnopril vs candesartan vs lisinopril	BP control and microalbunuria reduction	Superiority of combination confirmed
ONTARGET [68]	Hypertension +end organ damage (6 years)	Telmisartan+ramipril vs telmisartan vs ramipril	Proteinuria and renal failure improvement	Combination worsened renal failure
ORIENT [69]	Overt DN (3.2 years)	Olmesaran +ACEI vs ACEI	Proteinuria and renal failure improvement	Cobination did not improved
ADVANCE [70]	Hypertension (4.3 years)	Perindopril+ indapamide vs placebo	Macrro and microvascular events reduction	Confirm combined but not separetly
BENEDICT [71]	Hypertension +normoalbuminuria (3.0 years)	Trandolapril+verapamil vs trandolapril	Albuminuria prevention	Verapamil similar to placebo
AVOID [72]	Hypertension+microalbuminuria (6 months)	Aliskiren+losartan vs.losartan	Albuminuria reduction	Confirmed, independently of BP
Mehdi (2009) [73]	Hypertension+Overt DN (48 weeks)	Spironolactone+lisino. vs losartan+lisino. vs lisinopril	Albuminuria reduction	Combination with spironolactone is superior

Abbreviations: ACEI, angiotensin-converting enzyme inhibitor; BP, blood pressure; CV,cardio vascular; DN, diabetic nephropathy;.Lisino, lisinopril. Clinical studies: ABCD, The normotensive Appropriate Blood pressure Control in Diabetes; AVOID, Aliskiren in the Evaluation of Proteinuria in diabetes ; ADVANCE, Action in Diabetes and Vascular disease: PreterAx and DiamicroN MR Controlled Evaluation; BENEDICT, Bergamo Nephrologic Diabetes Complications Trial CALM, candesartan and lisinopril microalbuminuria; DETAIL, Diabetics Exposed to Telmisartan And enalaprIL; DIRECT, Diabetic Retinopathy Candesartan Trials; IRMA-2, Irbesartan Microalbuminuria in Hypertensive Patients with Type 2 Diabetes; MARVAL,MicroAlbuminuria Reduction With VALsartan ; ONTARGET, Ongoing telmisartan alone and in combination with ramipril global endpoint trial; ORIENT, Olmesartan Reducing Incidence of Endstage Renal Disease in Diabetic Nephropathy Trial; ROADMAP, Randomized Olmesartan and Diabetes Microalbuminuria Prevention

Table 1. The benefit of ACEI and ARBS in reducing proteinuria and renal preservation in DN, summary of studies.

11 140 patients with type 2 diabetes were randomised to treatment. After a mean of 4.3 years of follow-up, patients assigned to therapy had a mean reduction in systolic blood pressure of 5.6 mm Hg and diastolic blood pressure of 2.2 mm Hg. The relative risk of a major macrovascular or microvascular event was reduced by 9% (861 [15.5%]active vs 938 [16.8%]placebo; hazard ratio 0.91, 95% CI 0.83-1.00, p=0.04). The separate reductions in macrovascular and microvascular events were similar but were not independently significant (macrovascular 0.92; 0.81-1.04, p=0.16; microvascular 0.91; 0.80-1.04, p=0.16). The relative risk of death from

http://dx.doi.org/10.5772/56434

cardiovascular disease was reduced by 18% (211 [3.8%] active vs 257 [4.6%] placebo; 0.82, 0.68-0.98, p=0.03) and death from any cause was reduced by 14% (408 [7.3%] active vs 471 [8.5%] placebo; 0.86, 0.75-0.98, p=0.03) [70]. Bergamo Nephrologic Diabetes Complications Trial (BENEDICT) evaluated the effect of calcium channel blockers to prevent albuminuria alone or along with ACEI. studied 1204 subjects, who were randomly assigned to receive at least three years of treatment with trandolapril (at a dose of 2 mg per day) plus verapamil (sustained-release formulation, 180 mg per day), trandolapril alone (2 mg per day), verapamil alone (sustained-release formulation, 240 mg per day), The primary end point was the development of persistent microalbuminuria (overnight albumin excretion,>or =20 ucg per minute at two consecutive visits). The primary outcome was reached in 5.7 percent of the subjects receiving trandolapril plus verapamil, 6.0 percent of the subjects receiving trandolapril, 11.9 percent of the subjects receiving verapamil, and 10.0 percent of control subjects receiving placebo. The estimated acceleration factor (which quantifies the effect of one treatment relative to another in accelerating or slowing disease progression) adjusted for predefined baseline characteristics was 0.39 for the comparison between verapamil plus trandolapril and placebo (P=0.01), 0.47 for the comparison between trandolapril and placebo (P=0.01), and 0.83 for the comparison between verapamil and placebo (P=0.54). Trandolapril plus verapamil and trandolapril alone delayed the onset of microalbuminuria by factors of 2.6 and 2.1, respectively. Serious adverse events were similar in all treatment groups. The effect of verapamil alone was similar to that of placebo [71]. Aliskiren is an direct renin inhibitor blocks the conversion from angiotensinogen to angiotensin I. In the AVOID (Aliskiren in the Evaluation of Proteinuria in Diabetes) study 599 patients with hypertension and type 2 diabetes with nephropathy were randomized to receive aliskiren (150 mg daily for 3 months, followed by an increase in dosage to 300 mg daily for another 3 months) or placebo, in addition to losartan. The primary outcome was a reduction in the ratio of albumin to creatinine. The mean urinary albumin-to-creatinine ratio was reduced by 20% (95% confidence interval, 9 to 30; P<0.001), with a reduction of 50% or more in 24.7% of the patients who received aliskiren as compared with 12.5% of those who received placebo (P<0.001). Aliskiren may have renoprotective effects that are independent of its blood-pressure-lowering effect in patients with hypertension, type 2 diabetes, and nephropathy who are receiving the recommended renoprotective treatment [72]. Aldosterone receptor antagonist, such as spironolactone, has been shown to to reduce proteinuria, when added to ACEI or ARBS. A double-blind, placebo-controlled trial investigated 81 patients with diabetes, hypertension, and albuminuria (urine albumin-to-creatinine ratio > or =300 mg/g) who all received lisinopril (80 mg once daily). The patients were assigned to placebo, losartan (100 mg daily), or spironolactone (25 mg daily) for 48 wk. Compared with placebo, the urine albumin-to-creatinine ratio decreased by 34.0% (95% CI, -51.0%, -11.2%, P = 0.007) in the group assigned to spironolactone and by 16.8% (95% CI, -37.3%, +10.5%, P = 0.20) in the group assigned to losartan [73]. An interesting study assessed the effect of die tary sodium restriction on the efficacy of losartan in hypertensive subjects with type 2 diabetes and albumin excretion rates of 10-200 ucg/min. 20 subjects were randomized to losartan 50 mg/day (n = 10) or placebo (n = 10). Drug therapy was given in two 4-week phases separated by a washout period. In the last 2 weeks of each phase, patients were assigned to low- or regular-sodium diets, in random order. In each phase, 24-h ambulatory blood pressure, urinary albumin-to-creatinine ratio (ACR), and renal hemodynamics were measured. Achieved urinary sodium on a low-sodium diet was 85 +/- 14 and 80 +/- 22 mmol/day in the losartan and placebo groups, respectively. In the losartan group, the additional blood pressure-lowering effects of a low-sodium diet compared with a regular-sodium diet for 24-h systolic, diastolic, and mean arterial blood pressures were 9.7 mmHg (95% confidence interval [CI], 2.2-17.2; P = 0.002), 5.5 mmHg (2.6-8.4; P = 0.002), and 7.3 mmHg (3.3- 11.3; P = 0.003), respectively. In the losartan group, the ACR decreased significantly on a low-sodium diet versus on a regular-sodium diet (-29% [CI -50.0 to -8.5%] vs. + 14% [-19.4 to 47.9%], respectively; P = 0.02). There was a strong correlation between fall in blood pressure and percent reduction in the ACR (r = 0.7, P = 0.02). In the placebo group, there were no significant changes in blood pressure or ACR between regular- and low-sodium diets [74].

13. Glycemic control

Poor glycemic control is a risk factor for both the development of microalbuminuria and for progression to macroalbuminuria in patients with type 2 diabetes. Strict glycemic control is recommended in all patients because of its beneficial effects on the microvascular complications. Whilst the benefits of intensive glycemic therapy for people with diabetes and microalbuminuria have been well established, controversy remains as to whether intensive therapy slows the progression of established DN, particularly among individuals who have a reduced glomerular filtration rate. In addition, severe hypoglycemia has been associated with intensive glycemic therapy, raising safety concerns that may be of particular relevance for patients with decreased kidney function [75].

14. The ADVANCE study

The ADVANCE study investigated a strategy of intensive glucose control, involving gliclazide (modified release) and other drugs as required, that lowered the glycated hemoglobin value to 6.5% yielded a 10% relative reduction in the combined outcome of major macrovascular and microvascular events, primarily as a consequence of a 21% relative reduction in nephropathy. 11,140 patients with type 2 diabetes were assigned to undergo either standard glucose control or intensive glucose control, defined as the use of gliclazide (modified release) plus other drugs as required to achieve a glycated hemoglobin value of 6.5% or less. Primary end points were composites of major macrovascular events (death from cardiovascular causes, nonfatal myocardial infarction, or nonfatal stroke) and major microvascular events (new or worsening nephropathy or retinopathy), assessed both jointly and separately. Intensive control reduced the incidence of combined major macrovascular and microvascular events (18.1%, vs. 20.0% with standard control; hazard ratio, 0.90; 95% confidence interval [CI], 0.82 to 0.98; P=0.01), as well as that of major microvascular events (9.4% vs. 10.9%; hazard ratio, 0.86; 95% CI, 0.77 to 0.97; P=0.01), primarily because of a

http://dx.doi.org/10.5772/56434

reduction in the incidence of nephropathy (4.1% vs. 5.2%; hazard ratio, 0.79; 95% CI, 0.66 to 0.93; P=0.006), with no significant effect on retinopathy (P=0.50) [76].

15. UKPDS

In UKPDS the effects of intensive blood-glucose control with either sulphonylurea or insulin and conventional treatment on the risk of microvascular and macrovascular complications in patients with type 2 diabetes in a randomised controlled trial. 3867 newly diagnosed patients with type 2 diabetes, median age 54 years (IQR 48-60 years), who after 3 months' diet treatment had a mean of two fasting plasma glucose (FPG) concentrations of 6.1-15.0 mmol/L were randomly assigned intensive policy with a sulphonylurea (chlorpropamide, glibenclamide, or glipizide) or with insulin, or conventional policy with diet. The aim in the intensive group was FPG less than 6 mmol/L. In the conventional group, the aim was the best achievable FPG with diet alone; drugs were added only if there were hyperglycaemic symptoms or FPG greater than 15 mmol/L. Three aggregate endpoints were used to assess differences between conventional and intensive treatment: any diabetes-related endpoint (sudden death, death from hyperglycaemia or hypoglycaemia, fatal or non-fatal myocardial infarction, angina, heart failure, stroke, renal failure, amputation [of at least one digit], vitreous haemorrhage, retinopathy requiring photocoagulation, blindness in one eye, or cataract extraction); diabetes-related death (death from myocardial infarction, stroke, peripheral vascular disease, renal disease, hyperglycaemia or hypoglycaemia, and sudden death); all-cause mortality. Over 10 years, haemoglobin A1c (HbA1c) was 7.0% (6.2-8.2) in the intensive group compared with 7.9% (6.9-8.8) in the conventional group--an 11% reduction. There was no difference in HbA1c among agents in the intensive group. Compared with the conventional group, the risk in the intensive group was 12% lower (95% CI 1-21, p=0.029) for any diabetes-related endpoint; 10% lower (-11 to 27, p=0.34) for any diabetes-related death; and 6% lower (-10 to 20, p=0.44) for all-cause mortality. Most of the risk reduction in the any diabetes-related aggregate endpoint was due to a 25% risk reduction (7-40, p=0.0099) in microvascular endpoints, including the need for retinal photocoagulation [77].

16. Veterans affairs cooperative study

Veterans Affairs Cooperative Study proved that intensive glycemic control retards microalbuminuria in patients who have had type 2 diabetes for several years but may not lessen the progressive deterioration of glomerular function. 153 male patients to either intensive treatment (INT) (goal HbA(1c) 7.1%) or to standard treatment (ST) (goal HbA(1c) 9.1%; P = 0.001), and data were obtained during a 2-year period. Mean duration of known diabetes was 8 years, mean age of the patients was 60 years, All patients were treated with insulin. INT retarded the progression of microalbuminuria during the 2-year period: the changes in albumin:creatinine ratio from baseline to 2 years of INT versus ST were 0.045 vs. 0.141, respectively (P = 0.046). Retardation of progressive urinary albumin excretion was most pronounced in those patients who entered the study with microalbuminuria and were randomized to INT. Patients entering with microalbuminuria had a deterioration in creatinine clearance at 2 years regardless of the intensity of glycemic control.The unexplainined finding was that in the group entering without microalbuminuria, the subgroup receiving ST had a lower percentage of patients with a macrovascular event (17%) than the subgroup receiving INT (36%) (P = 0.03) [78].

17. ACCORD

ACCORD study concluded that microvascular benefits of intensive therapy should be weighed against the increase in total and cardiovascular disease-related mortality, increased weight gain, and high risk for severe hypoglycaemia. 10251 patients were randomly assigned, 5128 to the intensive glycaemia control group and 5123 to standard group. Intensive therapy was stopped before study end because of higher mortality in that group, and patients were transitioned to standard therapy. At transition, the first composite outcome was recorded in 443 of 5107 patients in the intensive group versus 444 of 5108 in the standard group (HR 1.00, 95% CI 0.88-1.14; p=1.00), and the second composite outcome was noted in 1591 of 5107 versus 1659 of 5108 (0.96, 0.89-1.02; p=0.19). Results were similar at study end (first composite outcome 556 of 5119 vs 586 of 5115 [HR 0.95, 95% CI 0.85-1.07, p=0.42]; and second 1956 of 5119 vs 2046 of 5115, respectively [0.95, 0.89-1.01, p=0.12]). Intensive therapy did not reduce the risk of advanced measures of microvascular outcomes, but delayed the onset of albuminuria and some measures of eye complications and neuropathy [79].

18. VADT

VADT study investigated the intensive glucose control in patients with poorly controlled type 2 diabetes had no significant effect on the rates of major cardiovascular events, death, or microvascular complications with the exception of progression of albuminuria (P = 0.01). 1791 military veterans (mean age, 60.4 years) who had a suboptimal response to therapy for type 2 diabetes were assigned to receive either intensive or standard glucose control. The goal in the intensive-therapy group was an absolute reduction of 1.5 percentage points in the glycated hemoglobin level, as compared with the standard-therapy group. The primary outcome was the time from randomization to the first occurrence of a major cardiovascular event, a composite of myocardial infarction, stroke, death from cardiovascular causes, congestive heart failure, surgery for vascular disease, inoperable coronary disease, and amputation for ischemic gangrene. The median follow-up was 5.6 years. Median glycated hemoglobin levels were 8.4% in the standard-therapy group and 6.9% in the intensive-therapy group. The primary outcome occurred in 264 patients in the standard-therapy group and 235 patients in the intensive-therapy group (hazard ratio in the intensive-therapy group, 0.88; 95% confidence interval [CI], 0.74 to 1.05; P=0.14). There was no significant difference between the two groups in any component of the primary outcome or in the rate of death from any cause (hazard ratio, 1.07;

95% CI, 0.81 to 1.42; P=0.62). No differences between the two groups were observed for microvascular complications. The rates of adverse events, predominantly hypoglycemia, were 17.6% in the standard-therapy group and 24.1% in the intensive-therapy group [80].

19. Kumato study

Kumato study investigated a total of 110 Japanese patients with type 2 diabetes (55 with no retinopathy [the primary prevention cohort] and 55 with simple retinopathy [the secondary intervention cohort]) in an 8-year prospective study. The patients were randomly assigned to multiple insulin injection therapy (MIT) groups and administered three or more daily insulin injections or assigned to conventional insulin injection therapy (CIT) groups and administered one or two daily intermediate-acting insulin injections. Worsening of microvascular complications was regularly assessed during 8 years. In both primary prevention and secondary intervention cohorts, the cumulative percentages of worsening in retinopathy and nephropathy were significantly lower ($P < 0.05$) in the MIT group than in the CIT group. In neurological tests after 8 years, the MIT group showed significant improvement ($P < 0.05$) in the median nerve conduction velocities (motor and sensory nerves), whereas the CIT group showed significant deterioration ($P < 0.05$) in the nerve conduction velocities and vibration threshold. From this study, the glycemic threshold to prevent the onset and progression of diabetic microvascular complications was as follows: HbA1c < 6.5%, fasting blood glucose concentration < 110 mg/dl, and 2-h postprandial blood glucose concentration < 180 mg/dl [81]. Moreover, antihypertensive therapy and improved glycaemic control were independent predictors for remission. 151 patients with type 2 diabetes and microalbuminuria at baseline in whom GFR was measured at least three times during 7.8 years of follow-up were divided into three groups according to the level of albuminuria during follow-up. Overt nephropathy was diagnosed as a UAER>300 mg/24 h and remission to normoalbuminuria was defined as an UAER<30 mg/24 h at the last examination. During follow-up, 46 patients achieved remission to normoalbuminuria, 58 remained microalbuminuric and 47 patients progressed to overt nephropathy. The mean (+/- SE) yearly decline in GFR was lowest (2.3+/-0.4 ml/min/year) in patients who obtained remission, in comparison with patients remaining microalbuminuric, in whomthe decline was 3.7+/-0.4 ml/min/year, and patients progressing to overt nephropathy, who had a decline in GFR of 5.4+/-0.5 ml/min/year (ANOVA, P<0.001). Start of antihypertensive treatment during follow-up was strongly associated with remission to normoalbuminuria [odds ratio: 2.32; 95% confidence interval (CI): 1.09-4.93] whereas a decrease in HbA(1c) by 1% increased the probability for remission (odds ratio: 1.48; 95% CI: 1.11-1.97) [82]

20. Other diabetic treatment strategies

Other treatments were developed in addition to blood pressure control, glucose control and renin-angiotensin system blockade to slow kidney function deterioration. We will briefly discuss some of them.

- Vitamin D receptor (VDR) agonists. The main sources of vitamin D3 are diet and skin under the influence of solar ultraviolet action. Vitamin D3 is activated to 1,25dihydroxyvitamin D3 [1,25(0H)2 D3] by liver and kidney. VDR agonists are renal protective in diabetic patients. VDR agonists slow renal fibrosis through RAS blockade and have synergic effects in combinations ACE inhibitors or ARBS [83]. Two of VDR agonists, doxercalciferol and paricalcitol decrease proteinuria. Doxercalciferol effect was investigated in diet-induced obesity mice Proteinuria,, renal mesangial expansion and podocytes injury were slowed by doxercalciferol. Doxercalciferol also diminished oxidative stress, macrophage infiltration and profibrotic growth factors [84]. Paricalcitol was investigated in Vital study. Paricalcitol had a synergic effect with ACE inhibitors and ARBs and reduced proteinuria in type 2 diabetic patients [85].

- Farnesoid X receptor agonists (FXR). The hydrophobic bile acid, chenodeoxycholic acid, activates FXR and has an important role in preventing atherosclerosis, and controlling metabolic and bile acid homeostasis [86]. FXR was detected in kidney and other organs like liver and adrenal gland [87]. FXR agonists was investigated in FXR knockout mice. The studies proved that FXR agonists diminished proteinuria, glomerulosclerosis, tubulointerstital fibrosis and macrophage infiltration [85,88].

- AGEs inhibitors. The clinical utility of these agents remain to be proven. Studies with aminoguanidine (pimagenide) were interrupted due to safety concern. AGE breakers (N-phenacylthiazodium bromide and alagebrium chloride), anti-RAGE antibodies were used only in experimental models. Pyridoxamine (vitamin B6 derivate), an AGEs inhibitor, reduced proteinuria in several studies [89,90].

Pirfenidone and Bartoxolone. Pirfenidone [5-methyl-1-phenyl-2(1H)-pyrodone] is a synthetic antifibrotic agent. Pirfenidone blocks TGF- β promoter and secretron and reduces tubular and glomerural lesions in experimental models [91]. Bardoxolone has an antiinflamatory effect and acts through Nrf2 pathway. Nrf2 is a transcription factor controlling antioxidant genes that help maintain redox homeostasis. A phase 2, double-blind, randomized, placebo-controlled trial investigated the role of bardoxolone. 227 adults with CKD (defined as an estimated glomerular filtration rate [GFR] of 20 to 45 ml per minute per 1.73 m(2) of body-surface area) in a 1:1:1:1 ratio were assigned to receive placebo or bardoxolone methyl at a target dose of 25, 75, or 150 mg once daily. The primary outcome was the change from baseline in the estimated GFR with bardoxolone methyl, as compared with placebo, at 24 weeks; a secondary outcome was the change at 52 weeks. Patients receiving bardoxolone methyl had significant increases in the estimated GFR, as compared with placebo, at 24 weeks (with between-group differences per minute per 1.73 m(2) of 8.2±1.5 ml in the 25-mg group, 11.4±1.5 ml in the 75-mg group, and 10.4±1.5 ml in the 150-mg group; P<0.001). The increases were maintained through week 52, with significant differences per minute per 1.73 m^2 of 5.8±1.8 ml, 10.5±1.8 ml, and 9.3±1.9 ml, respectively. Muscle spasms, the most frequent adverse event in the bardoxolone methyl groups, were generally mild and dose-related. Hypomagnesemia, mild increases in alanine aminotransferase levels, and gastrointestinal effects were more common among patients receiving bardoxolone methyl [92].

21. Conclusion

Microalbuminuria and proteinuria are common complications among patients with type 2 diabetes. Proteinuria is a predictive factor for cardiovascular events, and cardiovascular and all-cause mortality. Microalbuminuria is defined as persistent urinary albumin excretion between 30 and 300 mg/day (20 to 200 µg/min). Macroalbuminuria refers to albumin excretion above 300 mg/day (200 µg/min). Patients with diabetes mellitus type 2 must be screened annually for proteinuria, starting at diagnosis. Measurement of the albumin:creatinine ratio in a first-morning void is the superior method to predict renal events in patients with type 2 diabetes and nephropathy, but the difference compared to spot urine samples at other times was not significant. Intervention studies in microalbuminuric type 2 diabetic patients have demonstrated that it is possible to avoid progression to overt diabetic nephropathy and even to achieve regression to normoalbuminuria. The best therapeutic strategy is a multifactorial approach including glycemic control, blood pressure control, renin-angiotensin inhibition and lifestyle modification.

Author details

Relu Cernes[1] and Reuven Zimlichman[2]

1 Department of Nephrology and The Brunner Institute for Cardiovascular Research, Wolfson Medical Center and Tel Aviv University, Israel

2 Chief Department of Medicine and The Brunner Institute for Cardiovascular Research, Wolfson Medical Center and Tel Aviv University, Israel

References

[1] Wild S, Roglic G, Green A, Sicree R, King H. Global prevalence of diabetes: estimates for the year 2000 and projections for 2030. Diabetes Care. 2004; 27(5):1047-53.

[2] Zimmet P, Alberti KG, Shaw J. Global and societal implications of the diabetes epidemic. Nature. 2001; 414(6865):782-7.

[3] Plantinga LC, Crews DC, Coresh J, MIller ER 3rd, Saran R, Yee J, Hedgeman E, Pavkov M, Eberhardt MS, Williams DE, Powe NR; CDC CKD Surveillance Team. Prevalence of chronic kidney disease in US adults with undiagnosed diabetes or prediabetes. Clin J Am Soc Nephrol. 2010;5(4):673 – 682.

[4] Ruggenenti P, Remuzzi G. Nephropathy of type-2 diabetes mellitus. J Am Soc Nephrol 1998; 9(11):2157.

[5] Eknoyan G, Hostetter T, Bakris GL, Hebert L, Levey AS, Parving HH, Steffes MW, Toto R. Proteinuria and other markers of chronic kidney disease: a position statement of the national kidney foundation (NKF) and the national institute of diabetes and digestive and kidney diseases (NIDDK). Am J Kidney Dis. 2003; 42(4):617-22.

[6] Adler AI, Stevens RJ, Manley SE, Bilous RW, Cull CA, Holman RR; UKPDS GROUP. Development and progression of nephropathy in type 2 diabetes: the United Kingdom Prospective Diabetes Study (UKPDS 64). Kidney Int. 2003; 63(1):225-32.

[7] García-Donaire JA, Segura J, Cerezo C, Ruilope LM. A review of renal, cardiovascular and mortality endpoints in antihypertensive trials in diabetic patients. Blood Press. 2011; 20(6):322-34

[8] Sarnak MJ, Levey AS, Schoolwerth AC, Coresh J, Culleton B, Hamm LL McCullough PA, Kasiske BL, Kelepouris E, Klag MJ, Parfrey P, Pfeffer M, Raij L, Spinosa DJ, Wilson PW; American Heart Association Councils on Kidney in Cardiovascular Disease, High Blood Pressure Research, Clinical Cardiology, and Epidemiology and Prevention. Kidney disease as a risk factor for development of cardiovascular disease: A statement from the American Heart Association Councils on Kidney in Cardiovascular Disease, High Blood Pressure Research, Clinical Cardiology, and Epidemiology and Prevention. Circulation. 2003;108(17):2154 – 2169.

[9] Weir MR. Microalbuminuria and cardiovascular disease. Clin J Am Soc Nephrol. 2007;2(3):581 – 590.

[10] McCullough PA, Li S, Jurkovitz CT, Stevens L, Collins AJ,Chen SC, Norris KC, McFarlane S, Johnson B, Shlipak MG, Obialo CI, Brown WW, Vassalotti J, Whaley-Connell AT, Brenner RM, Bakris GL; KEEP Investigators.. Chronic kidney disease, prevalence of premature cardiovascular disease, and relationship to short-term mortality. Am Heart J. 2008;156(2):277 – 283.

[11] Agrawal V, Marinescu V, Agarwal M, McCullough PA. Cardiovascular implications of proteinuria: An indicator of chronic kidney disease. Nat Rev Cardiol. 2009;6(4):301 – 311.

[12] Chronic Kidney Disease Prognosis Consortium, Matsushita K, van der Velde M, Astor BC, Woodward M, Levey AS, de Jong PE, Coresh J, Gansevoort RT. Association of estimated glomerular fi ltration rate and albuminuria with all-cause and cardiovascular mortality in general population cohorts: A collaborative meta-analysis.Lancet. 2010; 375(9731):2073 – 2081.

[13] Bilous R. Microvascular disease: what does the UKPDS tell us about diabetic nephropathy? Diabet Med. 2008; 25 Suppl 2:25-9.

[14] Pan CY, Ho LT, Soegondo S, Prodjosudjadi W, Suwanwalaikorn S, Lim SC, Chan TM, Chow KW, Thoenes M, Choi DS; DEMAND Study InvestigatorsPrevalence of albuminuria and cardiovascular risk profile in a referred cohort of patients with type 2 diabetes: an Asian perspective. Diabetes Technol Ther. 2008; 10(5):397-403.

[15] Freeman JS. Treating Hispanic patients for type 2 diabetes mellitus: special considerations. J Am Osteopath Assoc. 2008; 108(5 Suppl 3):S5-13.

[16] Gall ML, Hougaard P, Borch-Johnsen K, Parving HH. Significant risk factors for development of microalbuminuria and diabetic nephropathy in patients with non-insulin-dependent diabetes. Ugeskr Laeger. 1998; 160(31):4524-7.

[17] Araki S, Haneda M, Sugimoto T, Isono M, Isshiki K, Kashiwagi A, Koya D. Factors associated with frequent remission of microalbuminuria in patients with type 2 diabetes. Diabetes. 2005;54(10):2983-7.

[18] Abbate M, Zoja C, Remuzzi G. How does proteinuria cause progressive renal damage? J Am Soc Nephrol. 2006; 17(11):2974-84.

[19] Salmon AH, Neal CR, Harper SJ. New aspects of glomerular filtration barrier structure and function: five layers (at least) not three. Curr Opin Nephrol Hypertens. 2009; 18(3):197-205.

[20] Heathcote KL, Wilson MP, Quest DW, Wilson TW : Prevalence and duration in exercise induced albuminuria in healthy people. Clin Invest Med 2009;32(4): E261-E265

[21] Romanelli G, Giustina A, Bossoni S, Caldonazzo A, Cimino A, Cravarezza P, Giustina G. Short-term administration of captopril and nifedipine and exercise-induced albuminuria in normotensive diabetic patients with early-stage nephropathy. Diabetes. 1990; 39(11):1333-8.

[22] Kagami S, Border WA, Miller DE, Noble NA. Angiotensin II stimulates extracellular matrix protein synthesis through induction of transforming growth factor-beta expression in rat glomerular mesangial cells. J Clin Invest. 1994;93(6):2431-7.

[23] Hilgers KF, Veelken R. Type 2 diabetic nephropathy: never too early to treat? J Am Soc Nephrol 2005; 16(3):574.

[24] Thomas MC. Pathogenesis and Progression of Proteinuria,. Lai KN, Tang SCW (eds): Diabetes and the Kidney. Contrib Nephrol. 2011; 170: 48–56 .

[25] Singh A, Satchell SC, Neal CR, McKenzie EA, Tooke JE, Mathieson PW. Glomerular endothelial glycocalyx constitutes a barrier to protein permeability. J Am Soc Nephrol. 2007; 18(11):2885-93.

[26] Dalla Vestra M, Saller A, Bortoloso E, Mauer M, Fioretto P. Structural involvement in type 1 and type 2 diabetic nephropathy. Diabetes Metab. 2000; 26 Suppl 4:8-14.

[27] Welsh GI, Hale LJ, Eremina V, et al. Insulin signaling to the glomerular podocyte is critical for normal kidney function. Cell Metab 2010; 12(4):329.

[28] Fornoni A .Proteinuria, the podocyte, and insulin resistance. N Engl J Med 2010; 363(21):2068

[29] Gagliardini E, Conti S, Benigni A, Remuzzi G, Remuzzi A. Imaging of the porous ultrastructure of the glomerular epithelial filtration slit. J Am Soc Nephrol. 2010; 21(12): 2081-9.

[30] Forbes JM, Bonnet F, Russo LM, Burns WC, Cao Z, Candido R, Kawachi H, Allen TJ, Cooper ME, Jerums G, Osicka TM. Modulation of nephrin in the diabetic kidney: association with systemic hypertension and increasing albuminuria. J Hypertens. 2002; 20(5):985-92.

[31] Peti-Peterdi J, Sipos A. A high-powered view of the filtration barrier. J Am Soc Nephrol. 2010; 21(11):1835-41.

[32] Thomas MC, Burns WC, Cooper ME. Tubular changes in early diabetic nephropathy. Adv Chronic Kidney Dis. 2005; 12(2):177-86.

[33] Osicka TM, Houlihan CA, Chan JG, Jerums G, Comper WD. Albuminuria in patients with type 1 diabetes is directly linked to changes in the lysosome-mediated degradation of albumin during renal passage. Diabetes. 2000; 49(9):1579-84.

[34] Monnier VM, Sell DR, Nagaraj RH, Miyata S, Grandhee S, Odetti P, Ibrahim SA. Maillard reaction-mediated molecular damage to extracellular matrix and other tissue proteins in diabetes, aging, and uremia. Diabetes. 1992; 41 Suppl 2:36-41.

[35] Thomas MC. Advanced glycation end products. Contrib Nephrol. 2011;170:66-74.

[36] Coughlan MT, Thorburn DR, Penfold SA, Laskowski A, Harcourt BE, Sourris KC, Tan AL, Fukami K, Thallas-Bonke V, Nawroth PP, Brownlee M, Bierhaus A, Cooper ME, Forbes JM. RAGE-induced cytosolic ROS promote mitochondrial superoxide generation in diabetes. J Am Soc Nephrol. 2009;20(4):742-52.

[37] Flyvbjerg A, Denner L, Schrijvers BF, Tilton RG, Mogensen TH, Paludan SR, Rasch R. Long-term renal effects of a neutralizing RAGE antibody in obese type 2 diabetic mice. Diabetes. 2004; 53(1):166-72.

[38] Singh AK, Mo W, Dunea G, Arruda JA. Effect of glycated proteins on the matrix of glomerular epithelial cells. J Am Soc Nephrol 1998; 9(5):802-10.

[39] G Nguyen. Renin/prorenin receptors. Kidney International 2006; 69(9), 1503–1506.

[40] Ichihara A, Suzuki F, Nakagawa T, Kaneshiro Y, Takemitsu T, Sakoda M, Nabi AH, Nishiyama A, Sugaya T, Hayashi M, Inagami T. Prorenin receptor blockade inhibits development of glomerulosclerosis in diabetic angiotensin II type 1a receptor-deficient mice. J Am Soc Nephrol. 2006; 17(7):1950-61.

[41] Khoury CC, Ziyadeh FN. Angiogenic factors. Contrib Nephrol. 2011;170:83-92.

[42] Mironidou-Tzouveleki M, Tsartsalis S, Tomos C. Vascular endothelial growth factor (VEGF) in the pathogenesis of diabetic nephropathy of type 1 diabetes mellitus. Curr Drug Targets. 2011; 12(1):107-14.

[43] Woolf AS. Angiopoietins: vascular growth factors looking for roles in glomeruli. Curr Opin Nephrol Hypertens. 2010;19(1):20-5.

[44] Lan HY, Chung AC. Transforming growth factor-β and Smads. Contrib Nephrol. 2011;170:75-82.

[45] KDOQI. KDOQI Clinical Practice Guidelines and Clinical Practice Recommendations for Diabetes and Chronic Kidney Disease. Am J Kidney Dis. 2007; 49(2 Suppl 2):S12-154.

[46] Lambers Heerspink HJ, Gansevoort RT, Brenner BM, Cooper ME, Parving HH, Shahinfar S, de Zeeuw D. Comparison of different measures of urinary protein excretion for prediction of renal events. J Am Soc Nephrol. 2010; 21(8):1355-60.

[47] Mattix HJ, Hsu CY, Shaykevich S, Curhan G. Use of the albumin/creatinine ratio to detect microalbuminuria: implications of sex and race. J Am Soc Nephrol. 2002; 13(4): 1034-9.

[48] Newman DJ, Mattock MB, Dawnay AB, Kerry S, McGuire A, Yaqoob M, Hitman GA, Hawke C. Systematic review on urine albumin testing for early detection of diabetic complications. Health Technol Assess. 2005; 9(30):iii-vi, xiii-163.

[49] Ting RZ, Luk AO, Chan JC. Treatment and landmark clinical trials for renoprotection. Contrib Nephrol. 2011;170:184-95.

[50] Rodbard HW, Blonde L, Braithwaite SS, Brett EM, Cobin RH, Handelsman Y, Hellman R, Jellinger PS, Jovanovic LG, Levy P, Mechanick JI, Zangeneh F; AACE Diabetes Mellitus Clinical Practice Guidelines Task Force. American Association of Clinical Endocrinologists medical guidelines for clinical practice for the management of diabetes mellitus. Endocr Pract. 2007; 13 Suppl 1:1-68.

[51] Bakris GL. Recognition, pathogenesis, and treatment of different stages of nephropathy in patients with type 2 diabetes mellitus. Mayo Clin Proc. 2011; 86(5):444-56.

[52] Kuznik A, Mardekian J. Trends in utilization of lipid- and blood pressure-lowering agents and goal attainment among the U.S. diabetic population, 1999-2008. Cardiovasc Diabetol. 2011;10:31.

[53] Garcia-Touza M, Sowers JR. Evidence-based hypertension treatment in patients with diabetes. J Clin Hypertens (Greenwich). 2012; 14(2):97-102.

[54] SHEP Cooperative Research Group. Prevention of stroke by antihypertensive drug treatment in older persons with isolated systolic hypertension in the Elderly Program. JAMA. 1991;265(24):3255–3264.

[55] ALLHAT Officers and Coordinators for the ALLHAT Collaborative Research Group. Major outcomes in high-risk hypertensive patients randomized to angiotensin-converting enzyme inhibitor or calcium channel blocker vs diuretic: the Antihyperten-

sive and Lipid Lowering Treatment to Prevent Heart Attack Trial. JAMA. 2002;288(23): 2981–2997.

[56] Nissen SE, Tuzcu EM, Libby P, et al. Effect of antihypertensive agents on cardiovascular events in patients with coronary disease and normal blood pressure: the CAMELOT study: a randomized controlled trial. JAMA. 2004;292(18):2217–2225.

[57] Ravid M, Savin H, Jutrin I, Bental T, Katz B, Lishner M. Long-term stabilizing effect of angiotensin-converting enzyme inhibition on plasma creatinine and on proteinuria in normotensive type II diabetic patients. Ann Intern Med. 1993;118(8):577.

[58] Ravid M, Brosh D, Levi Z, Bar-Dayan Y, Ravid D, Rachmani R Use of enalapril to attenuate decline in renal function in normotensive, normoalbuminuric patients with type 2 diabetes mellitus. A randomized, controlled trial. Ann Intern Med. 1998;128(12 Pt 1):982.

[59] Parving HH, Lehnert H, Bröchner-Mortensen J, Gomis R, Andersen S, Arner P, Irbesartan in Patients with Type 2 Diabetes and Microalbuminuria Study Group The effect of irbesartan on the development of diabetic nephropathy in patients with type 2 diabetes. N Engl J Med. 2001;345(12):870.

[60] EijkelkampWBA Zhang Z Remuzzi G , Parving,HH,Cooper ME,_ KeaneWF , Shahinfar G, Gleim GW,. Weir MR, Brenner BM, de Zeeuw D. Albuminuria is a target for renoprotective therapy independent from blood pressure in patients with type 2 diabetic nephropathy: post hoc analysis from the Reduction of Endpoints in NIDDM with the Angiotensin II Antagonist Losartan (RENAAL) trial. J Am Soc Nephrol 2007; 18(5): 1540–1546.

[61] Viberti G, Wheeldon NM, MicroAlbuminuria Reduction With VALsartan (MARVAL) Study Investigators Microalbuminuria reduction with valsartan in patients with type 2 diabetes mellitus: a blood pressure-independent effect. Circulation. 2002;106(6):672.

[62] Haller H, Ito S, Izzo JL Jr, Januszewicz A, Katayama S, Menne J, Mimran A, Rabelink TJ, Ritz E, Ruilope LM, Rump LC, Viberti G, ROADMAP Trial Investigators Olmesartan for the delay or prevention of microalbuminuria in type 2 diabetes. N Engl J Med. 2011;364(10):907.

[63] Lindholm LH, Ibsen H, Dahlöf B, Devereux RB, Beevers G, de Faire U, Fyhrquist F, Julius S, Kjeldsen SE, Kristiansson K, Lederballe-Pedersen O, Nieminen MS, Omvik P, Oparil S, Wedel H, Aurup P, Edelman J, Snapinn S, LIFE Study Group Cardiovascular morbidity and mortality in patients with diabetes in the Losartan Intervention For Endpoint reduction in hypertension study (LIFE): a randomised trial against atenolol. Lancet. 2002;359(9311):1004.

[64] Bilous R, Chaturvedi N, Sjølie AK, Fuller J, Klein R, Orchard T, Porta M, Parving HH of candesartan on microalbuminuria and albumin excretion rate in diabetes: three randomized trials. Ann Intern Med. 2009;151(1):11.

[65] Schrier RW, Estacio RO, Esler A, Mehler P Effects of aggressive blood pressure control in normotensive type 2 diabetic patients on albuminuria, retinopathy and strokes. Kidney Int. 2002;61(3):1086.

[66] Barnett A. Preventing renal complications in type 2 diabetes: results of the diabetics exposed to telmisartan and enalapril trial. J Am Soc Nephrol. 2006; 17(4 Suppl 2):S132-5.

[67] Mogensen CE, Neldam S, Tikkanen I, Oren S, Viskoper R, Watts RW, Cooper ME Randomised controlled trial of dual blockade of renin-angiotensin system in patients with hypertension, microalbuminuria, and non-insulin dependent diabetes: the candesartan and lisinopril microalbuminuria (CALM) study. BMJ. 2000;321(7274):1440.

[68] Mann JF, Schmieder RE, McQueen M, Dyal L, Schumacher H, Pogue J, Wang X, Maggioni A, Budaj A, Chaithiraphan S, Dickstein K, Keltai M, Metsärinne K, Oto A, Parkhomenko A, Piegas LS, Svendsen TL, Teo KK, Yusuf S; ONTARGET investigators. Renal outcomes with telmisartan, ramipril, or both, in people at high vascular risk (the ONTARGET study): a multicentre, randomised, double-blind, controlled trial. Lancet. 2008; 372(9638):547-53.

[69] Imai E, Chan JC, Ito S, Yamasaki T, Kobayashi F, Haneda M, Makino H; ORIENT study investigators. Effects of olmesartan on renal and cardiovascular outcomes in type 2 diabetes with overt nephropathy: a multicentre, randomised, placebo-controlled study. Diabetologia. 2011; 54(12):2978-86.

[70] Patel A, ADVANCE Collaborative Group, MacMahon S, Chalmers J, Neal B, Woodward M, Billot L, Harrap S, Poulter N, Marre M, Cooper M, Glasziou P, Grobbee DE, Hamet P, Heller S, Liu LS, Mancia G, Mogensen CE, Pan CY, Rodgers A, Williams B Effects of a fixed combination of perindopril and indapamide on macrovascular and microvascular outcomes in patients with type 2 diabetes mellitus (the ADVANCE trial): a randomised controlled trial.Lancet. 2007;370(9590):829.

[71] Ruggenenti P, Fassi A, Ilieva AP, Bruno S, Iliev IP, Brusegan V, Rubis N, Gherardi G, Arnoldi F, Ganeva M, Ene-Iordache B, Gaspari F, Perna A, Bossi A, Trevisan R, Dodesini AR, Remuzzi G, Bergamo Nephrologic Diabetes Complications Trial (BENEDICT) Investigators Preventing microalbuminuria in type 2 diabetes N Engl J Med. 2004;351(19):1941.

[72] Parving HH,Persson F, Lewis JB, Lewis EJ, Hollenberg NK: Aliskiren combined with losartan in type 2 diabetes and nephropathy. N Engl J Med 2008;358(23):2433-2446.

[73] Mehdi UF, Adams-Huet B, Raskin P, Vega GL, Toto RD. Addition of angiotensin receptor blockade or mineralocorticoid antagonism to maximal angiotensin-converting enzyme inhibition in diabetic nephropathy. J Am Soc Nephrol. 2009; 20(12):2641-50.

[74] Houlihan CA, Allen TJ, Baxter AL, Panangiotopoulos S, Casley DJ, Cooper ME, Jerums G. A low-sodium diet potentiates the effects of losartan in type 2 diabetes. Diabetes Care. 2002; 25(4):663-71.

[75] Jun M, Perkovic V, Cass A. Intensive glycemic control and renal outcome. Contrib Nephrol. 2011;170:196-208.

[76] ADVANCE Collaborative Group, Patel A, MacMahon S, Chalmers J, Neal B, Billot L, Woodward M, Marre M, Cooper M, Glasziou P, Grobbee D, Hamet P, Harrap S, Heller S, Liu L, Mancia G, Mogensen CE, Pan C, Poulter N, Rodgers A, Williams B, Bompoint S, de Galan BE, Joshi R, Travert F. Intensive blood glucose control and vascular outcomes in patients with type 2 diabetes. N Engl J Med. 2008 12;358(24):2560-72.

[77] [No authors listed] Intensive blood-glucose control with sulphonylureas or insulin compared with conventional treatment and risk of complications in patients with type 2 diabetes (UKPDS 33). UK Prospective Diabetes Study (UKPDS) Group. Lancet. 1998; 352(9131):837-53.

[78] Levin SR, Coburn JW, Abraira C, Henderson WG, Colwell JA, Emanuele NV, Nuttall FQ, Sawin CT, Comstock JP, Silbert CK. Effect of intensive glycemic control on microalbuminuria in type 2 diabetes. Veterans Affairs Cooperative Study on Glycemic Control and Complications in Type 2 Diabetes Feasibility Trial Investigators. Diabetes Care. 2000; 23(10):1478-85.

[79] Ismail-Beigi F, Craven T, Banerji MA, Basile J, Calles J, Cohen RM, Cuddihy R, Cushman WC, Genuth S, Grimm RH Jr, Hamilton BP, Hoogwerf B, Karl D, Katz L, Krikorian A, O'Connor P, Pop-Busui R, Schubart U, Simmons D, Taylor H, Thomas A, Weiss D, Hramiak I; ACCORD trial group. Effect of intensive treatment of hyperglycaemia on microvascular outcomes in type 2 diabetes: an analysis of the ACCORD randomised trial. Lancet. 2010; 376(9739):419-30.

[80] Duckworth W, Abraira C, Moritz T, Reda D, Emanuele N, Reaven PD, Zieve FJ, Marks J, Davis SN, Hayward R, Warren SR, Goldman S, McCarren M, Vitek ME, Henderson WG, Huang GD; VADT Investigators. Glucose control and vascular complications in veterans with type 2 diabetes. N Engl J Med. 2009; 360(2):129-39.

[81] Shichiri M, Kishikawa H, Ohkubo Y, Wake N. Long-term results of the Kumamoto Study on optimal diabetes control in type 2 diabetic patients. Diabetes Care. 2000; 23 Suppl 2:B21-9.

[82] Gaede P, Tarnow L, Vedel P, Parving HH, Pedersen O Remission to normoalbuminuria during multifactorial treatment preserves kidney function in patients with type 2 diabetes and microalbuminuria. Nephrol Dial Transplant. 2004;19(11):2784

[83] Levi M, Wang X, Choudhury D. Nuclear hormone receptors as therapeutic targets. Contrib Nephrol. 2011;170:209-16.

[84] Jiang T, Wang Z, Proctor G, Moskowitz S, Liebman SE, Rogers T, Lucia MS, Li J, Levi M. Diet-induced obesity in C57BL/6J mice causes increased renal lipid accumulation and glomerulosclerosis via a sterol regulatory element-binding protein-1c-dependent pathway. J Biol Chem. 2005; 280(37):32317-25.

[85] de Zeeuw D, Agarwal R, Amdahl M, Audhya P, Coyne D, Garimella T, Parving HH, Pritchett Y, Remuzzi G, Ritz E, Andress D. Selective vitamin D receptor activation with paricalcitol for reduction of albuminuria in patients with type 2 diabetes (VITAL study): a randomised controlled trial. Lancet. 2010;376(9752):1543-51.

[86] Wang H, Chen J, Hollister K, Sowers LC, Forman BM. Endogenous bile acids are ligands for the nuclear receptor FXR/BAR. Mol Cell. 1999; 3(5):543-53.

[87] Lefebvre P, Cariou B, Lien F, Kuipers F, Staels B. Role of bile acids and bile acid receptors in metabolic regulation. Physiol Rev. 2009; 89(1):147-91.

[88] Miyazaki-Anzai S, Levi M, Kratzer A, Ting TC, Lewis LB, Miyazaki M .Farnesoid X receptor activation prevents the development of vascular calcification in ApoE-/- mice with chronic kidney disease. Circ Res. 2010; 106(12):1807-17.

[89] Mathew A, Cunard R, Sharma K. Antifibrotic treatment and other new strategies for improving renal outcomes. Contrib Nephrol. 2011;170:217-27.

[90] Tanimoto M, Gohda T, Kaneko S, Hagiwara S, Murakoshi M, Aoki T, Yamada K, Ito T, Matsumoto M, Horikoshi S, Tomino Y. Effect of pyridoxamine (K-163), an inhibitor of advanced glycation end products, on type 2 diabetic nephropathy in KK-A(y)/Ta mice. Metabolism. 2007; 56(2):160-7.

[91] RamachandraRa0000000o SP, Zhu Y, Ravasi T, McGowan TA, Toh I, Dunn SR, Okada S, Shaw MA, Sharma K. Pirfenidone is renoprotective in diabetic kidney disease. J Am Soc Nephrol. 2009; 20(8):1765-75.

[92] Pergola PE, Raskin P, Toto RD, Meyer CJ, Huff JW, Grossman EB, Krauth M, Ruiz S, Audhya P, Christ-Schmidt H, Wittes J, Warnock DG; BEAM Study Investigators. Bardoxolone methyl and kidney function in CKD with type 2 diabetes. N Engl J Med. 2011; 28;365(4):327-36.

Chapter 10

Diabetes and Cancer

Subhashini Yaturu

Additional information is available at the end of the chapter

http://dx.doi.org/10.5772/56419

1. Introduction

Diabetes and cancer are two common conditions. Many epidemiological studies suggest frequent co-occurrence of diabetes and cancer. Meta-analyses and the summary of recommendations from the American Diabetes Association (ADA) and American Cancer Society suggest association of cancer and diabetes including liver, pancreas, endometrial, colorectal, breast and bladder cancers.[1] Diabetes appears to protect against prostate cancer based on decreased incidence of prostate cancer in subjects with diabetes. Lung cancer appears not to be associated with diabetes, and data is inconclusive for renal cell cancer and lymphoma.[1] Most of the association data is on the relation of cancer to type 2 diabetes. The major concern is that type 2 diabetes is associated with three of the five leading causes of cancer mortality such as carcinoma of the colon [2], pancreas [3] and breast (postmenopausal) [4]. The excess risk for each cancer is ~30% (colon), ~50% (pancreas) and ~20% (breast). The majority of the epidemiological data on cancer incidence and mortality had been obtained in type 2 diabetic patients. A cohort study to examine cancer incidence among 29,187 patients in Sweden who were hospitalized for type 1 diabetes from 1965 through 1999, observed 355 incident cases of cancer and which corresponded to a 20% increase in overall cancer incidence among type 1 diabetes patients (RR:1.2; CI: 1.0 to 1.3) [5]. Patients with type 1 diabetes had elevated risks of cancers of the stomach (RR: 2.3; CI: 1.1 to 4.1), cervix (R: 1.6; CI: 1.1 to 2.2), and endometrium (RR: 2.7; CI: 1.4 to 4.7) [5]. Hyperinsulinemia most likely favors cancer in diabetic patients as insulin is a growth factor with pre-eminent metabolic as well as mitogenic effects. Insulin action in malignant cells is favored by mechanisms acting at both the receptor and post-receptor level. Obesity, hyperglycemia, and increased oxidative stress may also contribute to increased cancer risk in diabetes [6]. There are reports of concern of hypoglycemic therapies on cancer risk, especially with insulin analogue-Glargine. A growing body of evidence suggests that metformin potentially reduces the risk of cancer. Aspirin and non-aspirin non-steroidal anti-inflammatory drugs appear to reduce recurrence of adenomas and incidence of advanced adenomas in individuals with an increased risk of colorectal adenomas and colorectal cancer, and calcium may reduce recurrence of adenomas [7, 8]. In this chapter we will include epidemiological evidence of association of diabetes and cancer, possible mechanisms and the effect of hypoglycemic agents in relation to cancer.

2. Epidemiology of diabetes and cancer risk

The Centers for Disease Control and Prevention (CDC) reports that 25.8 million people (8.3% of the U.S. population) have diabetes. Among them, 18.8 million people have diagnosed diabetes and 7.0 million people have undiagnosed diabetes. http://www.cdc.gov/diabetes/pubs/estimates11.htm#1. Three hundred and forty six million people worldwide have diabetes. Type 2 diabetes comprises 90% of people with diabetes around the world, and is largely the result of excess body weight and physical inactivity. http://www.who.int/mediacentre/factsheets/fs312/en/index.html. The incidence of diabetes is increasing globally. The estimated incidence of 12.7 million new cancer cases in 2008 will rise to 21.4 million by 2030, with nearly two thirds of all cancer diagnoses occurring in low- and middle-income countries. http://www.who.int/nmh/publications/ncd_report_chapter1.pdf. A series of recent studies and meta-analyses confirm that the risk for several solid and hematologic malignancies (including liver, pancreas, colorectal, kidney, bladder, endometrial and breast cancers, and non-Hodgkin's lymphoma) is increased in patients with diabetes [6]. Here the discussion follows on each malignancy with increased frequency in diabetes.

2.1. Pancreatic cancer

Type 2 diabetes mellitus is considered to be the third modifiable risk factor for pancreatic cancer after cigarette smoking and obesity. Based on the meta-analysis of 36 case–control and cohort studies, Everhart and Wright reported that the age and sex adjusted odds ratio for the development of pancreatic cancer in people with diabetes was 1.8 (CI of 1.7–1.9) [9]. They also noted that increased frequency of pancreatic cancer occurs with long-standing diabetes, especially those with the duration of at least 5 years with a RR of 2.0 with CI of 1.2 to 3.2 [9]. Gallo *et al* [10] from Italy reported that 40.2% of patients with pancreatic cancer and diabetes were diagnosed concomitantly or 15.9% were diagnosed within two years prior to diagnosis of cancer. Based on the data, the authors concluded increased prevalence of diabetes is related to pancreatic cancer and the diabetes is caused by the tumor [10]. A causal relationship between diabetes and pancreatic cancer is also supported by findings from pre-diagnostic evaluations of glucose and insulin levels in prospective studies. Data show that up to 80% of patients with pancreatic cancer are either hyperglycemic or diabetic. Diabetes has been shown to improve after pancreatic-cancer resection, suggesting that diabetes is caused by the cancer [11]. Pannala *et al* suggest new-onset diabetes may indicate subclinical pancreatic cancer, and patients with new-onset diabetes may constitute a population in whom pancreatic cancer can be detected early [11]. A meta-analysis of three cohorts and six case-control studies revealed even a two-fold risk in type 1 diabetes patients [12]. A meta-analysis of 36 studies was carried out by Huxley and associates that included17 case-control and 19 cohort or nested case-control studies with information on 9220 individuals with pancreatic cancer [3]. They noted that individuals with recent diagnosis of diabetes (< 4 years) had a 50% greater risk of the malignancy compared with individuals who had diabetes for ≥ 5 years (OR 2.1 vs. 1.5; $p = 0.005$).

2.2. Colorectal cancer

Increasing evidence suggests that a history of diabetes mellitus (DM) may be associated with an increased risk of colorectal cancer (CRC). In 2005, meta-analyses of 15 studies (six case-control and nine cohort studies) in the USA and Europe, including 2 593 935 participants, Larsson and associates found that diabetes was associated with an increased risk of colorectal cancer, compared with no diabetes (RR: 1.30; CI: 1.20–1.40] [2]. These results were said to be consistent between case-control and cohort studies and across the United States and Europe. The association did not differ significantly by sex, or by cancer sub-site. Diabetes was positively associated with colorectal cancer mortality. Results from a meta analysis of 41 cohorts was reported to support that diabetes was associated with an increased incidence of CRC (RR: 1.27;1.21-1.34) [13]. In a recent systematic review and meta-analysis, twenty-four studies including eight case-control and 16 cohort studies, with a total of 3,659,341 participants were included [14]. Meta-analysis of the 24 included studies indicated that diabetes was associated with an increased risk of colorectal cancer, compared with no diabetes (RR: 1.26; CI: 1.20-1.31), without heterogeneity between studies (p (heterogeneity) = 0.296). Sub-group analyses found that these results were consistent between case-control and cohort studies and among studies conducted in different areas. The association between diabetes and colorectal cancer incidence did not differ significantly by sex and sub-sites. Insulin therapy was also positively associated with risk of colorectal cancer (RR = 1.61; 1.18-1.35), with evidence of heterogeneity between studies (p (heterogeneity) = 0.014).

2.3. COX-2 and colon cancer

Although COX-2, the inducible isoform, is regularly expressed at low levels in colonic mucosa, its activity increases dramatically following mutation of the adenomatous polyposis coli (APC) gene, suggesting that β-catenin/T cell factor-mediated Wnt signaling activity may regulate COX-2 gene expression. In addition, hypoxic conditions and sodium butyrate exposure may also contribute to COX-2 gene transcription in human cancers [15]. Because of its role in carcinogenesis, apoptosis, and angiogenesis, it is an excellent target for developing new drugs with selectivity for prevention and/or treatment of human cancers [16].

2.4. Breast cancer

Meta-analyses of 20 studies (5 case-control and 15 cohort studies) by Larsson and associates found that women with diabetes had a statistically significant 20% increased risk of breast cancer (RR, 1.20; CI:1.12-1.28) compared with no diabetes [4]. The summary estimates were similar for case-control studies (RR, 1.18; CI: 1.05-1.32) and cohort studies (RR, 1.20; CI: 1.11-1.30). Meta-analysis of 5 cohort studies on diabetes and mortality from breast cancer yielded a summary RR of 1.24 and CI of 0.95-1.62 for women with versus without diabetes. Findings from this meta-analysis indicate that diabetes is associated with an increased risk of breast cancer [4]. In the

Nurses' Health Study, a total of 87,143 postmenopausal women, aged 30 to 55 years and free of cancer, were followed up for up to 26 years (1976-2002) and evaluated for the incidence of invasive breast cancer with increase in weight of at least 25.0 kg or more since age 18 years. Eliassen and associates noted an increased risk of breast cancer (RR: 1.45; CI: 1.27-1.66; *p* <. 001), with a stronger association among women who have never taken postmenopausal hormones (RR, 1.98; CI: 1.55-2.53). Data suggest that weight gain during adult life, specifically since menopause, increases the risk of breast cancer among postmenopausal women, whereas weight loss after menopause is associated with a decreased risk of breast cancer [17].

1. Non-modifiable risk factors:
a. Age
b. Sex
c. Ethnicity
2. Modifiable risk factors:
a. Overweight/obesity
b. Physical activity
c. Diet
3. Biological links:
a. Hyperglycemia
b. Insulin
c. IGF-1
d. Estrogen and androgen bioavailability
e. Cytokines

Table 1. Risk factors common to both diabetes and cancer

3. Pathophysiology

3.1. Hyperinsulinemia and cancer

Hyperinsulinemia most likely favors cancer in diabetic patients as insulin is a growth factor with pre-eminent metabolic but also mitogenic effects, and its action in malignant cells is favored by mechanisms acting at both the receptor and post-receptor level. Obesity, hyperglycemia, and increased oxidative stress may also contribute to increased cancer risk in diabetes [6].

3.2. Insulin

Insulin resistance and hyperinsulinemia are important factors in the development of type 2 diabetes. Insulin is known to stimulate cell proliferation and injection of insulin in rats

http://dx.doi.org/10.5772/56419

promoted carcinogen-induced colon cancer [18]. Insulin/insulin-like growth factor 1(IGF-1) receptors and G protein-coupled receptors (GPCR) signaling systems are implicated in autocrine-paracrine stimulation of a variety of malignancies, including ductal adenocarcinoma of the pancreas. Metformin, the most widely used drug in the treatment of type 2 diabetes, activates AMP kinase (AMPK), which negatively regulates mammalian target of rapamycin (mTOR) complex 1 (mTORC1) [19]. Metformin was shown to significantly decrease the growth of pancreatic cancer cells xenografted into the flank of nude mice by interrupting the G protein-coupled receptor (GPCR), insulin receptor signaling by down-regulating the mTOR pathway [20]. The GPCR and insulin receptor pathways are associated with increased DNA synthesis and pancreatic cancer cell growth. By negatively regulating GPCR and insulin receptor signally, and interrupting their cross talk, metformin is shown to decrease pancreatic cancer cell growth in mice. In a meta-analysis of epidemiological studies on markers of hyperinsulinemia and cancer, Pisani reported that subjects who develop colorectal and pancreatic cancers have increased pre-diagnostic blood levels of insulin and glucose [21]. High insulin levels have also been shown to be associated with risk of endometrial cancer independent of estradiol [22]. A link between breast cancer risk and hyperinsulinemia (measured by fasting C-peptide levels) has been shown mainly in postmenopausal breast cancer. Insulin levels were positively associated with endometrial carcinoma [HR: 2.33, CI: 1.13-4.82] among women not using hormone therapy [23].

3.3. Insulin resistance

The term insulin resistance denotes that action of insulin is impaired in peripheral target tissues that include skeletal muscle, liver, and adipose tissue. Recent literature supports the hypothesis that insulin resistance is a high risk for cancers. The molecular mechanisms for this association and the role in the neoplastic transformation process are being explored. Insulin is a major anabolic hormone that can stimulate cell proliferation. Adiposity induces adverse local and systemic effects that include adipocyte intracellular lipid accumulation, endoplasmic reticulum and mitochondrial stress, and insulin resistance, with associated changes in circulating adipokines, free fatty acids, and inflammatory mediators. Insulin resistance and associated hyperglycemia, hyperinsulinemia, and inflammation have been suggested to be the underlying mechanisms contributing to development of diabetes-associated pancreatic cancer. Hyperinsulinemia, insulin resistance and proinflammatory cytokines have been linked to neoplastic proliferation of various organ cells (Fig. 1).

In a study of the Polyp Prevention Trial of insulin and fasting glucose and risk of recurrent colorectal adenomas, Flood et al. noted the association of increased risk of adenoma recurrence and risk for recurrence of advanced adenomas with increased insulin [24].

3.4. Insulin-like Growth Factor-1 (IGF-1) and cancer

The IGF (insulin-like growth factor) system is essential for physiological growth. The IGF complex includes IGF-1 and IGF-2, their corresponding receptors (IGFR-1 and IGFR-2), IGF binding proteins 1–6 (IGFBPs), insulin receptor substrate (IRS). The signaling pathway of IGF plays a critical role in cellular proliferation and inhibition of apoptosis. Though growth

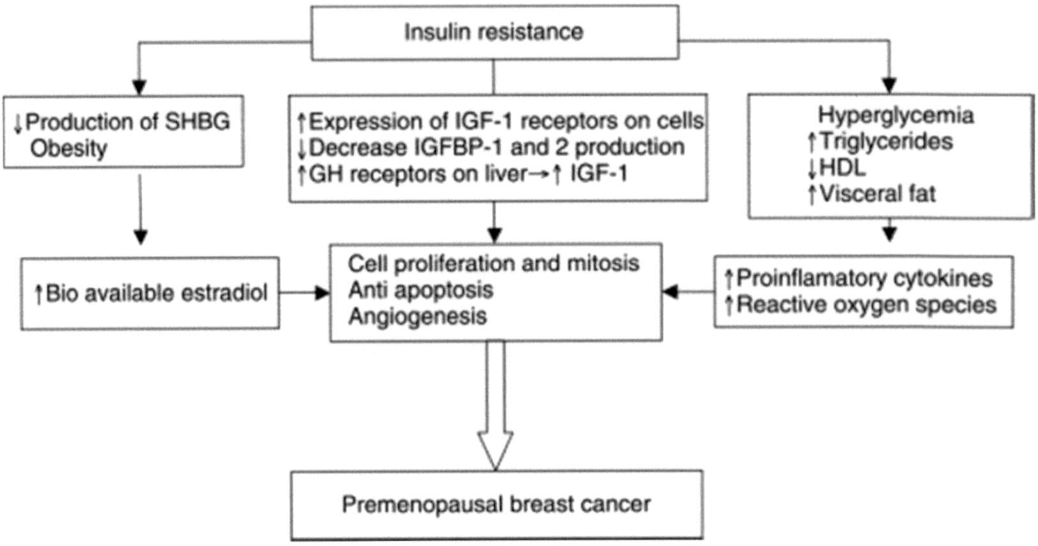

Figure 1. Insulin resistance and premenopausal breast cancer. Abbreviations: SHBG, sex hormone-binding globulin; IGF, insulin-like growth factor; GH, growth hormone; HDL, high-density lipoprotein cholesterol.

hormone is the primary stimulus for IGF-1 production in the liver and insulin can increase the IGF-1 production by up-regulating growth hormone receptors in the liver, hyperinsulinemia can also increase IGF-1 bioavailability by decreasing hepatic secretion of IGF-binding protein (IGFBP)-1 and −2 [25]. IGF-R, a tyrosine kinase receptor for IGF-I and IGF-II is said to play a role in malignant transformation, progression, protection from apoptosis, and metastasis as documented in cell culture, animal and human studies [26]. Since the expression of IGF-1 receptors occurs in several cancers, the effects of insulin on cancer cell proliferation *in vivo* may involve IGF-1 stimulation and indirectly stimulate cancers. The IGF signaling pathway is involved in cell proliferation and differentiation and inhibits apoptosis. Increased expression of IGF-1, IGF-2, IGF-1R, or combinations have been documented in various malignancies including glioblastomas, neuroblastomas, meningiomas, medulloblastomas, carcinomas of the breast, malignancies of the gastrointestinal tract, such as colorectal and pancreatic carcinomas, and ovarian cancer [27]. Higher IGF-1 levels were reported to be associated with increased colorectal adenoma risk (ORs = 1.58; 1.16-2.16),[28] and inversely associated with endometrial carcinoma (HR: 0.53; 0.31-0.90) [23].

3.5. Adiponectin and cancer

Adiponectin, which is also referred to as ACP30 (Acrp30), is secreted predominantly by white adipose tissue [29]. Circulating concentrations of adiponectin are reduced in obesity and type 2 diabetes [30-32]. Adiponectin is considered to have beneficial antineoplastic effects, which are believed to be due to anti-proliferative, anti-inflammatory effects, along with antagonizing insulin resistance [33]. Adiponectin has been found to be an important negative regulator of hematopoiesis and the immune system as adiponectin was shown to suppress the growth of myelomonocyte cell lines *in vitro* by inducing apoptosis in myelomonocytic progenitor cells (leukaemia lines) and modulating expression of apoptosis-related genes and down regulating Bcl-2 gene expression [34]. Epidemilogical data have also shown a link between low adiponectin levels and renal cell cancer [35, 36]; especially large tumor size [37, 38]. Adiponectin was inversely associated with non-Hodgkin lymphoma and acute myeloblastic leukaemia (OR: 0.56; 0.34-0.94), but not with acute lymphoblastic leukaemia of B or T cell [39]. In a number of epidemiological studies, adiponectin levels have been linked to breast cancer and are believed to inhibit breast cancer cell proliferation *in vivo*. This effect may be due to adiponectin-triggered cellular apoptosis in MDA-MB-231 breast cancer cells in the presence of 17β-estradiol. These findings may suggest that a cross-talk between adiponectin and estrogen receptor signaling exists in breast cancer cells and that adiponectin effects on the growth and apoptosis of breast cancer cells *in vitro* are dependent on the presence of 17β-estradiol [40]. Low serum adiponectin is associated with colon, prostate and breast cancer [41]. In a recent study, plasma adiponectin level was associated with decreased colorectal cancer risk [42].

Adiponectin and colorectal cancer: Adiponectin was shown to act on preneoplastic colon epithelial cells to regulate cell growth by inducing autocrine IL-6 production and trans-IL-6 signaling. In a prospective case control study, men with low plasma adiponectin levels were said to have a higher risk of colorectal cancer than men with higher levels [43]. Meta analysis of 13 studies in patients with colorectal cancer and adenoma, though there was significant heterogeneity among studies, noted that there was a negative dose response relationship between levels of adiponectin and the risk of colorectal neoplasm in men [44].

Adiponectin and Endometrial cancer: Circulating adiponectin concentrations are inversely correlated with the incidence of endometrial carcinoma in epidemiological studies. In a study that investigated the direct effects of adiponectin on two endometrial carcinoma cell lines, HEC-1-A and RL95–2, adiponectin treatment led to suppression of cell proliferation in both cell types, which was primarily believed to be due to the significant increase of cell populations at G_1/G_0 phase and secondary to the induction of apoptosis [45].

3.6. Obesity and cancer

Accumulating epidemiologic evidence shows that obesity is associated with an increased risk of several common adult cancers. The risk of diabetes increases linearly with BMI; the prevalence of diabetes increased from 2% in those with a BMI of 25 to 29.9 kg/m2, to 8% in those with a BMI of 30 to 34.9 kg/m2, and finally to 13% in those with a BMI greater than 35 kg/m2 [46]. Similarly, an association between obesity or an incremental increase in body mass index (BMI) and an increased cancer risk have been reported for colon cancer (men and women) and rectal cancer (men only),[47] colon cancer,[48] liver cancer,[49] gall bladder cancer,[50] multiple myeloma, non-Hodgkin's lymphoma,[51] pancreatic cancer,[52] leukemia,[53] ovarian cancer,[54] breast cancer,[55] and endometrial cancer [56, 57]. In a population based prospective study of more than 900,000 U.S. adults, the reported relative risk of cancers in overweight and obesity was 1.52 for men and 1.62 for women [18]. A study from the United

Kingdom showed that increasing BMI was associated with an increased incidence of endometrial cancer (RR:2.89, CI: 2.62–3.18), adenocarcinoma of the esophagus (RR:2.38;CI: 1.59–3.56), kidney cancer (RR:1.53, CI: 1.27–1.84), leukemia (RR:1.50, CI:1.23–1.83), multiple myeloma (RR:1.31;CI: 1.04–1.65), pancreatic cancer (RR:1.24;CI: 1.03–1.48), non-Hodgkin's lymphoma (RR:1.17; CI: 1.03–1.34), ovarian cancer (RR: 1.14; CI: 1.03–1.27), all cancers combined (RR:1.12; CI:1.09–1.14), breast cancer in postmenopausal women (RR: 1.40; CI: 1.31–1.49), and colorectal cancer in premenopausal women (RR:1.61; CI: 1.05–2.48) [58]. It is not surprising to note that increased adiposity may have a negative effect on treatment outcome and ultimate survival, because obesity has been found to be a negative prognostic factor for breast cancer[59] and colon cancer [60, 61].

3.7. Cyclooxygenase and cancers

Cyclooxygenase-2 (COX-2) over expression has been found in several types of human cancers, such as colon, breast, prostate, and pancreas, and appears to control many cellular processes. The contribution of COX-2 to carcinogenesis and the malignant phenotype of tumor cells have been thought to be related to its abilities to: (1) increase production of prostaglandins, (2) convert procarcinogens to carcinogens, (3) inhibit apoptosis, (4) promote angiogenesis, (5) modulate inflammation and immune function, and (6) increase tumor cell invasiveness [62].

3.8. Proinflammatory cytokines

Adipocytes secrete a number of proinflammatory cytokines. These cytokines are known to promote insulin resistance and increase circulating TG, features of the metabolic syndrome. Several cytokines, reactive oxygen species (ROS), and mediators of the inflammatory pathway, such as activation of nuclear factor-κB (NF-κB) and COX-2, lead to an increase in cell proliferation, survival, and inhibition of the proapoptotic pathway, ultimately resulting in tumor angiogenesis, invasion, and metastasis [16]. Proinflammatory cytokines implicated in carcinogenesis include IL-1, IL-6, IL-15, colony-stimulating factors, TNF-α, and the macrophage migration inhibitory factor.

Macrophage inhibitory cytokine-1 (MIC-1), also known as prostate-derived factor (PDF), is a molecule of the TGF-β super family and has been associated with the progression of various types of diseases including prostate cancer [63]. Collectively, cytokines are considered as a linker between inflammation and cancer. Cytokines, ROS, and mediators of the inflammatory pathway (e.g., NF-κB and COX-2) have been shown to increase cell cycling, cause loss of tumor suppressor function, and stimulate oncogene expression and lead to cancers. Positive feedback mechanisms between estrogens and inflammatory factors may exist in the breast and contribute to hormone-dependent breast cancer growth and progression [64]. Prostaglandin E synthase (PTGES) is also up-regulated by the proinflammatory cytokines TNF-α or IL-1β. Cytokines can enhance estrogen receptor (ER) activity and PTGES expression through the NF-κB pathway and cytokines can act to up-regulate aromatase expression as well as 17β-hydroxysteroid dehydrogenase activity in breast tissue, thereby leading to a further increase in E2 production [64].

http://dx.doi.org/10.5772/56419

4. Diabetes therapies and cancer

Diabetes is associated with increased risks of bladder, breast, colorectal, endometrial, kidney, liver and pancreatic cancer and a lower risk of prostate cancer. Diabetes treatments may influence the risk of cancer independently of their effect on glycemia. This may complicate the issues in investigation of the association between diabetes and cancer. Epidemiologic studies have suggested a protective role for metformin. On the other hand, Glargine, the most widely used long-acting insulin analogue, may confer a greater risk than other insulin preparations, particularly for breast cancer. In general, diabetes therapies that are said to be associated with increased risk of cancer include, use of insulin, sulfonyl urea and DPP4 inhibitors. Diabetes therapies that are shown benefit by decreasing the cancer risk include use of metformin and thiazolidinediones. Here we will discuss association of cancer risk with each of the diabetes therapeutic agents.

4.1. Thiazolidinedione (TZD) and cancer risk in type 2 diabetes

TZDs are reported to decrease in cancer both in clinical data series and in vitro studies. In addition pioglitazone, one of the TZDs, was shown to increase the risk of bladder cancer in those with the use for more than 24 months. Based on the randomized clinical trials of rosiglitazone with duration of >24 weeks that includes eighty trials enrolling 16,332 and 12,522 patients in the rosiglitazone and comparator groups, Monami and associates reported that the incidence of malignancies was significantly lower with the use of rosiglitazone than in control groups (RR: 0.23; CI: 0.19–0.26) vs. RR of 0.44(CI:0.34–0.58) cases/100 patient-years; $p < 0.05$) [65]. In a study using the diabetes registry of Hong Kong, Yang and associates reported that TZD usage was associated with 83% reduction in cancer risk in Chinese patients with type 2 diabetes in a dose–response manner [66]. Using the Taiwan National Health Insurance claims database, significantly lower risk of liver cancer incidence was found for any use of rosiglitazone or pioglitazone; use of rosiglitazone but not pioglitazone was associated with decreased incidence of colorectal cancer [67].

4.2. Pioglitazone and bladder cancer

Using the Kaiser Permanente Northern California diabetes registry with 193,099 patients who were ≥40 years of age between 1997 and 2002, excluding those with prior bladder cancer, 30,173 patients treated with pioglitazone were identified. In this cohort of patients with diabetes, short-term use of pioglitazone was not associated with an increased incidence of bladder cancer, but use for more than 2 years was weakly associated with increased risk [68].

Using the general practice research database in the United Kingdom, use of pioglitazone more than 24 months was reported to be associated with an increased risk of incident bladder cancer among people with type 2 diabetes [69. Using data from the French national health insurance information system, in a population based study, pioglitazone use of more than 24 months was reported significantly associated with increased risk of bladder cancer [70].

4.3. Metformin

Studies of patients with T2DM on metformin have demonstrated a lower risk of cancer [71-74]. In a recent study of the influence of treatment with metformin on survival after cancer diagnosis by Currie and associates, metformin was shown to be associated with survival benefit both in comparison with other treatments for diabetes and in comparison with a non-diabetic population [75]. An observational cohort study from the United Kingdom suggested that metformin use may be associated with a reduced risk of cancer (HR:0.63 (0.53-0.75) [72]. The study noted that the reduced risk was after adjusting for sex, age, BMI, A1C, smoking, and other drug use [72]. In a different database study from UK general practices, metformin use was reported to be associated with lower risk of cancer of the colon or pancreas, but did not affect the risk of breast or prostate cancer [71]. Metformin use was associated with survival benefit in comparison with other treatments for diabetes and also in comparison with a non-diabetic population [75]. Metformin has been associated with reduced risk of pancreatic cancer in diabetics and recognized as an antitumor agent with the potential to prevent and treat this cancer [76]. A retrospective cohort study to investigate the survival benefit of metformin in patients with diabetes and pancreatic malignancy, from the MD Anderson Cancer Center from 2000 to 2009, reported that metformin users have a significant survival benefit compared to non-users (the median survival 16.6 *vs.* 11.5 months; $p = 0.0044$) [77]. They also report a 33% decrease risk of death in patients who used metformin (HR: 0.67; $p = 0.005$) [77]. This implies that metformin may have some beneficial effects on slowing the progression of pancreatic malignancy. However, specific pathogenesis is unclear and would have to be further explored. In an interesting finding from a data base study from Hong Kong, nonusers of metformin with low HDL cholesterol had an adjusted hazard ratio of 5.75 (CI: 3.03-10.90) compared with HDL cholesterol ≥ 1.0 mmol/L plus use of metformin [78]. The reduction in cancer risk with the use of metformin in patients with type 2 diabetes is said to be dose related [74]. In a Canadian population-based cohort study, Bowker and associates noted that patients with type 2 diabetes exposed to sulfonylureas and exogenous insulin had a significantly increased risk of cancer-related mortality compared with patients exposed to metformin [79]. In addition they also noted that, the sulfonylurea cohort had greater cancer-related mortality compared with the metformin cohort after multivariate adjustment [79]. There are several *in vitro* and *in vivo studies* from cell lines and animal models support the benefit of metformin against cancer. There are several ongoing trials to examine the clinical outcomes.

4.3.1. Metformin and individual cancers

Long term use of metformin was shown to decrease risk of breast cancer in female patients with type 2 diabetes [80]. In a case-control study using the U.K.-based General Practice Research Database, metformin use was associated with an adjusted odds ratio of 0.44 (CI: 0.24-0.82) for developing breast cancer compared with no use of metformin [81]. In a similar study from the UK, long-term use of ≥ 40 prescriptions (>5 years) of metformin, based on 17 exposed case patients and 120 exposed control patients, was associated with an adjusted odds ratio of 0.44 (95% CI 0.24-0.82) for developing breast cancer compared with no use of metformin [80]. A meta-analysis of 17 case-control studies and 32 cohort studies of diabetes and hepatocellular carcinoma, metformin treatment was potentially protective [82]. In a meta- analysis of five studies comprising 108,161 patients with type 2 diabetes, metformin therapy appears to be associated with a significantly lower risk of colorectal cancer in patients with type 2 diabetes [82].

4.3.2. Mechanism of metformin in reducing cancer

It has been postulated that the effect of metformin on cancer development and progression may be a result of decreased levels of insulin [83] and insulin resistance. However, the possible anticancer effect of metformin is believed to be mediated by the inhibition of mitochondrial oxidative phosphorylation leading to activated AMPK pathway or independent of non-AMPK pathway. Human breast cancer cells treated with metformin demonstrate inhibited proliferation and colony formation and increased cell cycle arrest [84]. Studies have shown that metformin also has a direct effect on tumor cell proliferation [85]. As stated previously, metformin activates AMPK. The AMPK/mTOR axis is modulated by liver kinase B1 (LKB1). LKB1 is a tumor suppressor that activates AMPK, leading to mTOR inhibition, resulting in inhibited cell growth [85]. In vitro studies have shown that treatment with metformin inhibits cancer cell lines such as breast cancer breast cancer cells,[86] prostate cancer cell lines,[87, 88] glioma,[89] and fibro sarcoma cell lines [90].

4.4. Therapeutic consideration

4.4.1. Therapeutic considerations in general

Therapeutic considerations need to focus on reduction of the risk factors. Various therapeutic interventions for weight reduction and healthy life style have been linked to a reduced cancer risk in the general population. Therapeutic strategies to decrease chronic hyperinsulinemia and insulin resistance may offer a general approach to prevention of cancer. Metformin is the insulin sensitizer used primarily in the treatment of type 2 diabetes mellitus.

In a retrospective study of long term benefits of bariatric surgery, a significant decrease in mortality from cancer-related deaths in the bariatric surgery group compared both with all subjects and matched subjects with a decrease of 60% for cancer at mean follow-up of 7.1 years. Anticytokine vaccines, inhibitors of proinflammatory NF-κB and COX-2 pathways, thiazolidinediones, and antioxidants are potentially useful for the prevention or treatment of pancreatic cancer. Similarly epidemiologic studies have documented a 40–50% reduction in the incidence of colorectal cancer in individuals taking nonsteroidal anti-inflammatory drugs (NSAIDs). The long-term use of COX-2-selective inhibitors has, unfortunately, demonstrated cardiovascular toxicity, so their use in cancer prevention and therapy is currently questionable. However, there is evidence suggesting that further development of novel COX-2-selective agents is needed for the prevention and/or treatment of human cancers, especially pancreatic cancer. Targeting PGE_2 signaling by EP receptor antagonists holds promise for the development of targeted therapy for the treatment of cancer [91]. PPARs also play a role in the regulation of cancer cell growth. Recent evidence suggests that PPAR modulators may have beneficial effects as chemopreventive agents [92].

Recent clinical studies with IGF-1R inhibitors have revealed several obstacles to successful use in cancer therapy. Strategies to inhibit IGF-1R signaling such as tyrosine kinase inhibitors also disrupt IR signaling, resulting in hyperglycemia and hyperinsulinemia. Several strategies being considered are based on biomarkers that could identify subpopulations most likely to be responsive to IGF targeting. The combination therapies with other targeted drugs could maximize the therapeutic effects of IGF inhibitors [93].

4.4.2. Chemoprevention of colorectal cancer

Of cancers affecting both men and women, colorectal cancer (cancer of the colon and rectum) is the second leading cancer killer in the United States and the incidence increases with age. The U.S. Preventive Services Task Force report on the effectiveness of aspirin (ASA), non-aspirin non steroidal anti-inflammatory drugs (non-ASA NSAIDs), and cyclooxygenase-2 inhibitors (COX-2 inhibitors) for the chemoprevention of colorectal cancer indicate that aspirin and non-ASA NSAIDs appear to be effective at reducing the incidence of CRAs and CRC [7]. The report also stated that more information is required to clarify the optimal dose, starting age, and duration of use of ASA since observational studies suggest that higher doses and prolonged use improve chemo-preventative efficacy. In a recent systematic review and meta-analysis for randomized controlled trials (RCTs) from United Kingdom, Cooper and associates identified 44 relevant RCTs and six ongoing studies [8]. They reported that there was a statistically significant 21% reduction in risk of adenoma recurrence (RR: 0.79; CI: 0.68 to 0.92) in an analysis of aspirin versus no aspirin in individuals with a history of adenomas or CRC. In the general population, a significant 26% reduction in CRC incidence was demonstrated in studies with a 23-year follow-up (RR: 0.74; CI: 0.57 to 0.97). In individuals with a history of adenomas there was a statistically significant 34% reduction in adenoma recurrence risk (RR: 0.66; CI: 0.60 to 0.72) and a statistically significant 55% reduction in advanced adenoma incidence (RR 0.45; CI: 0.35 to 0.58). No studies assessed the effect of non-aspirin NSAIDs in the general population. There was said to be no significant effect of folic acid versus placebo on adenoma recurrence (RR: 1.16; CI: 0.97 to 1.39) or advanced adenoma incidence in individuals with a history of adenomas. In the general population there was said to be no significant effect of folic acid on risk of colorectal cancer (RR: 1.13; CI: CI: 0.77 to 1.64), although studies were of relatively short duration. Calcium use by familial adenomatous polyposis (FAP) patients was reported to have no significant reduction in polyp number or disease progression. In individuals with a history of adenomas there was said to be a statistically significant 18% reduction in risk of adenoma recurrence (RR: 0.82; CI: 0.69 to 0.98) and a non-significant reduction in risk of advanced adenomas (RR: 0.77; CI: 0.50 to 1.17). Though these studies are not selective for subjects with diabetes, prevention of colorectal cancer in subjects with diabetes is important and relevant.

Acknowledgements

The author receives salary support from Veterans Health Administration. Appreciate Barbara Youngberg for her efforts in an excellent proof reading.

Author details

Subhashini Yaturu*

Address all correspondence to: Subhashini.Yaturu@va.gov

Stratton Veterans Affairs Medical Center /Albany Medical College, Albany, NY, USA

References

[1] Giovannucci, E, et al. Diabetes and cancer: a consensus report. Diabetes Care, (2010). , 1674-1685.

[2] Larsson, S. C, Orsini, N, & Wolk, A. Diabetes mellitus and risk of colorectal cancer: a meta-analysis. J Natl Cancer Inst, (2005). , 1679-1687.

[3] Huxley, R, et al. Type-II diabetes and pancreatic cancer: a meta-analysis of 36 studies. Br J Cancer, (2005). , 2076-2083.

[4] Larsson, S. C, Mantzoros, C. S, & Wolk, A. Diabetes mellitus and risk of breast cancer: a meta-analysis. Int J Cancer, (2007). , 856-862.

[5] Zendehdel, K, et al. Cancer incidence in patients with type 1 diabetes mellitus: a population-based cohort study in Sweden. J Natl Cancer Inst, (2003). , 1797-1800.

[6] Vigneri, P, et al. Diabetes and cancer. Endocr Relat Cancer, (2009). , 1103-1123.

[7] Rostom, A, Dube, C, & Lewin, G. (2007).

[8] Cooper, K, et al. Chemoprevention of colorectal cancer: systematic review and economic evaluation. Health Technol Assess, (2010). , 1-206.

[9] Everhart, J, & Wright, D. Diabetes mellitus as a risk factor for pancreatic cancer. A meta-analysis. JAMA, (1995). , 1605-1609.

[10] Gullo, L, Pezzilli, R, & Morselli-labate, A. M. Diabetes and the risk of pancreatic cancer. N Engl J Med, (1994). , 81-84.

[11] Pannala, R, et al. New-onset diabetes: a potential clue to the early diagnosis of pancreatic cancer. Lancet Oncol, (2009). , 88-95.

[12] Stevens, R. J, Roddam, A. W, & Beral, V. Pancreatic cancer in type 1 and young-onset diabetes: systematic review and meta-analysis. Br J Cancer, (2007). , 507-509.

[13] Jiang, Y, et al. Diabetes mellitus and incidence and mortality of colorectal cancer: a systematic review and meta-analysis of cohort studies. Eur J Epidemiol, (2011). , 863-876.

[14] Deng, L, et al. Diabetes mellitus and the incidence of colorectal cancer: an updated systematic review and meta-analysis. Dig Dis Sci, (2012). , 1576-1585.

[15] Dempke, W, et al. Cyclooxygenase-2: a novel target for cancer chemotherapy? J Cancer Res Clin Oncol, (2001). , 411-417.

[16] Sarkar, F. H, et al. Back to the future: COX-2 inhibitors for chemoprevention and cancer therapy. Mini Rev Med Chem, (2007). , 599-608.

[17] Eliassen, A. H, et al. Adult weight change and risk of postmenopausal breast cancer. JAMA, (2006). , 193-201.

[18] Calle, E. E, et al. Overweight, obesity, and mortality from cancer in a prospectively studied cohort of U.S. adults. N Engl J Med, (2003). , 1625-1638.

[19] Rozengurt, E, Sinnett-smith, J, & Kisfalvi, K. Crosstalk between insulin/insulin-like growth factor-1 receptors and G protein-coupled receptor signaling systems: a novel target for the antidiabetic drug metformin in pancreatic cancer. Clin Cancer Res, (2010). , 2505-2511.

[20] Kisfalvi, K, et al. Metformin disrupts crosstalk between G protein-coupled receptor and insulin receptor signaling systems and inhibits pancreatic cancer growth. Cancer Res, (2009). , 6539-6545.

[21] Pisani, P. Hyper-insulinaemia and cancer, meta-analyses of epidemiological studies. Arch Physiol Biochem, (2008). , 63-70.

[22] Lacey, J. V, et al. Insulin-like growth factors, insulin-like growth factor-binding proteins, and endometrial cancer in postmenopausal women: results from a U.S. case-control study. Cancer Epidemiol Biomarkers Prev, (2004). , 607-612.

[23] Gunter, M. J, et al. A prospective evaluation of insulin and insulin-like growth factor-I as risk factors for endometrial cancer. Cancer Epidemiol Biomarkers Prev, (2008). , 921-929.

[24] Flood, A, et al. Elevated serum concentrations of insulin and glucose increase risk of recurrent colorectal adenomas. Gastroenterology, (2007). , 1423-1429.

[25] Cowey, S, & Hardy, R. W. The metabolic syndrome: A high-risk state for cancer? Am J Pathol, (2006). , 1505-1522.

[26] Frasca, F, et al. The role of insulin receptors and IGF-I receptors in cancer and other diseases. Arch Physiol Biochem, (2008). , 23-37.

[27] Samani, A. A, et al. The role of the IGF system in cancer growth and metastasis: overview and recent insights. Endocr Rev, (2007). , 20-47.

[28] Gao, Y, et al. Serum IGF1, IGF2 and IGFBP3 and risk of advanced colorectal adenoma. Int J Cancer, (2012). , E105-E113.

[29] Scherer, P. E, et al. A novel serum protein similar to C1q, produced exclusively in adipocytes. J Biol Chem, (1995). , 26746-26749.

[30] Yaturu, S, et al. Plasma and urine levels of resistin and adiponectin in chronic kidney disease. Cytokine, (2007). , 1-5.

[31] Yaturu, S, et al. Resistin and adiponectin levels in subjects with coronary artery disease and type 2 diabetes. Cytokine, (2006). , 219-223.

[32] Yaturu, S, & Bridges, J. F. and D.R. Subba Reddy, Decreased levels of plasma adiponectin in prediabetes, Type 2 diabetes and coronary artery disease. Med Sci Monit, (2006). , CR17-CR20.

[33] Barb, D, et al. Adiponectin in relation to malignancies: a review of existing basic research and clinical evidence. Am J Clin Nutr, (2007). , s858-s866.

[34] Yokota, T, et al. Adiponectin, a new member of the family of soluble defense collagens, negatively regulates the growth of myelomonocytic progenitors and the functions of macrophages. Blood, (2000). , 1723-1732.

[35] Horiguchi, A, et al. Decreased serum adiponectin levels in patients with metastatic renal cell carcinoma. Jpn J Clin Oncol, (2008). , 106-111.

[36] Spyridopoulos, T. N, et al. Low adiponectin levels are associated with renal cell carcinoma: a case-control study. Int J Cancer, (2007). , 1573-1578.

[37] Kapoor, S. Re: Jehonathan H. Pinthus, Nir Kleinmann, Britton Tisdale, et al. Lower plasma adiponectin levels are associated with larger tumor size and metastasis in clear-cell carcinoma of the kidney. Eur Urol 2008;54:866-74. Eur Urol, (2009). , e52-e53.

[38] Pinthus, J. H, et al. Lower plasma adiponectin levels are associated with larger tumor size and metastasis in clear-cell carcinoma of the kidney. Eur Urol, (2008). , 866-873.

[39] Petridou, E, et al. Adiponectin in relation to childhood myeloblastic leukaemia. Br J Cancer, (2006). , 156-160.

[40] Pfeiler, G. H, et al. Adiponectin effects on human breast cancer cells are dependent on 17-beta estradiol. Oncol Rep, (2008). , 787-793.

[41] Fenton, J. I, et al. Adiponectin blocks multiple signaling cascades associated with leptin-induced cell proliferation in Apc Min/+ colon epithelial cells. Int J Cancer, (2008). , 2437-2445.

[42] Touvier, M, et al. Pre-diagnostic levels of adiponectin and soluble vascular cell adhesion molecule-1 are associated with colorectal cancer risk. World J Gastroenterol, (2012). , 2805-2812.

[43] Wei, E. K, et al. Low plasma adiponectin levels and risk of colorectal cancer in men: a prospective study. J Natl Cancer Inst, (2005). , 1688-1694.

[44] Xu, X. T, et al. Meta-analysis: circulating adiponectin levels and risk of colorectal cancer and adenoma. J Dig Dis, (2011)., 234-244.

[45] Cong, L, et al. Human adiponectin inhibits cell growth and induces apoptosis in human endometrial carcinoma cells, HEC-1-A and RL95 2. Endocr Relat Cancer, (2007)., 713-720.

[46] Harris, M. I, et al. Prevalence of diabetes, impaired fasting glucose, and impaired glucose tolerance in U.S. adults. The Third National Health and Nutrition Examination Survey, 1988-1994. Diabetes Care, (1998)., 518-524.

[47] Larsson, S. C, & Wolk, A. Obesity and colon and rectal cancer risk: a meta-analysis of prospective studies. Am J Clin Nutr, (2007)., 556-565.

[48] Dai, Z, Xu, Y. C, & Niu, L. Obesity and colorectal cancer risk: a meta-analysis of cohort studies. World J Gastroenterol, (2007)., 4199-4206.

[49] Larsson, S. C, & Wolk, A. Overweight, obesity and risk of liver cancer: a meta-analysis of cohort studies. Br J Cancer, (2007)., 1005-1008.

[50] Larsson, S. C, & Wolk, A. Obesity and the risk of gallbladder cancer: a meta-analysis. Br J Cancer, (2007)., 1457-1461.

[51] Wang, Y, et al. A prospective study of waist circumference and body mass index in relation to colorectal cancer incidence. Cancer Causes Control, (2008)., 783-792.

[52] Larsson, S. C, Orsini, N, & Wolk, A. Body mass index and pancreatic cancer risk: A meta-analysis of prospective studies. Int J Cancer, (2007)., 1993-1998.

[53] Larsson, S. C, & Wolk, A. Overweight and obesity and incidence of leukemia: a meta-analysis of cohort studies. Int J Cancer, (2008)., 1418-1421.

[54] Olsen, C. M, et al. Body size and risk of epithelial ovarian and related cancers: a population-based case-control study. Int J Cancer, (2008)., 450-456.

[55] Jensen, A, et al. Risk of breast cancer and gynecologic cancers in a large population of nearly 50,000 infertile Danish women. Am J Epidemiol, (2008)., 49-57.

[56] Patel, A. V, et al. The role of body weight in the relationship between physical activity and endometrial cancer: results from a large cohort of US women. Int J Cancer, (2008)., 1877-1882.

[57] Mccourt, C. K, et al. Body mass index: relationship to clinical, pathologic and features of microsatellite instability in endometrial cancer. Gynecol Oncol, (2007). , 535-539.

[58] Reeves, G. K, et al. Cancer incidence and mortality in relation to body mass index in the Million Women Study: cohort study. BMJ, (2007)., 1134.

[59] Carmichael, A. R. Obesity and prognosis of breast cancer. Obes Rev, (2006)., 333-340.

[60] Dignam, J. J, et al. Body mass index and outcomes in patients who receive adjuvant chemotherapy for colon cancer. J Natl Cancer Inst, (2006). , 1647-1654.

[61] Haydon, A. M, et al. Effect of physical activity and body size on survival after diagnosis with colorectal cancer. Gut, (2006). , 62-67.

[62] Xu, X. C. COX-2 inhibitors in cancer treatment and prevention, a recent development. Anticancer Drugs, (2002). , 127-137.

[63] Dubey, S, et al. Inflammation-associated regulation of the macrophage inhibitory cytokine (MIC-1) gene in prostate cancer. Oncol Lett, (2012). , 1166-1170.

[64] Frasor, J, et al. Synergistic up-regulation of prostaglandin E synthase expression in breast cancer cells by 17beta-estradiol and proinflammatory cytokines. Endocrinology, (2008). , 6272-6279.

[65] Monami, M, et al. Rosiglitazone and risk of cancer: a meta-analysis of randomized clinical trials. Diabetes Care, (2008). , 1455-1460.

[66] Yang, X, et al. Use of thiazolidinedione and cancer risk in Type 2 diabetes: the Hong Kong diabetes registry. Diabetes Res Clin Pract, (2012). , e13-e17.

[67] Chang, C. H, et al. Association of thiazolidinediones with liver cancer and colorectal cancer in type 2 diabetes mellitus. Hepatology, (2012). , 1462-1472.

[68] Lewis, J. D, et al. Risk of bladder cancer among diabetic patients treated with pioglitazone: interim report of a longitudinal cohort study. Diabetes Care, (2011). , 916-922.

[69] Azoulay, L, et al. The use of pioglitazone and the risk of bladder cancer in people with type 2 diabetes: nested case-control study. BMJ, (2012). , e3645.

[70] Neumann, A, et al. Pioglitazone and risk of bladder cancer among diabetic patients in France: a population-based cohort study. Diabetologia, (2012). , 1953-1962.

[71] Currie, C. J, Poole, C. D, & Gale, E. A. The influence of glucose-lowering therapies on cancer risk in type 2 diabetes. Diabetologia, (2009). , 1766-1777.

[72] Libby, G, et al. New users of metformin are at low risk of incident cancer: a cohort study among people with type 2 diabetes. Diabetes Care, (2009). , 1620-1625.

[73] Jiralerspong, S, et al. Metformin and pathologic complete responses to neoadjuvant chemotherapy in diabetic patients with breast cancer. J Clin Oncol, (2009). , 3297-3302.

[74] Evans, J. M, et al. Metformin and reduced risk of cancer in diabetic patients. BMJ, (2005). , 1304-1305.

[75] Currie, C. J, et al. Mortality after incident cancer in people with and without type 2 diabetes: impact of metformin on survival. Diabetes Care, (2012). , 299-304.

[76] Li, D, et al. Antidiabetic therapies affect risk of pancreatic cancer. Gastroenterology, (2009). , 482-488.

[77] Sadeghi, N, et al. Metformin use is associated with better survival of diabetic patients with pancreatic cancer. Clin Cancer Res, (2012). , 2905-2912.

[78] Yang, X, et al. Low HDL cholesterol, metformin use, and cancer risk in type 2 diabetes: the Hong Kong Diabetes Registry. Diabetes Care, (2011). , 375-380.

[79] Bowker, S. L, et al. Increased cancer-related mortality for patients with type 2 diabetes who use sulfonylureas or insulin. Diabetes Care, (2006). , 254-258.

[80] Bodmer, M, et al. Long-term metformin use is associated with decreased risk of breast cancer. Diabetes Care, (2010). , 1304-1308.

[81] Keating, H. J. rd, Humanizing the intensive care unit. Del Med J, (1991). , 129.

[82] Wang, P, et al. Diabetes mellitus and risk of hepatocellular carcinoma: a systematic review and meta-analysis. Diabetes Metab Res Rev, (2012). , 109-122.

[83] Berstein, L. M. Metformin, insulin, breast cancer and more. Future Oncol, (2009). , 309-312.

[84] Alimova, I. N, et al. Metformin inhibits breast cancer cell growth, colony formation and induces cell cycle arrest in vitro. Cell Cycle, (2009). , 909-915.

[85] Ben SahraI., et al., Metformin, independent of AMPK, induces mTOR inhibition and cell-cycle arrest through REDD1. Cancer Res, (2011). , 4366-4372.

[86] Zakikhani, M, et al. Metformin is an AMP kinase-dependent growth inhibitor for breast cancer cells. Cancer Res, (2006). , 10269-10273.

[87] Chen, D, et al. Activation of AMP-Activated Protein Kinase by 3,3'-Diindolylmethane (DIM) Is Associated with Human Prostate Cancer Cell Death In Vitro and In Vivo. PLoS One, (2012). , e47186.

[88] Ben SahraI., et al., The antidiabetic drug metformin exerts an antitumoral effect in vitro and in vivo through a decrease of cyclin D1 level. Oncogene, (2008). , 3576-3586.

[89] Isakovic, A, et al. Dual antiglioma action of metformin: cell cycle arrest and mitochondria-dependent apoptosis. Cell Mol Life Sci, (2007). , 1290-1302.

[90] Hwang, Y. P, & Jeong, H. G. Metformin blocks migration and invasion of tumour cells by inhibition of matrix metalloproteinase-9 activation through a calcium and protein kinase Calpha-dependent pathway: phorbol-12-myristate-13-acetate-induced/extracellular signal-regulated kinase/activator protein-1. Br J Pharmacol, (2010). , 1195-1211.

[91] Wu, W. K, et al. Cyclooxygenase-2 in tumorigenesis of gastrointestinal cancers: an update on the molecular mechanisms. Cancer Lett, (2010). , 7-16.

[92] Tachibana, K, et al. The Role of PPARs in Cancer. PPAR Res, 2008. (2008). , 102737.

[93] Seccareccia, E, & Brodt, P. The role of the insulin-like growth factor-I receptor in malignancy: An update. Growth Horm IGF Res, (2012).

Chapter 11

Anemia of Chronic Kidney Disease — A Modifiable Risk Factor in a Growing High Cardiovascular Risk Population

Nadine Montemarano, Jennifer Guttman and
Samy I. McFarlane

Additional information is available at the end of the chapter

http://dx.doi.org/10.5772/56543

1. Introduction

Diabetes Mellitus (DM) has become a modern day epidemic, affecting millions of people around the globe. It has grown parallel to the rising epidemic of obesity, leading to increased cardiovascular disease (CVD) morbidity and mortality. Currently, DM is the most common cause of chronic kidney disease (CKD) and subsequent end stage renal disease (ESRD) requiring renal replacement therapy. Although statistics indicate a leveling off in the incidence of ESRD among diabetics, these statistics do not hold true for some of the most vulnerable populations such as minority populations.

CVD is the primary cause of death in people with DM who also possess traditional risk factors such as hypertension (HTN), obesity (particularly central obesity), dyslipidemia (decreased HDL, and elevated triglycerides), increased age, sedentary lifestyle and smoking. Nontraditional risk factors for CVD include increased inflammation, stimulation of the renin-angiotensin-aldosterone system (RAAS), increased fibrinogen, increased platelet activator inhibitor factor -1 (PAI-1) among others. Diabetic kidney disease (DKD) is a well established cause of CVD and currently, it is considered a cardiovascular equivalent. In fact, people with CKD generally die of CVD prior to the initiation of dialysis.

The exact cause of increased CVD risk in CKD is likely multifactorial but is largely unknown. Anemia has been shown to increase cardiovascular risk in this vulnerable population and prior studies have demonstrated that treatment of anemia reduces this risk and improves quality of life [5]. On the other hand, recent trials have shown an increased risk of CVD in those with higher hemoglobin values being treated with ESA [56]. It is unclear whether the ESA in large doses confers this harm or whether the correction of anemia to high hemoglobin levels is responsible. These uncertainties explain why many clinicians prefer transfusion therapy over the use of ESA. Several questions remain unanswered including the mechanisms by which anemia confers increased cardiovascular risk in CKD and dialysis patients. Another important issue surrounded by controversy is the degree to which anemia should be corrected with erythropoietic stimulating agents (ESA).

In this chapter, we discuss the relationship between DM and CKD and the associated CVD risk factors, highlighting the pathophysiologic mechanisms that link anemia and CVD. We also explore the therapeutic rationale behind the current guidelines provided by the National Kidney Foundation for the management of anemia. These guidelines are constantly updated as new randomized controlled trials continuue to emerge.

1.1. Definition and risk factors for anemia in CKD

According to the WHO criteria published in 1997, the Hemoglobin and Hematorcrit cutoffs for defining anemia are <13 g/dL and 39%, respectively, in men and <12 and 36%, respectively, in non pregnant women [1]. Newer research differentiates anemia cutoffs based on both race and age in addition to sex. Table 1 lists proposed lower limits of normal for hemoglobin concentration based on Scripps-Kaiser data for the 5th percentiles and the NHANES data published in 2006 [2].

White Men 20-59 yrs	13.7	White Men 60+ yrs	13.2
White Women 20-49 yrs	12.2	White Women 50+ yrs	12.2
Black Men 20-59 yrs	12.9	Black Men 60+ yrs	12.7
Black Women 20-49 yrs	11.5	Black Women 50+ yrs	11.5

Based on reference 3 Beutler et al.

Table 1. Lower Limits of normal Hemoglobin concentration (g/dL)

Multiple risk factors increase the risk of developing anemia. Among multiple factors, individuals with CVD, DM and CKD, HTN(HTN) and of African American race are at significantly high risk than the general population [4,5,6].

1.2. Postulated mechanisms of anemia in CKD, CVD and DM

CKD, CVD and DM are intricately interconnected with one another. CKD is extremely prevalent among the United States adult population. According to the Center for Disease Control (CDC), more than 35% of people aged 20 years or older with DM have CKD and more than 20% of people aged 20 years or older with HTN have CKD [9].

Regardless of the level of estimated glomerular filtration rate (e-GFR), anemia is both more frequent and more severe in diabetics compared to non-diabetic patients [10]. Diabetes types 1 and 2, are the leading cause of CKD in the western world, accounting for approximately 30-40% of cases. DM is therefore the most common cause of renal anemia [7,8]. A number of mechanisms contribute to the development of anemia in diabetics with CKD such as decreased red blood cell (RBC) life span, iron deficiency, nutritional folate deficiency, occult blood loss, systemic inflammation and what appears to be the most dominant causal factor, erythropoietin deficiency [11].

Renal anemia is associated with a reduction in the number of RBCs and with an increase in oxidative stress to RBCs [23]. RBC lifespan is reduced by approximately 50% in uremia. While this phenomenon has been recognized for over 50 years, the mechanism is not completely understood [12]. Some studies show that the decrease in RBC half life is partially caused by the uremic environment present in CKD patients. [13,14,15,16]. Studies have also shown that the RBCs in diabetics have multiple metabolic and functional abnormalities [17,18]. RBC properties are significantly modified by hyperglycemia. Prior reports suggest that increased levels of glucose decrease the activity of the RBC Na/K ATPase and generate multiple oxidative changes [19,20,21]. According to Manodori et al, as a result of these changes, RBC life span in diabetic patients is decreased compared to nondiabetic patients with similar degrees of renal impairment [22].

Iron homeostasis is altered in those with CKD. Transferrin is a protein that captures iron that has been absorbed from the GI tract and that has been released from macrophages and delivers it to maturing RBCs. In CKD, transferrin levels are decreased, impairing iron mobilization. As uremia leads to platelet dysfunction, CKD patients are at increased risk for bleeding and iron loss [24]. Hemodialysis patients are at particular risk because of the chance for blood loss during dialysis [25]. Diabetics with nephropathy are at an added risk for iron loss by urinary excretion as their proteinuria progresses [26].

Systemic Inflammation is one of the leading features of diabetics with CKD that appears to contribute to anemia. This inflammatory response is secondary to a variety of factors including elevated levels of inflammatory cytokines, volume overload and oxidative stress. Increased level of cytokines impair bone marrow function and significantly alter iron metabolism.

Erythropoietin (EPO) is a glycoprotein growth factor that is produced by the peritubular interstitial fibroblasts of the renal cortex and outer medulla [27]. The release of EPO is regulated by a complex feedback mechanism at the level of the kidney. in which. One major role of the kidney is to "sense" an imbalance between oxygen supply and demand. In response, it stimulates hematopoietic precursors through the production of EPO. EPO deficiency is currently considered a leading cause of anemia in patients with CKD. In this group, EPO deficiency is regarded as functional as it stems from a failure to increase EPO levels in response to a falling hemoglobin level, even though the absolute value of EPO may be within normal limits. EPO deficiency appears to contribute largely to the development of anemia in patients with diabetic nephropathy and CKD [28, 29]. Multiple explanations have been postulated to account for the EPO deficiency in this patient population including microvascular damage, chronic hypoxia, oxidative stress, and autonomic neuropathy. Damage to the tubulointerstitial cells has been observed in the early stages of diabetic nephropathy resulting in impairment of the signaling cascade that triggers transcription and release of EPO [29]. Unregulated activation of the Renin-Angiotensin-Aldosterone System (RAAS) in diabetics may also contribute to impaired erythropoietin release. Similarly, experimental models have illustrated that autonomic dysfunction, as seen in diabetics who tend to develop splanchnic nerve dysfunction, have impaired production of EPO [30].

CVD is a common co-morbidity among anemic patients with both DM and CKD. CVD, DM and CKD are strongly intertwined. Many of the same risk factors that contribute to DM, CKD and CVD, both independently and synergistically. These risk factors can be divided into two categories: traditional and non traditional. Some of the traditional risk factors include obesity, hypertension, dyslipidemia and smoking. Among the non traditional risk factors are anemia, chronic systemic inflammation, oxidative stress, hyperparathyroidism, hyperhomocysteinemia, endothelial dysfunction and prothrombin states [34].

Diabetic kidney disease, also known as diabetic nephropathy, is one of the major complications of type 2 diabetes. Elevated blood glucose levels activate various biochemical pathways within renal cells. The increased intracellular glucose leads to increased production of glucose intermediaries cycling through multiple metabolic pathways. This leads to the production of advanced glycation products (AGEs), activation of protein kinase C (PKC), increased expression of transforming growth factor-beta (TGF-beta), GTP-binding proteins, and the formation of reactive oxygen species (ROS) [64]. The ROS may also be responsible for the activation of the RAAS [65, 66]. In addition to these metabolic events, there is also a hemodynamic component to diabetic kidney disease. Hyperglycemia impairs glomerular circulation, mainly dilation of the afferent arteriole, which subsequently leads to increased glomerular capillary pressure [67, 68]. The culmination of these hyperglycemia induced metabolic and hemodynamic derangements sets off a cascade of aberrant cell growth, angiogenesis, extracellular matrix abnormalities, hyalinization of arterioles, proteinuria, and hyperfiltration, ultimately resulting in diabetic kidney injury [64].

Type 2 diabetes is the most common cause of CKD among the US adult population and both DM and CKD can cause anemia. The decreased oxygen carrying capacity associated with anemia may aggravate myocardial hypoxia, increase cardiac output, cause volume overload, increase heart rate, stimulate the RAAS, and can lead to left ventricular hypertrophy (LVH). The damage caused as a result produces myocyte loss, progressive fibrosis, coronary heart disease (CHD) and heart failure [32,33]. DM is both a CHD equivalent and the leading cause of CKD. Type 2 diabetes increases the risk of CHD events by at least by two- to three fold compared with non-diabetics [31]. Ultimately, patients with CKD are most likely to die from a cardiovascular event.

2. Epidemiology

Given the constant influx of immigrants to the western world, addressing the medical issues facing minorities holds critical relevance. Approximately one third of American population

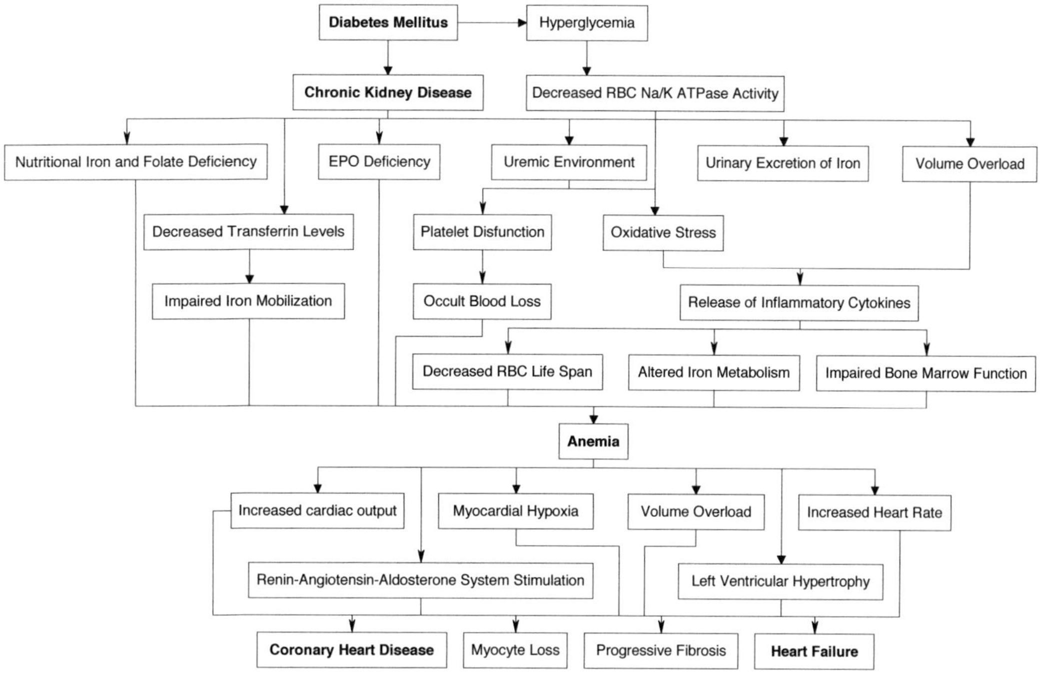

Figure 1. Highlights the postulated mechanisms of anemia in CKD, CVD and DM

currently identifies as minority, including Hispanics, African Americans, Asians, and Native Americans [35]. Between 2010 and 2050, this population is expected to grow geometrically, most markedly in the Asian and Hispanic American populations, which are both anticipated to double during this period [36].

2.1. Ethnic differences in CKD

ESRD is much more common among ethnic minorities with rates per million as high as 925 among blacks, 501 among Hispanics, and 465 among Native Americans compared with 276 among NHWs. ESRD as caused by HTN, the second leading cause, is also much more common in minorities with a nearly 11 times greater prevalence among blacks than whites [48]. On top of that, in patients with ESRD, the prevalence of HTN is greater in both Hispanic and NHBs compared with NHWs. Several biomarkers have been associated with this increased risk. Levels of C-reactive protein (CRP) and white blood cells are highest among blacks in this population, suggesting a role for inflammation in disease progression [49]. Elevated levels of CRP are associated with the development of Type 2 diabetes [50], an increased risk for coronary events [51] and symptomatic PAD [52] and may help to explain the increased prevalence of CKD in the black population.

CKD puts patients at greater risk for MI, stroke and death, with approximately 6 million Americans suffering from both CVD and CKD. According to NHANES, the prevalence of CVD is 63 percent in those with CKD stages 3–5, compared with 5.8 percent in those without kidney disease [48]. The risk for these cardiovascular endpoints is even higher among African Americans with CKD. One pooled analysis of several community based studies found that among subjects with CKD the hazard ratio for myocardial infarction, fatal CHD, stroke, and death was 1.76 in blacks compared with 1.13 in whites [53].

2.2. Ethnic differences in diabetic CKD

DM is significantly more prevalent among Non Hispanic Blacks (NHB) than among non-Hispanic whites (NHW). Whereas between 1980 and 2010, DM rose to a rate of 6.8 percent among white males and 5.4 percent among white females, it increased to 9.7 percent among black males and 9.5 percent among black females [37]. Because of the increased risk of Type 2 diabetes among blacks and among other ethnic minorities [38], the number of Americans with DM is expected to triple from 20 million [37] to more than 60 million over the next forty years [39].

In addition, the rate of DM induced ESRD is growing faster among blacks than among whites. Among those aged 30–39, the rate of ESRD in diabetics has risen by 69 percent between 2000 and 2010 whereas it has dropped by one percent in age matched whites. Similarly, Native Americans in this age group have seen an increase of ESRD by 30.1 percent during this period. This contrasts with rates of ESRD in diabetics older than sixty where ESRD has dropped more dramatically among ethnic minorities than among whites.

2.3. Ethnic differences in CKD as one of diabetic CVD complications

DM is also linked with a greatly increased risk of CVD. The rise in prevalence of both coronary heart disease (CHD) and peripheral arterial disease (PAD) ranges between double and quadruple the risk of the general population [40]. The risk of PAD increases by 28 percent with each one percent increase in glycosylated hemoglobin, a marker for blood glucose levels [41].

Furthermore, NHBs are at significantly greater risk of both PAD and CVD than NHWs [39]. Based on the third National Health and Nutrition Examination Survey (NHANES III), 5 million US adults above age 40 have PAD. Among NHBs older than 40, the prevalence of PAD is 7.9 percent compared with a prevalence of 4.3 percent among age matched NHWs [42]. Furthermore, NHBs have a 1.5 times greater rate of heart disease related deaths and a 1.8 times greater rate of fatal stroke relative to NHWs [43]. According to the NAACP, NHB males have a 30 percent greater chance of dying from heart disease than NHW males [44].

The development and the worsening of CKD as a complication of diabetic CVD is the result of a number of interacting pathways. These include enhanced levels of oxidative stress, inflammation, endothelial dysfunction, and RAAS activation [48]. In addition, hypertriglyceridemia, associated with CVD, promotes lipid accumulation in renal cells and consequent dysfunction [49]. Furthermore, vascular calcification in CVD is commonplace among the renal vessels, fostering CKD progression [63]. The intersection of CVD CKD, and DM is complex with each player exacerbating one another. Thus, ethnic minorities are more likely to develop these conditions both independently and as part of cardiorenal syndrome.

Part of the racial discrepancy in CKD, diabetic CKD and the associated complications may be explained by an increase in metabolic risk factors among minorities. Based on a three-year, cross-sectional sample of 15,826 patients with Type 2 diabetes, both Hispanics and NHBs were found to have higher body mass index, HbA1c, and LDL values in comparison with NHWs. NHBs also had significantly higher blood pressures compared to NHWs [45]. Moreover, ethnic minorities are both less physically active and have worse dietary behaviors compared to NHWs [46]. Minorities are also less likely to have health insurance coverage or to have a regular doctor [44]. As a result of the lower levels of glycemic control and the higher prevalence of both vascular disease and metabolic risk factors, rates of mortality from DM are persistently higher among NHBs than among NHWs [47].

The difference in the prevalence of cardiovascular disease in those with DM and CKD among different ethnicities is striking. It is likely a result of genetic susceptibility exacerbated by lifestyle differences. As health disparities continue to grow, a closer investigation into the root of these ethnic differences will help clinicians to create a more targeted approach.

3. Therapeutic rationale

Anemia is a risk factor for cardiovascular morbidity and mortality that is reversible [54]. According to the national Kidney Foundation Guidelines published in 2007, erythropoeisis stimulating agents (ESAs) should be used when the hemoglobin falls below the target range of 11-12 g/dL in both dialysis and non-dialysis patients. The goal for those receiving ESAs should be no greater than 13 g/dL. There are currently two Food and Drug Administration (FDA) approved ESAs in the United States, Epoetin alfa (Epogen, Procrit) and Darbepoetin alfa (Aranesp).

According to the Kidney Foundation Guidelines, all patients with CKD should be screened at least annually for anemia with a set of labs that include a complete blood count (CBC), a hemoglobin concentration (MCHC), iron studies, folate and Vitamin B12. Their stool should also be analyzed for occult blood loss [7]. Patients found to be iron deficient need to be started on iron supplementation, especially hemodialysis patients who may lose up to 3-5g of iron per year. Patients who qualify for ESAs should also receive iron therapy.

The Correction of Hemoglobin and Outcomes in Renal Insufficiency (CHOIR) and Cardiovascular Risk Reduction by Early Anemia Treatment with Epoetin Beta (CREATE), both landmark studies, provide an analysis of all-cause mortality and adverse cardiovascular events in patients with CKD with a therapeutic target of a hemoglobin greater than 13.0 g/dL compared with lower targets. None of the trials showed a benefit in those subjects with hemoglobin levels of greater than 13.0 g/dL. Investigators in the CHOIR study found that the 13.5g/dL target resulted in increased cardiovascular risk and no improvement in quality of life [58]. The CREATE study divided subjects with mild to moderate anemia (11-12.5 g/dl) into two groups. In one population, the goal was to raise the hemoglobin into the normal range (13-15g/dl) and while among the other subjects, the aim was to increase their hemoglobin to subnormal values (10.5-11.5g/dl). During this three year study complete correction of anemia did not affect the likelihood of a first cardiac death. There was no significant incidence of adverse events between the two groups. Investigators concluded that in patients with CKD, early complete correction of anemia does not reduce the risk of cardiovascular events [59].

According the Anemia Correction in DM (ACORD) study, in diabetics with mild to moderate anemia and moderate LVH, correction of hemoglobin target level of 13 to 15 g/dL (130 to 150 g/L) does not decrease left ventricular mass index. However, normalization of the hemoglobin value prevented any further increase in LVH [55]. The Trial to Reduce Cardiovascular Events with Aranesp Therapy (TREAT) trial in 2009 is randomized, double blind placebo controlled trial that was conducted to evaluate whether increasing the hemoglobin level with the use of darbepoetin would lower the rate of death, cardiovascular events or end stage renal disease in patients with type 2 diabetes and CKD. 2,012 patients were randomly assigned to receive darbepoetin in order to achieve a hemoglobin level of approximately 13g/dL, while 2,026 patients received a placebo, with administration of rescue darbepoetin when the hemoglobin level dropped below 9g/dL. Darbepoetin did not reduce the primary endpoints of death, cardiovascular events or ESRD in patients with DM and CKD. There was also an increased incidence of stroke to 2.1 percent in the darbepoetin arm compared with a 1.1 percent incidence in the placebo group [56].

In 2011, McMurray et al. published an analysis of TREAT, which aimed to examine predictors of cardiovascular morbidity and mortality in those patients with DM, CKD and anemia. They concluded that in this particularly high risk population, CVD risk is most strongly predicted by age, history of heart failure, CRP, urinary protein/creatinine ratio, abnormal electrocardiogram, and 2 specific cardiac biomarkers, serum N-terminal pro B-type natriuretic peptide and troponin T. Their findings brought to light several important ways to improve CVD risk stratification [57].

A 2012 update to the National Kidney Foundation clinical practice guidelines for DM and CKD was recently published to address new evidence that has emerged since the release of the 2007 guidelines. Recommendations include [58]:

1. Target hemoglobin A1c (HbA1c) of approximately 7.0 percent to prevent or delay the progression of the microvascular complications of DM including kidney disease

2. Use of Low density Lipoprotein cholesterol (LDL-C) lowering medicines, such as statins or statin/ezetimibe combination to reduce risk of major atherosclerotic events in patients with DM and CKD given that LDL-C with statin based therapies reduce the risk of major atherosclerotic events but not all-cause mortality in patients with CKD including those with DM

3. Use of an angiotensin converting enzyme inhibitor (ACE-I) or an angiotensive receptor Blocking agent (ARB) in normotensive patients with DM and albuminuria levels >30 mg who are at high risk for both the development of and the worsening of DKD

4. Conclusion

Anemia in CKD is a modifiable risk factor for CVD. If the anemia is addressed in its early stages, the risk of complications can be significantly reduced, especially those related to cardiovascular morbidity and mortality among the diabetic population. In addition, appropriate and timely treatment can improve the quality of life for these patients. It is important that physicians screen patients who are at risk for developing anemia as per accepted guidelines. This is especially important given that based on data collected from 1998-2008, NHANES found that the prevalence of DKD has steadily been increasing. The latest United States Renal Data System (USRDS) reported a 30 percent increase in the incidence of ESRD in diabetics in the United States between 1992 and 2008 [59, 60]. These figures indicate that anemia as caused by CKD in diabetics is an ongoing and ever-increasing problem in which all of the risk factors involved need to be addressed as part of regular preventative health measures.

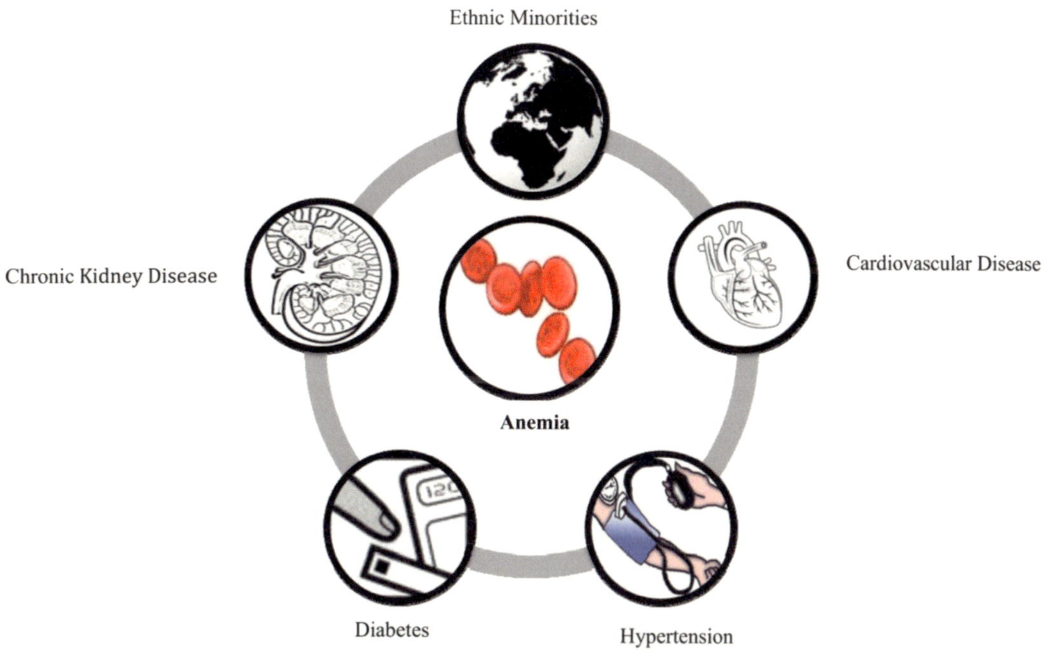

Figure 2. Highlights risk factors for anemia in this patient population.

Summary

1. With the rising epidemic of obesity in the western world, CVD, DM and CKD are becoming significant public health problems and each serves as risk factors for developing anemia.

2. Anemia is a modifiable risk factor for cardiovascular morbidity and mortality.
3. There are multiple postulated mechanisms for the development of anemia in diabetics with CKD such as decreased RBC life span, iron deficiency, nutritional folate deficiency, occult blood loss, systemic inflammation and erythropoietin deficiency, which appears to be the most dominant factor.
4. CVD is very common in patients with DM and CKD. The risk of developing CVD is significantly increased in diabetics with CKD compared with non-diabetics with CKD.
5. Regardless of the level of e-GFR, anemia is more frequent and severe in a diabetic compared to a non-diabetic patient.
6. Patients with CKD should be screened annually for anemia.
7. Patients who are found to be iron deficient need to be started on iron supplementation, especially hemodialysis patients.
8. ESAs are the mainstay of therapy for anemia in patients with CKD. Patients receiving ESA therapy should also be started on iron supplementation.
9. Correcting the hemoglobin level in this patient population to values greater than 13g/dL showed no benefit. It did, however, infer greater cardiac risk with no improvement in quality of life.
10. Guidelines currently recommend maintaining a hemoglobin level of 11-12 g/dL.

Author details

Nadine Montemarano, Jennifer Guttman and Samy I. McFarlane

*Address all correspondence to: smcfarlane@downstate.edu

Department of Medicine, State University of New York, Downstate Medical Center/ Kings County Hospital Center, Brooklyn, New York, USA

References

[1] National Kidney Foundation Practice Guidelines for Chronic Kidney Disease: Evaluation, Classification, and Stratification Andrew S. Levey, MD; Josef Coresh, MD, PhD; Ethan Balk, MD, MPH; Annamaria T. Kausz, MD, MS; Adeera Levin, MD; Michael W. Steffes, MD, PhD; Ronald J. Hogg, MD; Ronald D. Perrone, MD; Joseph Lau, MD; and Garabed Eknoyan, MD. Ann Intern Med. 2003;139:137-147.

[2] Rebecca J. Stoltzfus Michele L. Dreyfuss. Guidelines for the Use of Iron Supplements to Prevent and Treat Iron Deficiency Anemia. World Health Organization (WHO), United Nations Childrens Fund (UNICEF). 1998. ISBN: 1-57881-020-5 (ILSI Press)

[3] Beutler E, Waalen J. The definition of anemia: what is the lower limit of normal of the blood hemoglobin concentration? Blood. 2006 March 1; 107(5): 1747–1750.

[4] McFarlane SI, Chen SC, Whaley-Connell AT et al. Prevalence and associations of anemia of CKD: Kidney Early Evaluation Program (KEEP) and National Health Nutrition Examination Survey(NHANES)1999-2004. Am J Kidney Dis 51;S46-55, 2008.

[5] Dharawhat A, Golderberg T, Alam A, Atat Ali, Moore Alexis, McFarlane SI. Cardiovascular disease associated with anemia in diabetic patients with chronic kidney disease. International Diabetes Monitor 21:171-178, 2009.

[6] Beutler E, West C. Hematologic differences between African-Americans and whites: the roles of iron deficiency and alpha-thalassemia on hemoglobin levels and mean corpuscular volume. Blood 106:740-745, 2005.

[7] National Kidney Foundation: KDOQI Clinical Practice Guidelines and Clinical Practice Recommendations for Diabetes and Chronic Kidney Disease. Am J Kidney Dis 49:S12-154, 2007 (suppl 2)

[8] US Renal Data System: USRDS 2006 Annual Data Report. Bethesda, MD, The National Institutes of Health, National Institute of Diabetes and Digestive and Kidney Diseases, 2006.

[9] Centers for Disease Control and Prevention. www.cdc.gov/diabetes.

[10] Ritz E, Haxsen V. Diabetic nephropathy and anaemia. Eur J Clin Invest. 2005 Dec;35 Suppl 3:66-74.

[11] Merlin Thomas, Con Tsalamandri, et al. Anaemia in Diabetes: An Emerging Complication of Microvascular Disease. Current Diabetes Reviews, 2005, 1, 107-126.

[12] Ly J, Marticorena R, Donnelly S. Red blood cell survival in chronic renal failure. Am J Kidney Dis 2004; 44:715–719.

[13] McClellan W, Aronoff SL, Bolton WK, et al. The prevalence of anemia in patients with chronic kidney disease. Curr Med Res Opin 2004; 20:1501–1510.

[14] Ifudu O, Feldman J, Friedman EA. The intensity of hemodialysis and the response to erythropoietin in patients with end-stage renal dis- ease. N Engl J Med 1996; 334:420–425.

[15] Depner TA: Uremic toxicity: Urea and beyond. Semin Dial 14: 246–251, 2001

[16] Meyer TW, Hostetter TH: Uremia. N Engl J Med 357: 1316–1325, 2007

[17] Jennings PE, Wilkins MR, West MJ, Kendall MJ, Barnett AH. Sodium transport across erythrocyte membranes in diabetes mellitus. Diabetes Res 1986; 3: 407-10.

[18] Testa I, Rabini RA, Fumelli P, Bertoli E, Mazzanti L. Abnormal membrane fluidity and acetylcholinesterase activity in erythrocytes from insulin-dependent diabetic patients. J Clin Endocrinol Metab 1988; 67: 1129-33.

[19] Baldini P, Incerpi S, Lambert-Gardini S, Spinedi A, Luly P. Membrane lipid alteration and Na-pumping activity in erythrocytes from IDDM and NIDDM subjects. Diabetes 1989; 38: 825-31.

[20] Bryszewska M, Watala C, Torzecka W. Changes in fluidity and composition of erythrocyte membranes and in composition of plasma lipids in type I diabetes. Br J Haematol 1986; 62: 111-6.

[21] Resmi H, Akhunlar H, Temiz Artmann A, Guner G. In vitro effects of high glucose concentrations on membrane protein oxidation, G- actin and deformability of human erythrocytes. Cell Biochem Funct 2004.

[22] Manodori AB, Kuypers FA. Altered red cell turnover in diabetic mice. J Lab Clin Med. 2002; 140: 161-5.

[23] Grune T, Sommerburg O, Siems WG. Oxidative stress in anaemia. Clin Nephrol 2000; 53: S18–S22.

[24] Goodnough LT, Skikne B, Brugnara C. Erythropoietin, iron, and eryth- ropoiesis. Blood 2000; 96:823–833.

[25] Replacement of Renal Function by Dialysis.1996, Section II, 333-379, DOI: 10.1007/978-0-585-36947-1_14

[26] Kanauchi M, Akai Y, Hashimoto T. Transferrinuria in type 2 diabetic patients with early nephropathy and tubulointerstitial injury. Eur J Intern Med 2002; 13: 190-193.

[27] Erslev AJ. Erythropoietin. N Engl J Med 1991; 324:1339.

[28] Winkler AS, Marsden J, Chaudhuri KR, Hambley H, Watkins PJ. Erythropoietin depletion and anaemia in diabetes mellitus. Diabet Med 1999; 16: 813-9.

[29] Inomata H, Itoh M, Imai H, Sato T. Serum erythropoietin levels as a novel marker of the severity of diabetic nephropathy. Nephron 1997; 75: 426 –9.

[30] Finne PH, Skoglund RW. Erythropoietin production in the rat following splanchnic neurectomy. J Lab Clin Med 1970; 76: 103-6.

[31] Laakso M: Diabetes and cardiovascular disease in type 2 diabetes: challenge for treatment and prevention. J Intern Med 249 : 225 –235,2001

[32] Silverberg D, Blum M, Peer G, Iaina A. Anaemia during the predialysis period: a key to cardiac damage in renal failure. Nephron 1998; 80: 1–5.

[33] Levin A, Thompson CR, Ethier J, et al. Left ventricular mass index increase in early renal disease: impact of decline in haemoglobin. Am J Kidney Dis 1999; 34: 125-34.

[34] Vlagopoulos PT, Sarnak MJ. Traditional and nontraditional cardiovascular risk factors in chronic kidney disease. Med Clinic North Americ 89:587-611, 2005.

[35] US Census Bureau. 2009 Population Estimates. www.factfinder.census.gov. Accessed September 2, 2010.

[36] U.S. Census Bureau. (2009). Projections of the population by sex, race, and Hispanic origin for the United States: 2010 to 2050.

[37] . Centers for Disease Control and Prevention, National Center for Health Statistics. (2009). Age-adjusted percentage of civilian, noninstitutionalized population with diagnosed diabetes, by race and sex, United States, 1980–2009. Data from the National Health Interview Survey, at http://www.cdc.gov/diabetes/statistics/prev/national/figraceethsex.htm

[38] Cowie, C. C., Rust, K. F., Byrd-Holt, D. D., Gregg, E. W., Ford, E. S., Geiss, L. S., et al. (2010). Prevalence of diabetes and high risk for diabetes using A1C criteria in the U.S. population in 1988–2006. Diabetes Care, 33, 562–568.

[39] Boyle, J. P., Thompson, T. J., Gregg, E. W., Barker, L. E., & Williamson, D. F. (2010). Projection of the year 2050 burden of diabetes in the US adult population: dynamic modeling of incidence, mortality, and prediabetes prevalence. Popul Health Metrics, 8, 29.

[40] Newman AB, Siscovick DS, Manolio TA, Polak J, Fried LP, Borhani NO, et al. Ankle-arm index as a marker of atherosclerosis in the cardiovascular health study. Circulation 1993; 88:837–45.

[41] UK Prospective Diabetes Study (UKPDS) Group. Intensive blood-glucose control with sulphonylureas or insulin compared with conventional treatment and risk of complications in patients with type 2 diabetes (UKPDS 33). Lancet 1998; 352:854–65.

[42] Prevalence of and Risk Factors for Peripheral Arterial Disease in the United States : Results From the National Health and Nutrition Examination Survey, 1999 -2000. Elizabeth Selvin and Thomas P. Erlinger. Circulation. 2004;110:738-743.

[43] Mensah GA, Mokdad AH, Ford ES, et al. State of disparities in cardiovascular health in the United States. Circulation. 2005;111:1233-1241.

[44] Health Care Fact Sheet. National Association for the Advancement of Colored People. http://www.naacp.org/pages/health-care-fact-sheet (10.28.2012).

[45] Holland AT, Beinan ZA, Wong EC, Choi SE, Wong ND, Palaniappan LP. Racial/ethnic differences in control of cardiovascular risk factors among type 2 diabetes patients in an insured, ambulatory care population. Journal of Diabetes and Its Complications. Accepted 17 August 2012.

[46] August, K. J., & Sorkin, D. H. (2011). Racial/ethnic disparities in exercise and dietary behaviors of middle-aged and older adults. Journal of General Internal Medicine, 26,245–250.

[47] Writing Group Members for the American Heart Association Statistics Committee and Stroke Statistics Subcommittee Heart Disease and Stroke Statistics—2009 Update: A Report From the American Heart Association Statistics Committee and Stroke Statistics Subcommittee. Circulation. 2009:119: e21-e181.

[48] U.S. Renal Data System. USRDS 2012 Annual Data Report: Atlas of End-Stage Renal Disease in the United States.: National Institutes of Health.

[49] Nguyen HT and Stack AG. Ethnic Disparities in Cardiovascular Risk Factors and Coronary Disease Prevalence among Individuals with Chronic Kidney Disease: Findings from the Third National Health and Nutrition Examination Survey. Accepted March 23, 2006. ISSN: 1046-6673/1706-1716.

[50] Hackam DG, Anand SS. Emerging risk factors for atherosclerotic vascular disease: a critical review of the evidence. JAMA. 2003 Aug 20;290(7):932-40.

[51] Vidula H, Tian L, Liu K, Criqui M, Ferrucci L, Pearce W, et al. Biomarkers of inflammation and thrombosis as predictors of near-term mortality in patients with peripheral arterial disease: a cohort study. Ann Intern Med 2008; 148:85–93.

[52] Li J, Li JJ, Li Q, Li Z, Qian HY. A rational connection of inflammation with peripheral arterial disease. Med Hypotheses 2007; 69:1190–5.

[53] Weiner DE, Tighiouart H, Amin MG, et al. Chronic kidney disease as a risk factor for cardiovascular disease and all-cause mortality: A pooled analysis of community-based studies. J Am Soc Nephrol. 2004;15:1307-1315.

[54] Foley R. Cardiac disease in diabetic patients with renal disease. Acta Diabetol 39: S9-14, 2002.

[55] Ritz, E, et al. Target level for hemoglobin correction in patients with diabetes and CKD: primary results of the Anemia Correction in Diabetes (ACORD) Study. Am J Kidney Dis. 2007 Feb;49(2):194-207.

[56] Pfeffer MA, et al. TREAT Investigators: A trial of darbepoetin alfa in type 2 diabetes and chronic kidney disease. N Engl J Med 361: 2019–2032, 2009

[57] McMurray JJ, et al. Predictors of fatal and nonfatal cardiovascular events in patients with type 2 diabetes mellitus, chronic kidney disease, and anemia: an analysis of the Trial to Reduce cardiovascular Events with Aranesp (darbepoetin-alfa) Therapy (TREAT). Am Heart J. 2011 Oct;162(4):748-755.e3.

[58] KDOQI CLINICAL PRACTICE GUIDELINE FOR DIABETES AND CKD: 2012 UPDATE Am J Kidney Dis. 2012;60(5):850-886

[59] de Boer IH, Rue TC, Hall YN, Heagerty PJ, Weiss NS, Himmelfarb J. Temporal trends in the prevalence of diabetic kidney disease in the United States. JAMA. Jun 22 2011;305(24): 2532-2539.

[60] US Renal Data System. USRDS 2011 Annual Data Report: Atlas of Chronic Kidney Disease and End-Stage Renal Disease in the United States. Am J Kidney Dis. 2012;59(1)(suppl 1):e1-e420.

[61] Schiffrin EL, Lipman ML, Mann JF. Chronic kidney disease: Effects on the cardiovascular system. Circulation 116: 85–97, 2007.

[62] Zoccali C, Bode-Boger S, Mallamaci F, Benedetto F, Tripepi G, Malatino L, Cataliotti A, Bellanuova I, Fermo I, Frolich J, Boger R. Plasma concentration of asymmetrical dimethylarginine and mortality in patients with end-stage renal disease: A prospective study. Lancet 358: 2113–2117, 2001.

[63] Qunibi WY et al. Reducing the burden of cardiovascular calcification in patients with chronic kidney disease. J Am Soc Nephrol 16[suppl 2]: S95–S102, 2005.

[64] Kanwar YS et al. Diabetic nephropathy: mechanisms of renal disease progression. Exp Biol Med (Maywood). 2008 Jan;233(1):4-11.

[65] Wolf G. New insights into the pathophysiology of diabetic nephropathy: from hemodynamics to molecular pathology. Eur J Clin Invest 34:785–796, 2004.

[66] Jandeleit-Dahm K, Cooper ME. Hypertension and diabetes: role of renin-angiotensin system. Endocrinol Meab Clin North Am 35:469–490, 2006.

[67] Guinti S, Barit D, Cooper ME. Mechanisms of diabetic nephropathy: role of hypertension. Hypertension 48:519–526, 2006.

[68] Hostetter TH, Rennke HG, Brenner BM. Case for intrarenal hypertension in initiation and progression of diabetic and other glomerulopathies. Am J Med 72:375–380, 1982

Chapter 12

Diabetic Foot Ulcers — Treatment and Prevention

Jarrod Shapiro, Diane Koshimune and
Rebecca Moellmer

Additional information is available at the end of the chapter

http://dx.doi.org/10.5772/56400

1. Introduction

Diabetic foot ulcers are a growing problem in the diabetic community. Globally, diabetes mellitus has grown to pandemic proportions, affecting 194 million people worldwide and is expected to increase in prevalence to 344 million by the year 2030 [1]. Of these patients, between 2 and 6% will develop a diabetic foot ulcer (DFU) yearly [2]. The onset of a DFU often precipitates a complex chain of events that may lead to limb loss. The long-term outcome for a diabetic patient after a major limb amputation is grave, with 50% of these patients deceased at 5 years [3].

In the United States public discussion and much research money goes to the investigation and treatment of breast and prostate cancers. However, when the 5 year mortality percentages are analyzed, a diabetic neuropathic ulcer has a worse survival rate than each of these cancers. The same is true if a diabetic has had a prior amputation. Add peripheral arterial disease and the mortality statistics worsen. In fact having a neuropathic ulcer or prior amputation has the same poor survival rate as colon cancer [4]. It is unknown if the lower extremity complications themselves lead to greater mortality, but it may be assumed that complications such as a foot ulcer are indicators of more significant diabetic disease with its well-known increased risk of cardiovascular complications.

This chapter will focus on key concepts related to prevention and treatment of diabetic foot ulcers and their complications. A detailed discussion will cover pathogenesis and risk factors of diabetic foot ulcers; clinical presentation; initial evaluation; treatment methods, both nonsurgical and surgical care; and complication management, including infection of soft tissue and bone, Charcot neuroarthropathy, and limb preservation amputation. A rational approach to the evaluation and treatment of diabetic foot ulcers will be discussed, utilizing the most current research.

2. Pathogenesis of the diabetic foot ulcer

The diabetic foot ulcer is a complex multifactorial entity with a well-known etiologic pathway. The most common pathway is considered to be due to reduced peripheral sensation [5] coupled with increased shear and/or compressive pressure [6]. Brand discussed the concept of "tenderizing" the foot [7] in which peripheral neuropathy leads to a loss of function of two types of mechanoreceptors in the skin, responsible for delivering nociceptive signals. High threshold mechano-receptors, carried via A-delta fibers, normally become sensitized to increased repetitive pressures on healthy tissues. This sensitization lowers the pain threshold in the patient with normal sensation, carried by polymodal nociceptors, leading to altered behaviors which reduce pain and subsequent damage. In the neuropathic patient this sensitization system is absent, allowing tissue damage to occur without any pain response with the subsequent diabetic foot ulcer.

Diabetic peripheral neuropathy also causes motor and autonomic dysfunction. Motor dysfunction is seen in the form of weakness and atrophy [8]. As the intrinsic pedal musculature becomes poorly functional muscular imbalances occur causing deformity. This deformity allows for focal areas of increased pressure, becoming risk areas for ulceration. Autonomic neuropathy contributes via sudomotor dysfunction causing loss of sweat glands as well as loss of nutritive supply with subsequent dry skin that breaks down easily [5]. An ill-fitting pair of shoes may be all that was required for the shear forces to lead to an ulceration of a patient's foot who has diminished sensation.

If skin breakdown and wound formation occurs by a combination of high pressures in the insensate foot then wound chronicity is upheld by altered and inappropriately functioning biochemical pathways and chemical mediators. Various cytokines and matrix proteins have been implicated in the process of delayed wound healing. One of these mediators that has received much emphasis over the recent past is matrix metalloproteinase 8 (MMP-8), which is the primary collagenase in normal wounds [9]. In chronic wounds MMP-8 is upregulated due to reduction of its regulating enzyme TIMP-1 (tissue inhibitor of metalloproteinase 1). This overexpression of MMP-8 causes enzymatic destruction of the wound extracellular matrix, thus retarding wound healing. The diabetic foot ulcer may also be lacking growth factors such as platelet-derived growth factor (PDGF) and tumor growth factor beta (TGF-β) which stimulate fibroblast proliferation and synthesis and act as chemoattractants for neutrophils, smooth muscle cells, and macrophages [10] in the healthy wound. In diabetic wounds these factors may be diminished or absent.

3. Risk factors

Several clinical causal pathways have been researched, allowing the clinician to grade the primary risk factors associated with the onset of DFUs. Lavery et al, described an update to the clinical staging method previously proposed by the International Working Group for the Diabetic Foot [11, 12]. Table 1 demonstrates increasing trend of ulceration, infection, and amputation, with an extremely high risk of hospitalization with increasing stage. The presence of peripheral arterial disease and a history of prior ulceration or amputation greatly increases the risk of complications beyond the introducing factors of peripheral neuropathy or deformity.

The presence of peripheral neuropathy with loss of protective sensation is the sine qua non of diabetic foot ulceration, diagnosed using the 5.07 Semmes Weinstein monofilament. This simple, rapid test is easily performed in the primary or specialty clinic. The monofilament is constructed to produce a standard 10 grams of force when bent and has been found to accurately predict the presence of ulceration [13]. Ten sites are tested (plantar toes and metatarsal heads 1, 3, and 5; two points on the medial arch; one point on the heel; and one on the dorsum of the foot). If the patient is unable to feel 4 of 10 sites, he is diagnosed with peripheral neuropathy.

Stage	Description	Risk of Complications (by Odds Ratio)			
		Ulcer	Infection	Amputation	Hospitalization
0	No PN*, No PAD	N/A	N/A	N/A	N/A
1	PN, No PAD, no deformity	2.4	1.9	0	10
2a	PN and deformity, No PAD	1.2	2.3	10.9	13.6
2b	PAD	9.3	13.5	60.9	124.8
3a	Ulcer history	50.5	19.2	36.3	60.7
3b	Amputation	52.7	62.3	567.9	650.3

Table 1. IWGDF staging system for diabetic patients at risk for lower extremity complications. Adapted from Lavery, et al [11]. *PN = Peripheral Neuropathy; PAD = Peripheral Arterial Disease

4. Clinical presentation and initial evaluation

As in all medical conditions the initial evaluation of a patient with a diabetic foot ulcer begins with a detailed history. Important components of the history include length of time the ulcer has been present; etiology of the wound (if known); any self or professional treatment; prior ulcer, infection, or amputation history; personal medical history; allergies; medications; surgical history; family history; tobacco use; alcohol abuse; recreational drug use; and a detailed review of systems to elicit the presence of macrovascular or microvascular disease [14].

On physical examination one may appreciate the classic appearance of the diabetic plantar foot ulcer (Figure 1). This is most commonly a partial or full thickness wound underlying a bony prominence or area of deformity. When chronic low grade elevated plantar pressures are present the skin forms reactive hypertrophic tissue, indicated by hyperkeratotic callus, the tell-tale sign of the neuropathic ulcer. The wound should be examined for size, undermining (in which the edges of the wound overlap the base), general appearance, and the probe to bone test should be performed.

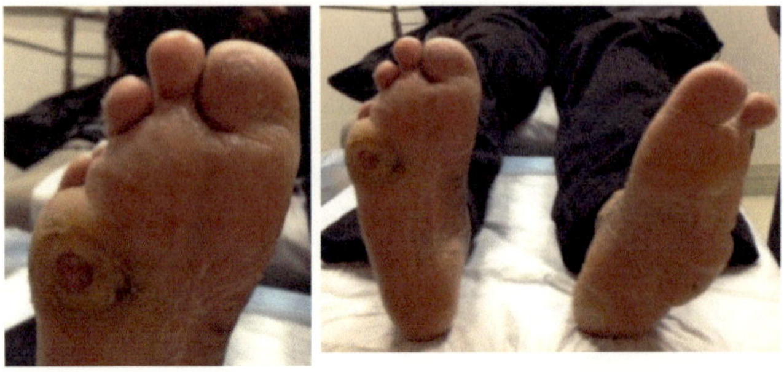

Figure 1. Classic appearance of the diabetic foot ulcer. Note the characteristic red, granular base and hyperkeratotic rim under an area of increased pressure as well as the contralateral foot with prior amputation of the 3rd, 4th, and 5th rays.

During this test the examiner uses a sterile metal probe (often the blunt end of a cotton swab is used) to gently but firmly push into the base of the wound. The examiner then determines the depth to which the probe may go, whether to subcutaneous, capsular, or bone layers. If the probe is able to touch bone this is considered a positive probe to bone test and is highly predictive of osteomyelitis. The predictive ability of this test differs based on the population studied. In patients with severe infection and a higher likelihood of osteomyelitis, this test has a positive predictive value of 89% [15]. However, in a patient population less likely to be infected, i.e. the outpatient wound clinic population, the positive predictive value is 57% but with a negative predictive value of 98% [16]. In this situation the inability to palpate bone with the probe indicates a low likelihood of osteomyelitis.

A thorough physical examination should also include an evaluation of arterial outflow and the presence of peripheral arterial disease (PAD). This includes palpation of all pulses in the lower extremity, including the dorsalis pedis/tibialis anterior, posterior tibial, popliteal, femoral, and abdominal aortic pulses. The absence or diminution of a peripheral pulse (specifically the dorsalis pedis or posterior tibial) has a sensitivity between 63% and 95% and a specificity between 73% and 99% for peripheral arterial disease [17-19]. Capillary refill time, in which the limb is elevated to heart level and pressure placed on multiple digits, counting the time for refill of the blanched skin, has a sensitivity of 28.3% and specificity or 85.3% [17]. Auscultation for femoral bruits may also be performed. However, this test has a low sensitivity (2-29%) but high specificity (95-96%) [19, 20]. Trophic changes of the skin may include atrophic, shiny appearance with loss of hair, coolness to touch, cyanosis, and thickened nails. Trophic changes generally have a lower sensitivity and specificity for PAD [17].

In the diabetic patient with a neuropathic foot ulcer and concomitant PAD the wound appearance may be slightly different. In some situations the wound will look similar to the well vascularized ulcer with the exception of a more pale or light pink appearance to the wound base instead of a red, granular appearance. In more advanced neuroischemic wounds the

http://dx.doi.org/10.5772/56400

appearance will be markedly different with a fibrous yellow appearance and an often irregular, sometimes punched out-appearing, shape (Figure 2).

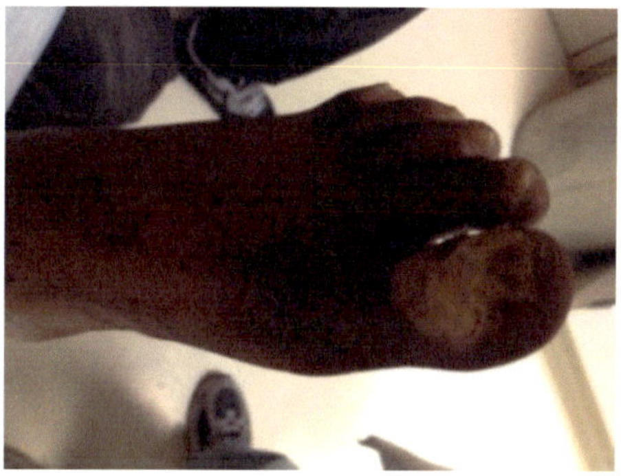

Figure 2. DFU with ischemic appearance demonstrating a yellow, fibrotic base and lack of healthy red granulation tissue.

The musculoskeletal examination is also fundamentally important to evaluate the patient with a diabetic foot ulcer. In the majority of patients an examination of the biomechanical contribution will reveal the cause of the ulcer. The common factor is a focal increased shear or vertical pressure. As such, a thorough examination for pedal deformity is of paramount importance. Overall appearance of the foot should be appreciated, followed by a detailed examination of specific deformities, including joint position, range of motion, and rigidity versus flexibility (Figure 3).

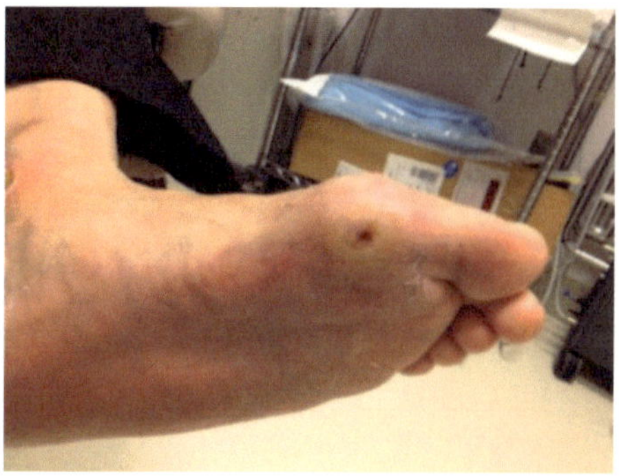

Figure 3. Diabetic neuropathic plantar foot ulceration underlying tibial sesamoid bone with involved hallux valgus deformity.

Functional compensation at one joint for lack of motion of another is also commonly seen. For example, lack of motion of the great toe joint (hallux limitus) often leads to a compensatory increased motion at the hallux interphalangeal joint. This compensation increases plantar pressures at the joint with a subsequent DFU (Figure 4).

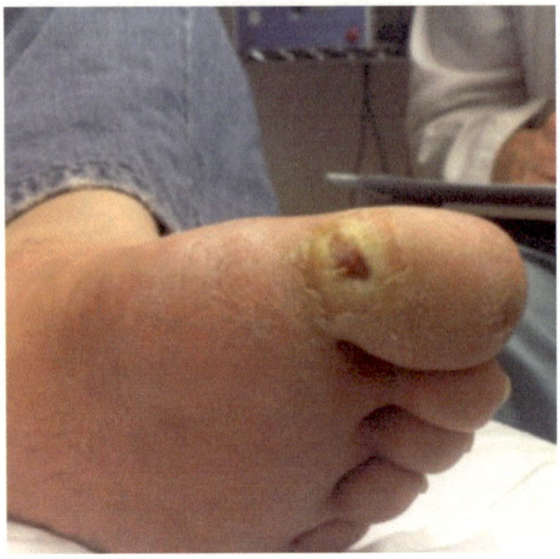

Figure 4. Diabetic foot ulcer located plantar to the hallux interphalangeal joint resulting from increased pressure after compensation at this joint for lack of motion at the first metatarsophalangeal joint.

Another highly important mechanical contributor to the creation of diabetic foot ulcers, especially those on the plantar forefoot area, is ankle joint equinus, or lack of dorsiflexion of the foot on the ankle during active walking. Plantar pressures have been shown to be increased three fold in diabetic patients with ankle equinus when compared with those without [21]. The relationship between callus and ulceration was confirmed by Murray and colleagues who found a relative risk of 11.0 for an ulcer developing under an area of callus [22]. As such, the relationship between ankle equinus, increased plantar pressures, and DFU is well established.

Upon completion of the physical examination, laboratory and imaging methods may be employed in certain circumstances to better appreciate the underlying anatomy and will be discussed below.

A simple, rapid examination of the foot takes no more than one to two minutes. From a clinical standpoint a significant sign of impending ulceration is the preulcerative callus. This is seen as hyperkeratotic tissue with visible hemorrhage within the epidermal or dermal skin layers.

Treatment of diabetic foot ulcerations can be intimidating and complex without a basic understanding of the treatment options available and a thorough evaluation of the ulcer's characteristics. Current literature suggests that, if the initial treatment plan does not reduce the size of the ulcer by 50% in four weeks that the course of treatment should be re-assessed [23-26]. Essential components of any initial or re-evaluated treatment plan should consist of debridement, moist wound healing environment, offloading and infection control [27]. Conservative options are typically employed initially [28] but if progress stalls, surgical components to the treatment plan may help to decrease time to healing or even promote healing. Characteristics of the diabetic foot ulcer are important to consider because they directly influence what treatment modalities are used. Evaluation of the diabetic foot ulcer's location, size and depth, tissue type, presence or absence of drainage, length of time the ulcer has been present, vascular supply, and any pathomechanics present are all important variables when formulating the treatment plan.

4.1. Debridement

The type of tissue found within the diabetic foot ulceration is an important treatment consideration. When yellow fibrotic tissue or dusky necrosis is noted, steps must be taken to covert the diabetic ulcer base to a beefy, red, healthy granular tissue. Surgical debridement of avascular tissue may improve rates of ulcer closure by removing the tissue that had served as a foreign body. Several types of debridement are commonly employed today but there is no scientific evidence suggesting that one type is superior to another [29, 30] only that diabetic foot ulcers receiving a regular debridement are found to heal faster [30]. Debridement is a necessary step that prepares the wound bed to promote healing [30] and is helpful when converting a chronic wound to an acute ulcer [25]. Sharp debridement is considered the gold standard [30, 31] and can be performed at the bedside or in the operating room [32]. Enzymatic debridement, such as collagenase for fibrotic tissue is a good option when the risk of debriding small quantities of healthy tissue is not acceptable or if the patient experiences pain with sharp debridement. Hydrosurgical debridement, as with Versajet® (Smith and Nephew corporation), demonstrates no statistically significant reduction in bacterial contamination [33] and was found only to decrease the duration of time spent debriding the ulcer [31]. Biologic debridement, using medically sterilized *Lucilia sericata* larvae, aims to rid the ulcer of necrotic tissue and pathogens [30, 34]. However, maggot therapy has not demonstrated improvement of healing rate or reduction of bacterial load as compared with hydrogel [29, 30]. Applying hydrogel or hydrocolloid dressings introduces moisture, and if placed under occlusion, serves as a form of autolytic debridement that allows the body's own enzymes to liquefy necrotic tissue. Hydrogel, additionally, has been found to increase the rate of healing as compared with plain gauze [29]. Mechanical debridement, also known as "non-selective debridement" is performed by applying saline moistened gauze to the ulcer and allowing it to dry before the dressing is periodically changed. The removal of the gauze mechanically removes both healthy and unhealthy tissue and is no longer considered the best dressing for diabetic foot ulcers [26].

The size and depth of the diabetic foot ulcer are important factors to evaluate because a deep ulcer may have avascular tissue such as tendon exposed. Instead of allowing the avascular tissues to desiccate and require debridement, potentially losing long-term function in the foot, immediate use of a negative pressure wound therapy (NPWT) system has been shown to increase volume of granulation tissue within the ulcer [29, 35, 36] which may possibly preserve that structure. NPWT has also been shown to significantly improve the rate of wound closure as compared to simple saline gauze dressings [26, 29, 37] and NPWT has demonstrated a reduced amputation incidence [26] and decreased hospital stay [38].

Ultrasound, lasers, electrical and electromagnetic therapies have been evaluated in laboratory research but there is insufficient evidence to suggest these have any effect on diabetic foot ulceration healing times [29].

4.2. Moist wound healing environment

The presence or absence of drainage helps to determine what type of adjunct dressing the diabetic foot ulcer may require. By converting a chronic diabetic foot ulcer to an acute wound and maintaining a moist wound bed, the inflammation, infection and exudate are controlled while increasing epithelial advancement [25, 34]. This prevents retardation of cellular proliferation and angiogenesis by eliminating the excessive levels of matrix metalloproteinase's, growth factors and cytokines [34] present in the chronic wound. Applying a hydrocolloid or hydrogel may help to introduce moisture. If excessive drainage is present an absorbent dressing should be used, such as a calcium alginate or another absorbent fiber. Other dressing components have been found to increase healing in small studies such as the use of topical and oral β-glucan [39]. In another study, comparison of various dressing options demonstrated no statistical difference in ulcer healing but did note that the basic wound contact dressing, was more cost-effective in healing diabetic foot ulcers than a fibrous hydrocolloid dressing [40].

If the diabetic foot ulcer has been present for 30-90 days [35] it is considered chronic. Chronicity may dictate whether or not to use bioengineered products that deliver fibroblasts superficially, such as Dermagraft® (Advanced Tissue Sciences), Apligraf (Organogenesis) or healthy doses of growth factors, such as platelet rich protein gel delivered superficially. Both, Dermagraft® and Apligraf®, used with effective offloading, have demonstrated decreased healing time [41, 42] and several studies suggest that utilization of near-physiological concentration of platelet rich protein gel on recalcitrant or chronic wounds demonstrate a rapid and consistent healing [32, 34, 35, 43] and is cost-effective [42]. A smaller study suggests that injected, rather than topical, epidermal growth factor at the lesion's base may result in improved healing [44] due to elimination of high levels of proteases that reduce levels of growth factors needed for healing [34].

4.3. Offloading

The location of the diabetic foot ulcer is commonly found overlying a bony prominence [25, 34] or involving a deformity (Figure 5). Early treatment may consist of pressure reduction. Total contact casting (TCC) (Figure6A), is considered the best method of offloading as compared to a removable walking cast [27]. However, when a total contact cast is unavailable or contraindicated, placing the patient in a wedge-type shoe (Figure 6B) or a walking boot (Figure 6C, 6D), using flexible and rigid casting tape [45], complete bed rest [28] or by using felt aperture padding have also been noted to reduce healing times [25, 35].

When these conservative means for offloading are ineffective, surgical resection of the underlying bony prominence, termed internal off-weighting, is an option [25]. This surgical treatment may entail bony procedures such as an exostectomy, condylectomy, arthroplasty [25, 36], metatarsal osteotomy [28] or arthrodesis [28]. Additionally, tendon transfers to rebalance the foot and amputation may also be applied as indicated (Figure 7).Surgical procedures should be chosen and performed by those with expertise in surgical reconstruction of the diabetic foot and ankle.

Pathomechanics of the patient's foot, such as gastrocnemius-soleus equinus or a taut plantar fascial ligament both leading to plantar forefoot ulcerations, may necessitate conservative offloading measures as previously mentioned. However, if the offloading attempts are ineffective, a surgical release (plantar fascial ligament resection [28, 46, 47]) or surgical lengthening (tendo-achilles lengthening [25, 28, 46, 48]) of the contracture may allow the forefoot to be more flexible when met with ground reactive forces thus healing the diabetic

http://dx.doi.org/10.5772/56400

plantar foot ulcer [49]. Mueller et al's randomized clinical trial found that patients treated with a tendo-achilles lengthening and a TCC were 12% more likely to heal a plantar foot ulcer than with a TCC alone. At two years post operatively, the group with both the TAL and TCC re-ulcerated at a rate of only 38% compared to 81% recurrence in the group with only a TCC [24, 49].

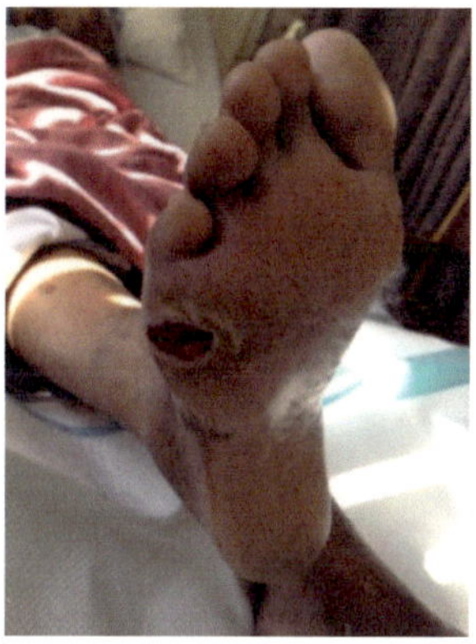

Figure 5. DFU overlying a prominent fifth metatarsal head deformity.

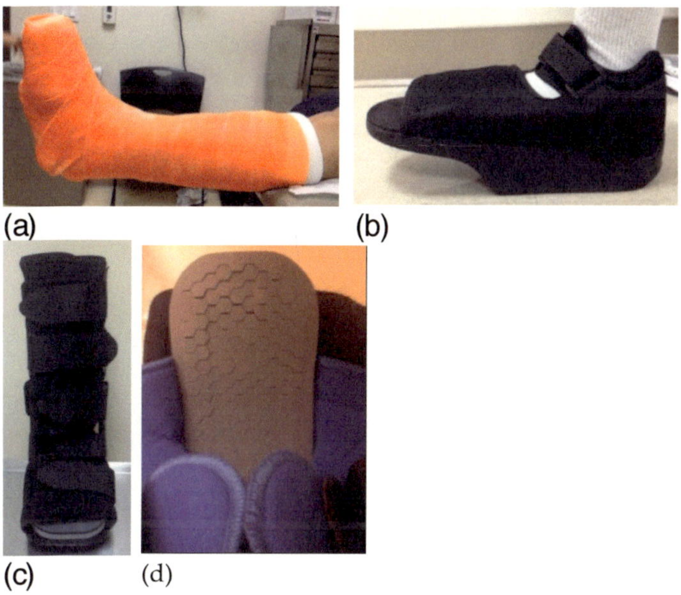

Figure 6. Off-loading devices; A – Total Contact Cast (TCC); B – Wedge type shoe to off-load the plantar forefoot; C – Darco® brand offweighting boot with removable hexagonal pegs for offweighting DFUs.

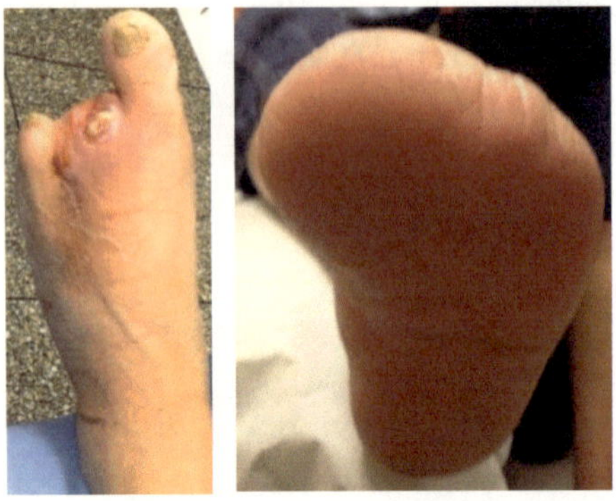

Figure 7. Nonfunctional foot with underlying osteomyelitis successfully treated with transmetatarsal amputation and percutaneous tendoachilles lengthening with 6 month follow-up (note lack of callus or recurrent ulceration).

4.4. Additional methods

Various types of skin grafts and flaps may assist with closure of the ulceration (Figure 8) as healing an ulcer by means of secondary intention represents a major burden to patients, health care professionals and the health care system [50]. Bioengineered skin grafts and split-thickness skin grafts do not show statistically significant success in healing diabetic foot ulcers [29] despite small studies suggesting grafts improve rates of healing and decreased evidence of amputations [51, 52]. Local muscle flaps have also been found to be successful in closing complicated diabetic foot wounds and are far superior as compared to the survival rates of amputees [53]. Despite an increased complication rate, pedicled flaps were found to have comparable limb salvage success as compared with free flaps [53]. A successful flap closure extends the life of an amputee [53].

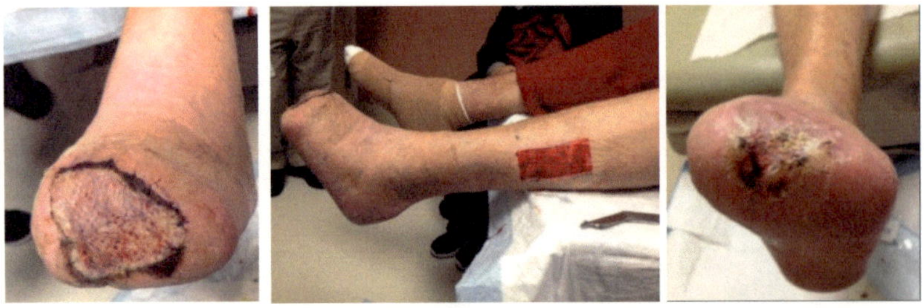

Figure 8. A. Complicated diabetic wound after guillotine-type trans-metatarsal amputation treated with split thickness skin graft. B. Donor site from lateral leg shown. C. Successful healing.

Hyperbaric oxygen (HBO) therapy systemically has been found to decrease the rate of major amputations [29] but not in the rate of minor amputations [54]. HBO therapy in diabetic foot ulcers has not yet demonstrated its cost effectiveness [29]. When a conservative treatment plan is found to improve the ulcer but does not heal it, utilizing HBO therapy may help to increase the partial pressure of oxygenation to tissues and help heal the wound [54, 55]. A study has demonstrated that the use of HBO facilitates wound closure when there is a change in transcutaneous oxygen measurements of ≥ 10 torr [56]. Topical hyperbaric oxygen therapy has not been found to decrease the rate of major amputations [29] and cannot be recommended for use in diabetic foot ulcers at this time.

When various treatment modalities are not successful, if possible, a limb salvage attempt is advised. External fixation is an additional option, boasting skeletal stability, easy access for soft tissue management, and assisting with plastic surgery wound closure techniques [36, 57]. If external fixation is not available or possible, there are many levels of amputations to consider [36]. While a trans-tibial amputation has the same long-term survivorship as some mid and rearfoot amputations (Symes, Lisfranc, calcanectomy or Chopart's) a partial foot amputation allows higher ambulatory levels and longer durability with less morbidity and mortality than trans-tibial amputations [51]. Allowing the patient to have a good quality of life, maintain as much function as possible and increase ease of prosthetic use following the amputation are important advantages to consider.

5. Complications

5.1. Infection

One of the earliest complications of diabetic foot ulcerations is infection [58] and if not treated adequately, may require amputation. This of particular concern because the 3 year survival rate following a lower limb amputation is 50%, decreasing to only 40% after 5 years [59].

All skin surfaces, and thus all wounds, have a certain level of bacteria on the surface at baseline, referred to as surface *contaminants*, defined as bacteria which are present but do not multiply. When those bacteria multiply, they are referred to as *colonizers*. Whether the bacteria are able to surmount a response from the host immune system will dictate whether there is an *infection*. Some believe that observing 10^5 bacteria per 1 gram of tissue is the threshold between a colonizer and an established infection. However, depending on the bacterial species or strain, an infection can result with far fewer than the 10^5 bacteria per 1 gram of tissue. Take for example β-hemolytic *streptococci*, which produce enzymes that promote tissue invasion and cause progressive infections without the same bacterial burden as other organisms [58, 60-62].

Risk factors for infection include a non-healing ulcer, advanced age, male sex, black race and a history of smoking in addition to sensory and autonomic neuropathy [63]. Diabetic foot infections are difficult to manage due to the associated comorbidities affecting the patient such as neuropathy, peripheral vascular disease, immunopathy and nephropathy [59]. Organisms such as methicillin resistant strains of *Staphylococcus aureus*, among others, pose a challenge to healthcare providers. Several factors such as prolonged hospital stays, exposure to surfaces and personnel who may have come into contact with resistant strains, and prolonged or prior antibiotic treatment can result in infections with these organisms. Many patients with chronic ulcerations have a history of recurrent ulcerations and infections that place them at high risk for infection with resistant organisms [65]. Immunopathy increases a patient's susceptibility to infection. Poor glycemic control has been connected to impairment in leukocyte phagocytosis and chemotaxis, which increase the risk for infection. Infections lead to hyperglycemia which potentiates in a vicious feedback loop [59, 62, 66, 67].

5.2. Clinical findings

Patients with infections typically present with erythema, edema, purulent drainage, malodor, calor, induration, lymphangitis, soft tissue edema and occasionally gangrene or necrotic tissue (Figure 9). Complaints of pain in an insensate patient should raise suspicion for an infection. Patients also complain of recalcitrant hyperglycemia and other constitutional symptoms such as fevers, malaise and chills, sometimes referred to as the 'diabetic flu', which should raise suspicion for a deep infection [59, 61, 68].. Due to the immunopathy however, some patients may not present with any constitutional signs or symptoms [59, 66].

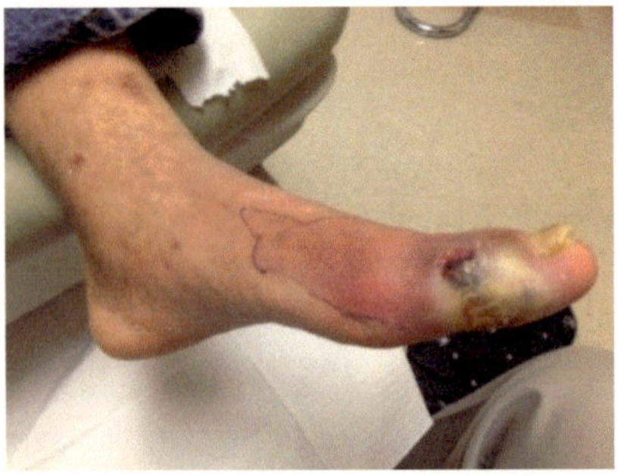

Figure 9. Diabetic patient with acute infection—notice the lymphangitis and local erythema.

Infections can be categorized by anatomical location and severity of illness. Superficial infections typically show no signs of systemic toxicity and glycemic levels remain unaffected. Deep foot infections, in contrast, result in contiguous spread of erythema and edema with accompanying constitutional symptoms such as fever, chills, malaise, and occasionally blood glucose elevations. When necrosis of tissue or skin is encountered, this signals impaired arterial supply, either from systemic arterial disease or from local vascular impairment [6] (Figure 10).

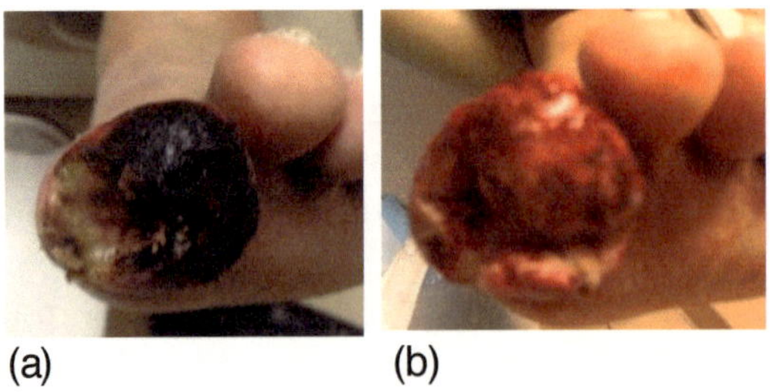

Figure 10. Diabetic patient with an infected hallux; A – at presentation, note necrotic and gangrenous tissue; B – after debridement.

5.3. Diagnosis

Identification of infecting organisms for diabetic foot wounds is of great interest, particularly when considering antibiotic therapies. Depending on the chronicity of the wound there can be a slight difference in the organisms that can be isolated from a wound culture. Acute wounds typically grow gram positive cocci while chronic wounds are polymicrobial, with a mixture of gram positive cocci, gram negative bacilli and anaerobic organisms (Table 2) [58, 69, 70]. Those patients who have been previously hospitalized or have had prolonged antibiotic therapy can have an altered profile of organisms. Patients who have not been on any recent antibiotics typically grow gram positive organisms with a greater likelihood of gram negative organisms and organisms that are resistant to antibiotics [65].

Performing a surface swab evaluation has been deemed diagnostically unreliable. Instead, deep tissue specimens should be taken from the wound after a sharp debridement either with a scalpel or curette. Alternatively, in the presence of an abscess, aspiration of the abscess can provide more accurate information regarding the infecting organisms [58, 61, 63, 64].

Chronicity	Organisms	Examples
Acute	Gram + cocci	*S. aureus, β-hemolytic streptococcus* (A, B, C and G)
Chronic	Gram + cocci	Staphylococcus, Streptococcus, Enterococcus
	Gram - bacilli	Enterobacter, E. coli, Proteus, Klebsiella, P. aeruginosa
	Anaerobe	Peptococcus, Peptostretococcus, Clostridium, Fusobacterium, Bacterioides

Table 2. Typical organisms found in Diabetic foot infections, acute vs. chronic. [58]

Laboratory testing can also help to guide or evaluate the effectiveness of therapy. The difficulty with diabetic patients is their lack of systemic response due to immunopathy, where leukocytosis may be absent. However, in a subset of patients elevation of white blood cells (WBC) may be found at initial presentation. Recent studies have shown that C-reactive protein (CRP) is the most sensitive and specific lab test to distinguish between grade 2 and grade 1 ulcers [71].

Plain radiographs can provide useful information in the presence of a diabetic foot ulcer when there is suspected soft tissue emphysema. Advanced imaging techniques such as magnetic resonance imaging (MRI) can provide information regarding the extent of tissue and bone involvement [58, 61, 63, 69]. The imaging techniques will be discussed to a greater extent in the osteomyelitis section.

5.4. Treatment

The consensus from multiple studies and practice guidelines is to utilize a multi-disciplinary approach, including providers from primary care, endocrinology (diabetologist), podiatry, vascular surgery, plastic surgery, infectious disease, microbiology, wound specialty nursing, physical therapy, orthotist and prosthetists [43, 58, 59, 61, 63, 69, 72, 73]. However, there is no evidence-based consensus on specific treatment algorithms for soft tissue infections. Unfortunately any attempt at making such a consensus based on existing data is challenged by inconsistent definitions of infection, improvement and cure, and patient to patient variability. Therapy is typically guided by knowledge of likely pathogens, based on history and clinical presentation and spectrum of available antibiotics that can reliably provide coverage [58].

Patients who have a Grade 2 non-limb threatening infection should be treated on an outpatient basis, covering for gram-positive cocci, and reassessed in 48-72 hours. If the infection has not improved the patient should be admitted for parenteral antibiotics and possible incision and drainage. Patients with grade 3-4 infections that are considered limb- or life- threatening should be admitted for parenteral antibiotics and incision and drainage. Caution should be exercised as approximately half of the patients in this category will not mount an immune response. Therapy should be broad spectrum, including coverage for gram negative rods and anaerobes [59] in addition to gram positive cocci.

A familiarity with antibiotics available in specific hospital formularies and profiles of microbial resistance patterns (via antibiogram) will improve targeted therapies. It was previously thought that parenteral antibiotics were necessary initially for all severe infections. However studying the high serum concentrations achieved with oral forms of some antibiotics such as Linezolid and trimethoprim-sulfamethoxazole, for example, suggest that intravenous administrations may not always be necessary [58]. Recommendations regarding the duration of therapy also vary. Mild infections warrant a short course of 1-2 weeks, while moderate to severe infections can require up to 2-4 weeks of targeted therapy. Inflammatory markers such as CRP and erythrocyte sedimentation rate (ESR) are used to define duration of therapy [58].

The SIDESTEP study published by Lipsky et al. in 2005 compared ertapenem to piperacillin/tazobactam in the treatment of diabetic foot infections in a prospective, randomized, controlled, double-blinded study, with a study population of 576 initial enrollees and 445 available for follow up. Although ertapenem did not provide specific coverage for *Pseudomonas* or *Enterococcus* species, at the end of the therapy period the success rate for both groups of patients was similar. This raises the question of whether certain bacteria such as *Pseudomonas* and *Enterococcus* require antibiotic coverage. These organisms are colonizers and become primary pathogens in very specific instances, acting as opportunistic pathogens. In order to prevent further propagation of multi-drug resistant organisms, practitioners should choose antibiotics with slightly narrower coverage [58, 60, 74].

Occasionally soft tissue infections accompanied by abscess, substantial necrosis or necrotizing fasciitis require surgical debridement in addition to broad spectrum, followed by targeted, antibiotic therapy. Vascular status must be evaluated and restored if possible. For moderate to severe diabetic foot infections, surgical intervention is often the key to limb salvage [69]. The incision should be centered on the abscess and extended proximally until there is no evidence of infection. Non-viable tissues can be debrided, and exposed tendons and bone can be removed in preparation for eventual closure [72].

There are three methods for wound closure: primary, delayed primary and closure by secondary intention. Primary closure can be achieved when the surgeon is confident the necrotic tissue and infection has been removed using a combination of sharp debridement and lavage. However, in cases of severe infection or when there is suspicion for additional drainage to be encountered, a wound may be left open initially then closed several days later when it is free of any signs of infection –delayed primary closure. Finally, for those wounds with significant undermining or other potential complicating factors, closure by secondary intention may be undertaken in which a wound is left open and allowed to granulate or contract, often with the help of advanced modalities such as NPWT, split thickness skin grafting or other synthetic graft materials [59, 72].

Ultimately, the goal in treatment is tissue preservation and restoration of foot function. When superficial infections are encountered physicians should aggressively treat them to prevent progression and involvement of deeper or wider margins of tissue. Some infections warrant early surgical debridement, which can reduce morbidity and cost [63]. When amputations are considered, they should be performed as far distal as possible as there are higher energy expenditures and disturbance to quality of life with proximal amputations. In paraplegic and quadriplegic patients or other patients who are otherwise non-ambulatory, surgical planning should take into account the future risk of complications such as decubitus or neuropathic ulcerations, contractures or infection [59]. Caution should be taken in patients with peripheral arterial disease. Debridement and amputations should be conservative, with later definitive amputations after revascularization for optimal healing [59].

Following amputation, the patient will have altered biomechanics and plantar pressures that will require bracing, orthotics, custom shoegear or adjunctive surgical procedures to avoid future complications [59].

6. Osteomyelitis

Occasionally, soft tissue infections can be severe and deep, involving underlying bony structures. When there is a break in the soft tissue, and the infective organisms have entered the bone directly, this is referred to as contiguous or direct extension osteomyelitis [15, 61, 75]. Infections most commonly will involve soft tissue but about 20% will extend to bone [64]. Other types of osteomyelitis include hematogenous osteomyelitis which is seen in prepubescent children and in elderly patients in which spread occurs through the blood [75].

6.1. Pathogenesis

Infections in the bone are initiated by adhesion of bacteria in the acute osteitis phase followed by firm attachment, which is the chronic phase. The adhesions are formed through a polysaccharide capsule that links strongly to the bone matrix. The bacteria are then protected from antibiotics and macrophages. Bacteria such as *S. aureus* create surface proteins after about 1 week that are osteolytic, resulting in a decrease in bone matrix production. In reaction to the bacterial antigens, the body will also produce interleukin-1 (IL-1) and tumor necrosis factor-α (TNF-α) which result in an increase in osteoclast-mediated osteolysis [60, 62].

As mentioned above, emergence of drug resistant organisms is a large problem facing healthcare providers today. It has been shown that gradual exposure of antibiotics through the biofilm layers can result in resistance as the organisms are able to tolerate 10-1000 times higher levels of antimicrobial agents in comparison to the minimum inhibitory concentration. *S. aureus*, the most common infecting organism, is able to survive within osteoblasts. When osteoblasts die, the bacteria are released and infect new osteoblasts. Small colonies of *S. aureus* with lower metabolic rates can exist latent for indefinite periods, resulting in chronic osteomyelitis [60, 75].

6.2. Diagnosis

6.2.1. Clinical evaluation

Thorough history of patients who present with suspected osteomyelitis should be performed in addition to a thorough physical exam as previously discussed.

6.2.2. Lab evaluation

Complete blood count is of limited usefulness in diagnosing osteomyelitis as leukocytosis is infrequent [62, 75]. ESR and CRP may be more sensitive, but is of questionable specificity [62, 75]. Unlike in metastatic or metabolic bone diseases, the serum calcium, phosphate and alkaline phosphatase all remain normal [75].

6.2.3. Microbiologic evaluation

Similar to the evaluation of infections, surface wound swabs are unreliable for identification of infecting organisms [58, 63, 75]. Specimens of deep tissue obtained from areas adjacent to bone in question can also grow different bacterial isolates [62, 63]. Therefore, bone biopsy is considered the gold standard for diagnosis [59, 60, 62]. Because osteomyelitis is a focal disease, multiple specimens of bone should be taken to provide a representative sample. The specimens can be obtained through core sample with CT guidance through uninvolved skin or tissue. Alternatively, surgical excision can also be performed [62]. Any systemic antibiotics should be discontinued for at least 3 drug half-lives, prior to biopsy [60]. Bone specimens should be sent for gram stain, culture and sensitivity and histology. In some instances, fungal and AFB may also be considered [60, 75].

Similar to infections above, osteomyelitis is also polymicrobial with an average of 2.25 pathogens per patient. The most commonly isolated organisms include *S. aureus*, *S. epidermidis*, *Streptococcus* and *Enterococcus* species. Wounds that are long standing with necrotic tissue and a foul odor should be tested specifically for anaerobic organisms [62].

6.3. Imaging

X-rays of the foot are the most readily available modality and is most cost effective, except they have a low sensitivity in early cases of osteomyelitis. Focal osteopenia and cortical erosions as well as periosteal reactions suggest osteomyelitis. Unfortunately, these changes can also be observed in patients with Charcot neuroarthropathy, which will be discussed in detail later. There can be a delay of 10-20 days before acute changes are detected on radiographs, when

http://dx.doi.org/10.5772/56400

40-70% resorption has occurred. Therefore, x-rays have a higher utility when used serially, once the diagnosis has been established [59, 62, 63, 75].

Technetium 99 bone scintigraphy has also been cited as a useful tool in identifying osteomyelitis. Although the sensitivity is very high, nearly 100% in some studies, the specificity for osteomyelitis is quite low. Other examinations such as the Tc99 –HMPAO (Tc-Hexamethylpropyleneamine oxime) leukocyte scan (also known as *Ceretec* ™scan) has been shown to have both high sensitivity and specificity for osteomyelitis. It is also considered to be more cost effective in comparison to the Indium scan.

CT can be utilized to reveal medullary destruction, periosteal reaction, cortical destruction and articular damage, even when plain radiographs appear normal [76]. Soft tissue structures can be better observed with MRI, which has been reported to have sensitivities as high as 90-100% with specificities between 80 and 100% [75]. Typically in the presence of osteomyelitis, there will be decreased signal intensity on T1 images in the bone marrow. There is also increased signal intensity on T2 weighted images due to edema (Figure 11). Unfortunately, these findings can also be observed in fractures, tumors, inflammatory arthritis, Charcot and post-operative changes. Therefore, clinical correlation is required [62].

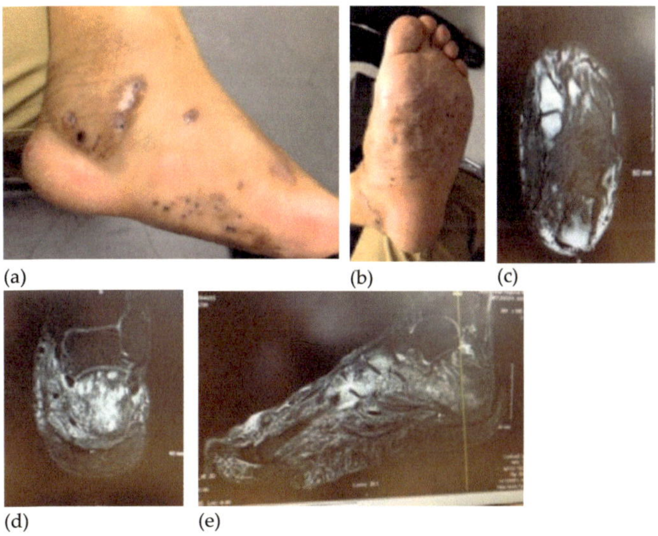

Figure 11. Patient with long-term chronic osteomyelitis; A-B – clinical images showing previous ulceration site; C – T1 transverse image, note low intensity signal throughout midfoot; D – T2 coronal image, note high intensity signal through calcaneus; E – T2 sagittal image, note high intensity signal throughout midfoot structures and calcaneus. Images courtesy of Jacqueline Truong, DPM.

Positron Emission Tomographic scans, particularly those with fluorine-18-fluoro-D-dehoxyglucose (FDG), can provide information as uptake of the agent occurs specifically in inflammatory cells such as macrophages and leukocytes. Combining PET scans and CT scanning can help to distinguish between osteomyelitis and Charcot neuroarthropathy [75].

6.4. Treatment

As with soft tissue infections, a team approach should be employed to improve outcomes [58, 59, 61, 63, 69, 72, 73, 77]. Optimization of patient health status including glycemic control, vascular status, nutritional status, and smoking cessation should be managed [4]. Control of hyperglycemia has been shown to increase leukocyte function. Wound healing has also been shown to improve when nephropathy, nutrition and smoking status are addressed [62].

Medical treatment following any necessary surgical debridement of necrotic tissue must take into account the most likely infective organisms. The most effective treatment includes coverage for both aerobic and anaerobic organisms. Side effects to medications as well as renal dosing and measuring trough levels as appropriate must be taken into account when employing antibiotic therapies. As soon as culture and sensitivity results are available, transition to targeted therapy must take place [63].

There is wide debate between whether to treat medically with antibiotics or surgically with debridement and primary amputations. Some authors are proponents of timely surgical intervention to prevent spread of infection, further necrosis of tissue, and bone [58-60, 62]. There are, however, some who argue that surgical debridement is not necessary to treat osteomyelitis. In fact, with the advent of newer drugs with high serum to bone ratios, they are able to penetrate through biofilms and enter eukaryotic cells better than drugs of the past. In a retrospective study by Faglia and colleagues (2012), however, each day of delay of surgical debridement increased the risk for major amputation [69]. The decision between surgical and non-surgical treatment for chronic osteomyelitis will likely continue to be debated over time [60].

The goal of surgical intervention is to salvage the foot and retain the greatest amount of foot after surgery. The harsh reality is only about 60% of diabetic patients ambulate with a prosthesis following a trans-tibial amputation. And, 50% of those patients develop an infection in the remaining limb requiring additional amputation. Every effort must be made to salvage the greatest amount of the limb as possible [62]. Following surgery, adjunctive procedures and protective devices such as bracing, orthotics and specialty shoegear must be provided in order to prevent further complications [62].

7. Charcot neuroarthropathy

Charcot neuroarthropathy is defined as a progressive joint dislocation with pathologic fracture resulting in debilitating deformity causing disruption to the bony architecture [68]. This disorder can be caused by a multitude of disorders that involve neuropathy such as diabetes, leprosy, syphilis, spina bifida, cerebral palsy, meningomyelocele, syringomyelia and alcohol abuse. Of the list, the most common associated disorder with Charcot neuroarthropathy is diabetes [78-83].

7.1. Pathogenesis

Early theories include the neurotraumatic and neurovascular theories. The *neurotraumatic theory* (also referred to as the German theory) is based on the notion that a neuropathic foot results in abnormal plantar pressures, in addition to intrinsic minus foot leading to pedal architectural changes due to overpowering by long extensor or flexor tendons during function. The repetitive trauma from activities of daily living causes extension of ligaments, joint distension and eventually microfractures and dislocations of the bones. The *neurovascular theory* (also referred to as the French theory) on the other hand focuses more on autonomic neuropathy resulting in a hyperemic state. Arteriorvenous shunts cause an increase in vascular flow leading to osteopenia and bone resorption. Microtrauma from activities of daily living cause microfractures and dislocations in the weakened bone. Although both of these theories are attractive, they do not account for why the problem commonly presents unilaterally [76, 78, 80-84].

The most recent accepted theory describes an increased expression of the receptor activator of nuclear factor KB/ostopotegerin (RANK-L/OPG), resulting in changes we see with Charcot neuroarthropathy. Some triggering event such as minor trauma that is unrecognized by the patient, vascular or orthopedic surgery results in localized inflammation which causes localized osteolysis. RANK-L is increased as it is potentiated by free radicals and hyperlipidemia, hyperglycemia and advanced glycation end-products, all of which exist in diabetics. Antagonists to RANK-L include nerve derived peptides and insulin which are low in diabetics [78, 85]. The breakdown in bone results in an up-regulation of TNF-α and IL-1β, which are both seen following fracture. TNF-α and IL-1β both increase RANK-L expression, causing maturation of osteoclasts, which are responsible for continuing to weaken the bone. A sensate patient would recognize a problem and seek treatment, such as immobilization at this point, which would help to decrease inflammation, and thus break the cycle. Unfortunately, these patients have profound insensitivity, peripheral sympathetic dysfunction and normal arterial outflow, resulting in bony destruction [68, 73, 78, 80, 85].

In 2011, La Fontaine and colleagues published a study comparing bone specimens from patients without diabetes, those with diabetes but without peripheral neuropathy and those with Charcot neuroarthropathy. Through histologic and histomorphometric evaluation, they concluded that bone in diabetic patients is more fragile and increases the risk for fracture. Whether a patient results in a fracture or dislocation appears to depend on the bone mineral density. Those with lower bone mineral density appear to have a greater propensity towards fracture, while those with normal bone mineral density result in a combined pattern of fracture and dislocation [79].

7.2. Clinical presentation

A thorough history and physical examination including dermal, vascular, neurological and musculoskeletal components should be performed for patients who present with a suspected Charcot foot. Affected feet typically exhibit warmth and swelling with occasional pain that is typically seen unilaterally, although bilateral cases have been reported [68, 73]. An infrared dermal thermometer can be used to show a difference in the temperature between the involved foot and the contralateral limb, ranging between 3-6 °C [86]. Although this is sensitive, it is not specific and thus can only be used to evaluate the progression of disease after diagnosis has been established [86]. Most patients have bounding pulses in the acute phase, owing to vascular sympathetic denervation, although patients with chronic Charcot may have elements of vascular compromise. In cases with concurrent ulcerations or if considering surgical therapy, it may be beneficial to perform the ankle brachial index (ABI), arterial Doppler, and transcutaneous pulse oximetry (TcPO2) [73, 81, 87]. Special attention should be paid to the neurologic examination where extent of neuropathy can be assessed. If a previously neuropathic patient begins to complain of pain, clinical suspicion should be raised [81]. The patient should also be evaluated for ankle equinus, particularly in cases where midfoot breakdown is present. The signs and symptoms are not specific to Charcot, thus a thorough evaluation to rule out infection or other disease process must be undertaken [73, 78, 88].

Patients may present at any point in the disease process, with varying structural abnormalities that result. In chronic midfoot Charcot neuroarthropathy, the medial arch may collapse or prolapse resulting in a rocker bottom foot-type with a varus or valgus deviation of the forefoot. Hindfoot or ankle involvement can result in frontal plane alterations of the calcaneus [78]. With proper, timely intervention, limited deformity may be observed, with resolution of the acute phase, which will be discussed in more detail later [81].

7.3. Lab evaluation

Complete blood cell count with differential, ESR, CRP, blood cultures, albumin, pre-albumin, chemistry panel, and glycosylated hemoglobin concentration (HbA1c) should be collected to rule out infection and determine metabolic competence. As was mentioned above, these values may be normal even in the presence of infection due to immunopathy secondary to diabetes [87]. If planning for surgical intervention, these values can also help to predict outcomes [87].

7.4. Imaging

Diagnosis can be delayed on average 29 weeks in Charcot neuroarthropathy [86, 89]. Plain radiography is universally available and inexpensive. In the first stage, the findings include debris formation, fragmentation at subchondral bone and capsular distention (Figure 12). In subsequent stages, the debris becomes absorbed in stage 2 with fusion of large fragments and sclerosis of bone ends. Finally, in the reconstruction phase, the bone ends are rounded [68, 73, 82, 89]. The most common joint to see destruction is the tarsometatarsal joint, likely secondary to equinus at the ankle resulting in midfoot collapse. Medial calcific sclerosis (*Mönckeberg's medial calcific sclerosis*) may also be visible on plain film studies in these patients as RANK-L is suspected to increase calcifications to the vascular smooth muscle wall [89].

CT and MRI can also be utilized particularly for early detection of Charcot neuroarthropathy. On CT, pseudocysts can also be revealed. Although the CT studies can provide useful information, it is more applicable for surgical reconstruction planning [89]. MRI will demonstrate similar findings as described above for osteomyelitis. However, osteomyelitis typically occurs through contiguous spread. Therefore, absence of an ulcer can increase suspicion for

Charcot. Osteomyelitis typically affects one bone while Charcot arthropathy is polyarticular. Deformity is common in Charcot, but the same is not observed in osteomyelitis. Location of effect also differs in that osteomyelitis typically affects the digits and forefoot while Charcot typically affects the midfoot [89]. MRI is superior to CT because it can provide earlier changes, even in stage 0, with edema of bone, soft tissue and joint effusion [89].

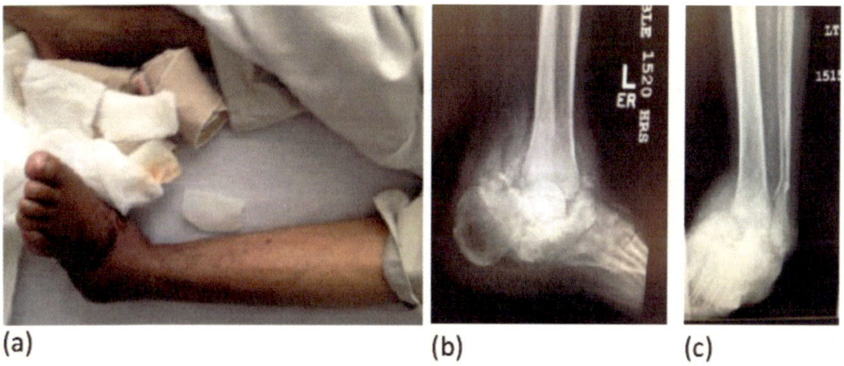

Figure 12. Acute Charcot ankle (6 weeks old) in a patient with peripheral arterial disease after sustaining a nondisplaced fibular fracture initially treated with cast immobilization. Patient eventually underwent transtibial amputation; A – Clinical images showing the collapse of normal architecture; B-C – plain radiography showing the debris formation, fragmentation and dislocation that is classic for stage 1 Charcot neuroarthropathy; also note the Monckeberg's medial calcinosis that is prominent throughout the images.

Bone scintigraphy including Tc99, Gallium, Indium, Ciprofloxacin-labeled scan, Leukocyte labeled Tc HMPAO (*Ceretec*™) scan and sulfur colloid bone scans have been described for use in diagnosing Charcot. The standard Tc99 scan has high sensitivity but low specificity. Indium scans are both sensitive and specific for osteomyelitis and can help to distinguish between Charcot and osteomyelitis. *Ceretec*™ scans provide high sensitivity and specificity for osteomyelitis but is very time consuming [89]. As for osteomyelitis, F-FDG-PET scan with glucose radiolabeling has also been described for use with Charcot. The primary disadvantage is poor anatomic resolution. CT and PET scans can be combined to provide better resolution [89].

7.5. Classification

There are several classification systems that have been introduced to define Charcot neuroarthropathy, including the Eichenholz system, Sanders and Frykberg classification, Schon et al and Brodsky's anatomical classification (Tables 6-8) [73, 80, 86, 88-90]. The Eichenholz system is based on radiographic findings, while the Sanders and Frykberg and Brodsky classifications are based on anatomical location [73, 78, 79, 81-84, 86].

7.6. Differential diagnoses

The clinical presentation for Charcot and osteomyelitis is often very similar with a red, hot, swollen foot [62]. Examples of differential diagnoses include cellulitis, DVT, acute gout and pseudogout, osteonecrosis and osteomyelitis. Patients who are suspected to have Charcot neuroarthropathy may have ulcerations that can confuse the diagnosis [62, 79]. However, in the acute situation, a foot which is warm, erythematous, and edematous without ulceration or known site of pathogen entry must be considered Charcot neuropathic until proven otherwise.

7.7. Treatment

Extensive patient and family education is crucial to the successful treatment of Charcot neuroarthropathy [78, 86, 88]. As discussed above, a team approach is necessary to provide timely, appropriate care for these patients. In the active phase (stage 1), the affected limb should be immobilized in a cast, with the goal to minimize stress to the foot by reducing shear forces and peak plantar pressures and maintain a stable, plantigrade foot [68, 73, 81, 84, 92]. Choices often utilized include a TCC, instant total contact cast (iTCC), and removable CAM walker although the gold standard is considered the TCC. [84, 88, 90].

The duration of immobilization is on average 3-6 months but can vary based on the anatomical location that is involved [78, 81, 86]. When the skin temperature differential becomes less than 1-2 °C, the patient should be transitioned into a Charcot restraint orthotic walker (CROW) device or removable CAM walker and finally into a custom molded shoe with orthotics [68, 81, 83, 88, 93]. Patellar tendon bearing orthotics can also be considered [80]. Some researchers recommend partial weight bearing instead of strict non-weight bearing in a protective device to avoid disuse osteopenia [86, 93]. Skin temperatures should be evaluated regularly.

Medications as an adjunctive therapy to immobilization have been gaining popularity over the last several years, starting with bisphosphonates [41, 73, 80]. Some studies have shown that with even a single dose administration of bisphosphonates clinical and radiologic improvements may be seen with a decreased bony turnover, evaluated as an increase in bone mineral density on dual-energy X-ray absorptiometry (DEXA-scan), and reductions in alkaline phosphatase levels in acute phase Charcot [41, 80, 94]. Salmon calcitonin, which has been shown to decrease osteoclastic activity, is another antiresorptive agent that has been gaining attention recently. It also has been shown to be associated with reduction in bone specific alkaline phosphatase [78, 80, 86, 88]. With the new information regarding the pathophysiology, TNF-α specific antagonists and RANK-L antagonists have been suggested to decrease the duration of time to resolution [78, 80].

Surgical therapies can range and selection is based on the needs of the patient, stability of the joint and the anatomical location involved as well as patient specific characteristics. Acute dislocations or instability should be reduced and possibly primarily fused. Alternatively, in a stable foot, an exostectomy or osteotomy can be performed to aid in ulcer healing [82, 88, 91]. Indications to surgery include recurring ulceration, joint instability, pain with malalignment, prominent exostoses, potential skin complications from bracing and non-platigrade foot. An area of controversy with surgical intervention is timing. It was once believed that performing any surgery during the acute phase was not recommended as further destruction of bone and joints would occur, making fixation nearly impossible. However, increasing numbers of surgeons are advocating for earlier surgery, even in the acute phase to prevent deformity. As with any procedure, benefits should outweigh the risks involved [73, 81, 90-92, 95, 96].

Considerations should be made to the patient's expectations with assessment of willingness to comply with post-operative recommendations before performing surgery [87, 92].

The procedures can be divided by anatomic location. The midfoot deformity reconstructions typically involve wedge shaped osteotomies or exostectomies [81, 82, 95]. Achilles tendon lengthening or tenotomy may be necessary to restore appropriate calcaneal sagittal position [73, 79, 82, 87, 95]. Hindfoot procedures are also approached with a mixture of fixation devices including screws, plates, intramedullary rodding and external fixators.

Arthrodesis in patients with poor bone stock can be challenging to fixate. Some surgeons advocate using an external fixator to provide constant compression during the post-operative period [82, 88]. Others use internal fixation alone with screws and plates or intramedullary rods [82, 90, 95]. Superconstructs, where fixation is extended to involve normal bone, are being described to improve the long term stability following surgical repair [79, 87, 90, 91]. Still others advocate for combinations of internal and external fixation or doubling the amount of internal fixation to decrease the likelihood for non-union [82, 87]. With the advent of locking plates, significant improvements in the strength of fixation have been demonstrated, even with osteopenic bone [79, 88].

Regardless of the location, the goals of surgery are the same, to prevent further deformity, increase stability in near anatomic alignment, while prevent subsequent ulcerations [73, 82, 95]. Occasionally, in severe deformities, the procedure can be staged for better anatomical correction without neurovascular compromise [95]. The proper alignment for surgical correction is to place the heel under the mechanical axis of the leg with the forefoot perpendicular to the rearfoot [95]. When concomitant midfoot deformity is seen with hindfoot pathology, an intramedullary nail in combination with external fixator has been shown to be beneficial for correction [96]. Surgical templates and use of 3-D reconstruction CT imaging should be utilized to plan the corrections [88, 91].

Bone growth stimulation is considered another adjunctive therapy that can be used with immobilization, medications or following surgery. Studies using electrical or ultrasound stimulators have shown statistically significant decreases of consolidation times [73, 87]. With severe deformities, bone deficits can result following osteotomies, particularly with angular corrections. In these instances, grafting may be necessary to fill the void. Several options exist including autogenous grafting from the fibula, iliac crest, proximal tibia, or decorticated osteotomized material [97]. Orthobiologic products can be used as an alternative to improve bone healing; e.g. demineralized bone matrix (DBM), osteoconductive and osteoinductive allografts, calcium phosphate, calcium sulfate and hydroxyapatite substitutes, bone marrow aspirates and platelet rich plasma [95, 97].

Post-operative complications are similar to any surgical intervention involving osseous work, including wound dehiscence, infection, osteomyelitis, delayed union, nonunion, malunion, fracture and failure of hardware. When external fixators are employed pin tract infections can also be observed. Meticulous surgical technique, pre-operative planning, patient education, wound care and pin care can all contribute to decreasing the rate of complications that may result in amputation [82, 88].

8. Conclusion / Prevention

As important as the treatment of immediate pedal complications are, prevention is the key to long term increases in survival rates and reduction of morbidity. In addition, an interprofessional patient-centered approach garners the greatest opportunity for success. For example, recent research shows a seven fold decreased risk of amputation in diabetic patients when treated using a vascular surgery-podiatry team approach with a 5 year rate of avoiding limb loss of 83% [62]. A multi-disciplinary approach [60, 62-64] is helpful to first confirm that the patient has adequate lower extremity blood flow for healing [60, 62], good glycemic control [60, 62, 65], adequate nutritional status [66] and that the ulcer is not infected [62]. A team of specialists may be better equipped to resolve any of these concerns prior to attempted treatment plans. A multi-disciplinary team may help avoid diabetic foot ulcerations with careful evaluation and preventative measures [63]. Without first addressing any above abnormalities, it may prove difficult to heal the diabetic foot ulcer.

Early recognition with timely treatment are emphasized to curb the development of permanent deformities [79]. Practitioners should maintain a high index of suspicion when treating neuropathic patients. No one diagnostic technique can provide both sensitive and specific conclusions. Incorporating history, clinical findings, and results of diagnostic imaging together will provide the most accurate diagnosis. There are many options to consider when treating patients with diabetic foot ulcers and their complications. Unfortunately, simple algorithms for treatment cannot be applied to all patients with these presentations. Post-intervention compliance plays a large role in the ultimate success of treatment, requiring buy in from the patient and care-givers [79]. Adherence to the evidence-based guidelines presented in this chapter will decrease patient morbidity and greatly improve clinical outcomes.

Author details

Jarrod Shapiro*, Diane Koshimune and Rebecca Moellmer

*Address all correspondence to: jshapiro@westernu.edu

Western University of Health Sciences, College of Podiatric Medicine, Pomona, California, USA

References

[1] Rathmann, W, & Giani, G. Global prevalence of diabetes: estimates for the year 2000 and projections for 2030. Diabetes care. (2004). author reply 9. Epub 2004/09/29., 27(10), 2568-9.

[2] Ramsey, S. D, Newton, K, Blough, D, Mcculloch, D. K, Sandhu, N, Reiber, G. E, et al. Incidence, outcomes, and cost of foot ulcers in patients with diabetes. Diabetes care. (1999). Epub 1999/03/31., 22(3), 382-7.

[3] Moulik, P. K, Mtonga, R, & Gill, G. V. Amputation and mortality in new-onset diabetic foot ulcers stratified by etiology. Diabetes care. (2003). Epub 2003/01/28., 26(2), 491-4.

[4] Armstrong, D. G, Wrobel, J, & Robbins, J. M. Guest Editorial: are diabetes-related wounds and amputations worse than cancer? International wound journal. (2007). Epub 2007/12/25., 4(4), 286-7.

[5] Nwomeh BC, Yager DR, Cohen IK. Physiology of the chronic wound. Clinics in plastic surgery. 1998;25(3):341-56. Epub 1998/08/11.

[6] Davis BL. Foot ulceration: hypotheses concerning shear and vertical forces acting on adjacent regions of skin. Medical hypotheses. 1993;40(1):44-7. Epub 1993/01/01.

[7] Brand PW. Tenderizing the foot. Foot & ankle international / American Orthopaedic Foot and Ankle Society [and] Swiss Foot and Ankle Society. 2003;24(6):457-61. Epub 2003/07/12.

[8] Andersen H. Motor dysfunction in diabetes. Diabetes/metabolism research and reviews. 2012;28 Suppl 1:89-92. Epub 2012/02/01.

[9] Armstrong DG, Jude EB. The role of matrix metalloproteinases in wound healing. Journal of the American Podiatric Medical Association. 2002;92(1):12-8. Epub 2002/01/18.

[10] Falanga V. Growth factors and wound healing. Dermatologic clinics. 1993;11(4): 667-75. Epub 1993/10/01.

[11] Lavery LA, Peters EJ, Williams JR, Murdoch DP, Hudson A, Lavery DC. Reevaluating the way we classify the diabetic foot: restructuring the diabetic foot risk classification system of the International Working Group on the Diabetic Foot. Diabetes care. 2008;31(1):154-6. Epub 2007/10/16.

[12] Peters EJ, Lavery LA. Effectiveness of the diabetic foot risk classification system of the International Working Group on the Diabetic Foot. Diabetes care. 2001;24(8): 1442-7. Epub 2001/07/27.

[13] Kumar S, Fernando DJ, Veves A, Knowles EA, Young MJ, Boulton AJ. Semmes-Weinstein monofilaments: a simple, effective and inexpensive screening device for identifying diabetic patients at risk of foot ulceration. Diabetes research and clinical practice. 1991;13(1-2):63-7. Epub 1991/08/01.

[14] C HLaH. Linking risk factors: the role of history in predicting outcome. The Diabetic Foot. 2004;7(3):114-22.

[15] Grayson ML, Gibbons GW, Balogh K, Levin E, Karchmer AW. Probing to bone in infected pedal ulcers. A clinical sign of underlying osteomyelitis in diabetic patients.

JAMA : the journal of the American Medical Association. 1995;273(9):721-3. Epub 1995/03/01.

[16] Lavery LA, Armstrong DG, Peters EJ, Lipsky BA. Probe-to-bone test for diagnosing diabetic foot osteomyelitis: reliable or relic? Diabetes care. 2007;30(2):270-4. Epub 2007/01/30.

[17] Boyko EJ, Ahroni JH, Davignon D, Stensel V, Prigeon RL, Smith DG. Diagnostic utility of the history and physical examination for peripheral vascular disease among patients with diabetes mellitus. Journal of clinical epidemiology. 1997;50(6):659-68. Epub 1997/06/01.

[18] Christensen JH, Freundlich M, Jacobsen BA, Falstie-Jensen N. Clinical relevance of pedal pulse palpation in patients suspected of peripheral arterial insufficiency. Journal of internal medicine. 1989;226(2):95-9. Epub 1989/08/01.

[19] Stoffers HE, Kester AD, Kaiser V, Rinkens PE, Knottnerus JA. Diagnostic value of signs and symptoms associated with peripheral arterial occlusive disease seen in general practice: a multivariable approach. Medical decision making : an international journal of the Society for Medical Decision Making. 1997;17(1):61-70. Epub 1997/01/01.

[20] Criqui MH, Fronek A, Klauber MR, Barrett-Connor E, Gabriel S. The sensitivity, specificity, and predictive value of traditional clinical evaluation of peripheral arterial disease: results from noninvasive testing in a defined population. Circulation. 1985;71(3):516-22. Epub 1985/03/01.

[21] Lavery LA, Armstrong DG, Boulton AJ. Ankle equinus deformity and its relationship to high plantar pressure in a large population with diabetes mellitus. Journal of the American Podiatric Medical Association. 2002;92(9):479-82. Epub 2002/10/17.

[22] Murray HJ, Young MJ, Hollis S, Boulton AJ. The association between callus formation, high pressures and neuropathy in diabetic foot ulceration. Diabetic medicine : a journal of the British Diabetic Association. 1996;13(11):979-82. Epub 1996/11/01.

[23] Snyder RJ, Cardinal M, Dauphinee DM, Stavosky J. A post-hoc analysis of reduction in diabetic foot ulcer size at 4 weeks as a predictor of healing by 12 weeks. Ostomy/wound management. 2010;56(3):44-50. Epub 2010/04/07.

[24] Sheehan P, Jones P, Caselli A, Giurini JM, Veves A. Percent change in wound area of diabetic foot ulcers over a 4-week period is a robust predictor of complete healing in a 12-week prospective trial. Diabetes care. 2003;26(6):1879-82. Epub 2003/05/27.

[25] Bergin SM, Gurr JM, Allard BP, Holland EL, Horsley MW, Kamp MC, et al. Australian Diabetes Foot Network: management of diabetes-related foot ulceration - a clinical update. The Medical journal of Australia. 2012;197(4):226-9. Epub 2012/08/21.

[26] Vig S, Dowsett C, Berg L, Caravaggi C, Rome P, Birke-Sorensen H, et al. Evidence-based recommendations for the use of negative pressure wound therapy in chronic

wounds: steps towards an international consensus. Journal of tissue viability. 2011;20 Suppl 1:S1-18. Epub 2011/11/29.

[27] Kashefsky H, Marston W. Total contact casting combined with human fibroblast-derived dermal tissue in 15 DFU patients. Journal of wound care. 2012;21(5):236, 8, 40, 42-3. Epub 2012/05/16.

[28] Besse JL, Leemrijse T, Deleu PA. Diabetic foot: the orthopedic surgery angle. Orthopaedics & traumatology, surgery & research : OTSR. 2011;97(3):314-29. Epub 2011/04/16.

[29] Gottrup F, Apelqvist J. Present and new techniques and devices in the treatment of DFU: a critical review of evidence. Diabetes/metabolism research and reviews. 2012;28 Suppl 1:64-71. Epub 2012/02/01.

[30] Haycocks S, Chadwick P. Debridement of diabetic foot wounds. Nurs Stand. 2012;26(24):51-2, 4, 6 passim. Epub 2012/03/27.

[31] Sainsbury DC. Evaluation of the quality and cost-effectiveness of Versajet hydrosurgery. International wound journal. 2009;6(1):24-9. Epub 2009/03/18.

[32] Akingboye AA, Giddins S, Gamston P, Tucker A, Navsaria H, Kyriakides C. Application of autologous derived-platelet rich plasma gel in the treatment of chronic wound ulcer: diabetic foot ulcer. The Journal of extra-corporeal technology. 2010;42(1):20-9. Epub 2010/05/05.

[33] Bowling FL, Stickings DS, Edwards-Jones V, Armstrong DG, Boulton AJ. Hydrodebridement of wounds: effectiveness in reducing wound bacterial contamination and potential for air bacterial contamination. Journal of foot and ankle research. 2009;2:13. Epub 2009/05/12.

[34] Panuncialman J, Falanga V. The science of wound bed preparation. The Surgical clinics of North America. 2009;89(3):611-26. Epub 2009/05/26.

[35] de Leon JM, Driver VR, Fylling CP, Carter MJ, Anderson C, Wilson J, et al. The clinical relevance of treating chronic wounds with an enhanced near-physiological concentration of platelet-rich plasma gel. Advances in skin & wound care. 2011;24(8): 357-68. Epub 2011/07/20.

[36] Stone C, Smith N. Resection arthroplasty, external fixation, and negative pressure dressing for first metatarsophalangeal joint ulcers. Foot & ankle international / American Orthopaedic Foot and Ankle Society [and] Swiss Foot and Ankle Society. 2011;32(3):272-7. Epub 2011/04/12.

[37] Yarwood-Ross L, Dignon AM. NPWT and moist wound dressings in the treatment of the diabetic foot. Br J Nurs. 2012;21(15):S26, S8, S30-2. Epub 2012/08/10.

[38] Ulusal AE, Sahin MS, Ulusal B, Cakmak G, Tuncay C. Negative pressure wound therapy in patients with diabetic foot. Acta orthopaedica et traumatologica turcica. 2011;45(4):254-60. Epub 2011/09/13.

[39] Karaaslan O, Kankaya Y, Sungur N, Kocer U, Sedat Cuzdan S, Sahin B, et al. Case series of topical and orally administered beta-glucan for the treatment of diabetic wounds: clinical study. Journal of cutaneous medicine and surgery. 2012;16(3):180-6. Epub 2012/06/21.

[40] Dumville JC, Deshpande S, O'Meara S, Speak K. Hydrocolloid dressings for healing diabetic foot ulcers. Cochrane Database Syst Rev. 2012;2:CD009099. Epub 2012/02/18.

[41] Anderson JJ, Woelffer KE, Holtzman JJ, Jacobs AM. Bisphosphonates for the treatment of Charcot neuroarthropathy. The Journal of foot and ankle surgery : official publication of the American College of Foot and Ankle Surgeons. 2004;43(5):285-9. Epub 2004/10/14.

[42] Buchberger B, Follmann M, Freyer D, Huppertz H, Ehm A, Wasem J. The evidence for the use of growth factors and active skin substitutes for the treatment of non-infected diabetic foot ulcers (DFU): a health technology assessment (HTA). Experimental and clinical endocrinology & diabetes : official journal, German Society of Endocrinology [and] German Diabetes Association. 2011;119(8):472-9. Epub 2011/08/04.

[43] Driver VR, Hanft J, Fylling CP, Beriou JM. A prospective, randomized, controlled trial of autologous platelet-rich plasma gel for the treatment of diabetic foot ulcers. Ostomy/wound management. 2006;52(6):68-70, 2, 4 passim. Epub 2006/06/27.

[44] Berlanga-Acosta J. Diabetic lower extremity wounds: the rationale for growth factors-based infiltration treatment. International wound journal. 2011;8(6):612-20. Epub 2011/09/14.

[45] Malone M, Gannass AA, Bowling F. Flexible and rigid casting tape as a novel approach to offloading diabetic foot ulcers. Journal of wound care. 2011;20(7):335-6, 8-9. Epub 2011/08/16.

[46] Greenhagen RM, Johnson AR, Bevilacqua NJ. Gastrocnemius recession or tendo-achilles lengthening for equinus deformity in the diabetic foot? Clinics in podiatric medicine and surgery. 2012;29(3):413-24. Epub 2012/06/26.

[47] Kim JY, Hwang S, Lee Y. Selective plantar fascia release for nonhealing diabetic plantar ulcerations. The Journal of bone and joint surgery American volume. 2012;94(14): 1297-302. Epub 2012/07/20.

[48] Kim PJ, Attinger CE, Evans KK, Steinberg JS. Role of the podiatrist in diabetic limb salvage. Journal of vascular surgery. 2012;56(4):1168-72. Epub 2012/10/03.

[49] Cunha M, Faul J, Steinberg J, Attinger C. Forefoot ulcer recurrence following partial first ray amputation: the role of tendo-achilles lengthening. Journal of the American Podiatric Medical Association. 2010;100(1):80-2. Epub 2010/01/23.

[50] Braumann C, Guenther N, Menenakos C, Muenzberg H, Pirlich M, Lochs H, et al. Clinical experiences derived from implementation of an easy to use concept for treatment of wound healing by secondary intention and guidance in selection of appropriate dressings. International wound journal. 2011;8(3):253-60. Epub 2011/03/16.

[51] Brown ML, Tang W, Patel A, Baumhauer JF. Partial foot amputation in patients with diabetic foot ulcers. Foot & ankle international / American Orthopaedic Foot and Ankle Society [and] Swiss Foot and Ankle Society. 2012;33(9):707-16. Epub 2012/09/22.

[52] Lullove E. Acellular fetal bovine dermal matrix in the treatment of nonhealing wounds in patients with complex comorbidities. Journal of the American Podiatric Medical Association. 2012;102(3):233-9. Epub 2012/06/05.

[53] Ducic I, Attinger CE. Foot and ankle reconstruction: pedicled muscle flaps versus free flaps and the role of diabetes. Plastic and reconstructive surgery. 2011;128(1): 173-80. Epub 2011/03/15.

[54] Kranke P, Bennett MH, Martyn-St James M, Schnabel A, Debus SE. Hyperbaric oxygen therapy for chronic wounds. Cochrane Database Syst Rev. 2012;4:CD004123. Epub 2012/04/20.

[55] Tiaka EK, Papanas N, Manolakis AC, Maltezos E. The role of hyperbaric oxygen in the treatment of diabetic foot ulcers. Angiology. 2012;63(4):302-14. Epub 2011/08/30.

[56] Grolman RE, Wilkerson DK, Taylor J, Allinson P, Zatina MA. Transcutaneous oxygen measurements predict a beneficial response to hyperbaric oxygen therapy in patients with nonhealing wounds and critical limb ischemia. The American surgeon. 2001;67(11):1072-9; discussion 80. Epub 2001/12/04.

[57] Belczyk RJ, Rogers LC, Andros G, Wukich DK, Burns PR. External fixation techniques for plastic and reconstructive surgery of the diabetic foot. Clinics in podiatric medicine and surgery. 2011;28(4):649-60. Epub 2011/09/29.

[58] Roberts AD, Simon GL. Diabetic foot infections: the role of microbiology and antibiotic treatment. Seminars in vascular surgery. 2012;25(2):75-81. Epub 2012/07/24.

[59] Frykberg RG, Wittmayer B, Zgonis T. Surgical management of diabetic foot infections and osteomyelitis. Clinics in podiatric medicine and surgery. 2007;24(3):469-82, viii-ix. Epub 2007/07/07.

[60] Kosinski MA, Joseph WS. Update on the treatment of diabetic foot infections. Clinics in podiatric medicine and surgery. 2007;24(3):383-96, vii. Epub 2007/07/07.

[61] Cavanagh PR, Lipsky BA, Bradbury AW, Botek G. Treatment for diabetic foot ulcers. Lancet. 2005;366(9498):1725-35. Epub 2005/11/18.

[62] Shank CF, Feibel JB. Osteomyelitis in the diabetic foot: diagnosis and management. Foot and ankle clinics. 2006;11(4):775-89. Epub 2006/11/14.

[63] Tan JS, File TM, Jr. Diagnosis and treatment of diabetic foot infections. Bailliere's best practice & research Clinical rheumatology. 1999;13(1):149-61. Epub 2000/08/23.

[64] Lavery LA, Armstrong DG, Wunderlich RP, Mohler MJ, Wendel CS, Lipsky BA. Risk factors for foot infections in individuals with diabetes. Diabetes care. 2006;29(6): 1288-93. Epub 2006/05/30.

[65] Day MR, Armstrong DG. Factors associated with methicillin resistance in diabetic foot infections. The Journal of foot and ankle surgery : official publication of the American College of Foot and Ankle Surgeons. 1997;36(4):322-5; discussion 31. Epub 1997/07/01.

[66] Armstrong DG, Lavery LA, Sariaya M, Ashry H. Leukocytosis is a poor indicator of acute osteomyelitis of the foot in diabetes mellitus. The Journal of foot and ankle surgery : official publication of the American College of Foot and Ankle Surgeons. 1996;35(4):280-3. Epub 1996/07/01.

[67] Faglia E, Clerici G, Caminiti M, Curci V, Somalvico F. Prognostic difference between soft tissue abscess and osteomyelitis of the foot in patients with diabetes: data from a consecutive series of 452 hospitalized patients. The Journal of foot and ankle surgery : official publication of the American College of Foot and Ankle Surgeons. 2012;51(1):34-8. Epub 2011/12/27.

[68] Boulton AJM. The diabetic foot. Medicine. 2010;38(12):644-8.

[69] Joseph WS, Lipsky BA. Medical therapy of diabetic foot infections. Journal of vascular surgery. 2010;52(3 Suppl):67S-71S. Epub 2010/09/10.

[70] Nielsen MD, Mendicino RW, Catanzariti AR. The use of ertapenem for the treatment of lower extremity infections. The Journal of foot and ankle surgery : official publication of the American College of Foot and Ankle Surgeons. 2009;48(2):135-41. Epub 2009/02/24.

[71] Richard JL, Sotto A, Jourdan N, Combescure C, Vannereau D, Rodier M, et al. Risk factors and healing impact of multidrug-resistant bacteria in diabetic foot ulcers. Diabetes & metabolism. 2008;34(4 Pt 1):363-9. Epub 2008/07/18.

[72] Fisher TK, Scimeca CL, Bharara M, Mills JL, Sr., Armstrong DG. A step-wise approach for surgical management of diabetic foot infections. Journal of vascular surgery. 2010;52(3 Suppl):72S-5S. Epub 2010/09/10.

[73] Burns PR, Wukich DK. Surgical reconstruction of the Charcot rearfoot and ankle. Clinics in podiatric medicine and surgery. 2008;25(1):95-120, vii-viii. Epub 2008/01/01.

[74] Lipsky BA, Armstrong DG, Citron DM, Tice AD, Morgenstern DE, Abramson MA. Ertapenem versus piperacillin/tazobactam for diabetic foot infections (SIDESTEP):

prospective, randomised, controlled, double-blinded, multicentre trial. Lancet. 2005;366(9498):1695-703. Epub 2005/11/18.

[75] Lew DP, Waldvogel FA. Osteomyelitis. Lancet. 2004;364(9431):369-79. Epub 2004/07/28.

[76] La Fontaine J, Shibuya N, Sampson HW, Valderrama P. Trabecular quality and cellular characteristics of normal, diabetic, and charcot bone. The Journal of foot and ankle surgery : official publication of the American College of Foot and Ankle Surgeons. 2011;50(6):648-53. Epub 2011/06/28.

[77] Driver VR, Fabbi M, Lavery LA, Gibbons G. The costs of diabetic foot: the economic case for the limb salvage team. Journal of vascular surgery. 2010;52(3 Suppl):17S-22S. Epub 2010/09/10.

[78] Nielson DL, Armstrong DG. The natural history of Charcot's neuroarthropathy. Clinics in podiatric medicine and surgery. 2008;25(1):53-62, vi. Epub 2008/01/01.

[79] Crim BE, Lowery NJ, Wukich DK. Internal fixation techniques for midfoot charcot neuroarthropathy in patients with diabetes. Clinics in podiatric medicine and surgery. 2011;28(4):673-85. Epub 2011/09/29.

[80] Molines L, Darmon P, Raccah D. Charcot's foot: newest findings on its pathophysiology, diagnosis and treatment. Diabetes & metabolism. 2010;36(4):251-5. Epub 2010/06/24.

[81] Sella EJ, Barrette C. Staging of Charcot neuroarthropathy along the medial column of the foot in the diabetic patient. The Journal of foot and ankle surgery : official publication of the American College of Foot and Ankle Surgeons. 1999;38(1):34-40. Epub 1999/02/24.

[82] Yablon CM, Duggal N, Wu JS, Shetty SK, Dawson F, Hochman MG. A review of Charcot neuroarthropathy of the midfoot and hindfoot: what every radiologist needs to know. Current problems in diagnostic radiology. 2010;39(5):187-99. Epub 2010/08/03.

[83] Hanft JR, Goggin JP, Landsman A, Surprenant M. The role of combined magnetic field bone growth stimulation as an adjunct in the treatment of neuroarthropathy/ Charcot joint: an expanded pilot study. The Journal of foot and ankle surgery : official publication of the American College of Foot and Ankle Surgeons. 1998;37(6): 510-5; discussion 50-1. Epub 1999/01/08.

[84] Crews RT, Wrobel JS. Physical management of the Charcot foot. Clinics in podiatric medicine and surgery. 2008;25(1):71-9, vii. Epub 2008/01/01.

[85] Jeffcoate WJ, Game F, Cavanagh PR. The role of proinflammatory cytokines in the cause of neuropathic osteoarthropathy (acute Charcot foot) in diabetes. Lancet. 2005;366(9502):2058-61. Epub 2005/12/13.

[86] Stanley JC, Collier AM. Charcot osteo-arthropathy. Current Orthopaedics. 2008;22(6): 428-33.

[87] Stapleton JJ, Belczyk R, Zgonis T. Revisional Charcot foot and ankle surgery. Clinics in podiatric medicine and surgery. 2009;26(1):127-39. Epub 2009/01/06.

[88] Bevilacqua NJ, Rogers LC. Surgical management of Charcot midfoot deformities. Clinics in podiatric medicine and surgery. 2008;25(1):81-94, vii. Epub 2008/01/01.

[89] Rogers LC, Bevilacqua NJ. Imaging of the Charcot foot. Clinics in podiatric medicine and surgery. 2008;25(2):263-74, vii. Epub 2008/03/19.

[90] Sammarco VJ. Superconstructs in the treatment of charcot foot deformity: plantar plating, locked plating, and axial screw fixation. Foot and ankle clinics. 2009;14(3): 393-407. Epub 2009/08/29.

[91] Stapleton JJ, Zgonis T. Surgical reconstruction of the diabetic Charcot foot: internal, external or combined fixation? Clinics in podiatric medicine and surgery. 2012;29(3): 425-33. Epub 2012/06/26.

[92] Pinzur M. Surgical versus accommodative treatment for Charcot arthropathy of the midfoot. Foot & ankle international / American Orthopaedic Foot and Ankle Society [and] Swiss Foot and Ankle Society. 2004;25(8):545-9. Epub 2004/09/15.

[93] Christensen TM, Gade-Rasmussen B, Pedersen LW, Hommel E, Holstein PE, Svendsen OL. Duration of off-loading and recurrence rate in Charcot osteo-arthropathy treated with less restrictive regimen with removable walker. Journal of diabetes and its complications. 2012;26(5):430-4. Epub 2012/06/16.

[94] Moreno M, Gratacos J, Casado E, Galisteo C, Orellana C, Larrosa M. [Usefulness of Pamidronate in the Treatment of Charcot's Arthropathy]. Reumatologia clinica. 2007;3(6):257-61. Epub 2007/11/01. Utilidad del pamidronato en el tratamiento de la artropatia de Charcot.

[95] Zgonis T, Roukis TS, Lamm BM. Charcot foot and ankle reconstruction: current thinking and surgical approaches. Clinics in podiatric medicine and surgery. 2007;24(3):505-17, ix. Epub 2007/07/07.

[96] DeVries JG, Berlet GC, Hyer CF. A retrospective comparative analysis of Charcot ankle stabilization using an intramedullary rod with or without application of circular external fixator--utilization of the Retrograde Arthrodesis Intramedullary Nail database. The Journal of foot and ankle surgery : official publication of the American College of Foot and Ankle Surgeons. 2012;51(4):420-5. Epub 2012/05/15.

[97] Ramanujam CL, Facaros Z, Zgonis T. An overview of bone grafting techniques for the diabetic charcot foot and ankle. Clinics in podiatric medicine and surgery. 2012;29(4):589-95. Epub 2012/10/10.

Chapter 13

The Diabetic Charcot Foot – New Insights on Treatment

Fernando Grover Páez, Sylvia Elena Totsuka Sutto,
Sara Pascoe González,
Ernesto G. Cardona Muñóz and
Carlos Enrique Medina García

Additional information is available at the end of the chapter

http://dx.doi.org/10.5772/56399

1. Introduction

The association between Charcot neuroarthropathy (CN) and diabetes mellitus was first described by Jordan in 1936 (Jordan WR, 1936). Since that time numerous treatment protocols have been proposed for this potentially devastating condition. Early diagnosis and swift care are the keys to reducing amputation risk in this patient population. Conservative management remains efficacious for certain clinical scenarios. Treatment of the patient should take into account the stage of CN, site(s) of involvement, presence or absence of ulceration, presence or absence of infection, overall medical status, and level of compliance. The most commonly used classification is the three-staged system described by Eichenholtz: Stage I is the developmental or acute phase, Stage II is the coalescent or quiescent phase, and Stage III is the consolidation or reconstruction and reconstitution phase (Eichenoltz SN, 1966). Involvement of the midfoot is most common in the diabetic population and this site tends to be more amenable to conservative options versus hindfoot or ankle CN. Generally, conservative care for the CN foot and ankle has been recommended for the following scenarios: joints in the acute phase, deformities that are clinically stable and that do not compromise the soft tissue envelope, stable deformities without soft tissue or bone infection, patients who do not have adequate arterial perfusion to support surgical reconstruction, and those patients who are extremely high risk for anesthesia and surgical intervention due to the presence of multiple severe comorbid conditions. In this chapter we present an overview of evidence-based non-operative treatment for CN with an emphasis on the most recent developments in therapy.

2. Clinical presentation

Acute diabetic neuroarthropathy may evolve slowly over many months or develop rapidly within weeks (Rajbhandari SM et al., 2002; Pogonowska MJ et al., 1967). The process begins with a hyperemia usually following trauma to the foot or ankle (Yu GV & Hudson JR, 2002). The trauma is often mild and may not even be recalled by the patient (Sanders LJ & Frykberg RG, 1993; Rajbhandari SM et al., 2002; Armstrong DG & Peters EJG, 2002; Armstrong DG et al., 1997). Not infrequently there may be a delay of several months between the trauma and the incipient neuroarthropathy (Sanders LJ & Frykberg RG, 1993).

Classical clinical findings are an edematous, warm foot with bounding pulses and a severe peripheral neuropathy. The normal architecture of the foot may be disturbed and plantar ulceration at the site of deformity may be present. Most patients complain of pain, but the complaints are usually less than would be expected from the clinical findings (Sanders LJ & Frykberg RG, 1993; Rajbhandari SM et al., 2002; Armstrong DG & Peters EJG, 2002). Men and women are equally affected. Most patients are in the mid-fifties, but neuroarthropathy can occur at any age (Sanders LJ & Frykberg RG, 1993). Unilateral development is most common, but a significant number of patients can develop bilateral involvement (Sanders LJ & Frykberg RG, 1993; Fabrin J et al., 2000). Patients with long-standing (>10 years) and poorly controlled diabetes, neuropathy, history of ulceration, recent history of trauma, prior neuroarthropathy, or renal transplantation are high risk and should be watched closely since early clinical findings may be mild (Sanders LJ & Frykberg RG, 1993).

However, the acute phase of CN often goes unnoticed, resulting in a delayed positive diagnosis and progression to the chronic phase, with irreversible deformation. The main problem is that, at this stage of the disease, not only is the clinical diagnosis not easy to make, but standard radiography often cannot distinguish acute CN from other conditions. Indeed, X-ray radiography may fail to document any evidence of fracture and/or dislocation. Radioisotope technetium (Tc-99m) bone scintigraphy has good sensitivity, but poor specificity, for osseous pathology and only shows increased focal uptake during the bony phase.

Only magnetic resonance imaging (MRI) is capable of revealing, in greater detail, the nature of the bony damage and evidence of inflammation in the bone (subchondral bone-marrow oedema with or without microfracture) as well as in the adjacent soft tissues (Edmonds ME et al., 2005; Chantelau E & Poll LW, 2006). MRI is particularly useful in the earliest stages of the disease, as there is a significant correlation between the intensity of bone-marrow oedema and clinical parameters such as soft-tissue oedema or pain (Schlossbauer T et al., 2008).

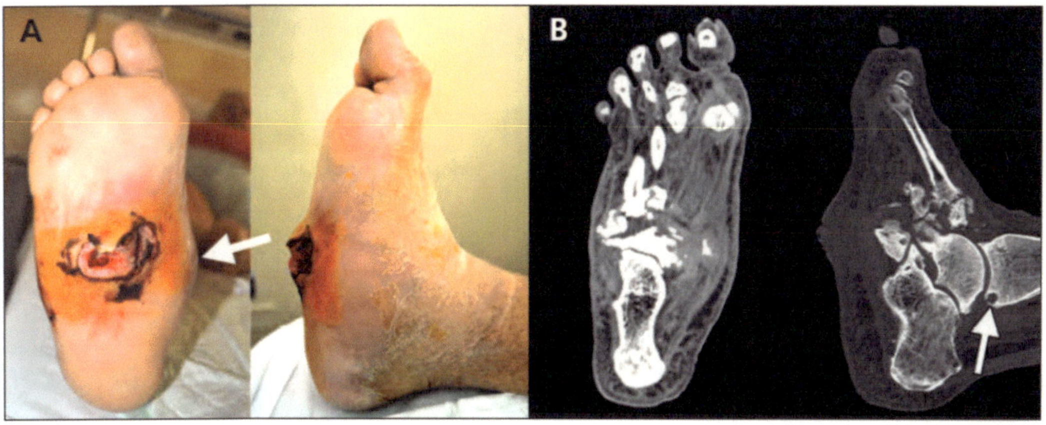

Figure 1. The right foot (plantar and lateral views) of a 59-year-old man with diabetic neuropathy showing collapse of the internal arch (arrow) and a large neuropathic ulcer on the midplantar surface. (B) Computed tomographic images (dorsoplantar and lateral views) of the patient's right foot showing a subchondral cyst (arrow), fragmentation, disorganization, and loss of normal architecture of the talus, calcaneus, tarsal bones and bases of the metatarsals. (Nicola Mumoli MD & Alberto Camaiti MD, 2012).

3. Classification

Different systems have been proposed to classify CN, and the one most commonly used is an anatomically based system, the Sanders–Frykberg anatomical classification that divides the foot into five zones, according to the joints involved (Sanders LJ & Frykberg RG, 1991):

Type I: involves the metatarsophalangeal and interphalangeal joints

Type II: involves the tarsometatarsal joints

Type III: involves the tarsal joints

Type IV: involves the subtalar joints

Type V: involves the calcaneum.

This classification has proved especially helpful in predicting prevalence and prognosis. Types I and II are the most common types, while types II and III are particularly associated with the risk of abnormal friction and ulceration, and types IV and V carry poor prognoses due to the effects of weight distribution during walking as shown in table 1, (Edmonds ME et al., 1985).

The most common classification of Charcot osteo-arthropathy follows the natural history of Charcot and was originally described by (Sidney Eichenholtz S.N, 1966). This classification incorporates both a clinical and a radiographic evaluation of the patient Table 2:

Pattern	Location	% of cases	Common findings
I	Forefoot	35	Atrophic destruction: resorption of metatarsal and phalangeal shafts, osteolysis, subluxation of metatarsophalangeal joints, plantar ulceration
II	Tarsometatarsal joint	30	Subluxation of metatarsal bases, Rocker-bottom deformity, plantar ulceration, chronic instability
III	Talonavicular, calcaneocuboid and naviculocuneiform joint	25	Osteolysis of naviculocuneiform joint, Rocker-bottom deformity, often found in conjunction with Pattern II
IV	Ankle joint	9	Extensive joint destruction, severe deformity and instability, risk of high level amputation
V	Calcaneus	1	No joint involvement, calcaneal insufficiency avulsion fracture

Table 1. Sanders-Frykberg anatomical classification of neuroarthorpathy.

Pattern	Location	% of cases	Common findings
I	Forefoot	35	Atrophic destruction: resorption of metatarsal and phalangeal shafts, osteolysis, subluxation of metatarsophalangeal joints, plantar ulceration
II	Tarsometatarsal joint	30	Subluxation of metatarsal bases, Rocker-bottom deformity, plantar ulceration, chronic instability
III	Talonavicular, calcaneocuboid and naviculocuneiform joint	25	Osteolysis of naviculocuneiform joint, Rocker-bottom deformity, often found in conjunction with Pattern II
IV	Ankle joint	9	Extensive joint destruction, severe deformity and instability, risk of high level amputation
V	Calcaneus	1	No joint involvement, calcaneal insufficiency avulsion fracture

Table 2. Add caption

Stage 0 has been added to the classification by Schon and Marks in 1995 in an attempt to indicate the high risk of developing an acute Charcot osteo-arthropathy following a traumatic event. (Schon LC et al., 1998; Brodsky JW, 1999).

4. Pathogenesis

The Charcot foot has been documented to occur as a consequence of various peripheral neuropathies; however, diabetic neuropathy has become the most common etiology. The interaction of several component factors (diabetes, sensory-motor neuropathy, autonomic neuropathy, trauma, and metabolic abnormalities of bone) results in an acute localized inflammatory condition that may lead to varying degrees and patterns of bone destruction, subluxation, dislocation, and deformity.

This inflammation leads to osteolysis and is indirectly responsible for the progressive fracture and dislocation (Uccioli L et al., 2010; La Fontaine J et al., 2008). When a bone is fractured, the release of proinflammatory cytokines including tumor necrosis factor- α and interleukin-1β leads to increased expression of the polypeptide receptor activator of nuclear factor-Kb ligand (RANKL) from any of a number of local cell types. RANKL triggers the synthesis of the nuclear transcription factor nuclear factor-kb (NF-kb), and this in turn stimulates the maturation of osteoclasts from osteoclast precursor cells. At the same time, NF-kb stimulates the production of the glycopeptide osteoprotegerin (OPG) from osteoblasts. This "decoy receptor" acts as an effective antagonist of RANKL (Mabilleau G et al., 2008). It has been suggested that this results in continual production of proinflammatory cytokines, RANKL, NF-kb, and osteoclasts, which in turn leads to continuing local osteolysis (La Fontaine J et al., 2008). Osteoclasts generated in vitro in the presence of macrophage colony-stimulating factor and RANKL from patients with active CN have been shown to be more aggressive and exhibit an increase in their resorptive activity that peptides normally secreted from nerve terminals are also important in the underlying pathophysiology. Of these, calcitonin gene-related peptide (CGRP) is a likely candidate because it is known to antagonize the synthesis of RANKL.

The receptor activator of the nuclear factor-ligand (RANKL)-activated peripheral blood monocytes have been found to induce a significant increase in bone resorption in Charcot patients (Mabilleau G et al., 2008; Jeffcoate W et al., 2004).

A possible link between proinflammatory cytokines and neuroarthropathy in the context of an exaggerated inflammatory response to trauma has been mentioned (Jeffcoate WJ et al, 2005), and the inability of the Charcot patient to control the intensity and the length of the local inflammatory response would lead to increased expression of tumor necrosis factor-α (TNF-α) and interleukin-1(IL-1) which, in turn, would trigger increased expression of RANKL leading to maturation of osteoclast and subsequent bone changes (Lam J et al., 2002; Boyle WJ et al., 2003).

The immune phenotype of monocytes was assessed by testing spontaneous and induced production of proinflammatory and anti-inflammatory cytokines by measuring the expression of surface molecules (CD40, CD80, and CD86), which enable monocytes to became competent co-stimulatory cells and to activate T lymphocytes responses (Jenkins MK et al 2001; Kuchroo VK et al., 1995; Yang Yet al., 1996), and by studying the ability of monocytes to undergo apoptosis, an important homeostatic mechanism that contributes to regulate the intensity and length of the inflammatory response (Gonzalez-Mejia ME & Doseff AI, 2009). Patients with acute Charcot, in both the active and recovered phase, peripheral monocytes acquire a proinflammatory immune phenotype characterized by increased production of proinflammatory cytokines, reduced secretion of anti-inflammatory cytokines, increased expression of co-stimulatory surface molecules, and increased resistance to apoptosis. Monocytes play a pivotal role in the development and maintenance of the inflammatory response. These cells are the major source of proinflammatory (TNF- α, IL-1, and IL-6) as well as anti-inflammatory cytokines (IL-4 and IL-10) (Kiener PA et al., 1995; Gautam SC et al., 1992; De Waal Malefyt R et al., 1991).

Alterations in the correct timing, intensity, and balance of expression of proinflammatory versus anti-inflammatory cytokines by monocytes result in pathologic modulation of the inflammatory response. Thus, the activation of inflammatory and suppression of anti-inflammatory cytokines that we have found in patients with acute Charcot is consistent with the abnormally intense and prolonged inflammatory response that characterizes the acute phase of this disease. A growing body of evidence is now supporting the possibility that this inflammatory response plays a pivotal pathogenetic role in the changes in bone and joints that develop in this disorder (Jeffcoate WJ et al., 2005). Indeed, TNF-α and IL-1, released during the inflammatory process, trigger increased expression of RANKL (Lam J et al., 2002; Xu J et al., 2009).

This leads to activation of NFk-b and maturation of osteoclasts (Hofbauer LC et al 2000; Boyle WJ et al 2003). The effect of IL-6 on bone formation/resorption is more controversial. Indeed, several reports support the possibility that IL-6 could in fact induce an osteocytic phenotype (Chipoy C et al., 2004). As opposed, there is evidence that IL-6 can stimulate osteoclasts differentiation and bone resorption by an indirect mechanism, increasing interactions between osteoblasts and osteoclasts (Palmqvist Pet al 2002; Sinistro A et al., 2008).

The proinflammatory alterations we have found in the phenotype of monocytes from acute Charcot patients appear to be specific to this condition. Indeed, both the phenotype of monocytes from diabetic patients with uncomplicated neuropathy and that of monocytes from diabetic patients with neuropathy and osteomyelitis-associated foot inflammation was not different from that of cells from healthy control subjects. This indicates that neither diabetes nor neuropathy or inflammation, per se, is associated with any modulation of the inflammatory response of monocytes. Interestingly, we found that all the modification of the immune phenotype of monocytes disappeared after recovery in patients with acute Charcot. This suggests that the initiating cause that triggers the inflammatory response in patients with acute Charcot acts in an environment where mechanisms that physiologically control the intensity and duration of inflammation are lacking. calcitonin gene-related peptide (CGRP), a 37-amino acid peptide widely distributed in the central and peripheral nervous systems and mainly in sensory nerves (Poyner DR et al., 1992), has been shown to inhibit proinflammatory cytokine production and augment the release of IL-10 by monocytes (Feng Y et al., 1997).

On the other hand, pathogenetic knowledge has focused on purely mechanical theories for some time. Two theories, initially thought to be competing concepts, are now considered to be overlapping to varying degrees. On the one hand, the neurotraumatic theory proposes that, in the presence of sensorimotor neuropathy, abnormal plantar pressure occurs. This is supported by the amyotrophy of intrinsic muscles, and the imbalance between the extensor and flexor muscles. In addition, the bones and joints lose their protective sensory capacity, allowing repetitive trauma that, in turn, leads to excessive extension of the ligaments, and microfractures and more joint dislocation. On the other hand, the neurovascular theory suggests that the autonomic neuropathy leads to a hyperaemic state, with an increase in blood flow to the lower limbs due to the development of arteriovenous shunts. The hyperaemia appears to cause osteopenia, bone resorption and bone weakening. Ultimately, it is on this weakened foot that, either spontaneously or due to minor trauma, microfractures and dislocations occur.

Although both these theories are attractive, they are not able to explain some of the typical features of acute Charcot neuro-osteoarthropathy (CN) and, in particular, why the condition is unilateral while neuropathy is most often bilateral, why CN is so infrequent while neuropathy is a common complication of diabetes, and what is the link with the inflammatory reaction that is initially observed.

There is no singular cause for the development of the Charcot foot, but there are factors that predispose to its development, as well as a number of likely precipitating events. The current belief is that once the disease is triggered in a susceptible individual, it is mediated through a process of uncontrolled inflammation in the foot. This inflammation leads to osteolysis and is indirectly responsible for the progressive fracture and dislocation that characterizes its presentation (Jeffcoate WJ et al, 2005).

However, as mentioned before, the common link is the local inflammation (Baumhauer et al, 2006) that is associated with the release of proinflammatory cytokines such as interleukin (IL)-1β and tumour necrosis factor (TNF)-α, which are known mediators of bone resorption *via* excess osteoclactic activity (Petrova et al, 2007).

Interestingly, a dissociation between the local inflammatory response related to the increased proinflammatory cytokine secretion and lack of systemic inflammatory response has been found in patients with CN (Jeffcoate WJ, 2004).

At the same time, NF-κB induces the increased expression of the glycoprotein osteoprotegerin (OPG), which acts as a decoy receptor for RANK-L to effectively neutralize its effect and so avoid excess osteolysis (Fig. 1) (Boyle WJ, 2003).

The role of this pathway in acute CN pathogenesis is supported by the fact that the same RANK/RANK-L/OPG system is also involved in the process of medial arterial calcification, a feature that is strongly associated with both the distal symmetrical neuropathy of diabetes (Jeffcoate WJ, 2009) and CN (Sinha S et al., 1972; Clouse ME et al., 1974).

Nevertheless, a traumatic triggering factor causes the release of inflammatory cytokines that increase the expression of RANK-L, thereby resulting in clinical signs of inflammation, osteoclast maturation and activation, and osteolysis. Physiologically, this process is limited by immobilization in response to the pain caused by local inflammation. However, when pain perception is reduced due to sensory neuropathy, there is no protective suppression, thereby allowing the inflammatory process to continue which, in turn, ultimately leads to osteolysis and bone breakdown. The result is the establishment of a vicious circle of inflammation and worsening structural damage to the foot (Frykberg RG et al, 2000).

4.1. Diferential diagnosis

While cellulitis may seem to be the likely diagnosis, if a patient with long-standing diabetes, a history of poor glycemic control, and peripheral neuropathy presents with a red, hot, swollen

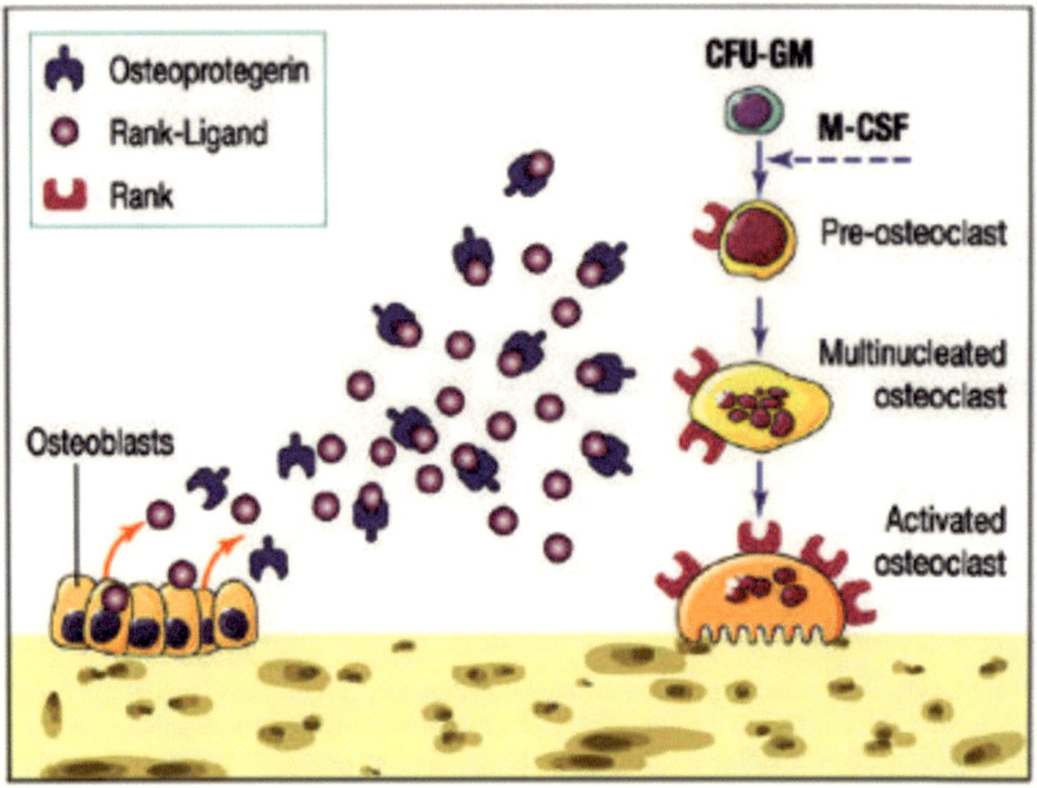

Figure 2. Diagrammatic representation of the RANK/RANK-L/OPG signalling pathway in the process of bone resorption. On the one hand, RANK-L (receptor activator of nuclear factor-_B ligand), a surface-bound molecule found on osteoblasts and bone-marrow stromal cells, binds to its specific membrane-bound receptor RANK (receptor activator of nuclear factor-_B) at the surface of preosteoclasts and other cells of this lineage. The binding subsequently triggers a kinase cascade that promotes osteoclast differentiation, activation and survival. On the other hand, OPG (osteoprotegerin), which is also expressed by osteoblasts, acts as a decoy receptor to bind and effectively neutralize RANK-L which, in turn, limits excess osteoclastogenesis and osteolysis. CFU-GM: colony-forming unit granulocyte–macrophage; M-CSF: monocyte colony-stimulating factor. (L. Molines et al, 2010)

foot with no history of open ulceration, then Charcot neuroarthropathy should be at the top of the list in the differential diagnosis. Other possibilities include osteomyelitis, acute gout, cellulitis, abscess, neuropathic fracture, and deep venous thrombosis. However, if the patient has no open ulceration or history of an open wound, infection is probably not the culprit. Most diabetic foot infections begin with a direct inoculation through an opening in the skin, such as a diabetic neuropathic foot ulcer.

4.2. Laboratory tests

There are no laboratory criteria for the diagnosis of Charcot neuroarthropathy and no hematologic markers, but laboratory testing can help narrow the differential diagnosis. Leukocytosis, an elevated C-reactive protein and erythrocyte sedimentation rate, and recent unexplained hyperglycemia suggest infection. However, unremarkable results on clinical tests in this population may not com- prehensively exclude infection.

4.3. Imaging studies

Radiographs are the primary initial imaging method for evaluation of the foot in diabetic patients. Easily available and inexpensive, they provide information on bone structure, alignment, and mineralization. X-rays may be normal or show subtle fractures and dislocations or later show more overt fractures and subluxations.

In later stages, the calcaneal inclination angle is reduced and the talo-first metatarsal angle is broken.

However, radiographic changes of Charcot neuropathic osteoarthropathy (CN) are typically delayed and have low sensitivity (Morrison WB et al., 2002).

Magnetic resonance imaging (MRI) allows detection of subtle changes in the early stages of active Charcot neuropathic osteoarthropathy when X-rays could still be normal. MRI primarily images protons in fat and water and can depict anatomy and pathology in both soft tissue and bone in great detail. Because of its unique capability of differentiating tissues with high detail, MRI has a high sensitivity and specificity for osteomyelitis and has become the test of choice for evaluation of the complicated foot in diabetic patients (Morrison WB et al., 2001).

Although not required for diagnosis when X-rays are diagnostic for Charcot bone and joint changes, MRI is very useful in making the diagnosis at its earliest onset before such changes become evident on plain films. Nuclear medicine includes a number of exams based on the use of radioisotopic tracers. Three-phase bone scans, based on technetium-99m (99mTc), are highly sensitive for active bone pathology. However, diminished circulation can result in false-negative exams and, perhaps more importantly, uptake is not specific for osteoarthropathy. Labeled white blood cell scanning (using 111In or 99mTc) provides improved specificity for infection in the setting of neuropathic bone changes but it can be difficult to differentiate soft tissue from bone (Keidar Z et al., 2005; Palestro CJ et al., 1998)

More recently, positron emission tomography scanning has been recognized as having potential for diagnosis of infection and differentiating the Charcot foot from osteomyelitis (Hopfner S et al., 2005). However, this remains investigational at this time. Evaluation of bone mineral density (BMD) may be useful in those with diabetes to assess onset of CN as well as fracture risk. BMD can be assessed using dual-energy X-ray absorptiometry or calcaneal ultrasound. (Frykberg RG et al., 2010).

Experts agree that radiographs are important as the first exam in virtually all settings (Hopfner S et al., 2005;). However, a negative result obviously should not offer any confidence regarding lack of disease.

The MRI is very effective at excluding osseous disease. If the patient has anulceration with a high likelihood of deep infection, MRI is the best diagnostic modality. The decision of nuclear imaging versus MRI is largely based on personal preference, availability, and local experience.

In general, if metal is present in the foot, nuclear medicine exams are preferred, whereas diffuse or regional ischemia makes MRI the preferred exam.

The diagnosis of active Charcot foot is primarily based on history and clinical findings but should be confirmed by imaging. Inflammation plays a key role in the pathophysiology of the Charcot foot and is the earliest clinical finding. The X-rays should be the initial imaging performed, and one should look for subtle fractures or subluxations if no obvious pathology is visible. MRI or nuclear imaging can confirm clinical suspicions in the presence of normal-appearing radiographs. (Lee C et al., 2011).

In the other hand, Positron emission tomography (PET) with fluorine-18 fluorodeoxyglucose is also gaining support, especially when combined with computed tomography (CT). This PET-CT hybrid has better anatomic localization than PET alone.

PET-CT is very reliable for differentiating Charcot neuroarthropathy from osteomyelitis, a distinction that can be difficult to make when Charcot neuroarthropathy is complicated by adjacent loss of skin integrity. The sensitivity of PET-CT in this situation has been reported as 100%, and its sensitivity 93.8%.22.

5. Treatment

The goals of treatment for acute or quiescent Charcot neuroarthropathy should be to maintain or achieve structural stability of the foot and ankle, to prevent skin ulceration, and to preserve the plantigrade shape of the foot so that prescription footwear can be used.

Immobilization: A total-contact cast is worn until the redness, swelling, and heat subside, generally 8 to 12 weeks, after which the patient should use removable braces or a Charcot restraint orthotic walker for a total of 4 to 6 months of treatment. Many physicians also recommend elastic stockings (eg, Stockinette) or an elastic tubular bandage (eg, Tubigrip) to reduce edema under the cast.

6. Drug therapy

Due to bone mineral density alterations in CN patients manifested by localized osteopenic changes, bisphosphonates have been tested for their benefit with off-loading in Stage I. Bisphosphonates are pyrophosphate analogs that inhibit osteoclastic bone resorption and are commonly used in treatment of conditions characterized by abnormal bone turnover. Pamidronate is the most commonly used and acts by attaching onto hydroxyapatite crystals in newly synthesized bone matrix, blocking access of osteoclast precursors to this matrix. (Jude EB et al., 2001) performed a randomized double-blind placebo-controlled 39 patients with active Charcot in which a single 90 mg pamidronate infusion was administered and standard off-loading provided while foot temperatures, symptoms, and bone turnover markers were measured over 1-year. There was a statistically significant reduction in bone turnover,

http://dx.doi.org/10.5772/56399

symptoms, and disease activity. Similarly, (Pitocco et al., 2005) showed significant reduction in bone resorption markers with the use of another bisphosphonate alendronate and noted clinical improvements in the CN foot at 6 months. Some clinicians also prescribe bisphosphonates in the early stages of treatment, as the bone mineral density of the affected foot is low. Unfortunately, while these drugs can significantly reduce the levels of bone turnover markers, temperature, and pain, evidence of clinical benefit such as an earlier return to ambulation or radiographic improvement is weak at best.

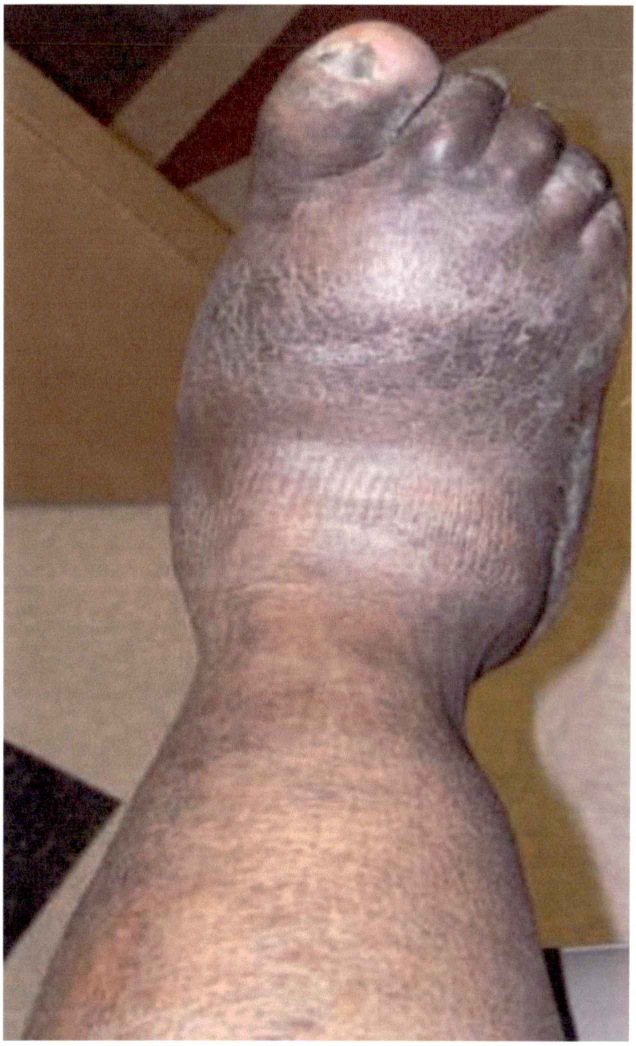

Figure 3. Neuro-osteoarthropathy of Charcot foot

Surgery is reserved for severe ankle and midfoot deformities that are susceptible to skin ulcerations and that make braces and orthotic devices difficult to use.

7. New insights on treatment

Similarly, use of calcitonin and non-steroidal anti-inflammatory drugs has been reported as adjunct treatment to conventional therapy. Recently, new anti-inflammatory therapeutic agents such as corticosteroids, TNF-α antagonists (infliximab, etanercept) and RANK-L antagonists (denosumab) have been proposed, but further research is needed.

Another potential therapeutic agents that also have a direct effect on the RANK-L/OPG system in addition to calcitonin are inhibitors of tumor necrosis factor- α (TNF- α), glucocorticoids and non-steroidal anti-inflammatories, (Jeffcoate WJ et al., 2005) has also mentioned other future options including synthetic OPG and RANK-L antagonists and other inhibitors of NF-kB and TNF-α like diacerein.

Diacerein is another medication used frequently in the treatment of some articular diseases as a result of its effect on the inflammatory process. Diacerein decreases cytokine concentrations, in particular, TNF- α and IL-1b and it could be one of the most promising strategies in the current treatment of the acute phase of the diabetic Charcot foot.

Diacerein (9,10-dihydro-4,5-bis(acetyloxy)9,10-dioxo-2-anthracene carboxylic acid) is one of symptomatic slow-acting drugs in osteoarthritis (SYSADOA) for the treatment of OA (Bruyère O et al., 2008). After oral administration, it is rapidly broken down and deacetylated into its active metabolite, rhein, (Spencer CM., 1997). The potential disease modifying properties of diacerein and its metabolite have been shown in vitro and in vivo models to be primarily due to potent inhibition of the production and activity of inflammatory cytokines and other catabolic cytokines expressed in OA and in CN, which are involved in cartilage catabolism and also may induce the apoptosis of chondrocytes (De Isla NG et al, 2008; Tamura T et al., 2001)

In addition to this, Briefly, activation of osteoclasts involved in osteolysis is accomplished by the nuclear transcription factor NF- kB. The expression of NF-kB is induced by the cytokine RANK-L, which is accompanied by increased production of osteoprotegerin (OPG). The RANK-L/OPG system's theoretical role in osteopenia associated with diabetic neuropathy led to the development and use of intranasal salmon calcitonin for treatment of acute CN. A randomized controlled trial by (Bem et al., 2006) was performed on 32 acute CN patients administered 200 IU daily, showing reduction in markers of bone turnover as well as a decreased time to healing. This therapy has shown fewer complications compared to bi-sphosphonate use.

8. Conclusion

Conservative options continue to evolve in their indications for the treatment of the CN foot and ankle. The modalities discussed within this chaspter provide a wide variety of options; yet, a further higher level of evidence studies is warranted. There is no doubt that there are specific indications for conservative management versus surgical. Regardless of the chosen treatment pathway, all protocols should be specific to the patient based on their lower extremity pathology, overall medical status, and ability to comply with the given therapy.

Author details

Fernando Grover Páez, Sylvia Elena Totsuka Sutto, Sara Pascoe González,
Ernesto G. Cardona Muñóz and Carlos Enrique Medina García

Department of Physiology, Cardiovascular Research Unit, University Center of Health Science, Universidad de Guadalajara, México

References

[1] Armstrong, D. G. Peters EJG. Charcot's arthropathy of the foot. J Am Podiatr Med Assoc (2002). , 92, 390-4.

[2] Armstrong, D. G, Todd, W. F, Lavery, L. A, Harkless, L. B, & Bushman, T. R. The natural history of acute Charcot's arthropathy in a diabetic foot specialty clinic. Diabetic Med (1997). , 14, 357-63.

[3] Baumhauer, J. F, Keefe, O, Schon, R. J, Pinzur, L. C, & Cytokine-induced, M. S. osteoclastic bone resorption in Charcot arthropathy: an immunohistochemical study. Foot Ankle Int (2006). , 27, 797-800.

[4] Bem, R, Jirkovska, A, Fejfarova, V, Skibova, J, & Jude, E. B. Intranasal calcitonin in the treatment of acute Charcot neuroosteoarthropathy: a randomized controlled trial. Diabetes Care (2006).

[5] Boyle, W. J, Simonet, W. S, & Lacey, D. L. Osteoclast differenciation and activation. Nature (2003). , 423, 337-42.

[6] Brodsky, J. W. The diabetic foot. In: Coughlin MJ, Mann RA, editors. Surgery of the foot and ankle. Mosby; (1999). , 895e969.

[7] Bruyère, O, Burlet, N, Delmas, P. D, Rizzoli, R, Cooper, C, & Reginster, J. Y. Evaluation of symptomatic slow-acting drugs in osteoarthritis using the GRADE system," BMC Musculoskeletal Disorders, article 165, (2008). , 9

[8] Chantelau, E, & Poll, L. W. Evaluation of the diabetic foot by MR imaging or plain radiography-an observational study. Exp Clin Endocrinol Diabetes (2006). , 114, 428-31.

[9] Chipoy, C, Berreur, M, Couillaud, S, Pradal, G, Vallette, F, & Colombeix, C. Re´dini F, Heymann D, Blanchard F. Downregulation of osteoblast markers and induction of

the glial fibrillary acidic protein by oncostatin M in osteosarcoma cells require PKCdelta and STAT3. J Bone Miner Res (2004). , 19, 1850-1861.

[10] Clouse, M. E, Gramm, H. F, Legg, M, & Flood, T. Diabetic osteoarthropathy: clinical and roentgenographic observations in 90 cases. Am J Roentgenol Radium Ther Nucl Med (1974). , 121, 22-33.

[11] De Isla, N. G, Mainard, D, Muller, S, & Stoltz, J. F. In vitro effects of diacerein on NO production by chondrocytes in response to proinflammatory mediators," Bio-Medical Materials and Engineering, supplement, (2008). , 18(1), S99-S104.

[12] De Waal Malefyt RAbrams J, Bennett B, Figdor CG, de Vries JE. Interleukin 10 (IL-10) inhibits cytokine synthesis by human monocytes: an autoregulatory role of IL-10 produced by monocytes. J Exp Med (1991). , 174, 1209-1220.

[13] Edmonds, M. E, Clarks, M. B, Newton, S, Barrett, J, & Watkins, P. J. Increased uptake of bone radiopharmaceutical in diabetic neuropathy. Q J Med (1985). , 57, 843-55.

[14] Edmonds, M. E, Petrove, N. L, & Elias, D. A. The earliest magnetic resonance imaging sign of mid-foot charcot osteoarthropathy is oedema of subchondral (subarticular) bone marrow which needs prompt therapeutic offloading. Diabet Med (2005). Suppl. 2):93. , 272.

[15] Eichenholtz, S. N. Charcot joints. Springfield, IL: Charles C. Thomas; (1966).

[16] Fabrin, J, Larsen, K, & Holstein, P. E. Long-term follow-up in diabetic Charcot feet with spontaneous onset. Diabetes Care (2000). , 23, 796-800.

[17] Feng, Y, Tang, Y, Guo, J, & Wang, X. Inhibition of LPS-induced TNF-_ production by calcitonin gene-related peptide (CGRP) in cultured mouse peritoneal macrophages. Life Sci (1997). , 61, 281-287.

[18] Frykberg, R. G, & Eneroth, M. Principles of conservative management. In The Diabetic Charcot Foot: Principles and Management. Frykberg RG, Ed. Brooklandville, MD, Data Trace Publishing Company, (2010). , 93-116.

[19] Frykberg, R. G, & Mendeszoon, E. Management of the diabetic Charcot foot. Diabetes Metab Res Rev (2000). Suppl. 1):S, 59-65.

[20] Gautam, S. C, Chikkala, N. F, & Hamilton, T. A. Anti-inflammatory action of IL-4: negative regulation of contact sensitivity to trinitrochlorobenzene. J Immunol (1992). , 148, 1411-1415.

[21] Gonzalez-mejia, M. E, & Doseff, A. I. Regulation of monocytes and macrophages cell fate. Front Biosci (2009). , 14, 2413-2431.

[22] Growth Factor Rev 2009; 20:7-17.

[23] Hofbauer, L. C, & Heufelder, A. E. The role of receptor activator of nuclear factor-ligand and osteoprotegerin in the pathogenesis and treatment of metabolic bone diseases. J Clin Endocrinol Metab (2000). , 85, 2355-2363.

[24] Hopfner, S, Krolak, C, Kessler, S, & Tiling, R. Preoperative imaging of Charcot neuroarthropathy. Does the additional application of 18F-FDG-PET make sense?. Nuklearmedizin (2005). , 45, 15-20.

[25] Jeffcoate, W. J, Game, F. L, & Cavanagh, P. R. The role of proinflammatory cytokines in the cause of neuropathic osteoarthropathy (acute Charcot foot) in diabetes. Lancet (2005). , 366, 2058-61.

[26] Jeffcoate, W. J, Rasmussen, L. M, Hofbauer, L. C, & Game, F. L. Medial arterial calcification in diabetes and its relationship to neuropathy. Diabetologia (2009). , 52, 2478-88.

[27] Jeffcoate, W. J. Charcot neuro-osteoarthropathy. Diabetes Metab Res Rev (2008). Suppl. 1):S, 62-5.

[28] Jeffcoate, W. J. Vascular calcification and osteolysis in diabetic neuropathy Is RANK-L the missing link? Diabetologia (2004). , 47, 1488-92.

[29] Jenkins, M. K, Khoruts, A, Ingulli, E, Mueller, D. L, Mcsorley, S. J, Reinhardt, R. L, Itano, A, & Pape, K. A. In vivo activation of antigenspecific CD4 T cells. Annu Rev Immunol (2001). , 19, 23-45.

[30] Jordan, W. R. Neuritic manifestations in diabetes mellitus. Arch Intern Med (1936). , 57, 307-66.

[31] Jude, E. B, Selby, P. L, Burgess, J, Lilleystone, P, Mawer, E. B, Page, S. R, et al. Bisphosphonates in the treatment of Charcot neuroarthropathy: a double-blind randomised controlled trial. Diabetologia (2001). , 44, 2032-7.

[32] Keidar, Z, Militianu, D, Melamed, E, Bar- Shalom, R, & Israel, O. The diabetic foot: initial experience with 18F-FDG PET/CT. J Nucl Med (2005). , 46, 444-449.

[33] Kiener, P. A, Moran-davis, P, Rankin, B. M, Wahl, A. F, Aruffo, A, & Hollenbaugh, D. Stimulation of CD40 with purified soluble gp39 induces proinflammatory responses in human monocytes. J Immunol (1995). , 155, 4917-4925.

[34] Kuchroo, V. K, Das, M. P, Brown, J. A, Ranger, A. M, Zamvil, S. S, Sobel, R. A, Weiner, H. L, Nabavi, N, & Glimcher, L. H. B. and B7-2 costimulatory molecules activate differentially the Th1/Th2 developmental pathways: application to autoimmune disease therapy. Cell (1995). , 80, 707-718.

[35] La Fontaine JHarkless LB, Sylvia VL, Carnes D, Heim-Hall J, Jude E. Levels of endothelial nitric oxide synthase and calcitonin gene-related peptide in the Charcot foot: a pilot study. J Foot Ankle Surg (2008). , 47, 424-429.

[36] Lam, J, Abu-amer, Y, Nelson, C. A, Fremont, D. H, Ross, F. P, & Teitelbaum, S. L. Tumor necrosis factor superfamily cytokines and the pathogenesis of inflammatory osteolisis. Ann Rheum Dis (2002). Suppl. 2):iiii83, 82.

[37] Lee, C. Rogers, Robert G. Frykberg, David G. Armstrong, Andrew J.M. Boulton, The Charcot Foot in Diabetes. Diabetes Care (2011). , 34, 2123-2129.

[38] Mabilleau, G, Petrova, N. L, Edmonds, M. E, & Sabokbar, A. Increased osteoclastic activity in acute Charcot's osteoarthropathy: the role of receptor activator of nuclear factor-ligand. Diabetologia (2008). , 51, 1035-1040.

[39] Molines, L, et al. Charcot's foot: Newest findings on its pathophysiology, diagnosis and treatment, Diabetes & Metabolism (2012). , 36, 251-255.

[40] Morrison, W. B, Ledermann, H. P, & Schweitzer, M. E. MR imaging of the diabetic foot. Magn Reson Imaging Clin N Am (2001). , 9, 603-613.

[41] Morrison, W. B, & Ledermann, H. P. Work-up of the diabetic foot. Radiol Clin North Am (2002). , 40, 1171-1192.

[42] Nicola Mumoli MD & Alberto Camaiti MDCharcot foot, CMAJ, (2012).

[43] Palestro, C. J, Mehta, H. H, Patel, M, et al. Marrow versus infection in the Charcot joint: indium-111 leukocyte and technetium-99m sulfur colloid scintigraphy. J Nucl Med(1998). , 39, 346-350.

[44] Palmqvist, P, Persson, E, Conaway, H. H, & Lerner, U. H. IL-6, leukemia inhibitory factor, and oncostatinMstimulate bone resorption and regulate the expression of receptor activator of NF-ligand, osteoprotegerin, and receptor activator of NF- in mouse calvariae. J Immunol (2002). , 169, 3353-3362.

[45] Pitocco, D, Ruotolo, V, Caputo, S, Mancini, L, Collina, C. M, Manto, A, et al. Six-month treatment with alendronate in acute Charcot neuroarthropathy: a randomized controlled trial. Diabetes Care (2005). , 28, 1214-5.

[46] Pogonowska, M. J, Collins, L. C, & Dobson, H. L. Diabetic osteopathy. Radiology (1967). , 89, 265-71.

[47] Poyner, D. R. Calcitonin gene-related peptide: multiple actions, multiple receptors. Pharmacol Ther (1992). , 56, 23-51.

[48] Rajbhandari, S. M, Jenkins, R. C, Davies, C, & Tesfaye, S. Charcot neuroarthropathy in diabetes mellitus. Diabetologia (2002). , 45, 1085-96.

[49] Sanders, L. J, & Frykberg, R. G. Charcot foot. In: Levin ME, O'Neal LW, Bowker JH, eds. The Diabetic Foot. St. Louis: Mosby, (1993). , 1993, 149-80.

[50] Sanders, L. J, & Frykberg, R. G. Diabetic neuropathic osteoarthropathy: the Charcot foot. In: Frykberg RG, editor. The high risk foot in diabetes mellitus. New York: Churchill Livingstone; (1991). , 297-333.

[51] Schlossbauer, T, Mioc, T, Sommerey, S, Kessler, S. B, Reiser, M. F, & Pfeifer, K. J. Magnetic resonance imaging in early stage charcot arthropathy: correlation of imaging findings and clinical symptoms. Eur J Med Res (2008). , 22, 409-14.

[52] Schon, L. C, Weinfeld, S. B, Horton, G. A, & Resch, S. Radiographic and clinical classification of acquired midtarsus deformities. Foot Ankle Int (1998). , 19(6), 394-404.

[53] Sinha, S, Munichoodappa, C, & Kozak, G. P. Neuro-arthropathy (Charcot joints) in diabetes mellitus: a clinical study of 101 cases. Medicine (Baltimore) (1972). , 51, 191-210.

[54] Sinistro, A, Almerighi, C, Ciaprini, C, Natoli, S, & Sussarello, E. Di Fino S, Calo-Carducci F, Rocchi G, Bergamini A. Downregulation of CD40 ligand response in monocytes from sepsis patients. Clin Vaccine Immunol (2008). , 15, 1851-1858.

[55] Spencer, C. M, & Wilde, M. I. Diacerein," Drugs, (1997). , 53(1), 98-108.

[56] Stanley & CollierCharcot osteo-arthropathy, Current Orthopaedics, (2008). , 22, 428-433.

[57] Tamura, T, Kosaka, N, Ishiwa, J, Sato, T, Nagase, H, & Ito, A. Rhein, an active metabolite of diacerein, down-regulates the production of pro-matrix metalloproteinases-1,-3,-9 and-13 and up-regulates the production of tissue inhibitor of metalloproteinase-1 in cultured rabbit articular chondrocytes," Osteoarthritis and Cartilage (2001).

[58] Uccioli LuigiAnna Sinistro, Cristiana Almerighi. Proinflammatory Modulation of the Surface and Cytokine Phenotype of Monocytes in Patients With Acute Charcot Foot. Diabetes Care (2010). , 33, 350-355.

[59] Vega, D, Maalouf, N. M, & Sakhaee, K. The role of receptor activator of nuclear factor-_B (RANK)/RANK Ligand/Osteoprotegerin: clinical implications. J Clin Endocrinol Metab (2007). , 92, 4514-21.

[60] Xu, J, & Wu, . . NF- modulators in osteolytic bone diseases. Cytokine

[61] Yang, Y, Wilson, J. M, & Ligand-dependent, C. D. T cell activation: requirement of B7- CD28 signaling through CD40. Science (1996). , 273, 1862-1864.

[62] Yu, G. V, & Hudson, J. R. Evaluation and treatment of stage 0 Charcot's neuroarthropathy of the foot and ankle. J Am Podiatr Med Assoc (2002). , 92, 210-20.

Section 3

Prevention and Treatments

Chapter 14

Screening for Diabetes in Family Practice: A Case Study in Ontario, Canada

Gina Agarwal

Additional information is available at the end of the chapter

http://dx.doi.org/10.5772/56463

1. Introduction

1.1. Prevalence and Incidence of Diabetes in Ontario, Canada

The scale of the problem of diabetes in family practice is described with respect to prevalence and incidence in family medicine.

Type 2 diabetes (T2DM) and prediabetes [impaired fasting glucose (IFG); impaired glucose tolerance (IGT); and / or both IFG and IGT] are common metabolic disturbances in Canada and worldwide, having long been recognized to be reaching close to epidemic proportions [1]. Indeed, the global prevalence of diabetes in 2011 was 8.3% [2]. According to the National Diabetes Surveillance System, in 2009, over 2 million Canadians were estimated to have T2DM; a prevalence of T2DM 6.4% [3]. As many as one in six people over the age of 65 years are currently estimated to have diabetes [4]. Adults from lower income groups are twice as likely to have diabetes as those in the highest income groups [4]. Estimates suggest that over 5 million Canadians had prediabetes in 2004; a prevalence of 23% for ages 40 to 74 years [5]. The prevalence of IFG is more frequent in women but both IFG and IGT increase in prevalence with age [6].

2. Predicted increase in numbers of people with diabetes

Alarmingly, diabetes prevalence is expected to increase significantly; this will be described in detail with respect to the effect on the primary care system.

The global prevalence for diabetes is predicted to be 9.9% in 2030, an increase of approximately 20% in 20 years [2]. Indeed, over time, the prevalence of Type 2 Diabetes (T2DM) in Ontario has increased at a much faster rate than anticipated. Adult diabetes prevalence in Ontario rose by 80%, from 5% in 1995, to 9% in 2005[6], thereby exceeding the global prevalence increase of T2DM of 6.4% projected for 2030 [7]. Following that, over a 6 year period, a 31% increase in yearly incidence occurred in Canada, from 6.6 per 1,000 in 1997 to 8.2 per 1,000 in 2003 [7]. The diabetes epidemic is not restricted to Canada, as 1 in 10 adults in the USA now have diabetes [8].

Increasing numbers of people with diabetes will result in more healthcare resources being utilised [5,6,7]. Current estimates suggest that people with diabetes use five-times as many health resources as those without [9]. Therefore, developing and testing effective strategies to increase detection of diabetes in the community is an important primary care and population health issue. Furthermore, up to one third of the people with diabetes are estimated to be undiagnosed [8,10] and may be developing diabetes-related complications which may also remain undiagnosed. Not only will the utilisation of healthcare resources be restricted to diabetes-related micro and macro vascular diseases, but other conditions as well. People with diabetes or dysglycemia are at over a twofold risk of developing cardiovascular disease compared to diabetes-free individuals [11,12,13]. These factors point to the seriousness of the diabetes epidemic and its potential impact.

3. Progression of prediabetes to diabetes

The speed at which prediabetes progresses to diabetes has serious implications for adequate healthcare. The scale of this will be discussed in depth.

Individuals with prediabetes are estimated to progress to type 2 diabetes at a rate of 10-12% per year; in total up to as much as 70% will progress [14-16]. Furthermore, individuals with both IFG and IGT develop type 2 diabetes at approximately twice the rate as those who have only one of these impairments [17]. The speed at which prediabetes progresses to diabetes has serious implications for adequate healthcare provision to the adult Canadian population aged 40 and over (which represented approximately 50% of the Canadian population in the 2006 census) [18].

Since diabetes is a multi-system metabolic chronic disorder, it causes complications that affect many organs including eyes, nerves and kidneys as well as other health related consequences. Specific complications of diabetes include macrovascular (i.e. coronary artery disease), and microvascular (i.e. renal damage, nerve damage and retinal damage) [19]. Treatment for diabetes consists of dietary and lifestyle changes, oral medication and injected insulin [19]. The healthcare system will be stretched having to care for an epidemic of people with diabetic complications.

However, pharmacological and lifestyle interventions could prevent or delay T2DM and thus decrease morbidity and mortality associated with its complications if individuals at risk of developing diabetes are detected early [20]. Unfortunately, only 49% of Canadians over 40 years old report ever having a diabetes screening blood test sometime during their life [21] and much diabetes and prediabetes remains undiagnosed [10]. Future treatment costs could possibly be avoided by increasing prevention and screening efforts.

4. Diagnosis of diabetes

This section will outline the many tests possible and the best choices for family physicians.

Prediabetes and diabetes can be diagnosed with inexpensive fasting blood tests [either a fasting plasma glucose (FPG) level or a 75-gram oral glucose tolerance test (OGTT). The WHO 2006 diagnostic criteria provide the appropriate cut-off points for blood tests interpretation (see Table 1) [22]. The FPG test is commonly used by Canadian physicians to identify those with prediabetes and diabetes [21].

Measurement of only a FPG misses 15% or more of people with IGT [23,24]; but, using the diagnostic criteria for IFG identifies a different and smaller group of people compared to using criteria for IGT [25,26]. Although the oral glucose tolerance test (OGTT) is the diagnostic gold standard, cost and impracticality limit its use as a screening test (overnight fasting and a 2-hour laboratory wait are required). In addition glycosylated hemoglobin or A1c is already being used as a diagnostic test by many physicians. The American Diabetes Association in 2010 recommended that A1c could be used as a screening test in non-pregnant individuals, and those without chronic kidney, liver or blood disorders which can all affect the hemoglobin levels [27]. Their recommendations state that an A1c of 6.5% (47 mmol/mol) or higher indicates diabetes and an A1c of 5.7% - 6.4% (39 - 46 mmol/mol) is indicative of prediabetes.

The Canadian Diabetes Association has also followed suit and recommended that A1c be used as a screening tool with the same limitations, and diagnostic for diabetes above 6.5%, however two separate readings (two of a combination of A1c or FPG) are required for diagnosis [28]. Increasingly, there is debate concerning the use of other laboratory tests since although the OGTT is the gold standard it may not be used frequently (Ontario data shows that less than 1% of people underwent an OGTT between 1995 and 2005) [29]. An increasing number of individuals without documented diabetes in Ontario have been tested using the A1c [1]. Additionally, many Ontarians receive serum blood glucose testing, which is either random or fasting (80% of women and 66% of men) [30].

	Fasting Plasma Glucose (mmol/l)	2 hour Post 75g Glucose Load (mmol/l)
T2DM	≥7.0	≥11.1
Isolated IGT	<6.1	7.8-11.0
Isolated IFG	6.1 – 6.9	<7.8
IGT and IFG	6.1 – 6.9	7.8-11.0
Normal	<6.1	<7.8

Table 1. Diagnostic Criteria for Diabetes and Prediabetes [22,31,32]

5. Screening for diabetes

The use of risk assessment tools in general practice will be discussed with reference to the literature.

Though T2DM can often remain undiagnosed and asymptomatic in its early stages [33], once diagnosed, it can be treated with lifestyle modification and medication, and some elements of the disease process may be reversible [14,16,34]. In light of this, early T2DM detection may be beneficial to both patients and society [35]. Screening may also detect people at high risk of developing diabetes; and thereby, determine the likelihood that a person may have a positive diagnosis of diabetes.

Screening for diabetes can be approached in 3 different ways; opportunistic, risk-based or universal. Opportunistic screening occurs where a health care practitioner will screen as part of routine medical care, whether this is part of a physical examination or other arising medical interaction [36]. Risk-based screening focuses on screening individuals at high risk of developing diabetes due to a health related trait that they have, such as obesity, age, positive family history [37]. Universal screening would screen everyone irrespective of characteristics [37] or just use age and gender criteria for screening.

Since the OGTT is the gold standard, including it in any screening program for diabetes and prediabetes may therefore be an important strategy [37], though impractical for universal screening. The challenge is how to improve the overall accuracy of diabetes screening, and to incorporate OGTT at a reasonable cost, by incorporating it as part of a multi-stage screening process. This two-step approach has already been tested and proven in Finland, and is now being implemented across many European countries as an emerging best practice. Literature demonstrates that non-laboratory based questionnaires (e.g. the FINRISK) to pre-identify individuals at risk of T2DM and prediabetes can be successful [38,39]. Screening questionnaires have similar diagnostic accuracy to laboratory screening tests and are inexpensive, simple to use and can also be used as educational tools for patients undergoing screening [38,39,40]. They can be used in conjunction with laboratory testing for universal screening.

An effectively screened population will have diabetes diagnosed 5–6 years earlier than a population without an organized screening program [41], offering opportunities for delaying diabetes and related complications [16]. The current screening tests of repeated serum glucose measurements are too costly and inconvenient to be offered at a population level in the form of a screening program. Furthermore, the organization of primary care in Canada is poorly designed to cope with the initiation and management of comprehensive diabetes screening for everyone over 40 years of age [36]. Existing diabetes prevention and lifestyle programs, designed for research and not community application, have unrealistic program costs, since they require all participants to have OGTTs [42,43]. However, sequential and selective screening of high-risk groups could increase efficiency [44] and reduce workload and screening costs for the healthcare system by reducing the number of individuals requiring a 'gold standard' diagnostic test, as compared to universal screening [45,46].

6. Role of family practitioners

This chapter will clarify what the best method of screening is for family physicians by examining the evidence and provide recommendations for current practice.

In light of the evidence for early treatment of diabetes, in the Canadian Diabetes Association (CDA) clinical practice guidelines [31,32], the recommendations are clear that individuals at high risk for developing diabetes should be screened to determine their dysglycemic status, in an attempt to be able to recommend changes to lifestyle which may prevent or delay the onset of diabetes. 'High risk' is defined as a person whose first degree relatives have diabetes, and/or who have other diabetes risk factors such as ethnic origin, obesity and dyslipidemia, and who have a FPG of 5.7-6.9 mmol/L. Though not explicitly stated, the implementation of this screening recommendation is the responsibility of family doctors, since traditionally they are the first point of access to health care in Canada. Family doctors usually have the opportunity to detect diabetes in their patients at annual health checks as long as the patient has a physical exam. However, at least 15% of the Canadian population does not have a family doctor and will not receive a physical examination [47]. Family doctors are a scarce resource and may not be able to initiate successful screening programs for all their patients. Indeed, evidence shows that they may be too busy [33], or resources too scarce to implement comprehensive screening either opportunistically or targeted, or to provide appropriate follow up to identified individuals. Therefore, opportunistic screening in this way may not be the best approach to effectively identify the individuals with diabetes. Other strategies may be more appropriate, but few have been tested or rigorously evaluated in family practice.

Rather than a universal screening program of everybody over the age of 40 years, selective screening of subgroups at high risk of having the disease may reduce the workload and the cost to the healthcare system by reducing the number of individuals who need a diagnostic test [48], while still identifying the vast majority of new cases. Involving patients themselves in the decision to attend screening may also lessen the burden on family physicians, since a consultation initiated for risk assessment alone, is likely to be more focused than one initiated for other reasons [49]. Taking into account these issues, a program utilising this philosophy, the Community Health Awareness of Diabetes program, was developed and piloted in Ontario. CHAD assessed risk of diabetes in the over 40 year old population using the Finnish Diabetes Risk Score [38] (for impaired glucose tolerance detection), the Cambridge Diabetes Risk Score [50] (for undiagnosed diabetes), fasting capillary blood glucose and a glycosylated hemoglobin level. Individuals were invited by their family doctors, for 'diabetes awareness and risk assessment' sessions delivered by specially trained community peers, in a network of local community pharmacies.

There were 588 participants in CHAD; of these, the majority that had received invitation letters were seniors and were females; 526 did not have pre-existing diabetes; and 16% of participants were identified as being at high risk for diabetes [51]. Those at high risk of diabetes had significantly more modifiable risk factors, including higher fat, fast food and salt intake, and higher systolic blood pressure. Satisfaction with the program was high. An audit of 1030 medical charts of individuals eligible to attend the CHAD program, from 28 family doctors' practices in Grimsby, Ontario. Of these, 387 charts were of patients who had attended the CHAD program and 643 charts were of individuals who did not attend the program but who met the program eligibility criteria. Overall, the difference between the rates of diabetes diagnosis before-and-after the program was not statistically different. The difference in rate of diabetes diagnosis annually in the attendee group was 20 per 1000 and in the non-attendee group was -2 (to be interpreted as 0) per 1000. In the community, the annual rate of new diabetes diagnosis was 27 per 1000 (95% CI = 17.90 – 39.00) in the year before the introduction of the CHAD program, and 45 per 1000 (95% CI = 33.00 – 59.80) in the year after.

The attendee and non-attendee groups were significantly different demographically in that the CHAD attendees were more likely to be female, retried and older than the random sample of eligible patients drawn from the same practices. Multi-level regression modeling showed that attending CHAD did seem to have a positive effect on whether diabetes was diagnosed; however, this effect was lessened both in statistical significance and magnitude when taking in to account the physician effect (clustering), patient gender, patient employment status and patient age. If found to be effective in both case detection and cost, a targeted community diabetes screening program should be recommended to Canadian Health Policy makers. Current literature shows that screening is more cost effective in hypertensive and obese groups and the costs of screening are offset in many groups by lower treatment costs [52].

7. Conclusions

The debate for or against screening and even the method of screening in the community therefore has not been fully resolved in Canada. Currently, though the Canadian Diabetes Association recommends screening all individuals over the age of 40 [31,32], the Canadian Task Force on Preventive Health Care (CTFPHC) recommends screening only for adults with hypertension or hyperlipidemia [46]. Both guidelines are under frequent review and revision. For now, health policy makers will need to assess their own communities' needs, which may vary based on the population mix, and assess whether or not local programs for screening (whether targeted or universal) could be initiated; an example of this is the Aboriginal Diabetes Initiative [53]. Through this program, targeting the Aboriginal population increased regular screening for early diagnosis using population-based and opportunistic screening methods is supported, with the use of mobile detection programs. It is possible that diabetes screening could be increased in communities predicted by population-based algorithms to have high rates of undiagnosed diabetes [54]. Researchers have used population based data (national registries and other such data) and developed and validated an algorithm to estimate the number of individuals who will develop diabetes over a 9-year period [54]. This algorithm could be applied to existing provincial data to decide where to focus diabetes screening strategies for greatest effect.

Those reading this chapter from other countries must evaluate the need for screening for diabetes or at the very least, risk-assessment for diabetes, in the primary care setting, which is the natural setting for such activities. Given the epidemic of diabetes worldwide, it is likely that many other countries will be able to use the case study example posed here, as a way of evaluating the need to screen in primary care or family medicine situations elsewhere.

Author details

Gina Agarwal

Department of Family Medicine, McMaster University, Canada

References

[1] Health Canada (1999) Diabetes in Canada: National Statistics and Opportunities for Improved Surveillance, Prevention, and Control. Catalogue No. H49-121/1999. Ottawa: Laboratory Centre for Disease Control, Bureau of Cardio-Respiratory Diseases and Diabetes.

[2] IDF 5th Diabetes Atlas: The Global Burden of Diabetes. http://www.idf.org/diabetesatlas/5e/the-global-burden accessed 12th December 2012).

[3] Dawson K G, Gomes D, Gerstein H, Blanchard J F, Kahler K H. The Economic Cost of Diabetes in Canada. Diab Care 1998;25:1303-7.

[4] Simpson SH, Corabian P, Jacobs P, et al. The cost of major comorbidity in people with diabetes mellitus. CMAJ 2003;168:1661-7.

[5] Goeree R, Morgan E. Lim, Rob Hopkins, et al. Prevalence, Total and Excess Costs of Diabetes and Related Complications in Ontario, Canada. CJD 2009;33(1):35-45.

[6] Lipscombe L, Hux J. Trends in diabetes prevalence, incidence and mortality in Ontario, Canada 1995-2005: a population-based study, Lancet 2007;369(9563):750-6.

[7] Wild S, Roglic G, Green A, Sicree R, King H. Global prevalence of diabetes: estimates for the year 2000 and projections for 2030. Diab Care 2004;27:1047-53.

[8] Centre for Disease Control and Prevention. Prevalence of Diabetes and Impaired fasting glucose in Adults – United States, 1999-2000 MMWR 2003;52.

[9] Hogan P, Dall T, Nikolov P; American Diabetes Association. Economic costs of diabetes in the US in 2002. Diab Care 2003;26(3):917-32.

[10] Leiter LA, Barr A, Belanger A, et al. Diabetes Screening in Canada (DIASCAN) Study: prevalence of undiagnosed diabetes and glucose intolerance in family physician offices. Diab Care 2001;24(6):1038-43.

[11] Fuller JH, Shipley MJ, Rose G, Jarrett RJ, Keen H. Coronary-heart-disease risk and impaired glucose tolerance. The Whitehall study. Lancet 1988;1:1373-6.

[12] Jarrett RJ, McCartney P, Keen H. The Bedford Survey: 10 year mortality rates in newly diagnosed diabetics, borderline diabetics and normoglycaemic controls and risk indices for coronary heart disease in borderline diabetics: Diabetologica 1982;22:79-84.

[13] Robins SJ, et al. The VA-HIT study Group. Relation of gemfibrozil treatment and lipid levels with major coronary events: VA-HIT: a randomized control trial. JAMA 2001 March;285(12):1585-91.

[14] Pan XR, Li GW, Hu YH, et al. Effects of diet and exercise in preventing NIDDM in people with impaired glucose tolerance. The Da Qing IGT and Diabetes Study. Diab Care 1997;20:537-44.

[15] Tuomilehto J, Lindstrom J, Eriksson JG, et al. Finnish Diabetes Prevention Study group. Prevention of type 2 diabetes mellitus by changes in lifestyle among subjects with impaired glucose tolerance. N Engl J Med 2001;344:1343-50.

[16] Knowler WC, Barrett-Conner E, Fowler SE, et al. Diabetes Prevention Program Research Group. Reduction in the incidence of type 2 diabetes with lifestyle intervention or metformin. N Engl J Med 2002;346;393-403.

[17] Larson H, Lindgarde F, Berglund G, Ahren B. Prediction of diabetes using ADA or WHO criteria in post-menopausal women: a 10-year follow- up study. Diabetologia 2004;43:1224-8.

[18] 2006 Census: Portrait of the Canadian Population in 2006, by Age and Sex: National portrait. Statistics Canada. Accessed November 8th 2010: http://www12.statcan.ca/census-recensement/2006/as-sa/97-551/p4-eng.cfm

[19] International Textbook of Diabetes Mellitus, 3rd Edition/2 Volume Set

[20] De Fronzo (Editor), Ele Ferrannini (Editor), Harry Keen (Editor), Paul Zimmet (Editor) Published by Wiley.

[21] Gillies C, Abrams K, Lambert P, et al. Pharmacological and lifestyle interventions to prevent or delay type 2 diabetes in people with impaired glucose tolerance: systematic review and meta-analysis. BMJ 2007;334:299.

[22] PHAC. PHAC Prediabetes and Diabetes Awareness in Canada (PADAC) Survey. 2009.

[23] WHO. Definition and diagnosis of diabetes mellitus and intermediate hyperglycemia. World Health Organization. 2006:1-50.

[24] Consequences of the new diagnostic criteria for DM in older men and women. The DECODE Study group. Diabetes Care 1999;22(10):1667-71.

[25] Gerstein H. Fasting versus Postload Glucose levels. Why the controversy? Diab Care 2001;24(11):1855-7.

[26] The DECODE-study group. Is fasting glucose sufficient to define diabetes? Epidemiological data from 20 European studies. European Diabetes Epidemiology Group. Diabetologica 2000;43(1):132-3.

[27] Tominaga M, Eguchi H, Manaka H, Igarashi K, Kato T, Sekikawa A. Impaired glucose tolerance is a risk factor for cardiovascular disease but not impaired fasting glucose: the Funagata Diabetes Study. Diab Care 1999;22(6):920-4.

[28] American Diabetes Association. Executive summary: standards of medical care in diabetes—2010. Diabetes Care 33: S4-S10.

[29] Goldenberg RM, Cheng AYY, Punthakee Z, Clement M. Position statement: Use of glycated hemoglobin (A1C) in the diagnosis of type 2 diabetes mellitus in adults. Can J Diabetes. 2011;35:247–249

[30] Wilson SE, Lipscombe LL, Rosella LC, Manuel DG: Trends in laboratory testing for diabetes in Ontario, Canada 1995-2005: A population-based study. BMC Hlth Serv Res 2009;9:41-47.

[31] Wilson SE, Rosella LC, Lipscombe LL, Manuel DG. The effectiveness and efficiency of diabetes screening in Ontario, Canada: a population-based cohort study. BMC Public Health 2010;10:506.

[32] Canadian Diabetes association [CDA] 2003 Clinical Practice Guidelines for the Prevention and Management of Diabetes in Canada. Cdn J Diabetes 2003;27:(s2).

[33] Canadian Diabetes Association Clinical Practice Guidelines Expert Committee. Canadian Diabetes Association 2008. Clinical practice guidelines for the prevention and management of diabetes in Canada. Can J Diabetes. 2008;32(suppl 1):S1-S201.

[34] Harris MI, Klein R, Welborn TA, Knuiman MW. Onset of NIDDM occurs at least 4-7 yr before clinical diagnosis. Diab Care 1992;15(7):815-9.

[35] Chiasson JL, Josse RG, Gomis R, Hanefeld M, Karasik A, Laakso M. Acarbose for prevention of type 2 diabetes mellitus: the STOP-NIDDM randomised trial. Lancet. 2002;359(9323):2072-7.

[36] Borch-Johnsen, Lauritzen T, Glumer C, Sandbaek A. Screening for Type 2 diabetes—should it be now? Diabet Med 2003;20:175–81.

[37] Ealovega MW, Tabaei BP, Brandle M, Burke R, Herman WH. Opportunistic screening for diabetes in routine clinical practice. Diab Care 2004;27(1):9-12.

[38] Alberti KG. Screening and diagnosis of prediabetes: where are we headed? Diabetes Obes Metab 2007;9 Suppl 1:12-6.

[39] Lindstrom J, Tuomilehto J. The Diabetes Risk Score. A practical tool to predict type 2 diabetes risk. Diab Care 2003;26:725-31.

[40] Kaczorowoski J, Robinson C, Nerenberg K. Development of the CANRISK quesitonnaire to screen for prediabetes and undiagnosed type 2 diabetes. Cdn J Diabetes 2009;33(4):318-85.

[41] Nerenberg K, Punthakee Z, Gerstein H. Systematic review of screening quesitonnaires for type 2 diabetes. Clinical Investigative Medicine. 2006;(29):314.

[42] Harris R, et al. Screening Adults for type 2 diabetes: a review of the evidence for the US preventive services task force. Annals of Int Med 2003;138(3);4.

[43] Tabaei BP, et al. Community based screening for diabetes in Michigan. Diab Care 2003;26(3):668-70.

[44] Lawrence JM, Bennet P, Young A, Robinson AM. Screening for diabetes in general practice: cross sectional population study. BMJ 2001;323(7312):548-51.

[45] Tsuyuki RT, Johnson JA, Teo KK, et al. A Randomized Trial of the Effect of Community Pharmacist Intervention on Cholesterol Risk Management: The Study of Cardiovascular Risk Intervention by Pharmacists (SCRIP). Arch Intern Med 2002;162:1149-55.

[46] Grant T, et al. Community based screening for cardiovascular disease and diabetes using HbA1c. Am J Prev Med 2004;26(4):271-5.

[47] Feig D, Palda VA, Lipscombe L with The Canadian Task Force on Preventive Health Care. Screening for type 2 diabetes mellitus to prevent vascular complications. CMAJ 2005;172(2):177-80.

[48] Gulli C, Lunau K. Adding Fuel to the Doctor Crisis: Five million Canadians are currently without a family doctor – and things are only getting worse.. Maclean's [Business Magazine], 14 January 2008, p. 62.

[49] Agarwal G. How to diagnose diabetes. CMAJ. 2005;172(5):615-6.

[50] Ciardulli LM, Goode JV. Using health observances to promote wellness in community pharmacies. J Am Pharm Assoc (Wash). 2003 Jan-Feb;43(1):13-6.

[51] Park P, Sargeant L, Griffin S, Wareham N. The performance of a risk score in detecting undiagnosed hyperglycemia. Diab Care June 2002;25(6):984-88.

[52] Agarwal G, Kaczorowski, J, Gerstein, H, Hanna S. Effectiveness of a community-based diabetes program to increase awareness and detection of diabetes. North American Primary Care Research Group (NAPCRG), Montreal, Quebec, Canada. November 2009. [Abstract]

[53] Waugh N, Scotland G, McNamee P, et al. Screening for type 2 diabetes: literature review and economic modelling. Health Technol Assess 2007;11(17):iii-iv, ix-xi, 1-125.

[54] Health Technology Assessment. HTA Reports and Publications. Health Technology Update. Issue 12; November 2009. Accessed Sept 28th 2010; http://www.cadth.ca/index.php/en/hta/reports-publications/health-technology-update/ht-update-12/diabetes-screening-and-diagnosis.

[55] Rosella LC, Manuel D, Burchill C, Stukel TA. A population-based risk algorithm for the development of diabetes: development and validation of the Diabetes Population Risk Tool (DPoRT). J Epidemiol Community Health 2011;65(7):613-20.

Chapter 15

Socio-Ecological Approach to Self-Management of Type 2 Diabetes: Physical Activity and Dietary Intervention

Rashid M. Ansari, John B. Dixon and
Colette J. Browning

Additional information is available at the end of the chapter

http://dx.doi.org/10.5772/56512

1. Introduction

The incidence of type 2 diabetes is increasing worldwide, resulting in large measure from the increasing prevalence of obesity (Yale, 2000). Diabetes mellitus is a pandemic disease and is one of the main threats to human health (Narayan, 2005). In 2003, 194 million people worldwide, ranging in age from 20 to 79 years, had diabetes. It is projected that this number will be increased by 72% to 333 million by 2025, and nearly 80% of these cases will be in the poorer industrialized countries (IDF, 2003).Type 2 diabetes is also a major public health problem in Pakistan as the middle-aged population in that country is overweight or obese, lack of physical activity, unhealthy food and eating habits exposing this population to a high risk of type 2 diabetes (Ansari, 2009). In the local context, prevalence of Type 2 diabetes in Pakistan for the year 2000 was 7.6 % (5.2 million populations) and for 2030 it will increase to around 15% (13.8 million populations) and as such Pakistan is ranked 7th on diabetes prevalence list (WHO, 2004). It was found by Jafar et al (2006) that on the age-specific prevalence of overweight and obesity, more than 40% of women and 30% of men aged 35–54 years were classified as overweight or obese.

Despite the high prevalence of diabetes and serious long term complications, there is still lack of established evidence-based guidelines for self-management (ADA, 2006) and translation of practice recommendations to care in Asian countries (Rayappa et al. 1998) and as well as in developed countries (Chin et al. 2000). Therefore, promoting an active lifestyle or regular exercise has become the highest public health priority in that country to overcome the onslaught of type 2 diabetes and in this context this project is very significant as it addresses this important problem of type 2 diabetes. There is a need for self-management approach for patients of type 2 diabetes and the assessment of quality of diabetes care in the community can help draw attention to the need for improving diabetes self-management and provide a benchmark for monitoring changes over time.

2. Brief literature review

A systematic review of the literature was carried out to cover socio-ecological approach to self-management of type 2 diabetes. Electronic databases were searched, including Cochrane library, Medline, Embase. References of all retrieved articles were checked for relevant studies.

The selection of studies was based on the following criteria:

Interventions: educational interventions compared with usual care, physical activity and diet interventions, behavioural intervention.

Participants: middle-aged population, aged 30-65 with poorly controlled type 2 diabetes.

Outcomes: Studies must report haemoglobin (HbA1c) or hypoglycemia episodes, diabetic complications, cardiovascular disease and quality of life.

Design: The studies related to socio-ecological approach to self-management of type 2 diabetes were included. The search key words were type 2 diabetes, socio-ecological intervention and self-management.

The literature survey revealed that diabetes self-management education is the cornerstone of diabetes care (Mensing et al. 2007). There are several studies indicated an association between diabetes self-management and improved diabetes knowledge and self-management behaviours and improved clinical outcomes (Norris et al. 2001; Philis-Tsimikas et al. 2004). However, authors of a meta-analysis of diabetes self-management programmes reported sharp declines in benefits within one month post intervention (Norris et al. 2001) suggesting that self-management interventions alone do not enable individuals to maintain behaviours changes. The improved outcomes were reported when diabetes self-management was carried out for a longer duration, community-based (CDC, 2001), included follow-up support (Norris et al. 2001), and provided culturally sensitive interventions (Philis-Tsimikas et al 2004; Brown et al. 2005), and addressed psychosocial issues (Mauldon et al. 2006; Norris et al. 2001).

In addition, the social interaction between the patients and doctors is of great significance. The patients of diabetes need to engage with a range of health professionals. Gaining knowledge of the patient's perspective builds on traditional models of physician-patient communication (Pendleton et al. 1984) provides greater clarity to the range of lay understandings that should be explored as a component of effective risk communication.

Fisher et al (2005) suggested that the quality clinical care and self management are compatible and dependent on each other and without sound care, individual's efforts may be misdirected and expert clinical care will fall far short of its potential, through patient failure to use prescribed medications to control his blood sugar or to implement its management plans (Fisher et al. 2005).

http://dx.doi.org/10.5772/56512

A framework for integrating the resources and supports for self-management with key components of clinical care was also provided by Wagner et al (1996) in their chronic care model. A number of studies have also suggested that patient understanding and beliefs about health and illness may be shaped by historical and local contexts (Macfarlane and Kelleher, 2002), whether respondents are thinking about health or behaviour in general or about their own (Blaxter, 1990; French et al. 2001), and personal experience and observation (Davison et al. 1991). The following figure 1 provides a conceptual framework of self-management of type 2 diabetes using the socio-ecological approach.

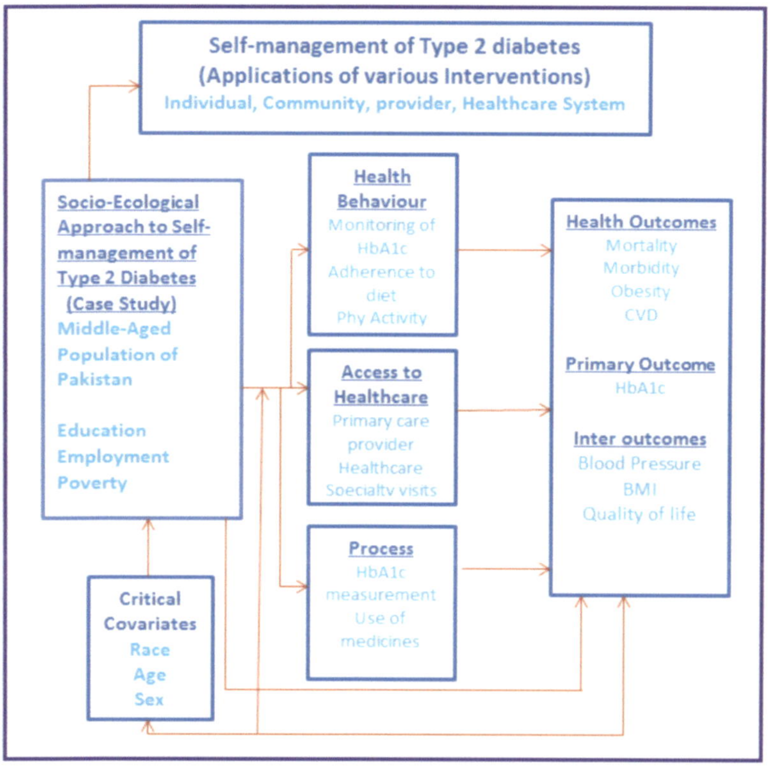

Figure 1. Conceptual framework of self-management of type 2 diabetes

3. Ecological approach to self-management

This case study would also demonstrate that the person is solely responsible to take care of his diabetes related problems and its management and therefore the issue of self-management becomes more important for those with chronic disease, where only the patient can be responsible for day to day care over the length of the illness (Lorig and Holman, 2003). It is generally agreed that self-management is required for control of chronic diseases and for prevention of disease complications; however, patients generally do not adhere to self-management recommendations (Sherbourne et al. 1992; Gochman, 1997; Glasgow and Eakin, 1998). The adherence to the recommendations and barriers are both problematic for "lifestyle" behaviour such as eating patterns and physical activity rather than medication adherence (Brown, 1990; Roter et al. 1998; Ansari, 2009). This is evident from the culture, tradition and life style behavior of the people of Pakistan that both the eating patterns and physical activity are posing a great deal of difficulties to middle-aged population with diabetes.

There is compelling evidence that higher levels of social support are related to better long-term self management and better health outcomes (Kaplan and Toshima, 1990; Uchino et al. 1996). There is also a significant relationship between support and health where support can be assessed from a variety of sources, including spouses, family, friends and neighbours (Dignam et al. 1986). The relationships between support and immunity (Cohen et al. 1997), health status and health behaviours (Glasgow and Toobert, 1988), mortality and quality of life (House et al. 1988; Glasgow et al. 1997) have also been reported in the literature. King et al (2010) has demonstrated that self-efficacy, problem solving, and social environment support are associated with diabetes self-management behaviours.

4. Health services in the local community

The health services in the community in Pakistan are not adequate and diabetes health management programme in the community health clinics does not provide enough help and support to the patients. Shortage of community doctors and expensive consultation with private doctors make the life of patients more difficult in terms of managing their diabetes in that region of Pakistan.

These clinics in Pakistan face special challenges to provide diabetes care to the poor patients as most of these clinics do not meet the evidence-based quality of care standards as compared to the targets established by the American Diabetes Association (ADA, 2000). Similar cases have been reported in several studies in diversified health care settings; including academic institutions (Peters et al. 1996), health maintenance organization (Miller and Hirsch, 1994), health centers (Chin et al. 2000) and medical providers (Chin et al. 1998) where substantial portion of diabetes care does not meet the evidence-based quality of standard care. Marshall et al (2000) have reported that community-based health clinics and their patients have fewer resources than the private clinics and the clinics often lack access to integrated delivery system, and their small size limits the financial feasibility of full-time teams devoted solely to diabetes care.

5. Interventions to improve health services in the community

The health services in the community can be improved by making use of on-going follow-up and support for the self-management of diabetes which has shown promising results (Norris

http://dx.doi.org/10.5772/56512

et al. 2002). For the poor patients in that region of Pakistan where access to the community doctors is not easy and private doctors are not affordable, support may be provided through telephone calls (Weinberger et al. 1995) or the internet (McKay et al. 1998). It has been reported that telephone monitoring of patients, combined with nurse follow-up and tailored information has been shown to reach low income patients and helped them managed their blood sugar level and reduced levels of depression (Piette et al. 1999; Piette et al. 2000).

Another strategy to improve the health services in the community is the group visit to medical clinics by the patients of diabetes (Beck et al. 1997) in which all the patients in a particular category visit the physicians for general check-up including the educational and supportive discussions. Evaluation of this type of strategy has indicated impressive effects on glycosylated hemoglobin and other measures to usual care (Trento et al. 2001).

6. Self-management approach in local context

In order to meet the main objective of this study, the socio-ecological approach to self-management of type 2 diabetes will be applied to middle-aged population of Pakistan using case study approach. The case study is most suitable as it integrates the skills and choices of individuals with the services and support they receive from (a) the social environment of family, friends, organizations and cultures (b) the physical and policy environments of neighbourhoods, communities and governments (Stokols, 1996). The self management from an ecological perspective requires access to a variety of resources, including services provided by professionals and support for the initiation and maintenance of healthy behaviours (Glasgow, 1995; Glasgow et al. 2000).

There is only one study conducted in Pakistan on diabetes knowledge, beliefs and practices among people with diabetes (Rafique et al. 2006). The study provided further evidence that there was a lack of information available to people with diabetes in Pakistan as the large population has never received any diabetes education at all (Rafique et al. 2006). Also, the study was conducted in an urban university hospital, where diabetes education may be more readily available as compared to rural areas where people have less access to information and will have even poorer diabetes perception and practices.

This case study would make a unique contribution to public health in the rural area of Pakistan. This will be first type detailed study of diabetes self-management among the population of Pakistan. It will address the issues and the ways in which diabetes in viewed and managed in that region. The study will also be useful for health care professionals suggesting that coping with diagnosis and living with diabetes is affected by a complex constellation of factors, including life circumstances, social support, gender roles and economy.

7. Aims and objectives

The main objective of this study is to examine the role of physical inactivity and obesity in the development of type 2 diabetes and its self-management in a middle-aged population living in rural area of Pakistan and to evaluate a lifestyle intervention (Physical Activity and Diet) in the management of type 2 diabetes. The study would use the qualitative health approach conducting one-on-one interviews with a sample of informants – patients of type 2 diabetes (n=210) and to explore patients perceptions and experiences of undertaking physical activity and eating behaviour as part of their diabetes self-management. In addition, the study would analyze how the health issue related to diabetes is viewed and addressed in the community and identify the barriers to diabetes care in community and healthcare clinics and would use the concepts of socio-ecological approach to self-management of type 2 diabetes.

This research protocol design addresses the lifestyle interventions for lowering hemoglobin (HbA1c) in this randomized controlled trial and determines whether the intervention of physical activity and diet in combination of usual medical care lowers HbA1c in patients with type 2 diabetes. These types of trials are critical and significant in determining if the culturally tailored interventions are effective in the practical world in which patients live as these patients with diabetes in sub-continent may have different characteristics than those in other western countries due to their eating of different foods and drinking habits.

In addition, this study will help to minimize the gap between the physician-patient understanding and management of diabetes and to identify the barriers to self management of diabetes and quality of life. This study will contribute to improving the quality health care for diabetes in health clinics in that region and would recommend a multifactorial approach emphasizing patient education, improved training in behavioural change for providers, and enhanced delivery system (Chin et al. 2000). The understanding of people about diabetes and susceptibility to diabetes is linked to family, community and society and therefore, this study will impress upon the need to recognize that in developing strategies and interventions to address diabetes, self-care, family support, community education and community ownership are important (Weeramanthri et al. 2003; Wong et al. 2005).

Research Questions: The research questions have been formulated as follows:

1. Will this study help to enhance the patient understanding of self-management of diabetes and will it minimize the gap between the physician-patient interactions?
2. Will hemoglobin (HbA1c) improve after the 90 days trial of lifestyle interventions in patients with poorly controlled type 2 diabetes?
3. Will physical activity and healthy diet lead to reducing the Body Mass Index (BMI) and consequently the risk of diabetes in patients of type 2 diabetes in that region?

Hypotheses: The following hypotheses are to be tested in this study:

1. The lifestyle interventions (physical activity and diet) in patients with poorly controlled diabetes will lead to reduction of 1% hemoglobin (HbA1c) in 90 days trial. (HbA1c as Primary outcome variable)

2. The self-management of type 2 diabetes will reduce 5% weight in patients in 90 days trial and consequently the BMI (BMI as secondary outcome variable)

8. Justification of hypotheses

The justification of the first hypothesis stem from the fact that the clinical complications are significantly associated with glycemia (Stratton et al. 2000) and it has been reported that that each 1% reduction in hemoglobin (HbA1c) is associated with reductions in risk of 21% for any end point related to diabetes, 21% for deaths related to diabetes, 14% for myocardial infarction and 37% for microvascular complications (DCCT, 1996; UKPDS, 1998). The second hypothesis is related to Body Mass Index (BMI) and weight reduction which are measures of obesity and linked to the development of problems in glycemic control and are major risk factors for the development of cardiovascular disease (Michael, 2007).

9. Study design and sampling method

The patients will be recruited from the diabetic medical centre in rural area of Peshawar conducting the study of management of type 2 diabetes among the population aged 30-65 years. The eligibility of patients will be subjected to further screening if their records will not be found in the clinic database. The patients with diabetes having HbA1c >7.0% will be included in this study and patients having coexisting liver, kidney or thyroid disorder will be excluded from this study. The Word Health Organization (WHO, 2006) diabetes criteria will be followed in the selection of the patients with diabetes as indicated in Table 1.

Condition	2 hour glucose	Fasting glucose
	mmol/l(mg/dl)	mmol/l(mg/dl)
Normal	<7.8 (<140)	<6.1 (<110)
Impaired fasting glycaemia	<7.8 (<140)	≥ 6.1(≥110) & <7.0(<126)
Impaired glucose tolerance	≥7.8 (≥140)	<7.0 (<126)
Diabetes mellitus	≥11.1 (≥200)	≥7.0 (≥126)

Table 1. World Health Organization (WHO, 2006). Diabetes Criteria for patients

All the participants will adhere to their usual medications as recommended by their doctors. In order to assess the effectiveness of this intervention, it was advised not to modify the medications during this trial. In addition, participants will be advised not to take any other new treatments for the management of type 2 diabetes during this study. All participants will be contacted again after 90 days (3-months) to give their blood sample for HbA1c testing, their weight will be taken and BMI will be calculated.

10. Study population and randomization

Initially 325 patients with type 2 diabetes will be invited to pre-randomized interview, out of which only 210 patients will be included in the actual trial. For the purpose of this trial, it is expected that out of the 325 patients, 93 patients will not meet the inclusion criteria and 22 patients might refuse to participate in the trial. In that case, two hundred and ten (210) patients will agree to participate and will be required to sign informed consent documents at the clinic where they usually visit for their usual medical care for diabetes. Therefore, 105 patients will be randomized to intervention group (Physical Activity and Diet) and 105 to the control group (usual medical care). Figure 2 shows their progress during the randomized controlled trial. This RCT trial will not be double-blinded as the participants receiving the education on lifestyle modifications in the community and healthcare clinics would know that they are on the active intervention.

Once the randomization phase is completed, all patients will be instructed to follow-up the usual medical care for their diabetes for the duration of the 90 days trial. The patients will not be allowed to adjust their usual medications and follow their previous prescriptions recommended by their doctors. In addition, each patient will be asked to go for blood test for HbA1c on day 1 and then return to give blood sample after 90 days. In addition, participants will be advised not to take any other new treatments for the management of type 2 diabetes during the trial periods.

Those patients randomized to adhere to physical activity and diet (intervention group) will receive education, advice, and behaviour modification skills to help them to maintain a low fat diet, lose weight (goal of 5% weight loss) and moderate intensity physical activity such as brisk walking for 150 minutes/week. Those patients randomized to usual medical care (control group) will be instructed to take their normal medicines and follow-up with their doctor as per their normal schedule.

All participants will be contacted again after 90 days (3-months) to give their blood sample for HbA1c testing, their weight will be taken and BMI will be calculated. At that time, a questionnaire will be sent via e-mail to participants in intervention group to assess the progress of the physical activity and diet intervention and to control group to assess the progress of the treatment with normal medical care only.

11. Measurement

The factors which will be measured in this study are the physical activity of participants (an intervention), hemoglobin (HbA1c – primary outcome variable), blood pressure and weight (secondary outcome) whereas the body mass index (BMI) is a calculated variable. The linear regression analysis will be performed after three months between HbA1c and on the blood glucose results to see the reliability of measurement data and to observe any relationship between the two variables.

http://dx.doi.org/10.5772/56512

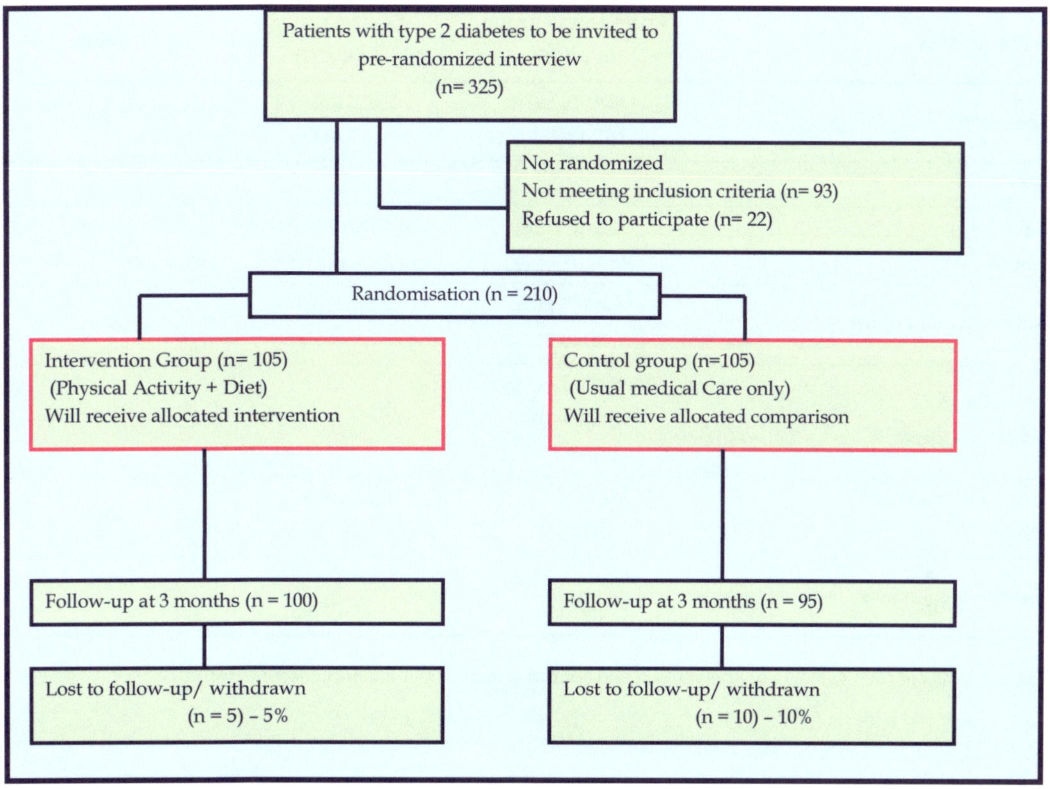

Figure 2. Flow chart describing Randomized Controlled Trial of lifestyle Interventions

Physical activity is a key component of lifestyle modification that can help individuals prevent or control type 2 diabetes. It is considered that diet is probably more important in the initial phases of weight loss, incorporating exercise as part of a weight loss regimen helps maintain weight and prevent weight regain (Klein et al. 2004). In this study, the message will be given to participants to do 30 minutes of moderate physical activity daily (approximately 8000 step count) and it may offer greater benefits to these patients in managing their diabetes (Wright and Royson, 1996).

For measurement of physical activity, the method of step count using pedometer will be used as it has been demonstrated to have a superior validity of step counts over a questionnaire approach in predicting health markers such as BMI and waist circumference (Ewald et al. 2008). The participants will be given pedometer for a week for the measurement of physical activities (step counts). These participants will be instructed to wear the pedometer on a waist belt, either side and wear it from the early morning till they go to bed in the night. The participants will record the start and end time for each day wearing the pedometer and in the evening record the step count showing on the display without resetting the counter. The participants will return a 7-day diary with a record of all the events. Table 2 shows the baseline characteristics of participants in intervention and control group.

Characteristics	Intervention Group (n = 105)	Control Group (n = 105)	P-value
Age (years)	Mean (62.5) ± SD (10.5)	Mean (59.5) ± SD (8.5)	0.78
Sex			
Male	55% (n = 58)	58% (n = 61)	
Female	45% (n = 47)	42% (n = 44)	
Body Mass Index (Kg/m2)	Mean (30.8) ± SD (6.5)	Mean (30.6) ± SD (6.5)	0.40
Physical Activity	95% (8000 steps)	-	
Adherence to diet	98% (n=103) 2% (n = 2)	-	
Baseline Hemoglobin (HbA1c) %	Mean (8.5) ± SD (1.6)	Mean (8.4) ± SD (0)	0.59
Diabetes Medications	Mean (1.75) ± SD (0.8)	Mean (1.82) ± SD (0.8)	0.15

Table 2. Baseline characteristics of intervention and control groups in RCT trial (ref: Medical Record)

12. Method of analysis

12.1. Statistical analysis

The primary outcome will be analysed by an un-paired sample t-test (mean difference between baseline and final HbA1c). The statistical analysis, using STATA will be carried out on an intention to treat basis and that will subject to the availability of data at follow up (after 90 days) as well as at entry level for individual patients. The linear regression analysis will be performed after three months between HbA1c and on the blood glucose results and it is expected that the HbA1c and the self-glucose monitoring via a glucometer will demonstrate a significant relationship ($P < 0.0001$) similar to the findings of Nathan et al. (2008) who reported that the linear regression analysis carried out between the HbA1c and blood glucose (BG) values provided the tightest correlations ($BG = 28.7 \times A1C - 46.7$, $R^2 = 0.84$, $P < 0.0001$), allowing calculation of an estimated average glucose for HbA1C values. The linear regression equations did not differ significantly across subgroups based on age, sex, diabetes type, race/ethnicity, or smoking status.

12.2. Data analysis method

In this study, the thematic analysis of data will be adopted for analysing the data because the method was developed to meet the needs of investigating the experiences, meanings and the reality of the participants (Braun and Clarke, 2006). The method also allows the study to adopt

http://dx.doi.org/10.5772/56512

the element from constructionist notions – to investigate the ways in which events, realities, meanings, experiences are the effects of a range of discourses operating within a society. There are five stages to complete this method – it follows the sequence of familiarization, generating initial codes, searching for themes, reviewing themes, defining and naming and preparing the report.

12.3. Sample size estimation

The study sample size was determined based on the assumption of the estimation of Standard Deviation (SD). Therefore, the study design was selected to detect an effect size of 0.5 SD lowering of HbA1c. It was assumed that 10% patients might be lost to follow-up in control group over the period of three months and only 5 % patients will be lost to follow-up in intervention group. This assumption was based on impact of education and advice on lifestyle behavioural modifications to patients and overall popularity of this approach among the diabetic patients in sub-continent to manage their glycemic control.

Taking into consideration all these factors, the following parameters were considered: α = Level of significance test = 0.05, Power = 0.8, m= the follow-up period 90 days (3 months), Standard Deviation (SD) = 0.5, the sample size was calculated for each group to detect an effect size of 0.5 SD. The sample size (N) for each group was =105; therefore, the total, N=210 patients were recruited to participate in both the groups. The figure 2 shows n=210 patients randomized to each group and their progress during double-blinded fenugreek randomized controlled trial.

12.4. Calculation of sample size — An alternate method

$$\text{Sample Size (N)}=\frac{P1\times(100-P1)+P2\times(100-P2)}{(P1-P2)^2}\times(\alpha,\beta)$$

Where,

P1 = % age success expected in intervention group

P2 = % age success on the control group, being different from P1

α = Level of significance test

β = type II error

Assuming that % age success P1 = 95 %, P2 = 90%,

and the factor f (α, β) = f (0.05, 0.5) = 3.8 (source: Table of f (α, β) – EPID6430 course notes)

$$\text{Sample Size (N)}=\frac{95\times(100-95)+90\times(100-90)}{(95-90)^2}\times(3.8)=209$$

13. Clinical settings in pakistan

Diabetic Medical Center, Ayub Medical College, Abbottabad – Pakistan

Patients = patients of type 2 diabetes visiting the medical center

Doctors = doctors working in medical center

14. Minimizing the bias

It is possible that the outcome measures associated with physical activity and diet interventions will be subject to bias particularly when treatment will be in progress or just afterwards. The main difference between usual medical care alone for the patients and usual medical care with physical activity and dietary interventions will occur after 3 months period of trial. In order to reduce the bias, the questionnaire will be sent to patients at home or via e-mail to minimize any chance that their answers might be affected by actual or perceived influence by medical practitioners at clinic.

15. Discussions

The results of this randomized controlled trial will support the research question that lifestyle interventions (physical activity and diet) with usual medical care for type 2 diabetes is more effective than the usual medical care alone. The higher % age of lost to follow up throughout this trial (Figure 2) in those patients with usual medical care (10%) than in those in intervention group (5%) suggests greater satisfaction with physical activity and dietary education and advice. The difference at 3 months follow up is the mean change in HbA1c levels for the intervention group minus the mean change of HbA1c for the control group. Therefore, the positive differences reflect more improvement in those patients following physical activity and dietary guidelines than in those patients with medical care only.

15.1. Testing hypothesis 1 (Primary outcome variable — HbA1c)

The expected changes in HbA1c from baseline values in patients with type 2 diabetes after 3 months will be calculated by unpaired sample t-test. At 3 months follow-up, the patients would show significantly greater improvement and lower values of HbA1c by 1%. This would support the hypothesis 1 that the lifestyle interventions (physical activity and diet) in patients with poorly controlled diabetes will lead to reduction of 1% hemoglobin (HbA1c) in 90 days trial.

These finding are in agreement with the studies by Stratton et al (2000) and the United Kingdom Prospective Diabetes Studies (UKPDS, 1998), suggesting that any reduction in HbA1c is likely to reduce the risk of complications, with the lowest risk being in those with HbA1c values in the normal range (< 6.0%). Therefore, the potential results of this trial which have shown improvement in patients of diabetes by lowering HbA1c by 1% might be expected to provide similar reductions in morbidity.

http://dx.doi.org/10.5772/56512

15.2. Testing Hypothesis 2 (Secondary outcome variable)

The hypothesis 2 will be supported if we can provide evidence that the type 2 diabetic patients after the 90 days trial would reduce 5% weight and consequently the BMI as compared to the these values at baseline. The polynomial regression analysis will be used to generate the reference range models as these models do not make assumptions about linearity of step count with age (Wright and Royson, 1996). It is expected to find a correlation of step count with BMI similar to one of the studies (Ansari, 2009) which provided evidence that relationship between physical activity and BMI was found to be statistically significant in a cross-sectional study of a large sample of population and it was also associated with reduced risk of type 2 diabetes with (RR=0.82; 95% CI=0.68-1.00; P =0.048). The changes in BMI from the base line values will determine the level of reduction in weight and BMI based on physical activity, diet and exercise.

16. Ethical consideration

The scientific validity of the study is a fundamental ethical protection and this study has a scientific merit and clinical value as it aims at using the socio-ecological approach to self-management of type 2 diabetes and will help diabetic patients to control their hemoglobin (HbA1c) and help them to understand the importance of physical activity and healthy diet and to enjoy a healthy lifestyle.

All the patients will be provided clear instruction about the study and informed consent will be obtained and ethical clearance will be taken from a legal authority before conducting this study.

Finally, the main contribution of this trial is to provide health professionals (diabetes care providers) and patients with type 2 diabetes an insight into the ways in which diabetes is viewed and managed in that region of Pakistan which will help them in the self-management and treatment of type 2 diabetes.

17. Conclusion

It has been demonstrated in this study that the level of HbA1c (primary outcome) will reduce by 1% in the patients of poorly controlled type 2 diabetes after the 90 days trial of physical activity and dietary interventions and hence will support the hypothesis and the research question. This study will enhance the relationship between the medical practitioner and the patients of diabetes and will improve the health care system in that region of the country in managing and treating the patients with chronic disease such as diabetes. This study will improve upon the overall functioning of community healthcare clinics to diabetes care in terms of recognizing the symptoms of diabetes to early detection and diagnosis, easy access to community doctors.

Author details

Rashid M. Ansari, John B. Dixon and Colette J. Browning

School of Primary Health Care, Faculty of Medicine, Nursing and Health Sciences, Monash University, Notting Hill, Australia

References

[1] American Diabetes Association ((2000). Clinical practice recommendations 2000. Diabetes Care 23 (Suppl. 1):SS116, 2000., 1.

[2] American Diabetes Association ((2006). Standards of medical care in diabetes. Diabetes Care. 29 (suppl. 1): SS42., 4.

[3] Ansari, R. M. (2009). Effect of physical activity and obesity on type 2 diabetes in middle-aged population. Journal of Environmental and Public Health, , 2009, 4-9.

[4] Beck, A, Scott, J, Williams, P, et al. (1997). A randomized trial of group outpatient visits for chronically older HMO members: the cooperative health care clinic. J Am Geriatr Soc. , 45(5), 543-549.

[5] Blaxter, M. (1990). Health and Lifestyles.London: Tavistock/Routledge.

[6] Brown, S. A. (1990). Studies of educational interventions and outcomes in diabetic adults: A meta-analysis revisited. Patient Education and Counselling, , 16, 189-215.

[7] Brown, S. A, & Hedges, L. V. (1994). Predicting metabolic control in diabetes: a pilot study using meta-analysis to estimate a linear model. Nurs Res , 43, 362-368.

[8] Brownson, R. C, Housemann, R. A, Brown, D. R, et al. (2000). Promoting physical activity in rural communities: walking trail access, use and effects. Am J Pre Med. , 18, 235-241.

[9] Chandler, M. J, Lalonde, C. E, Sokol, B. W, & Hallett, D. (2003). Personal persistence, identity development, and suicide: a study of Native and Non- native North American adolescents. Monogr Soc Res Child Dev.68 (2): vii-viii, , 1-130.

[10] Chin, M. H, Auerbach, S. B, Cook, S, Harrison, J. F, et al. (2000). Quality of diabetes care in community health centers. Am J Public Health , 90, 431-434.

[11] Chin, M. H, Zhang, J. X, Merrell, K, et al. (1998). Diabetes in the African-American Medicare population: morbidity, quality of care, and resource utilization. Diabetes Care , 21, 1090-1095.

[12] Cohen, S, Doyle, W. J, & Skoner, D. P. (1997). Social ties and susceptibility to the common cold. JAMA , 277, 1940-1944.

[13] Davison, C, Smith, G. D, & Frankel, S. (1991). Lay epidemiology and the prevention paradox. Sociol Health Illn , 13, 1-19.

[14] Dignam, J. T, Barrera, M, & West, S. G. (1986). Occupational stress, social support, and burnout among correctional officers. Am. J. COMMUN. Psychol. , 14, 177-193.

[15] Ewing, R, Schmid, T, & Killingsworth, R. (2003). Relationship between urban sprawl and physical activity, obesity, and morbidity. Am J Health Promot. , 18, 47-57.

[16] Fisher, E. B, Brownson, C. A, Tool, O, et al. (2005). Ecological approaches to self-management: The case of diabetes. American Journal of Public Health. , 95, 1523-1535.

[17] Frank, L. D, Engelke, P. O, & Schmid, T. L. (2003). Health and Community Design: The Impact of the Built Environment on Physical Activity. Washington, DC: Island Press.

[18] French, D. P, Senior, V, Weinman, J, et al. (2001). Causal attributions for heart disease: a systematic review. Psychol Health , 16, 77-98.

[19] Frumkin, H, Frank, L, & Jackson, R. (2004). Urban Sprawl and Public Health: Designing, Planning, and Building for Healthy Communities. Washington, DC: Island Press.

[20] Gaede, P, Vedel, P, Larsen, N, Jensen, G. V. H, et al. (2003). Multifactorial intervention and cardiovascular disease in patients with Type 2 diabetes. New England Journal of Medicine, , 348, 383-393.

[21] Glasgow, R. E, Strycker, L. A, Toobert, D, et al. (2000). The Chronic Illness Resources Surveys: A social-ecologic approach to assessing support for disease self-management. Journal of Behavioral Medicine. , 23, 559-583.

[22] Glasgow, R. E, & Eakin, E. G. (1998). Issues in diabetes self-management. In Shumaker, SA et al. (eds). The Handbook of Health Behaviour Change, Springer, New York, , 435-461.

[23] Glasgow, R. E, Toobert, D. J, & Gillette, C. D. (2001). Psychosocial barriers to diabetes self-management and quality of life. Diabetes Spectrum, , 14, 33-41.

[24] Glasgow, R. E, Ruggiero, L, Eakin, E. G, et al. (1997). Quality of life and associated characteristics in a large diverse sample of adults with diabetes. Diabetes Care, , 20, 562-567.

[25] Glasgow, R. E, & Toobert, D. J. (1988). Social environment and regimen adherence among Type II diabetic patients. Diabetes Care, , 11, 377-386.

[26] Glasgow, R. E, Wagner, E, Kaplan, R. M, et al. (1999). If diabetes is a public health problem, why not treat it as one? A population-based approach to chronic illness. Ann. Behav. Med. , 21, 1-13.

[27] Glasgow, R. E. (1995). A practical model of diabetes management and education. Diabetes Care. 18(1), 117-126.

[28] Glasgow, R. E, Orleans, C. T, Wagner, E. H, et al. (2001). Curry SJ, Solberg LI. Does the Chronic Care Model serve also as a template for improving prevention? Milbank Q. , 79(4), 579-612.

[29] Glasgow, R. E, Toobert, D. J, Barrera, M. J, et al. (2005). The Chronic Illness Resources Survey: cross-validation and sensitivity to intervention. Health Educ Res. , 402-409.

[30] Gochman, D. S. (1997). Handbook of Health Behaviour Research II, Plenum Press, NY.

[31] Haire-joshu, D. (1996). Management of Diabetes Mellitus: Perspectives of care across the lifespan. 2nd ed. St. Louis, Mo: C.V. Mosby Co.

[32] Hampson, S. E, Glasgow, R. E, & Strycker, L. (2000). Beliefs versus feelings: a comparison of personal models and depression for predicting multiple outcomes in diabetes. Br J Health Psychol. , 5, 27-40.

[33] House, J. S, Landis, K. R, & Umberson, D. (1988). Social relationships and health. Science , 241, 540-545.

[34] HughnerR.S & Schultz, KS ((2004). Views of Health in the Lay Sector: A Compilation & Review of How Individuals Think about Health. , 8, 395-422.

[35] Huston, S. L, Evenson, K. R, Bors, P, et al. (2003). Neighbourhood environment, access to places for activity, and leisure-time physical activity in a diverse North Carolina population. Am J Health Promot., 18, 58-69.

[36] International Diabetes Federation ((2003). Diabetes prevalence, available online from: http://www.idf.org/home/index.cfm

[37] Jafar, T. H, Chaturvedi, N, & Pappas, G. (2006). Prevalence of overweight and obesity and their association with hypertension and diabetes mellitus in an Indo-Asian population. CMAJ , 175(9), 1071-7.

[38] Johnston, M. E, Gibson, E. S, Terry, C. W, et al. (1984). Effects of labelling on income, work and social function among hypertensive employees. Journal of Chronic Disease, , 37, 417-423.

[39] Kahn, E. B, Ramsey, L. T, Brownson, R. C, et al. (2002). The effectiveness of interventions to increase physical activity: a systematic review. Am J Prev Med. , 22, 73-107.

[40] Kaplan, R. M, Ganiats, T. G, & Sieber, W. J. (1998). The quality of well being scale: Critical similarities and differences with SF-36. International Journal of Quality of Health Care. , 10, 509-520.

[41] Kaplan, R. M, & Toshima, M. T. (1990). The functional effects of social relationships on chronic illness and disability. In Sarason, BS, Sarason, I.G and Pierce, G.R (eds). Social Support: An International View, Wiley, New York, , 427-453.

[42] King, D. K, Glasgow, R. E, Toobert, D. J, et al. (2010). Self-efficacy, problem solving, and social environment support are associated with diabetes self-management behaviours. Diabetes Care , 33, 751-753.

[43] Kirmayer, L. J, Gregory, M, & Tait, L. (2000). The mental health of Aboriginal peoples: transformations of identity and community. Can J Psychiatry. , 45(7), 607-16.

[44] Lorig, K. R, & Holman, H. (2003). Self-management education: history, definition, outcomes, and mechanisms. Ann Behav Med. , 26, 1-7.

[45] Macfarlane, A, & Kelleher, D. (2002). Concepts of illness causation and attitudes to health care among older people in the Republic of Ireland. Soc Sci Med , 54, 1389-400.

[46] Marzilli, G. (1999). The Effects of Social Support on Eating Behaviour in Patients with Diabetes." Available: (http://insulin-pumpers.org/textlib/psyc353.pdf).Retrieved May 25, 2009.

[47] May, P. A, Serna, P, Hurt, L, & Debruyn, L. M. (2005). Outcome evaluation of a public health approach to suicide prevention in an American Indian tribal nation. Am J Public Health., 95(7), 1238-44.

[48] Mckay, H. G, Feil, E. G, Glasgow, R. E, et al. (1998). Feasibility and use of an internet support service for diabetes self-management. Diabetes Educ. , 24, 174-179.

[49] Miller, K. L, & Hirsch, I. B. (1994). Physicians' practices in screening for the development of diabetic nephropathy and the use of glycosy-lated hemoglobin levels. Diabetes Care , 17, 1495-1497.

[50] Narayan, K. M. V. (2005). The Diabetes Pandemic: Looking for the silver lining: Clinical diabetes. , 23, 51-52.

[51] National Health Survey of Pakistan ((1998). Health Profile of the people of Pakistan, Islamabad, Pakistan: Pakistan Medical Research Council., 1990-94.

[52] Norris, S. L, Lau, J, Smith, S. J, et al. (2002). Self-management education for adults with type 2 diabetes: a meta-analysis of the effect on glycemic control. Diabetes Care. , 25, 1159-1171.

[53] Pendleton, D, Schofield, T, & Tate, P. (1984). The Consultation: An Approach to Learning and Teaching. Oxford: Oxford University Press.

[54] Peters, A. L, Legorreta, A. P, Ossorio, R. C, et al. (1996). Quality of outpatient care provided to diabetic patients: a health maintenance organization experience. Diabetes Care, 19, 601-606.

[55] Piette, J. D, Weinberger, M, Kraemer, F. B, et al. (2001). Impact of automated calls with nurse follow-up on diabetes treatment outcomes in a Department of Veterans

Affairs Health care system: a randomized controlled trial. Diabetes Care. , 24, 202-208.

[56] Piette, J. D, Mcphee, S. J, Weinberger, M, et al. (1999). Use of automated telephone disease management calls in an ethnically diverse sample of low-income patients with diabetes. Diabetes Care. , 22, 1302-1309.

[57] Rayappa, P. H. Raju, KNM, Kapur, A et al ((1998). The impact of socio-economic factors on diabetes care. Int J Diab Dev Countries. , 19, 7-15.

[58] Rood, R. P. (1996). Patients and physician responsibility in the treatment of chronic illness: the case of diabetes. American Behavioral Scientist, , 39(6), 729-751.

[59] Roter, D. L, Hall, J. A, Mersica, R, et al. (1998). Effectiveness of interventions to improve patient compliance. Med. Care , 36, 1138-1161.

[60] Sherbourne, C. D, Hays, R. D, & Ordway, L. (1992). Antecedents of adherence to medical recommendations: Results from the medical outcomes study. J. Behav. Med. , 15, 447-468.

[61] Stokols, D. (1996). Translating social ecological theory into guidelines for community health promotion. Am J Health Promot. 10(4), 282-298.

[62] Thompson, S. J, & Gifford, S. M. (2000). Trying to keep a balance: the meaning of health and diabetes in an urban Aboriginal community. Social Science and Medicine, , 51, 1457-1473.

[63] Thompson, O. M, Ballew, C, Resnicow, K, et al. (2004). Food purchased away from home as a predictor of change in BMI z-score among girls. Int J Obes Relat Metab Disord., 28(2), 282-289.

[64] Trento, M, Passera, P, Tomalino, M, et al. (2001). Group visits improve metabolic control in type 2 diabetes: a 2-year follow-up. Diabetes Care. , 24, 995-1000.

[65] Uchino, B. N, Cacioppo, J. T, & Kiecolt-glaser, J. K. (1996). Relationship between social support and physiological processes: A review with emphasis on underlying mechanisms and implications for health. Psychol. Bull. , 119, 488-531.

[66] Wagner, E. H. (1998). Chronic disease management: What will it take to improve care for chronic illness? Effective Clinical Practice. , 1, 1-4.

[67] Wagner, E. H, Austin, B. T, & Von Korff, M. (1996). Organizing care for patients with chronic illness. Milbank Q. , 74, 511-544.

[68] Wagner, E. H, Glasgow, R. E, Davis, C, et al. (2001). Quality improvement in chronic illness care: a collaborative approach. Jt Comm J Qual Improv. 2001; , 27, 63-80.

[69] Weeramanthri, T, Hendy, S, Connors, C, Ashbridge, D, et al. (2003). The Northern Territory Preventable Chronic Disease Strategy- promoting an integrated and life

course approach to chronic disease in Australia. Australian Health Review , 26(3), 31-42.

[70] Wareham, N. J, Byrne, C. D, Williams, R, et al. (1999). Fasting proinsulin concentrations predict the development of type 2 diabetes. Diabetes Care, , 22, 262-270.

[71] Weinberger, M, Kirkman, M. A, Samsa, G. P, et al. (1995). A nurse-coordinated intervention for primary care patients with non-insulin-dependent diabetes mellitus: impact on glycemic control and health-related quality of life. J Gen Intern Med. , 10, 59-66.

[72] WHO Expert Consultation ((2004). Appropriate body-mass index for Asian populations and its implications for policy and intervention. Lancet. , 363, 157-63.

[73] Williams, R, Herman, W, Kinmonth, A. L, et al. (2002). Evidence Base for Diabetes Care. Wiley, Chichester.

[74] Wong, M, Haswell-elkins, M, Tamwoy, E, et al. (2005). Perspectives on clinic attendance, medication and foot-care among people with diabetes in the Torres Strait Islands and Northern Peninsula Area. Australian Journal of Rural Health , 13(5), 172-177.

Chapter 16

Lifestyle Modification Is the First Line Treatment for Type 2 Diabetes

Kazuko Masuo

Additional information is available at the end of the chapter

http://dx.doi.org/10.5772/56377

1. Introduction

The prevalence of diabetes, especially type 2 diabetes and hypertension are significantly increased with the prevalence of obesity (Figures 1, 2 and 3) [1, 2]. Type 2 diabetes, hypertension frequently associated with type 2 diabetes, and obesity are important risk factors for cardiovascular morbidity and mortality and cardiac- and renal complications. Hyperglycemia as well as hyperinsulinemia in type 2 diabetes is a cardiovascular risk by itself [3]. Type 2 diabetes, hypertension and obesity are characterized by stimulation of the renin-angiotensin-aldosterone system (RAAS), elevated sympathetic activity and insulin resistance. Importantly, these characteristics, themselves, are one of the cardiovascular risks. Therefore, pharmacological and non-pharmacological treatments for type 2 diabetes should be selected from favourable effects on stimulated RAAS, elevated sympathetic nervous system activity, insulin resistance and leptin resistance.

Weight loss is recommended to delay and prevent type 2 diabetes in obesity, and for the treatment. Lifestyle modification such as a caloric restricted diet, reducing sedentary behaviour and an increase in exercise form the basis of all therapy. Weight loss treated with lifestyle modification including calorie restriction and/or exercise causes normalization of stimulated RAAS, sympathetic activation, insulin resistance, and hyperleptinemia, which are usually observed in type 2 diabetes and obesity. Recently, Straznicky *et al.* [4] and Masuo *et al.* [5] have shown the low caloric diet and exercise have different effects on insulin resistance, the RAAS, and sympathetic nervous activity in obese hypertensive subjects, although similar weight loss was observed between both interventions. Straznicky *et al.* [4] reported that exercise had stronger effects of normalized the RAAS stimulation, sympathetic activation and insulin resistance compared to diet only, whereas Masuo *et al.* [5] showed mild calorie restriction and mild exercise has different mechanisms on weight loss (normalization on sympathetic

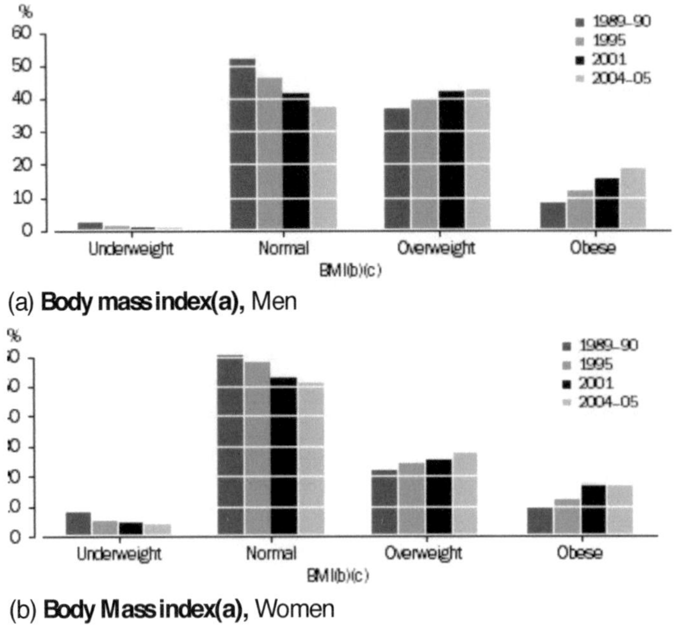

Source: National Health Survey, Australian Bureau of Statics in 2008.
Prevalence of overweight and obesity has increased in both genders.

Figure 1. Overweight/obesity has increased in both genders in Australia [Source. Australian Bureau of Statics. 4819.0. Released at 11:30 AM (CANBERRA TIME) 25/01/2008] Reference [1]

activation for mild calorie restriction, and normalization on insulin resistance for exercise). The observations, however, demonstrate that a combination therapy for weight loss with a low caloric diet and exercise is recommended for weight loss due to stronger suppression of insulin resistance and sympathetic activation, which both are known as strong risk factors for cardiovascular events. Although few studies have observed changes in body weight, blood pressure, neurohormonal changes over a long duration such as 2 years, Masuo *et al.* [6] observed more than 30% individuals who initially succeeded to significantly lose weight, had rebound weight gain over 2 years. Understanding mechanisms underlying both type 2 diabetes and obesity may help to achieve weight loss and maintenance of weight loss and the stricter blood glucose goal. Maintenance of weight loss is another key factor to reduce cardiovascular risks in type 2 diabetes in obesity [6].

In addition, most hypertensive patients with diabetes and obesity are very resistant to controlling hypertension and frequently require two or more types of medications to achieve blood pressure goals. Similarly, diabetic patients, especially type 2 diabetic patients with obesity, need higher dose of anti-diabetic medications such as metformin or insulin. However, pharmacological treatments for hypertension and diabetes with weight loss could reduce pharmacological treatment [7, 8].

http://dx.doi.org/10.5772/56377

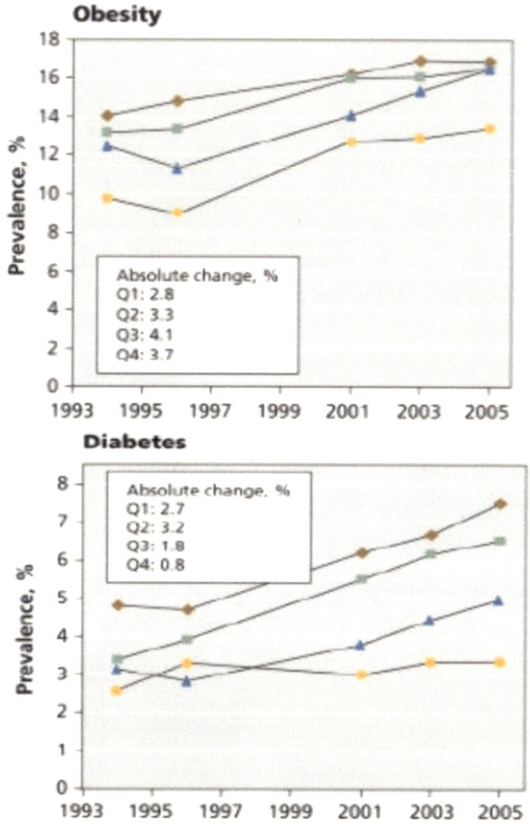

Figure 2. Prevalence of diabetes has increased in parallel with obesity. [Reference 2]

The purpose of this review is to provide, *i)* the importance of lifestyle modifications to delay and prevent type 2 diabetes, *ii*) Lifestyle modification to reduce cardiovascular risks in type 2 diabetes, and *iii)* weight loss for the better pharmacological control on type 2 diabetes and hypertension, which frequently co-exist with type 2 diabetes. *iv)* The mode of weight loss influences different physiological pathways, with calorie restriction and exercise program. *v*) Different mechanisms may contribute to reductions in blood pressure and cardiovascular risks associated with weight loss with the relevant physiological mechanisms at play being dependent on the mode of weight loss.

2. Type 2 diabetes versus Type 1 diabetes

Prevalence of diabetes has increased markedly over the last 20 years in parallel with obesity (Figures 2 and 3) [1, 2]. As of 2010 there are approximately 285 million people with the disease compared to around 30 million in 1985. Long-term complications from high blood sugar can include heart disease, strokes, renal failure, diabetic retinopathy, and diabetic neuropathy.

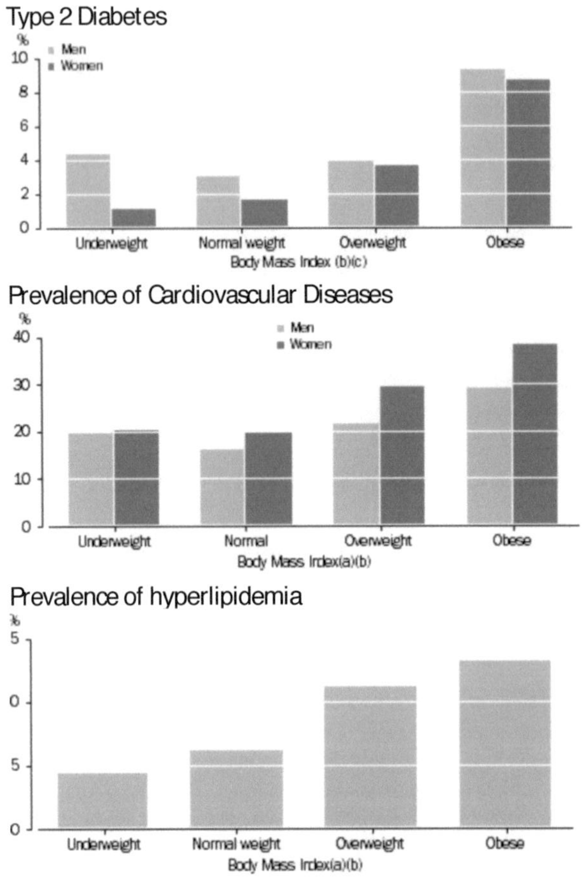

Figure 3. Prevalence of type 2 diabetes, cardiovascular disease and hyperlipidemia (hyper cholesterolemia) increased with obesity in both genders. [Source: National Health Survey, Australia, 2004-2005] Reference [1]

Diabetes mellitus includes type 2 diabetes (formerly noninsulin dependent diabetes), type 1 diabetes (formerly insulin dependent diabetes), and gestational diabetes. These 3 types of diabetes have different characteristics and progress [9]. Ninety percent of diabetic patients are type 2 diabetes and the other 10% are due primarily to diabetes mellitus type 1 and gestational diabetes.

2.1. Diabetes mellitus type 2 (Formerly noninsulin-dependent diabetes mellitus (NIDDM))

Type 2 diabetes is the most common form of diabetes, affecting 90% of all patients with diabetes. This type of diabetes is characterised by metabolic disorder with insulin resistance and relative insulin deficiency [10]. This is in contrast to type 1 diabetes, in which there is an absolute insulin deficiency due to destruction of islet cells in the pancreas [9, 11]. Obesity is thought to be the primary cause of type 2 diabetes in people who are genetically predisposed to the disease, and obesity has been found to contribute to approximately 55% of case of type 2 diabetes [12].

The disease is strongly genetic in origin but lifestyle factors such as excess weight, inactivity, high blood pressure and poor diet are major risk factors for its development. Symptoms may not show for many years and, by the time they appear, significant problems may have developed. People with type 2 diabetes are twice as likely to suffer cardiovascular disease. The classic symptoms are excess thirst, frequent urination, and constant hunger.

Type 2 diabetes is initially managed by increasing exercise and dietary modification. If blood glucose levels are not adequately lowered by these measures, medications such as metformin or insulin may be needed. In those on insulin, there is typically the requirement to routinely check blood sugar levels.

2.2. Type 1 diabetes (Insulin-dependent diabetes)

Type 1 diabetes is an auto-immune disease targeting on the insulin-producing beta cells in the pancreas. This type of diabetes, also known as juvenile-onset diabetes, accounts for approximately 10% of all people with the disease. In the majority of cases this type of diabetes appears before the patient is 40 years old, triggered by environmental factors such as viruses, diet or chemicals in people genetically predisposed. Patients with type 1 diabetes will require insulin therapy regularly, and should follow a careful diet and exercise plan.

2.3. Gestational diabetes mellitus

Gestational diabetes, or glucose intolerance, is first diagnosed during pregnancy through an oral glucose tolerance test. Between 5.5 and 8.8% of pregnant women develop gestational diabetes in Australia [13], and 2 to 10 percent of all pregnancies in USA [14]. The hormones produced during pregnancy increase the amount of insulin needed to control blood glucose levels. If the body can't meet this increased need for insulin, women can develop gestational diabetes during the late stages of pregnancy.

While the glucose intolerance usually returns to normal after the birth, the mother has a significant risk of developing permanent diabetes while the baby is more likely to develop obesity and impaired glucose tolerance and/or diabetes later in life [15]. Risk factors for gestational diabetes include a family history of diabetes, increasing maternal age, obesity, lack of sleep [16], and being a member of a community or ethnic group with a high risk of developing type 2 diabetes. Self-care and dietary changes are essential in treatment.

3. Prevalence of type 2 diabetes

The prevalence of type 2 diabetes has dramatically increased in parallel in rising prevalence of obesity (Figures 1 and 2), and it increases with obesity (Figure 3). Rates of diabetes in 1985 in worldwide were estimated at 30 million, increasing to 135 million in 1995 and 217 million

	Type 1 Diabetes	**Type 2 Diabetes**
Diagnosis:	Genetic, environmental and auto-immune factors, idiopathic	Genetic, obesity (central adipose), physical inactivity, high/low birth weight, GDM, poor placental growth, metabolic syndrome
Warning Signs:	Increased thirst & urination, constant hunger, weight loss, blurred vision and extreme tiredness, glycouria	Feeling tired or ill, frequent urination (especially at night), unusual thirst, weight loss, blurred vision, frequent infections and slow wound healing, asymptomatic
Target Groups:	Children/teens	Adults, elderly, ethnic groups
Prone ethnic groups:	All	more common in African American, Latino/Hispanic, indigenous, Asian or Pacific Islander
Bodily Effects:	Believed to be triggered autoimmune destruction of the beta cells; autoimmune attack may occur following a viral infection such as mumps, rubella cytomegalovirus	Appears to be related to aging, sedentary life-style, genetic influence, but mostly obesity
Common physical attributes found:	Mostly Normal or Thin	Mostly Overweight or Obese
You have this when:	Your body makes too little or no insulin.	Your body either cannot produce insulin or does not use it properly.
Estimated percentage of occurrence:	5% -10% of the 171 million of people affected by diabetes in 2000	90% - 95%-of total cases. Although the projected number of Americans that will have type II diabetes in the year 2030 will double from 171 million to 366 million cases
Affected age group:	Between 5 - 25 (maximum numbers in this age group; Type 1 can affect at any age)	Until recently, the only type of diabetes that was common in children was Type 1 diabetes, most children who have Type 2 diabetes have a family history of diabetes, are overweight, and are not very physically active. Usually develops around puberty
Glucose Channels/receptors:	Open and absorb glucose into cell to be utilized by processes after the induction of insulin	Are unable to open and absorb glucose, therefore glucose cannot be utilized by processes; as a result the glucose stays in the blood stream
Cure:	None	Physical exercise, healthy loss of weight & diet control
Treatment:	Insulin Injections, dietary plan, regular check up of blood sugar levels, daily exercise Goals: optimal glucose, prevent/treat chronic complications, enhance health with food/PA, individual nutrition needs	Diet, exercise, weight loss, and in many cases medication. Insulin Injections may also be used, SMBG
Dependency:	Insulin-dependent	Not insulin-dependent
Onset:	Rapid (weeks)	Slow (years)

[Reference, American Diabetes Association-Executive Summary-2012, A-348]

Table 1. Comparison between type 1 diabetes and type 2 diabetes

in 2005 [17]. This increase is believed to be primarily due to the global population aging, a decrease in exercise, and increasing rates of obesity [18].

The prevalence of diabetes is recognized as a global epidemic by the World Health Organization (WHO) [19]. The World Health Organization (WHO) has reported 346 million people worldwide had diabetes in 2004. Globally as of 2010 it was estimated that there were 285 million people with type 2 diabetes, and this is equivalent to about 6% of the world's adult population [18]. In 2010, diabetic patients were estimated as 316 million people worldwide, and this is equivalent to about 6% of the world's adult population. Importantly, the National Diabetes Fact Sheet 2011 by Centers for Disease Control and Prevention (CDC) pointed out 7.0 million American people (27% of those with diabetes) were not diagnosed and an estimated 79 million Americans have pre-diabetes, indication that much more of the population were affected by diabetes [20, 21]. An estimated 3.4 million people died from consequences of diabetes in 2004, which more than 80% of diabetes deaths occurs in low- and middle-income countries, and diabetes deaths will increase by double between 2005 and 2030 [22]. The five countries with the greatest number of people with diabetes as of 2000 are India, China, the United States, Indonesia, and Japan. Diabetes is common both in the developed and the developing world, but not in the underdeveloped world. Women seem to be at a greater risk as do certain ethnic groups such as South Asians, Pacific Islanders, Latinos, and Native Americans [18]. This may be due to enhanced sensitivity to a Western lifestyle in certain ethnic groups [23].

4. What causes type 2 diabetes?

Many epidemiological studies showed a strong association between obesity and type 2 diabetes, however it is also true that not all obese individuals have type 2 diabetes [20]. Majority of the onset and development of type 2 diabetes is caused by a combination of lifestyle and genetics. Other confounders are also reported to relate to the onset and development of type 2 diabetes: *i.e.* lack of sleep [16], which has been linked to type 2 diabetes through its effect on metabolism [15], nutritional status of a mother during fetal development may also play a role, with one proposed mechanism being that of altered DNA methylation [24]. While some are under personal control, such as diet and obesity, others, such as increasing age, female gender, and genetic susceptibility, is not. The followings are several causes known for type 2 diabetes.

4.1. Lifestyle

A number of lifestyle factors are known to be important to the development of type 2 diabetes, including obesity, lack of physical activity (sedentary life style) [12], poor diet, stress, and urbanization.

Excess body fat is associated with 30% of cases in type 2 diabetes of Chinese and Japanese descent, 60-80% of cases in those of European and African descent, and 100% of Pima Indians and Pacific Islanders [19, 23]. Interestingly, Pima Indians and Pacific Islanders have relatively higher waist-to-hip ratio even if they are not obese, suggesting that abdominal obesity and visceral fat is more important to cause type 2 diabetes.

Dietary factors also influence the risk of developing type 2 diabetes. Consumption of sugar-sweetened drinks in excess is associated with an increased risk. It has been demonstrated saturated fat and trans-fatty acids increase LDL cholesterol, the risk of type 2 diabetes, and cardiovascular risk. Poly-unsaturated, and monounsaturated fat decreasing the risk, but It is recommended to take both in a limited quantity. The American Heart Association has recommended that Americans should limit their intake of saturated fats to 7% of their total calories in a day, while unsaturated fats can form 30% of the calorie intake.

4.2. Genetics

Most cases of diabetes involve many genes, with each being a small contributor to an increased probability of becoming a type 2 diabetic. If one identical twin has diabetes, the chance of the other developing diabetes within his lifetime is greater than 90% while the rate for non-identical siblings is 25-50%. As of 2011, more than 36 genes have been found that contribute to the risk of type 2 diabetes. All of these genes together still only account for 10% of the total heritable component of the disease. The TCF7L2 allele, for example, increases the risk of developing diabetes by 1.5 times and is the greatest risk of the common genetic variants. Most of the genes linked to diabetes are involved in beta cell functions in pancreas.

There are a number of rare cases of diabetes that arise due to an abnormality in a single gene (known as monogenic forms of diabetes or "other specific types of diabetes"). These include maturity onset diabetes of the young (MODY), Donohue syndrome, and Rabson-Mendenhall syndrome, among others. Maturity onset diabetes of the young constitutes 1–5% of all cases of diabetes in young people.

4.3. Medical conditions

There are a number of medications, including glucocorticoids, thiazides, beta blockers, atypical antipsychotics, and statins that can predispose to diabetes [25].

Statins have beneficial effects on reductions of cardiovascular risks through lipids control, and mortality and morbidity in patients with high cardiac risk such as diabetes, coronary heart disease, ischemic heart disease, chronic kidney disease, chronic heart failure, and peripheral vascular disease [26, 27]. National and international clinical guidelines in the management of these cardiovascular disease conditions all advocate for the utilization of statins therapy in appropriate patients. The meta-analysis including 80,771 participants with low cardiac risk showed that all-cause mortality was significantly lower among patients receiving a statin than among controls with a 10-year risk of cardiovascular disease < 20% [28]. Patients in the statin group were also significantly less likely than controls to have nonfatal myocardial infarction, and nonfatal stroke, but the effects did not depend on high- and low-potency statins, or larger reductions in cholesterol. The JUPITER trial [27] and Atherosclerosis Risk in Communities (ARIC) Study [29] demonstrated that suppression of low-grade inflammation by statins improves these clinical outcomes.

Recently, concerns were raised regarding the onset and development of diabetes in statin-treated patients [30]. The meta-analysis studied by Coleman *et al.* [31] showed that statins, as a class, did not demonstrate a statistically significant positive or negative impact on a patient's risk of developing new-onset type 2 diabetes mellitus, whereas Satter *et al.* [32] observed that statin therapy is associated with a slightly increased risk of development of diabetes using meta-analysis, but the risk is low both in absolute terms and when compared with the reduction in coronary events. Clinical practice in patients with moderate or high cardiovascular risk or existing cardiovascular disease should not change. In 2012, two major studies have addressed the question of whether statins lead to an increase in diabetes, which included the meta-analysis of 33,000 participants enrolled in 5 major clinical trials using statins [33, 34], and analysed data from 153,840 postmenopausal women between 50 and 80 years in the Women Health Initiative Study [30]. The study showed women taking statins had a 48% increased risk of diabetes compared those without statins. The American Heart Association concluded in 2012 that the benefits of statins on lipids-lowering effects and resultant reductions in cardiovascular risks overweighted to the new onset or development of diabetes [35].

Combined bezafibrate/statin therapy is theoretically believed more effective in achieving a comprehensive lipid control and residual cardiovascular risk reduction [36, 37]. The ACCORD Study [38], however, showed that the combination of fenofibrate and simvastatin did not reduce the rate of fatal cardiovascular events, nonfatal myocardial infarction, or nonfatal stroke, as compared with simvastatin alone. Based on the beneficial effects of pan-PPAR agonist bezafibrate on glucose metabolism and prevention of new-onset diabetes, one could expect a neutralization of the adverse pro-diabetic effect of statins using the strategy of a combined statin/fibrate therapy [39, 40].

5. Type 2 diabetes mellitus as a risk factor for cardiovascular disease

Several epidemiological studies are available to understand that diabetes is a strong cardiovascular disease risks. A population-based European Prospective Investigation into Cancer and Nutrition (EPIC)-Potsdam study [41], which consisted of 23,455 participants (9,729 men and 15,438 women) followed up from 1994-1998 to 2006, showed that participants with a high risk of the development of diabetes had significantly higher risks of myocardial infarction and stroke than those with a low risk of diabetes development. Subjects at a high risk of diabetes development were also at considerably higher risks of developing cardiovascular complications in general.

The Framingham Heart Study [42] observed that both cardiovascular disease and non-cardiovascular disease mortality rates among individuals with diabetes mellitus were approximately 2-fold higher compared with individuals without diabetes. Non-cardiovascular disease mortality declined among women without diabetes mellitus, while no change in non-cardiovascular disease mortality was observed among women and men with diabetes between the "1950 to 1975" and "1976 to 2001" period. Importantly, individuals with diabetes were at a higher risk of all-cause mortality, especially cardiovascular disease mortality, in both the periods compared to those without diabetes. Another study has shown that diabetes is associated with a substantial increase in all cause and coronary heart disease mortality [43].

Regarding the gender differences in mortality and morbidity of cardiovascular complications, Kanaya *et al.* [44], in their meta-analysis, documented that absolute coronary heart disease death rates were higher in diabetic men compared with diabetic women at every age except the very oldest, however, the excess relative risk of coronary heart disease mortality in women versus men with diabetes was absent after adjusting for classic coronary heart disease risk factors (*i.e.* dyslipidemia, hypertension).

Recently, the Detection of Ischemia in Asymptomatic Diabetics (DIAD) study [45] was performed in 1,123 patients with type 2 diabetes and no symptoms of coronary heart disease using adenosine-stress radionuclide myocardial perfusion imaging from 2000 to 2007. The cumulative cardiac event rate in DIAD was 2.9% over a mean follow-up of 4.8 years for an average of 0.6% per year, which is higher compared to the general population.

The World Health Organization Multinational Study of Vascular Disease in diabetes [46, 47] examined the relationship between excess mortality and proteinuria/hypertension in a stratified random sample of 4,714 diabetic patients aged 35-55 years from 1975 to 1987. Even in the absence of proteinuria and hypertension, standardized mortality rates were significant higher in patients with both type 1 and type 2 diabetes compared to the general population. Standardized mortality was higher in those with type 1 diabetes compared with type 2 diabetes, and the standard mortality rate increased with increasing diabetes duration. In addition, both hypertension and proteinuria had a strikingly high mortality risk by 11-fold for men with type 1 diabetes, and 5 fold for men with type 2 diabetes, indicating that diabetes accompanying cardiovascular disease leads to even higher mortality risk.

Hypertension is twice as frequent in diabetic patients in the general population, and its prevalence is higher in type 2 diabetes than in type 1 diabetes. In type 2 diabetes, the onset of hypertension often precedes the diagnosis of diabetes, whereas in type 1 diabetes it is strictly related to the presence of nephropathy [48].

Further, many studies have shown the strong associations of myocardial infarction [49] and atherosclerosis [50-52]. A number of epidemiological studies provide evidence that diabetes mellitus is a significant risk factor for cardiovascular disease mortality and morbidity [53]. Longer duration of diabetes is a stronger predictor of mortality among diabetic patients. Therefore, people who have diabetes mellitus or strong lifestyle or dietary factors to predict the development of type 2 diabetes [54] should avoid the cardiovascular complications.

6. Neurohoromonal characteristics in type 2 diabetes: Insulin resistance and sympathetic activity

It is widely recognized that insulin resistance is a major mechanism of the onset of type 2 diabetes. Insulin resistance in children could predict future glucose intolerance and type 2 diabetes in 10 years [46, 55]. Reduced energy expenditure and resting metabolic rate are predictive of weight gain (obesity). The sympathetic nervous system participates in regulating energy balance through thermogenesis. Many epidemiological and clinical studies have shown a close relationship between sympathetic nervous system activity and insulin levels in obesity and in weight gain [56, 57]. Elevations of sympathetic nervous system activity and insulin levels during weight gain [58-60] and reductions of sympathetic activity and insulin levels during weight loss [61-64] are typically observed. In addition, The response of the sympathetic nervous system to changes in plasma insulin levels after oral glucose loading (oral glucose tolerance test) are different between subjects with and without insulin resistance [65], between nonobese and obese subjects [66], and between subjects with and without metabolic syndrome [67]. Those observations provide evidence of a strong linkage between the activity of the sympathetic nervous system and insulin levels over glucose metabolisms. Straznicky *et al.* [68] reported that the progress from metabolic syndrome to type 2 diabetes might be associated with increased central sympathetic drive, blunted sympathetic responsiveness, and altered norepinephrine disposition.

Acute hyperglycemia caused sympathetic activation and peripheral vasodilation. Moreover, both acute and chronic hyperglycemia and hyperinsulinemia may enhance adrenergic vasoconstriction and decrease vasodilation in animal models (pithed rats) [69, 70]. Insulin causes forearm vasoconstriction in obese, insulin-resistant hypertensive humans [71]. On the other hand, van Veen *et al.* [72] found that hyperglycemia in the forearm induced vasodilation, but this vasodilation was not modified by hyperinsulinemia.

Huggett *et al.* [66] examined muscle sympathetic nerve activity (MSNA) in four groups of subjects, patients with essential hypertension and type 2 diabetes, patients with type 2 diabetes alone, patients with essential hypertension alone, and healthy normotensive controls. They found higher MSNA in hypertensive-type 2 diabetic patients compared with hypertensive alone patients or type 2 diabetic alone patients, and higher MSNA in hypertensive alone patients or type 2 diabetic alone patients compared with healthy normotensive controls. Fasting insulin levels were greater in hypertensive-type 2 diabetic patients and type 2 diabetic patients compared to hypertensive patients or healthy normotensive subjects. These findings provided evidence that type 2 diabetic patients had elevated sympathetic nerve activity regardless of the prevailing blood pressure levels, and that the combination of hypertension and type 2 diabetes resulted in an augmentation in sympathetic nerve activity and levels of plasma insulin.

Moreover, stimulation of the renin-angiotensin-aldosterone system (RAAS) is frequently demonstrated in type 2 diabetes [73], and may be related to insulin resistance either via direct or indirect mechanisms [74].

7. Treatments for type 2 diabetes

Weight loss is recommended as the first line of treatment for type 2 diabetes and hypertension associated with obesity, because obesity is the primary cause for insulin resistance, metabolic syndrome and type 2 diabetes. Indeed, lifestyle modification including a low caloric diet, reducing sedentary behaviour and exercise form the foundation of all therapy. For the subjects who are more severely obese or unable to undertake an exercise program, bariatric surgery is recommended.

7.1. Lifestyle modification for weight loss

Weight loss is recommended as the first-line treatment for obesity-related type 2 diabetes and hypertension. The objective of treatment for obesity, type 2 diabetes and hypertension is both to reduce the high risk of cardiovascular events and to prevent or delay the onset of type 2 diabetes and complications. Lifestyle intervention with diet and exercise leading to weight loss prevents and delays the onset of type 2 diabetes or glucose intolerance [75]. Weight loss may also prevent cardiovascular- and renal-complications [76-79], and renal function and left ventricular hypertrophy as a marker for future cardiac events in obese individuals with metabolic syndrome and hypertension [77, 80]. The US Diabetes Prevention Program [81] and the Oslo Diet and Exercise Study [82] have shown marked clinical benefits with lifestyle intervention, and modest weight loss, on the resolution of the metabolic syndrome and type 2 diabetes. A limited number of epidemiological studies have shown that intentional weight loss may be associated with increased mortality and fat loss may reduce the all-cause mortality rate [83].

Cohort studies with lifestyle intervention [84] and case control studies with bariatric surgeries [85, 86] also provide some evidence that intentional weight loss has long-term benefits on all cause mortality in overweight adults. In a cohort of patients enrolled in a cardiac rehabilitation program, weight loss was associated with favourable long-term outcomes on the composite end-point of mortality and acute cardiovascular events (fatal and nonfatal myocardial infarction, fatal and nonfatal stroke, emergent revascularization for unstable angina pectoris, and congestive heart failure) [87].

Many clinical studies have demonstrated that weight loss associated with life-style modification adds to the first line treatment for diabetes mellitus and the efficacy of antihypertensive pharmacological treatments [8], however, maintaining weight loss is often the greatest challenge [5, 6, 88].

7.1.1. Calorie restricted diet versus aerobic exercise

The American Diabetes Association (ADA) has recommended for the maintenance of a healthy weight to prevent and control diabetes as following; (i) more than 2.5 hours of exercise per week, (ii) having a modest fat intake (approximately 30% of energy supply), and (iii) rating sufficient fiber [89]. Recently, several investigations [4, 5, 90] compared the effects on weight loss between calorie restriction (diet) and exercise. They showed that combined intervention with diet and exercise proved to be effective in weight reduction than diet alone or exercise alone. Masuo *et al.* [5] reported that the group with mild exercise alone had greater and faster loss of total body fat-mass compared to the diet alone group, whereas Toji *et al.* [90] reported that exercise intervention alone was not found to be effective on weight loss. There are discordant results on the effects of diet and exercise on weight loss and weight loss-induced blood pressure reductions, however many large cohort interventions and clinical studies have

http://dx.doi.org/10.5772/56377

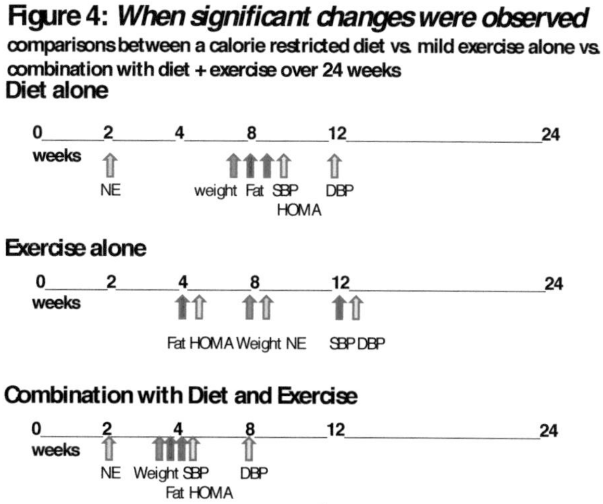

Reference [5]
NE, plasma norepinephrine as index of sympathetic activity;
HOMA, HOMA-IR (homeostasis model assessment of insulin resistance) as an index of insulin resistance; Weight, body weight; Fat, total body fat-mass; SBP, systolic blood pressure;
DBP, diastolic blood pressure.

Figure 4. When significant chages were observed comparisons between a calorie restricted diet vs. mild exercise alone vs. combination with diet + exercise over 24 weeks

shown combination weight loss regimens with mild calorie restriction and mild exercise was the most effective for significant weight loss compared to diet alone or exercise alone.

A low caloric diet and exercise exert different effects on insulin resistance, the RAAS, and sympathetic nervous activity in obese hypertensive subjects, even though similar weight loss was observed [4, 5]. Low caloric diet may be prominent for normalization of sympathetic nervous activity and exercise may be related more to normalization of insulin resistance [5, 88] (Figure 4). They previously observed that baseline plasma norepinephrine levels could predict future weight gain and weight gain-induced blood pressure elevation over 5 years in a longitudinal study [91], resistant weight loss by weight loss intervention with combination of calorie restriction and exercise intervention over 2 years. [6, 88] Similarly, Straznicky *et al.* [92] showed baseline sympathetic tone measured by muscle sympathetic nervous activity and nutritional responsiveness could predict the success of dietary weight loss, but not exercise, supporting the results including that the sympathetic nervous activity plays major mechanisms and roles on diet-induced weight loss pointed by Masuo, *et al.* [5]. Ribeiro *et al.* [93], Trombetta *et al.* [94] and Tonacio *et al.* [95] compared the effects of a low caloric diet and exercise on blood pressure lowering and forearm blood flow. They observed that only exercise, not diet, significantly increased forearm blood flow.

Santarpia *et al.* [96] reviewed the effectiveness of weight loss regimens and body composition after weight loss between diet and exercise. At a long term follow up (over one year), relatively high protein, moderately low calorie, low glycemic index diets, associated with a daily, moderate intensity, physical exercise (of at least 30 min), appear to be more successful in limiting long term rebound, maintaining fat-free-mass and achieving the highest fat loss. Diet alone or physical exercise alone does not produce similar results. Adequate dietetic advice plus regular physical exercise avoid the fat-free-mass loss usually observed in the rebound of the weight cycling syndrome and prevent the onset of sarcopenic obesity.

Exercise training is important for weight loss and to prevent rebound weight gain after significant weight loss. Public health interventions promoting walking are likely to be the most successful. Indeed, walking is unique because of its safety, accessibility, and popularity. It is noteworthy that there is a clear dissociation between the adaptation of cardiopulmonary fitness and the improvements in the metabolic risk profile such as insulin resistance and sympathetic activation, which can be induced by endurance training programs. Dumortier *et al.* [97] also reported that individualized low intensity endurance aerobic training improves lipid oxidation, body composition and insulin resistance. It appears that as long as the increase in energy expenditure is sufficient, low-intensity endurance exercise is likely to generate beneficial metabolic effects that would be essentially similar to those produced by high-intensity exercise [98]. The clinician should therefore focus on the improvement of the metabolic profile rather than on weight loss alone [98].

7.1.2. Dietary

7.1.2.1. Saturated fat versus unsaturated fat

Recently, several large cohort studies have shown that saturated fat, which comes mainly from animal sources of food, raises LDL cholesterol and links strongly to cardiovascular risk [99, 100]. Saturated fats are needed for the production of hormones, the stabilization of cellular membranes, the padding around organs, and for energy. A deficiency in the consumption of saturated fats can lead to age-related declines in white blood cell function, along with dysfunction of the immune system and cancer [101]; however, a high content of saturated fat can leads to coronary heart disease [102], ischemic heart disease, and atherosclerosis and increase the chances of stroke.

Consistent evidence from prospective observational studies of habitual trans fatty acids (TFA) consumption and retrospective observational studies using TFA biomarkers indicates that TFA consumption increases risk of clinical coronary heart disease, and other disease outcomes such as cancer [102].

Unsaturated fats are known to increase the levels of High Density Lipoprotein (HDL cholesterol) and hence decrease LDL and VLDL cholesterol. Both types of unsaturated fat- mono-unsaturated and poly-unsaturated fats can replace saturated fats in the diet. Substituting saturated fats with unsaturated fats help to lower levels of total cholesterol and LDL cholesterol in the blood. However, intake of unsaturated fats in very high amounts can also increase the risk of coronary heart diseases.

i. **Monounsaturated fat:** This is a type of fat found in a variety of foods and oils. Studies show that eating foods rich in monounsaturated fats (MUFAs) improves blood cholesterol levels, which can decrease the risk of heart disease. Research also shows that MUFAs may benefit insulin levels and blood sugar control, which can be especially helpful for type 2 diabetes.

ii. **Polyunsaturated fat (PUFAs):** This is a type of fat found mostly in plant-based foods and oils. The Swedish Mammography Cohort study including 34, 670 women with a mean follow-up of 10.4 years, showed that intake of long-chain omega-3 PUFAs is inversely associated with risk of stroke, whereas dietary cholesterol is positively associated with risk [103]. Similarly, Chowdhury *et al.* [104] observed in meta-analysis that moderate, inverse associations of fish consumption and long chain omega 3 fatty acids with cerebrovascular risk, but long chain omega 3 fatty acids measured as circulating biomarkers in observational studies or supplements in primary and secondary prevention trials were not associated with cerebrovascular disease. The beneficial effect of fish intake on cerebrovascular risk is likely to be mediated through the interplay of a wide range of nutrients abundant in fish. PUFAs decrease the risk of type 2 diabetes. One type of polyunsaturated fat, a long chain omega-3 fatty acids is especially beneficial to coronary heart disease.

iii. **Trans-fatty acids (TFA):** Growing evidence indicates that trans-fatty acids (TFA) adversely affect cardiovascular health. Controlled trials and observational studies provide concordant evidence that consumption of TFA from partially hydrogenated oils adversely affects multiple cardiovascular risk factors, and contributes significantly to increased risk of coronary heart disease events. The public health implications of ruminant TFA consumption appear much more limited. Nurses' health study showed that *trans*-fat intake was associated with increased risk of coronary heart disease, particularly for younger women [105]. Interestingly, incidence of insulin resistance is lowered with diets higher in monounsaturated fats (especially oleic acid), while the opposite is true for diets high in polyunsaturated fats (especially large amounts of arachidonic acid) as well as saturated fats. This relationship between dietary fats and insulin resistance is presumed secondary to the relationship between insulin resistance and inflammation, which is partially modulated by dietary fat ratios (Omega3/6/9) with both omega 3 and 9 thought to be anti-inflammatory, and omega 6 pro-inflammatory [106].

It is recommended to take both in a limited quantity. The American Heart Association has recommended that Americans should limit their intake of saturated fats to 7% of their total calories in a day, while unsaturated fats can form 30% of the calorie intake to reduced cardiovascular risks.

7.1.2.2. Special diet

i. **Low Carbohydrate Diet**

Low-carbohydrate diets are dietary programs that restrict carbohydrate consumption usually for weight control or for the treatment of obesity. The term "low-carbohydrate diet" is generally applied to diets that restrict carbohydrates to less than 20% of caloric intake, but can also refer to diets that simply restrict or limit carbohydrates. Recently, the low carbohydrate diets has been spotlighted due to strong effects on weight loss, but many investigations have also shown no benefits on the reductions on cardiovascular risk as the major aim of weight loss.

A study of more than 100,000 people over more than 20 years within "the Nurses' Health Study" observationally concluded that a low-carbohydrate diet high in vegetables, with a large proportion of proteins and oils coming from plant sources, decreases mortality with a hazard ratio of 0.8. In contrast, a low-carbohydrate diet with largely animal sources of protein and fat increases mortality, with a hazard ratio of 1.1, although there were criticisms on the methods [107]. A 2003 meta-analysis that included randomized controlled trials found that "low-carbohydrate, non-energy-restricted diets, appear to be at least as effective as low-fat, energy-restricted diets in inducing weight loss for up to 1 year [108]. Gardner *et al.* [109] compared the 4 special diet including the Atkins (a low-carbohydrate), Zone (by Barry Sears PhD, 40% carbohydrates, 30% protein, and 30% fats), Ornish (very low fat diet), and LEARN diets (55% to 60% energy from carbohydrate and less than 10% energy from saturated fat) to evaluate the effects of weight loss, metabolic effects and the risk over 1 year in 311 obese, non-diabetic, premenopausal women with randomized design. Weight loss was significantly greater for women in the Atkins diet group (low carbohydrate) compared with the other 3 diet groups at 12 months, and weight loss in the other 3 groups were similar, but at 12 months, secondary outcomes for the Atkins group were more favorable metabolic effects than the other diet groups. While questions remain about long-term effects and mechanisms, a low-carbohydrate, high-protein, high-fat diet may be considered a feasible alternative recommendation for weight loss. However, some investigators suggested that that one of the reasons people lose weight on low carbohydrate diet is related to the phenomenon of spontaneous reduction in food intake [110].

Previously, in routine practice a reduced-carbohydrate, higher protein diet was recommended approach to reducing the risk of cardiovascular disease and type 2 diabetes [111]. In 2004, the American Diabetes Association (ADA) affirmed its acceptance of carbohydrate-controlled diets as an effective treatment for short-term (up to one year) weight loss among obese people suffering from type 2 diabetes [112]. And the American Diabetes Association (ADA) revised their *"Nutrition Recommendations and Interventions for Diabetes in 2008"* to acknowledge low-carbohydrate diets as a legitimate weight-loss plan [113]. The recommendation, however, fell short of endorsing low-carbohydrate diets as a long-term health plan nor do they give any preference to these diets. On the other hand, the official statement from the American Heart Association (AHA) regarding these diets states categorically that the association doesn't recommend high-protein diets [35]. A science advisory from the AHA further states the association's belief that these diets are associated with increased risk for coronary heart disease [114, 115]. The AHA has been one of the most adamant opponents of low-carbohydrate diets. The American Heart Association supported low-fat and low-saturated-fat diets, but that a low-carbohydrate diet could not potentially meet AHA guidelines.

ii. Low fat diet

Recently, the effectiveness of low-fat high- protein and low-fat high-carbohydrate dietary advice on weight loss were compared using group-based interventions, among overweight people with type 2 diabetes. However, in a 'real-world' setting, prescription of an energy-reduced low-fat diet, with either increased protein or carbohydrate, results in similar modest losses in weight, waist circumference and metabolic benefits over 2 years [116].

Ebbeling *et al.* [117] investigated the effect of dietary composition on energy expenditure during weight-loss maintenance among the 3 different diet groups (low-fat diet, low-glycemic index diet, and very low carbohydrate diet) with a controlled 3-way crossover design involving 21 overweight and obese young adults each for 4 weeks. Resting energy expenditure (REE), total energy expenditure (TEE), hormone levels, and metabolic syndrome components at pre-weight-loss were compared. Decreases in REE and TEE following 10% or 15% weight loss were greatest with the low-fat diet, intermediate with the low-glycemic index diet, and least with the very low-carbohydrate diet, but metabolic or hormonal parameters were similar between 3 groups.

iii. Low glycemic index

The concept of the glycemic index was developed about 1981 by Dr. David Jenkins to account for variances in speed of digestion of carbohydrates. This concept classifies foods according to the rapidity of their effect on blood sugar levels – with fast digesting simple carbohydrates causing a sharper increase and slower digesting complex carbohydrates such as whole grains a slower one. The concept has been extended to include amount of carbohydrate actually absorbed as well, despite differences in glycemic index [118].

7.2. Pharmacological treatments for type 2 diabetes

If the individuals failed to improve glucose levels or HbA1c, pharmacological therapy is required. The first-line oral agents should minimize the degree of insulin resistance and suppress hepatic glucose production rather than increase plasma insulin concentrations. The decision to include thiazolidinediones (TZDs) and metformin as first-line therapy draws from the algorithm proposed by Wyne *et al.* [118]. Garber *et al.* [120] reported that Initial combination treatment with glyburide/metformin tablets produces greater improvements in glycemic control than either glyburide or metformin monotherapy.

The goal for glucose control is shown in Table 2 [11, 121]. Stimulating insulin secretion and minimizing insulin resistance both have the potential to bring a patient to goal, but it is theorized that bringing a patient to goal by reducing insulin resistance is more likely to reduce the macro-vascular complications and cardiovascular risks.

Based on several long-term, prospective studies which showed the significant reductions in cardiovascular risks associated with diabetes, the American Diabetes Association and American Association of Clinical Endocrinologists set forth standards and guidelines for the medical management of diabetes [11]. The recommendations clearly outline a multifactorial plan for managing diabetes and reducing complications [11], but they do not provide specific recommendations for selection and titration of pharmacological treatment. Pharmacological treatment for glucose control aims to reduce cardiovascular risk and to delay diabetic complications.

Glycemic control	A1C goal of < 7.0%	Measure every 3 months
Blood pressure control	< 130/80 mmHg	Every visit
Lipid control LDL	< 70 mg/dl†	Measure yearly or
Triglycerides	< 150 mg/dl	more frequently
HDL	> 45 mg/dl if	goals are not met
Urine protein Microalbuminuria	<30 mg/24 hours	Measure yearly

*American Diabetes Association Standards of medical care for patients with diabetesmellitus. *Diabetes Care* 26 (Suppl.):S33–S50, 2003.

†National Cholesterol Education Program: Implications of clinical trials for the ATP

Table 2. Diabetes Control Goals (by American Diabetes Association) Goals Endpoints Assessment

Pharmacological treatment for the management of obesity is primarily aimed at weight loss, weight loss maintenance and cardiovascular risk reduction. Anti-obesity agents decrease appetite, reduce absorption of fat or increase energy expenditure. Recently, anti-obesity drugs such as orlistat, sibtramine and rimonabant have been developed and placed on markets, however, the latter two were withdrawn from markets in the United States, Europe and Australia due to serious adverse events including psychiatric and cardiovascular related concerns. Recently, contrave, a combination of two approved drugs of bupropion and naltrexone, completed Phase III trials with significant weight loss and was approved by FDA in 2010, but subsequently the FDA declined to approve contrave due to serious cardiovascular adverse events in 2011 [122]. A contrave cardiovascular outcome trial, called "Light Study", is ongoing and is expected to be completed by the first quarter of 2013. Importantly, obesity is, at least, in part, determined by genetic backgrounds [123], suggesting that a genetic approach to limiting obesity may find a place in the future.

7.3. Bariatric surgery

Gastric bypass and adjustable gastric banding are the two most commonly performed bariatric procedures for the treatment of morbid obesity or obesity which is resistant to lifestyle modification such as a low caloric diet plus exercise. Multiple mechanisms contribute to the improved glucose metabolism seen after bariatric surgery, including caloric restriction, changes in the enteroinsular axis, alterations in the adipoinsular axis, release of nutrient-stimulated hormones from endocrine organs, stimulation from the nervous system, and psychosocial aspects including a dramatic improvement in quality of life [124]. Dixon *et al.* [86, 125] showed that gastric banding induced significant weight loss and resulted in better glucose control and less need for diabetes medication than conventional approaches to weight loss and diabetes control in a randomized controlled study in obese subjects with recently diagnosed type 2 diabetes. Koshy *et al.*[124] and other investigators [126, 127] compared the effects on weight loss, mortality, morbidity and changes in quality of life in subjects with either gastric bypass or gastric banding. The percent of excess weight loss at 4 years was higher in the gastric bypass group compared to the gastric banding group. Postoperative HOMA-IR correlated with % weight loss [126]. Concurrent with restoration of insulin sensitivity and decreases in plasma leptin were dramatic decreases in skeletal muscle at 3 and 9 months after gastric banding and a significant decrease in peroxisome proliferation activated receptor-alpha-regulated genes at 9 months. Gumbs *et al.* [128] speculated that a decrease in fat mass after bariatric surgery significantly affected circulating adipocytokines, which favourably influenced insulin resistance. Improvements in glucose metabolism and insulin resistance following bariatric surgery occur, in the short-term from decreased stimulation of the entero-insular axis by restricted calorie intake and in the long-term by decreased release of adipocytokines due to reduced fat mass. Leptin levels drop and adiponectin levels rise following laparoscopic adjustable gastric banding and gastric bypass. These changes correlate with weight loss and improvement in insulin sensitivity [128].

All forms of weight loss surgery lead to calorie restriction, weight loss, decrease in fat mass, and improvement in insulin resistance, type 2 diabetes mellitus, obesity and obesity-related hypertension [127]. Left ventricular relaxation impairment, assessed by tissue Doppler imaging, normalized 9 months after surgery [129]. Laparoscopic gastric bypass and gastric banding are both safe and effective approaches for the treatment of morbid obesity, but gastric bypass surgery seems to exert a better early weight loss and more rapid ameliorative effects on insulin resistance and adipocytokines, muscle metabolism and left ventricular function.

8. Conclusion

The prevalence of diabetes, especially type 2 diabetes and hypertension are significantly increased due, at least in part, to the increased prevalence of obesity. Type 2 diabetes is frequently associated with obesity, and is an important risk factor for cardiovascular morbidity and mortality and cardiac- and renal complications. Type 2 diabetes, hypertension and obesity are characterized by stimulation of the renin-angiotensin-aldosterone system (RAAS), elevated sympathetic activity and insulin resistance. Importantly, these characteristics, themselves, confer cardiovascular risk. Therefore, treatments for type 2 diabetes should be selected from favourable effects on stimulated RAAS, elevated sympathetic nervous system activity, insulin and leptin resistance.

Weight loss is recommended as the first line of treatment for type 2 diabetes and hypertension associated with type 2 diabetes in obesity. Lifestyle modification such as a caloric restricted diet, reducing sedentary behaviour and increases in exercise form the basis of all therapy. Weight loss treated with lifestyle modification including calorie restriction and/or exercise causes normalization of stimulated RAAS, sympathetic activation, insulin resistance, and hyperleptinemia. Recently, Masuo *et al.* [5] and Straznicky *et al.* [4] have shown that low caloric diet and exercise have different effects on insulin resistance, the RAAS, and sympathetic nervous activity in obese hypertensive subjects, even though similar weight loss was observed. Exercise had stronger effects on normalizing the RAAS stimulation, sympathetic activation and insulin resistance compared to diet only. The observations demonstrate that a combination therapy for weight loss with a low caloric diet and exercise is recommended for weight loss due to stronger suppression of insulin resistance and sympathetic activation, which both, themselves, are known as risk factors for cardiovascular events. Although few studies have observed changes in body weight, blood pressure, RAAS, sympathetic nervous activity, insulin resistance and leptin resistance over a long duration such as more than 2 years, Masuo *et al.* [6] observed more than 30% individuals who initially succeeded to significantly lose weight, had rebound weight gain over 2 years. Maintenance of weight loss is another key factor to delay and prevent type 2 diabetes and to reduce cardiovascular risks in type 2 diabetes in obesity.

In addition, special diets such as a low carbohydrate diet were reported as beneficial on weight loss previously, but it might cause an increase in cardiac risk. The official statement from American Heart Association reported that high-protein diet and low carbohydrate diet are not recommended diets due to increases in cardiovascular risk.

Gastric bypass and adjustable gastric banding are the two most commonly performed bariatric procedures for the treatment of morbid obesity or obesity which is resistant to lifestyle modification such as a low caloric diet plus exercise. Weight loss by bariatric surgery leads to improvement or normalization of glucose metabolisms from multiple mechanisms including caloric restriction, changes in the enteroinsular axis, alterations in the adipoinsular axis, release of nutrient-stimulated hormones from endocrine organs, stimulation from the nervous system, and psychosocial aspects including a dramatic improvement in quality of life.

Understanding the mechanisms underlying type 2 diabetes in obesity may help to achieve weight loss and maintenance of weight loss and resultant better control on type 2 diabetes, and delay and prevent the onset of type 2 diabetes or reduce complications.

This review provides information regarding, *i)* the importance of lifestyle medication on type 2 diabetes in obesity, *ii)* different effects of lifestyle modifications on weight loss and neurohormonal parameters between diet and exercise, and *iii)* the mode of weight loss and how it influences different physiological pathways. Different mechanisms may contribute to control in blood glucose levels and blood pressure and cardiovascular risks associated with weight loss with the relevant physiological mechanisms at play being dependent on the mode of weight loss.

Author details

Kazuko Masuo[1,2]

1 Nucleus Network Ltd., Baker IDI Heart & Diabetes Institute, Australia

2 Human Neurotransmitters Laboratory, Baker IDI Heart & Diabetes Institute, Australia

References

[1] Year Book Australia, 2012, 1301.0. Australian Bureau of Statistics. (24/5/2012)

[2] Mokdad AH, Ford ES, Bowman BA, Dietz WH, Vinicor F, Bales VS, Marks JS. Prevalence of obesity, diabetes, and obesity-related health risk factors, 2001. JAMA, 2003; 289(1): 76-79.

[3] The ORIGIN Trial Investigators. Basal insulin and cardiovascular and other outcomes in dysglycemia. N Engl J Med 2012;367(4):319-28. doi: 10.1056/NEJMoa1203858. Epub 2012 Jun 11.

[4] Straznicky NE, Grima MT, Eikelis N, et al. The effects of weight loss versus weight loss maintenance on sympathetic nervous system activity and metabolic syndrome components. J Clin Endocrinol Metab. 2011; 96(3): E503-8.

[5] Masuo K, Rakugi H, Ogihara T, Lambert GW. Different mechanisms in weight loss-induced blood pressure reduction between a calorie-restricted diet and exercise. Hypertens Res. 2012; 35(1): 41-7. doi: 10.1038/hr.2011.134.

[6] Masuo K, Katsuya T, Kawaguchi H, Fu Y, Rakugi H, Ogihara T, Tuck ML. Rebound weight gain as associated with high plasma norepinephrine levels that are mediated through polymorphisms in the beta2-adrenoceptor. Am J Hypertens. 2005; 18(11): 1508-16.

[7] Kumar AA, Palamaner Subash Shantha G, Kahan S, Samson RJ, Boddu ND, Cheskin LJ. Intentional weight loss and dose reductions of anti-diabetic medications--a retrospective cohort study. PLoS One. 2012; 7(2): e32395.

[8] Masuo K, Mikami H, Ogihara T, Tuck ML. Weight reduction and pharmacologic treatment in obese hypertensives. Am J Hypertens. 2001; 14(6 Pt 1): 530-8.

[9] merican Diabetes Association. Diagnosis and classification of diabetes mellitus. Diabetes Care. 2012; 35 Suppl 1: S64-71.

[10] Kumar H, Mishra M, Bajpai S, Pokhria D, Arya AK, Singh RK, Tripathi K. Correlation of insulin resistance, beta cell function and insulin sensitivity with serum sFas and sFasL in newly diagnosed type 2 diabetes. Acta Diabetol. 2011 Jun 22. [Epub ahead of print].

[11] American Diabetes Association. Executive Summary: Standards of Medical Care in Diabetes—2012. Diabetes Care 2012; 35: S4-S10; doi:10.2337/dc12-s004.

[12] Eckert K. Impact of physical activity and bodyweight on health-related quality of life in people with type 2 diabetes. Diabetes Metab Syndr Obes. 2012; 5: 303-11.

[13] Diabetes Australia website, http://www.diabetesaustralia.com.au/living-with-diabetes/gestational-diabetes/./ Last Update: 21/06/2012. (accessed 15 November 2012).

[14] National Diabetes Statistics, 2011. National Institute of Diabetes and Digestive and Kidney Diseases website. www.diabetes.niddk.nih.gov/dm/pubs/statistics/index.aspx. Updated February 2011. (accessed on 15 November 2012).

[15] Katon J, Maynard C, Reiber G. Attempts at weight loss in U.S. women with and without a history of gestational diabetes mellitus. Womens Health Issues. 2012 Sep; 22(5):e447-53. doi: 10.1016/j.whi.2012.07.004.(accessed 10 November 2012).

[16] O'Keeffe M, St-Onge MP. Sleep duration and disorders in pregnancy: implications for glucose metabolism and pregnancy outcomes. Int J Obes (Lond). 2012 Sep 4. doi: 10.1038/ijo.2012.142.

[17] Carulli L, Rondinella S, Lombardini S, Canedi I, Loria P, Carulli N. Review article: Duiabetes, genetic and ethnicity. Alimentary Pharmacology & Therapeutics. 2005; 22 Suppl 2: 16-9.

[18] Meetoo D, McGovern P, Safadi R. An epidemiological overview of diabetes across the world. British Journal of Nursing. 2007; 16(16): 1002-7.

[19] Wold S, Roglic G, Green A, Sicree R, King H. Global prevalence of diabetes: estimates for the year 2000 and projections for 2030. Diabetes Care. 2004; 27 (5): 1047-1055.

[20] Centers for Diseases Control and Prevention (CDC). National Diabetes Fact Sheet, 2011. 2011. www.cdc.gov/diabetes/pubs/pdf/ndfs_2011.pdf

[21] Cali AM, Caprio S. Prediabetes and type 2 diabetes in youth: an emerging epidemic disease? Curr Opin Endocrinol Diabetes Obes. 2008; 15(2):123-7.

[22] Khalil AC, Roussel R, Mohammedi K, Danchin N, Marre M. Cause-specific mortality in diabetes: recent changes in trend mortality. Eur J Prev Cardiol. 2012; 19(3): 374-81.

[23] Abate N, Chandalia M. Ethnicity and type 2 diabetes: focus on Asian Indians. J Diabetes Complicat. 2001; 15(6): 320-7.

[24] Christian P, Sterwart CP. Maternal micronutrient deficiency, fetal development, and the risk of chronic disease. J Nutr. 2010; 140(3): 437-45.

[25] Latry P, Molimard M, Dedieu B, Couffinhal T, Bégaud B, Martin-Latry K. Adherence with statins in a real-life setting is better when associated cardiovascular risk factors increase: a cohort study. BMC Cardiovasc Disord. 2011 Jul 26;11:46. doi: 10.1186/1471-2261-11-46.

[26] Lardizabal JA, Deedwania PC. Benefits of statin therapy and compliance in high risk cardiovascular patients. Vasc Health Risk Manag. 2010; 6: 843–853.

[27] Narla V, Blaha MJ, Blumenthal RS, Michos ED. The JUPITER and AURORA clinical trials for rosuvastatin in special primary prevention populations: perspectives, outcomes, and consequences. Vasc Health Risk Manag. 2009; 5: 1033–1042.

[28] Tonelli M, Lloyd A, Clement F, et al. for the Alberta Kidney Disease Network. Efficacy of statins for primary prevention in people at low cardiovascular risk: a meta-analysis;. CMAJ. 2011; 183(16): e1189–e1202.

[29] Yang EY, Nambi V, Tang Z, Virani SS, Boerwinkle E,Hoogeveen RC, et al. Clinical implications of JUPITER in a United States population: insights from the Atherosclerosis Risk in Communities (ARIC) Study. J Am Coll Cardiol. 2009; 54(25): 2388–2395.

[30] Culver AL, Ockene IS, Balasubramanian R, Olendzki BC, Sepavich DM, Wactawski-Wende J, et al. Statin use and risk of diabetes mellitus in postmenopausal women in the Women's Health Initiative.. Arch Intern Med. 2012; 172(2): 144-52.

[31] Coleman CI, Reinhart K, Kluger J, White CM. The effect of statins on the development of new-onset type 2 diabetes: a meta-analysis of randomized controlled trials. Curr Med Res Opin. 2008; 24(5): 1359-62.

[32] Sattar N, Preiss D, Murray HM, Welsh P, Buckley BM, de Craen AJ, et al. Statins and risk of incident diabetes: a collaborative meta-analysis of randomised statin trials. Lancet. 2010; 375(9716): 735-42.

[33] Preiss D, Seshasai SR, Welsh P, Murphy SA, Ho JE, Waters DD, et al. Risk of incident diabetes with intensive-dose compared with moderate-dose statin therapy: a meta-analysis.. JAMA; 305(24): 2556-64.

[34] McEvoy JW. Statin therapy dose and risk of new-onset diabetes. JAMA. 2011; 306(12):1325-6.

[35] American Heart Association statement on high-protein, low-carbohydrate diet study presented at scientific sessions. American Heart Association press release, Nov 19, 2012.

[36] Filippatos TD. A Review of Time Courses and Predictors of Lipid Changes with Fenofibric Acid-Statin Combination. Cardiovasc Drugs Ther. 2012 June; 26(3): 245–255.

[37] Uchechukwu K. Sampson, MacRae F. Linton, Sergio Fazio. Are statins diabetogenic? Curr Opin Cardiol. 2011; 26(4): 342–347.

[38] The ACCORD Study Group. Effects of Combination Lipid Therapy in Type 2 Diabetes Mellitus. N Engl J Med. 2010; 362(17): 1563-74.

[39] Tenenbaum A, Fisman EZ. Balanced pan-PPAR activator bezafibrate in combination with statin: comprehensive lipids control and diabetes prevention? Cardiovasc Diabetes. 2012; 11(1):140.

[40] Carmena R, Betteridge DJ. Statins and diabetes. Semin Vas Med. 2004; 4 (4): 321-332.

[41] Heidmann C, Boeing H, Pischon T, Nothlings U, Joost HG, Schulze MB. Association of a diabetes risk score with risk of myocardial infarction, stroke, specific types of cancer, and mortality: a prospective study in the European Prospective Investigation

into Cancer and Nutrition (EPIC)-Potsdam cohort. Eur J Epidemiol. 2009; 24(6): 281-8.

[42] Preis SR, Hwang SJ, Coady S, Pencina MJ, D'Agostino RB Sr, Savage DJ, et al. Trends in all cause and cardiovascular disease mortality among women and men with and without diabetes mellitus in the Framingham Heart Study, 1950 to 2005. Circulation. 2009; 119(13): 1728-35.

[43] Lutufo PA, Gaziano M, Chae CU, Ajani UA, Moreno-John G, Buring JE, et al. Diabetes and all-cause and coronary heart disease mortality among US male physicians. Arch Intern Med. 2001; 161(2): 242-7.

[44] Kanaya AM, Grady D, Barrett-Connor E. Explaining the sex difference in coronary heart disease mortality among patients with type 2 diabetes mellitus: a meta-analysis. Arch Intern Med. 2002; 162(15); 1737-45.

[45] Young LH, Wackers FJ, Chyun DA, Davay JA, Barrett EJ, Taillefer R, et al. for DIAD Investigators. Cardiac outcomes after screening for asymptomatic coronary artery disease in patients with type 2 diabetes: the DIAD study: a randomized controlled trial. JAMA. 2009; 301(15): 1547-55.

[46] Morrison JA, Glueck CJ, Horn PS, Schreiber GH, Wang P. Pre-teen insulin resistance patients weight gain, impaired fasting glucose, and type 2 diabetes at age 18-19: a 10-y prospective study of black and white girls. Am J Clin Nutr. 2008; 88(3): 778-88.

[47] Koska J, Ortega E, Bogardus C, Krakoff J, Bunt JC. The effect of insulin on net lipid oxidation predicts worsen of insulin resistance and development of type 2 diabetes mellitus. Am J Physiol Endocrinol Metab. 2007; 293(1): 1264-1269.

[48] Rossing P, Hougaard P, Parving HH. Risk factors for development of incipient and overt diabetic nephropathy in type 1 diabetic patients: a 10-year prospective observational study. Diabetes Care. 2002; 25(5): 859-864.

[49] Cho E, RimmEB, Stampfer MJ, Willett WC, Hu FB. The impact of diabetes mellitus and prior myocardial infarction on mortality from all causes and from coronary heart disease in men. J Am Coll Cardiol. 2002; 40(5): 954-60.

[50] Iglseder B, Cip P, Malaimare L, Ladurner G, Paulweber B. The metabolic syndrome is a stronger risk factor for early carotid atherosclerosis in women than in men. Stroke. 2005; 36(6): 1212-7.

[51] Kawamoto R, Tomita H, Ohtsuka N, Inoue A, Kamitani A. Metabolic syndrome, diabetes and subclinical atherosclerosis as assessed by carotid intima-media thickness. J Atheroscler Thromb. 2007; 14(2): 78-85.

[52] Bertoni A, Wong ND, Shea S, et al. Insulin resistance, metabolic syndrome, and subclinical atherosclerosis. The Multi-Ethnic Study of Atheroclerosis (MESA). Diabetes Care. 2007; 30: 2951-6.

[53] Held C, Gerstein HC, Yusuf S, Ma S, Liu K, Preethi S, et al. for the ONTARGET/ TRANSCEND investigators. Glucose levels predict hospitalization for congestive heart failure in patients at high cardiovascular risk. Circulation. 2007; 115(11): 1371-5.

[54] Schulze MB, Hoffmann K, Boeing H, Linseisen J, Rothmann S, Mohilg M, et al. An accurate risk score based on anthropometric, dietary, and lifestyle factors to predict the development of type 2 diabetes. Diabetes Care. 2007; 30(3): 510-15.

[55] Morrison JA, Glueck CJ, Umar M, Daniels S, Dolan LM, Wang P. Hyperinsulinemia and metabolic syndrome at mean age of 10 years in black and white schoolgirls and development of impaired fasting glucose and type 2 diabetes mellitus by mean age of 24 years. Metabolism. 2011; 60(1): 24-31.

[56] Masuo K. Obesity-related hypertension: Role of sympathetic nervous system, insulin, and leptin. Curr Hypertens Rep. 2002; 4(2): 112-8.

[57] Esler M, Straznicky N, Eikelis N, Masuo K, Lambert G, Lambert E. Mechanism of sympathetic activation in obesity-related hypertension. Hypertension. 2006; 48(5): 787-96.

[58] Masuo k, Mikami H, Ogihara T, Tuck ML. Weight gain-induced blood pressure elevation. Hypertension. 2000; 35(5): 1135-40.

[59] Gentile CL, Orr JS, Davy BM, Davy KP. Modest weight gain is associated with sympathetic neural activation in nonobese humans. Am J Physiol Regul Interg Comp Phisiol. 2007; 292(5); R1834-38.

[60] Barnes MJ, Lapanowski K, Conley A, Rafols JA, Jen KL, Dunbar JC. High fat feeding is associated with increased blood pressure, sympathetic nerve activity and hypothalamic mu opioid receptors. Brain Res Bull. 2003; 61(5): 511-9.

[61] Anderson B, Elam M, Wallin BG, Bjorntorp P, Anderson OK. Effect of energy-restricted diet on sympathetic muscle nerve activity in obese women. Hypertension. 1991; 18(6): 783-9.

[62] Straznicky NE, Lambert EA, Lambert GW, Masuo K, Esler MD, Nestle PJ. Effects of dietary weight loss on sympathetic activity and cardiac risk factors associated with the metabolic syndrome. J Clin Endocrinol Met. 2005; 90(11): 5998-6005.

[63] Tuck ML, Sowers JR, Dornfeld L, Whitfield L, Maxwell M. Reductions in plasma catecholamines and blood pressure during weight loss in obese subjects. Acta Endocrinol (Copenh). 1983; 102(2): 252-7.

[64] Grassi G, Seravalle G, Colombo M, Bolla G, Cattaneo BM, Cavagnini F, et al. Body weight reduction, sympathetic nerve traffic, and arterial baroreflex in obese normotensive humans. Circulation. 1998; 97(20): 2037-2042.

[65] Masuo K, Katsuya T, Ogihara T, Tuck ML. Acute hyperinsulinemia reduces plasma leptin levels in insulin sensitive men. Am J Hypertens. 2005; 18(2 Pt 1): 235-43.

[66] Huggett RJ, Scott EM, Gilbey SG, Stoker JB, Mackintosh AF, Mary DASG. Impact of type 2 diabetes mellitus on sympathetic neural mechanisms in hypertension. Circulation. 2003; 108(25): 3097-3101.

[67] Staznicky NE, Lambert GW, Masuo K, et al. Blunted sympathetic neural response to oral glucose in obese subjects with the insulin-resistant metabolic syndrome. Am J Clin Nutr. 2009; 89: 27-36.

[68] Straznicky NE, Grima MT, Sari CI, Eikelis N, Lambert EA, Nestel PJ, et al. Neuroadrenergic dysfunction along the diabetes continuum: a comparative study in obese metabolic syndrome subjects. Diabetes. 2012; 61(10): 2506-16.

[69] Takatori S, Zamami Y, Mio M, Kurosaki Y, Kawasaki H. Chronic hyperinsulinemia enhances adrenergic vasoconstriction and decreases calcitonin gene-related peptide-containing nerve-mediated vasodilation in pithed rats. Hypertens Res. 2006; 29(5): 361-368.

[70] Zamami Y, Takatori S, Yamawaki K, Miyashita S, Mio M, Kitamura Y, Kawasaki H. Acute hyperglycemia and hyperinsulinemia enhance adrenergic vasoconstriction and decrease calcitonin gene-related peptide-containing nerve-mediated vasodilation in pithed rats. Hypertens Res. 2008(5); 31: 1033-1044.

[71] Gudbjornsdottir S, Elam M, Sellgren J, Anderson EA. Insulin increases forearm vascular resistance in obese, insulin-resistant hypertensives. J Hypertens. 1996; 14(1): 91-7.

[72] van Veen S, Frolich M, Chang PC. Acute hyperglycemia in the forearm induces vasodilation that is not modified by hyperinsulinemia. J Human Hypertens. 1999; 13(4): 263-68.

[73] Thethi T, Kamiyama M, Kobori H. The link between the renin-angiotensin-aldosterone system and renal injury in obesity and the metabolic syndrome. Curr Hypertens Rep. 2012; 14(2): 160-9.

[74] Maser RE, Lenhard MJ, Kolm P, Edwards DG. Direct renin inhibition improves parasympathetic function in diabetes. Diabetes Obes Metab. 2013; 15(1): 28-34. 2012 Jul 27. doi: 10.1111/j.1463-1326.2012.01669.x.

[75] Kosaka K, Noda M, Kuzuya T. Prevention of type 2 diabetes by lifestyle intervention: a Japanese trial in IGT males. Diabetes Res Clin Pract. 2005; 67(2): 152-62.

[76] Masuo K, Rakugi H, Ogihara T, Esler MD, Lambert GW. Effects of weight loss on renal function in overweight Japanese men. Hypertens Res. 2011; 34(8): 915-21.

[77] Masuo K, Rakugi H, Ogihara T, Esler MD, Lambert GW. Cardiovascular and renal complications of type 2 diabetes in obesity: role of sympathetic nerve activity and insulin resistance. Curr Diabetes Rev. 2010; 6(2): 58-67.

[78] Straznicky NE, Grima MT, Lambert EA, et al. Exercise augments weight loss induced improvement in renal function in obese metabolic syndrome individuals. J Hypertens. 2011; 29(3): 553-64

[79] Masuo K, Lambert GW, Esler MD, Rakugi H, Ogihara T, Schlaich MP. The role of sympathetic nervous activity in renal injury and end-stage renal disease. Hypertens Res. 2010; 33(6): 521-8.

[80] Masuo K, Rakugi H, Ogihara T, Tuck ML. β1 (Arg389Gly, Ser49Gly)- and β2 (Arg16Gly)-adrenoceptor polymorphisms are related to left ventricular hypertrophy in middle-aged, nonobese,l normotensive men, but through different mechanisms. Circulation. 2008; 18 (119) Suppl 2: S1154.

[81] Orchard TJ, Temprosa M, Goldberg R, Haffner S, Ratner R, Marcovina S, Fowler S. The effect of metformin and intensive lifestyle intervention on the metabolic syndrome: The Diabetes Prevention Program randomized trial. Ann Intern Med. 2005; 142(8): 611-619.

[82] Anderssen SA, Carroll S, Urdal P, Holme I. Combined diet and exercise intervention reverses the metabolic syndrome in middle-aged males: results from the Oslo Diet and Exercise Study. Scand J Med Sci Sports. 2007; 17(6): 687-95.

[83] Allison DB, Zannolli R, Faith MS, Heo M, Piethobelli A, Vanltallie TB, et al. Weight loss increases and fat loss decreases all-cause mortality rate: results from two independent cohort studies. Int J Obes Relat Metab Disord. 1999; 23(6): 603-11.

[84] Poobalan AS, Aucott LS, Smith WCS, Avenell A, Jung R, Broom J. Long-term weight loss effects on all cause mortality in overweight/obese populations. Obes Rev. 2007; 8(6): 503-13.

[85] Sjostrom L, Narbro K, Sjostrom CD, Karason K, Larsson B, Nedei H, et al. Effects of bariatric surgery on mortality in Swedish obese subjects. N Engl J Med. 2007; 357(8): 741-52.

[86] Dixon JB, O'Brien PE, Playfair J, Chapman L, Schachter LM, Skiner S, et al. Adjustable gastric banding and conventional therapy for type 2 diabetes: a randomized controlled trial. JAMA. 2008; 299(3): 316-23.

[87] Sierra-Johnson J, Romeo-Corral A, Somers VK, Lopez-Jimenez F, Thomas RJ, Squires RW, Allison TG. Prognostic importance of weight loss in patients with coronary heart disease regardless of initial body mass index. Eur J Cardiovasc Prev Rehabil. 2008; 15(3): 336-40.

[88] Masuo K, Mikami H, Ogihara T, Tuck ML. Differences in mechanisms between weight loss-sensitive and -resistant blood pressure reduction in obese subjects. Hypertens Res. 2001; 24(4):371-6.

[89] American Diabetes Association. Evidence-Based Nutrition Principles and Recommendations for the Treatment and Prevention of Diabetes and Related Complications. Diabetes Care January 2002; 25 (suppl 1): s50-s60.

[90] Toji C, Okamoto N, Kobayashi T, Furukawa Y, Tanaka S, Ueji K, et al. Effectiveness of diet versus exercise intervention on weight reduction in local Japanese residents. Environ Health Prev Med. 2012; 17(4): 332-40.

[91] Masuo K, Kawaguchi H, Mikami H, Ogihara T, Tuck ML. Serum uric acid and plasma norepinephrine concentrations predict subsequent weight gain and blood pressure elevation. Hypertension. 2003; 42(4): 474-80.

[92] Straznicky NE, Eikelis N, Nestel PJ,Dixon JB, Dawood T, Grima MT, et al. Baseline sympathetic nervous system activity predicts dietary weight loss in obese metabolic syndrome subjects. J Clin Endocrinol Metab. 2012; 97 (2): 605-13.

[93] Ribeiro MM, Silva AG, Santos NS, Guazzalle I, Mates LN, Tronbetta IC, et al. Diet and exercise training restore blood pressure and vasodilatory responses during physiological maneuvers in obese children. Circulation. 2005; 111(15): 1915-23

[94] Trombetta IC, Batalha LT, Rondon MU, et al. Gly16 + Glu27 beta2-adrenoceptor polymorphisms cause increased forearm blood flow responses to mental stress and handgrip in humans. J Appl Physiol. 2005; 98(3): 787-94

[95] Tonacio AC, Trombetta IC, Rondon MU, Laterza MC, Frazzatto E, Alves MJ, et al. Effects of diet and exercise training on neurovascular control during mental stress in obese women. Braz J Med Biol Res. 2006; 39(1): 53-62.

[96] Santarpia L, Contaldo F, Pasanisi F. Body composition changes after weight-loss interventions for overweight and obesity. Clin Nutr. 2013; 32(2): 157-61.

[97] Dumortier M, Brandou F, Perez-Martin A, Fedou C, Mercier J, Brun JF. Low intensity endurance exercise targeted for lipid oxidation improves body composition and insulin sensitivity in patients with the metabolic syndrome. Diabetes Metab. 2003; 29(5): 509-18.

[98] Poirier P, Pespres JP. Exercise in weight management of obesity. Cardio Clin. 2001; 19(3): 459-470.

[99] Skilton MR, Mikkilä V, Würtz P, Ala-Korpela M, Sim KA, Soininen P, et al. Fetal growth, omega-3 (n-3) fatty acids, and progression of subclinical atherosclerosis: preventing fetal origins of disease? The Cardiovascular Risk in Young Finns Study. Am J Clin Nutr. 2013; 97(1): 58-65.

[100] Mozaffarian D, Abdollahi M, Campos H, Houshiarrad A, Willett WC. Consumption of trans-fats and estimated effects on coronary heart disease in Iran. Eur J Clin Nutr. 2007; 61(8): 1004-10.

[101] Whitman SC, Rateri DL, Szilvassy SJ, Yokoyama W, Daugherty A. Depletion of natural killer cell function decreases atherosclerosis in low-density lipoprotein receptor null mice. Arterioscler Thromb Vasc Biol. 2004; 24(6): 1049-54.

[102] Teegala SM, Willett WC, Mozaffarian D. Consumption and health effects of trans fatty acids: a review. J AOAC Int. 2009; 92(5): 1250-7.

[103] Larsson SC, Virtamo J, Wolk A. Dietary fats and dietary cholesterol and risk of stroke in women. Atherosclerosis. 2012; 221(1): 282-6.

[104] Chowdhury R, Stevens S, Gorman D, Pan A, Wamakula S, Chowdhury S, et al. Association between fish consumption, long chain omega 3 fatty acids, and risk of cerebrovascular disease: systematic review and meta-analysis. BMJ. 2012 Oct 30;345:e6698. doi: 10.1136/bmj.e6698.

[105] Oh K, Hu FB, Manson JAE, Stampfer MJ, Willett WC. Dietary Fat Intake and Risk of Coronary Heart Disease in Women: 20 Years of Follow-up of the Nurses' Health Study. Am. J. Epidemiol. 2005; 161 (7): 672-9.

[106] Storlien LH, Baur LA, Kriketos AD, Pan DA, Cooney GJ, Jenkins AB, et al. Dietary fats and insulin action. Diabetologia. 1996; 39(6):621-31.

[107] Halton TL, Willett WC, Liu S, Manson JE, Albert CM, Rexrode K, et al. Low-Carbohydrate-Diet Score and the Risk of Coronary Heart Disease in Women. N Engl J Med. 2006; 355(19):1991-2002.

[108] Samaha FF, Iqbal N, Seshadri P, Chicano KL, Daily DA, McGrory J, Williams T, Williams M, et al. "A Low-Carbohydrate as Compared with a Low-Fat Diet in Severe Obesity". New England Journal of Medicine 2003; 348(21): 2074–81.

[109] Gardner CD, Kiazand A,Alhassan S, Kim S, Stafford RS, Balise RR, et al. Comparison of the Atkins, Zone, Ornish, and LEARN diets for change in weight and related risk factors among overweight premenopausal women: the A TO Z Weight Loss Study: a randomized trial. JAMA. 2007; 297(9): 969-77.

[110] Boden G, Sargrad K, Homko C, Mozzoli M, Stein TP, Effect of a low-carbohydrate diet on appetite, blood glucose levels, and insulin resistance in obese patients with type 2 diabetes. Annals of Internal Medicine. 2005, 142(6):403-411.

[111] McAuley KA, Hopkins CM, Smith KJ, McLay RT, Williams SM, Taylor RW, Mann JI. Comparison of high-fat and high-protein diets with a high-carbohydrate diet in insulin-resistant obese women. Diabetologia. 2005; 48(1): 8-16.

[112] Klein S, Sheard NF, Pi-Sunyer X,Daly A, Wylie-Rosett J, Kulkarni K, et al. Weight Management Through Lifestyle Modification for the Prevention and Management of Type 2 Diabetes: Rationale and Strategies. A statement of the American Diabetes Association, the North American Association for the Study of Obesity, and the American Society for Clinical Nutrition. Diabetes Care. 2004; 27(8): 2067-2073.

[113] Bantle JP, Wylie-Rosett J, Albright AL, APovian CM, Clark NG, Franz MJ, et al. American Diabetes Association (2008) Nutrition recommendations and interventions for diabetes: a position statement of the American Diabetes Association. Diabetes care. 2008; 31 Suppl: S61-S78.

[114] Kones R. Low-fat versus low-carbohydrate diets, weight loss, vascular health, and prevention of coronary artery disease: the evidence, the reality, the challenge, and the hope. Nutr Clin Pract. 2010; 25(5): 528-41

[115] St. Jeor ST, Howard BV, Prewitt E, Bovee V, Bazzarre T, Eckel RH. Dietary Protein and Weight Reduction: A Statement for Healthcare Professionals From the Nutrition Committee of the Council on Nutrition, Physical Activity, and Metabolism of the American Heart Association, American Heart Association, 2001.

[116] Krebs JD, Elley CR, Parry-Strong A, et al. The Diabetes Excess Weight Loss (DEWL) Trial: a randomised controlled trial of high-protein versus high-carbohydrate diets over 2 years in type 2 diabetes. Diabetologia. 2012; 55(4): 905-14.

[117] Ebbeling CB, Swain JF, Feldman HA, Wong WW, Hachey DL, Garcia-Lago E, Ludwig DS, Effects of dietary composition on energy expenditure during weight loss maintenance. JAMA. 2012; 307(24):2627-34.

[118] Jenkins DJA, Kendall CWC, Augustin LSA, Francrschi S, Hamidi M, Marchie A, et al. Glycemic index: overview of implications in health and disease. Am J Clin Nutr. 2002; 76(1):266S-73S.

[119] Wyne KL, Drexler AJ, Miller JL, Bell DS, Braunstein S, Nuckolls JG: Constructing an algorithm for managing type 2 diabetes: focus on the role of the thiazolidinediones. Postgrad Med. 2003 May; 8 Spec.63–72.

[120] Garber AJ, Larsen J, Schneider SH, Piper BA, Henry D. The Glyburide/Metformin Initial Therapy Study Group[1.] Simultaneous glyburide/metformin therapy is superior to component monotherapy as an initial pharmacological treatment for type 2 diabetes. Diabetes, Obesity and Metabolism. 2002; 4(3): 201-8.

[121] Chitre MM, Burke S. Treatment Algorithms and the Pharmacological Management of Type 2 Diabetes. Diabetes Spectrum. 2006;19(4):249-255.

[122] Greenway FL, Fujioka K, Plodkowski RA, Mudaliar S, Guttadauria M, Erickson J, Kim DD, Dunayevich E; COR-I Study Group. Effect of naltrexone plus bupropion on weight loss in overweight and obese adults (COR-I): a multicentre, randomised, double-blind, placebo-controlled, phase 3 trial. Lancet. 2010; 376(9741): 595-605.

[123] Heal DJ, Gosden J, Smith SL. What is the prognosis for new centrally-acting anti-obesity drugs? Neuropharmacology. 2012; 63(1): 132-46.

[124] Koshy AA, Babe AM, Brady MJ. Potential mechanisms by which bariatric surgery improves systemic metabolism. Transl Res. 2012. doi: 10.1016/j.trsl.2012.09.004.

[125] Dixon JB, Murphy DK, Segel JE, Finkelstein EA. Impact of laparoscopic adjustable gastric banding on type 2 diabetes. Obes Rev. 2012; 13(1): 57-67. doi: 10.1111/j.1467-789X.2011.00928.x.

[126] Ballantyne GH, Wasielewski A, Saunders JK. The surgical treatment of type II diabetes mellitus: Changes in HOMA insulin resistance in the first year following laparoscopic Rou-en-Y gastric bypass (LRYGB) and laparoscopic adjustable gastric banding (LAGB). Obes Surg. 2009; 19(9): 1297-303. doi: 10.1007/s11695-009-9870-2.

[127] Trakhenbroit MA, Leichman JG, Algahim MF, Miller CC 3rd, Moody FG, Lux TR, Taegtmeyer H. Body weight, insulin resistance, and serum adipokine levels 2 years after 2 types of bariatric surgery. Am J Med. 2009; 122(5): 435-42. doi: 10.1016/j.amjmed.2008.10.035.

[128] Gumbs AA, Modlin IM, Ballantyne GH. Changes in insulin resistance following bariatric surgery: role of caloric restriction and weight loss. Obes Surg. 2005; 15(4): 462-73.

[129] Leichman JG, Wilson EB, Scarborough T, Aguilar D, Miller CC 3rd, Yu S, Algahim MF, Reyes M, Moody FG, Taegtmeyer H. Dramatic reversal of derangements in muscle metabolism and left ventricular function after bariatric surgery. Am J Med. 2008; 121(11): 966-73. doi: 10.1016/j.amjmed.2008.06.033.

Chapter 17

Control and Prevention of Obesity and Diabetes Type 2 Through Non-Pharmacological Treatments Based on Marine Products

Daniela Seelenfreund, Pilar Durruty, Nicolas Palou,
Sergio Lobos and Rodrigo González

Additional information is available at the end of the chapter

http://dx.doi.org/10.5772/56427

1. Introduction

Obesity is currently considered as the pandemic of the 21st century and is paradigmatic of non-transmissible chronic diseases, such as type 2 diabetes mellitus (DM2), cardiovascular disease and cancer. Thus, due to its extent, obesity is considered a public health problem that is constantly growing and globally affects both the developed world and developing countries (WHO Prevalence of Diabetes, 2010). In the United States of America (USA) over 30% of the adult population is obese, the numbers in Europe are between 15 and 20 % and in Chile, with a GDP close to $US 20,000 per year, the National Health Survey (Encuesta Nacional de Salud, ENS) of 2010, showed a total prevalence of obesity of 27.4 %, very similar to industrialized countries (ENS, 2010).

All epidemiologic studies show that obesity is greater in subjects with low education and less in individuals with higher education; in Chile, obesity reaches 35% in the former. Additionally, obesity increases with people's age, reaching its highest level in the group of those between 50 – 64 years. However, it is very important to mention the increase in obesity in children and adolescents observed in Europe, in Chile and practically throughout the world, and which is the main cause of the appearance in recent years of a constantly increasing number of type 2 diabetes cases in these age groups (ENS, 2010).

Obesity should be considered as a heterogeneous, multifactorial disease with a genetic base – more than 60 genes involved have been described – however, predisposition to obesity is not higher than 30% and environmental factors of individuals and populations account for 70%. The highest impact factor in the development of obesity is excess food intake and the quality of the diet with high contents of carbohydrates and fats, to which sedentary lifestyles and lack of physical activity are added, both at work and at leisure, a feature common to all populations nowadays.

Among the causes of obesity, mention should be made of aggressive marketing of non-healthy foods, the low price of the so-called "junk food", higher economic income, as well as higher availability of public transportation and of television sets, video games and internet, all of which lead to an increase in sedentary lifestyles at all ages. Obesity *per se* is an independent risk factor for coronary cardiopathy, whereby it has been included by the American Heart Association as a major risk factor. Two important investigations, the Framingham and the Finnish prospective study, confirm the direct association between obesity and coronary mortality.

Visceral obesity is the main causing factor of metabolic syndrome (MS), which has been defined as a group of metabolic risk factors (arterial hypertension, dyslipidemia, glucose intolerance), that are more than randomly interrelated with each other and which directly promote the development of DM2 and cardiovascular disease (CVD). In the USA, health surveys show a sustained increase in the prevalence of MS; thus, the National Health and Nutrition Examination Survey (NHANES) for 1988 – 94 showed a prevalence of 23.1%, while the same survey in 1999 – 2006 reported a worrying increase reaching 34%. The Chilean ENS for 2010 reported very similar figures of 35% (ENS, 2010), while in 2003 it was 22.6%.

Obesity and particularly android or visceral obesity is associated with type 2 diabetes. It should be highlighted that at diagnosis of DM2, 80% of the subjects are obese. While this is true for diabetes in general, it should be considered that 90 – 95% of diabetic patients suffer diabetes type 2 and only 5 to 10% correspond to diabetes type 1, of autoimmune pathogenesis not related to obesity. In our country, only 1% are type 1 diabetic patients.

There is a universal consensus in that obesity is the leading pathogenic factor of pre-diabetes and DM2. Obesity is a determinant of insulin resistance (IR) with compensatory hyperinsulinemia; DM2 becomes manifest when a relative deficiency of insulin secretion is produced.

The International Diabetes Federation estimated a world-wide DM2 prevalence rate of 8.3% for 2011, which will increase to 9.9% by 2030. Some populations, such as Pima Indians from the USA or Mexico and people from the Mauritius Islands with rates higher than 20 – 30% are exceptions. Prevalence is growing explosively, thus the WHO reported that in 2010 there existed 250,000,000 diabetic patients in the world and most remarkably predicted a figure of 333,000,000 for 2025. The same growth is shown in Chilean investigations, with a progressive increase from 5.3% in 1981 to 6.3 in 2003 and 9.4% in 2010. The Chilean survey also shows a clear parallel between prevalence of obesity and DM2 according to age groups (ENS, 2010). The same as with obesity, DM2 is present in higher rates in people with less education and socially more vulnerable groups, which confirms the close association with DM2. It also increases with age, reaching figures close to 20% in elderly subjects.

Mortality for diabetes due to its chronic complications, particularly macrovascular complications and especially coronary death, is among the 10 leading causes of death worldwide, and the seventh cause of death in Chile. Diabetic patients exhibit 8 to 15 time higher frequency of

http://dx.doi.org/10.5772/56427

cardiovascular disease (CVD) and 2 to 3 time higher cardiovascular disease mortality than the general population. In the last 40 years, mortality for this cause has decreased in the general population, but not in diabetics. In summary, coronary disease is the main cause of death in DM2 and hyperglycemia is a direct mortality risk factor.

From the above the strong association between obesity, metabolic syndrome and DM2 can be derived, which have common pathogenic mechanisms. It is widely accepted that for prevention of these three pathologies, the main control measures are similar: a healthy diet and increased physical activity.

2. Prevention of DM

It is well known that dietary strategies are needed in order to prevent the onset and control of DM2, at least 80% of the population with DM2 is obese, 75% suffers hypertension and approximately 50% of DM2 patients are dislipidemic (mainly low high-density lipoprotein cholesterol (HDL) and hypertriglyceridemia). General dietary prescriptions for both obese and DM2 patients include well known diets of controlled calorie intake and predominant consumption of certain food groups like vegetables, legumes, fruits and nuts, whole-grain cereals, olive oil, wine and fish.

Risk Prediction Factors for DM2. In 2007, the International Diabetes Federation (IDF) published a consensus on DM2 prevention and defined non-modifiable and modifiable risk factors (Alberti *et al.*, 2007). Among the first are genetic factors, age - at an older age frequency of DM2 is higher - and previous gestational diabetes (about 50% of women with a history of gestational diabetes present DM2 10 years after delivery). Other non-modifiable risk factors are low birth weight children (fetal undernutrition) and big for gestational age babies, who frequently develop obesity as adults and, consequently, diabetes. The main individual modifiable risk factor is obesity, particularly of the android type and, secondly, physical inactivity. There is uncertainty regarding the influence of certain dietary factors, such as a possible involvement of diets that are high in caloric content, saturated fatty acids and low in unsaturated fatty acids and fiber.

Physiopathology of DM2. An important fact for being able to prevent a disease is the existence of a long latency period, which allows the individual to take favorable actions. DM2 meets this requirement, as it has a slow progression and is preceded by identifiable, reversible stages. These begin with an insulin resistance (IR) state with compensatory insulin secretion sufficient to maintain normoglycemia, with hyperinsulinemia values. Subsequently, there begins a progressive fall in insulin levels, when the beta cell is no longer able to maintain hyperfunction, and as insulin secretion deficiency begins, glycemia levels increasingly rise. Initially post-prandial glucose is affected, and later fasting glucose, a state designated as "prediabetes". If no measures are taken, after approximately 10 years of the IR state, clinical DM2 develops. Other physiopathological alterations in DM2 patients that are still under study are the existence of an accelerated gastric emptying and defects in the regulation of feeding, which may explain obesity of these patients.

Search for individuals at risk for DM2. In 2007 international experts established the necessary steps for preventing DM2, based on controlling the modifiable risk factors (Alberti *et al.*, 2007). They defined two groups, separating persons at high risk of developing DM2 from the rest of individuals. Once the former have been identified, it is necessary to measure the risk level with a score, in order to take the necessary actions. For identifying persons over 18 years with a high risk for DM2, a questionnaire is applied which should include the following factors: (android) obesity, age, family history of DM, cardiovascular and in women of gestational diabetes, and the use of diabetogenic drugs (glucocorticoids, adrenergic beta antagonists, thiazides and thyroid hormones). For a precise risk measurement, some models have been proposed, such as the non-invasive, low cost Diabetes Risk Score by Lindström (Lindström & Tuomihleto, 2003), which does not include laboratory tests.

To date, evaluation guidelines recommended by the international organizations to establish with higher certainty a predictive score are still lacking, in order to mathematically select those individuals with higher risk for DM; in the future, this will be a very useful tool. There is no agreement regarding the search mode in children and adolescents, and the risk factors employed are those established for adults: obesity, sedentarism, family history of DM and, additionally, other factors pertaining to adolescents, such as the increase in growth hormone during puberty and presence of polycystic ovary syndrome or hyperandrogenism; in children, low birth weight and growth retardation could be important. A search mode for pregnant women at risk for DM has not been internationally defined either.

The IDF (Alberti *et al.*, 2007) establishes that once persons at risk for DM2 have been identified, the recommendation is to determine fasting and post-load glycemias, which allow detecting cases of glucose intolerance and non-diagnosed DM. In addition, in fasting glycemias ranging between 110-125 mg/dl (impaired fasting glucose, as defined by the IFG), the recommendation is to perform an Oral Glucose Tolerance Test (OGTT) with 75 g glucose. Those persons with glycemia of 140-200 mg/dl are glucose intolerant (GI). Both states are designated as prediabetes and, if no pharmacological and non-pharmacological measures are received, they will develop DM2 in the short term.

2.1. Interventions for preventing or delaying DM2

Prevention with changes in lifestyle. Since the Malmö study, Sweden 1991, there exists evidence demonstrating that changes in lifestyle may delay or prevent DM2, in prediabetic individuals and in those at high risk of developing the disease, even if glycemias are normal. Research carried out in different countries and mainly in Caucasian subjects (the Malmö study, the Finnish Diabetes Prevention Study (DPS) and the US Diabetes Prevention Program (DPP, 2002), achieve similar results, with a decrease in the relative risk (RR) of developing DM2 of 63%, 58% and 58%, respectively (**Table 1**). Studies performed in Chinese individuals, in the city of Da Qing, and in India, Indian Diabetes Prevention Program (IDPP), obtain a smaller risk reduction, of 40% and 29%, respectively. The most remarkable conclusion is that for all studied ethnic groups, it is possible to prevent DM2.

STUDY Country	n	Years of follow-up	Average age (years)	Average BMI (kg/m2)	↓Relative risk of developing DM2
DA QING China	577	6.0	45	25.6	40%
DPS Finland	522	3.2	55	31	58%
DPP USA	3234	2.8	51	34	58%
IDPP India	531	3.0	45.4	25.8	29%

Table 1. Studies on DM2 prevention with lifestyle changes

The five studies discussed have in common that the groups submitted to intervention received feeding advice for reducing weight, plans of structured physical exercise and periodic visits from the medical team for controlling compliance of the indications; on the contrary, the individuals who constituted control groups were only observed, without receiving any special indications. The results of the follow-up of DPS (Lindström *et al.*, 2006) after the end of the three-year intervention period in subjects who had not developed diabetes are very interesting to note, as a 43% reduction of the RR of incidence of DM2 was found. The authors believe that the final success obtained in prediabetic patients is due to the fact that these individuals permanently adopted a healthy lifestyle with greater physical activity, dietary changes and weight loss.

The Da Qing study published similar results to the DPS in an observational study of up to 20 years. It showed a risk reduction of 43% in intolerant patients who were followed for up to 14 years after the end of the 6-year intervention period. The beneficial preventive effect for DM2 does not disappear at the end of the study period, but extends for many more years, probably through permanent lifestyle modifications which were internalized by the individuals.

2.2. DM2 prevention with pharmacological measures

The success obtained in DM2 prevention with changes in lifestyle encouraged many researchers to perform pharmacological interventions in glucose intolerant patients, especially with pharmacological measures. In Table 2 we summarize findings from several reports on the use of antidiabetic drugs, indicating the number of subjects involved, the years of intervention and the results of these programs on lowering the RR of DM2.

The DPP study (2002) in which glucose intolerant individuals received the metformin but without indications for a change in lifestyle had a much lower efficacy in preventing DM2 (31%), than that obtained with non-pharmacological measures (58%). Very similar achievements were shown by the group with metformin of the IDPP, with the same design and methodology as the previous work. In spite of the relatively modest results with the use of

Study	Drug	n	Years of follow-up	Average age (years)	Average BMI (kg/m2)	↓Relative risk of developing DM2
DPP	Metformin	3234	2.8	51	34	31%
STOP NIDDM	Acarbose	682	3.3	55	31	25%
IDPP	Metformin	531	3.0	46	25.8	26%
ACT NOW	Pioglitazone	602	4.0	52.3	34.3	78%

Table 2. Studies on DM2 prevention with pharmacological interventions

metformin, this insulin-sensitizing medicament is the drug of choice for the pharmacological treatment of the prediabetes state, when additional high-risk factors exist. Presently, it is the drug recommended by the ADA, due to its low side effects and proven therapeutic action.

There are lesser benefits obtained with acarbose in the STOP- NIDDM study with a 25% decrease in RR, in addition to producing marked undesirable digestive side effects and premature drop-out in 31% of the subjects, due to said cause. The use of glitazones is under discussion: Troglitazone and Rosiglitazone have been withdrawn from the market due to cardiovascular risk, and the future of Pioglitazone, used in the ACT NOW study, is uncertain.

Myths or realities in DM2 prevention. Consumption of coffee is widespread throughout the world; it contains caffeine and magnesium which affect glucose metabolism; high coffee intake has been related to lesser risk of DM2 in the USA, Europe and Japan. The phytochemicals in coffee could have a positive effect in slowing down the development of DM2 (van Dam *et al.*, 2006). In Japanese individuals, it was found that consumption of green tea reduces the risk for DM2; flavonoids from vegetables and fruit - also contained in green tea - have insulin activity and increase the action of the hormone (Iso *et al.*, 2006).

One possibility for preventing DM2 would be the administration of vitamins E and C, which improve insulin sensitivity by inhibiting oxidative stress and inflammation, respectively. Rizzo *et al.* (2008), in a controlled study in older men with IFG, found that daily intake of 1000 mg of vitamin E combined with 1000 UI of vitamin C for four weeks, decreased inflammation and improved insulin action, by increasing non-oxidative glucose metabolism, glycemia, insulinemia and lipids. It has been proposed that, due to their potential anti-inflammatory and autoimmune effects, in humans calcium and vitamin D supplements would reduce the incidence of type 1 diabetes and possibly of DM2 (Danescu *et al.*, 2009). The above findings open new prospects for the pharmacological or non-pharmacological prevention of DM2.

DM2 prevention in primary health care. The IDF in its consensus of 2007 (Alberti *et al.*, 2007) addresses this issue and states that "intervention for delaying or preventing diabetes will cause an important reduction of its incidence, its complications and co-morbidities", and recommends controlling the modifiable risk factors:

http://dx.doi.org/10.5772/56427

- - in the whole population and
- - in individuals at high risk of presenting DM2.

For prevention in the population, the IDF suggests to organize National Plans of Diabetes Prevention, adapted to the cultural conditions of each country and supported by existing organized social groups, which might start in nurseries, pre-schools and schools. Programs must have a broad coverage and must be oriented to controlling the two main modifiable risk factors, obesity and sedentarism with the purpose of therapeutic emphasis directed to changes in lifestyle.

3. Dietary strategies for the control of diabetes

The goals of nutritional therapy for diabetes are to prevent and treat complications such as cardiovascular disease, hypertension, nephropathy, obesity and dyslipidemia, and include achieving and maintaining safe or normal blood glucose levels, a normal lipoprotein profile, and an improvement of health through a change of food choices and increased physical activity. A healthy and balanced diet should provide enough calories for daily energy requirements, in order to reduce and/or maintain an acceptable body weight.

3.1. Metabolic control of DM2

It is necessary to know the degree of metabolic control in the type 2 diabetic patient in order to make the proper decisions for his/her treatment (Redsalud, 2006). It has been shown that there is a direct correlation between chronic hyperglycemia and damage to the patient's target systems and organs. The main tests for metabolic control are: glycosylated hemoglobin A1c (HbA1c) and glycemia.

HbA1c. It is currently the best control parameter of glycaemia and reports retrospectively, the glycemia average for a period of 6 to 12 weeks. Two important studies, UKPDS and DCCT, which demonstrated the relationship between metabolic control and appearance or aggravation of microangiopathic complications, employed it as an indicator of the degree of metabolic control. The goal of the treatment is to achieve HbA1c <7%, with individualized variations, the recommendation being that the HbA1c levels should be "the closest to normal, with the least risk of hypoglycemia for the patient". The recommended frequency of check-ups is every 3 months. Considering the heterogeneity of the elderly, goals may be variable, with 7% in a patient in good conditions, to 8.0 - 8.5 % in a patient with limited life expectations due to co-morbidities or with scarce awareness of hypoglycemias.

Glycemia. All patients should be checked with periodic laboratory glycemias or glycemias measured by capillary blood monitors in the clinic. In DM2 patients, this check-up should be carried out every three months. The goals or targets required for pre-prandial and post-prandial glycemias appear in **Table 3.** Capillary glycemias assessed by the patient through self-monitoring are necessary only in DM2 patients on insulin treatment; the usefulness of self-monitoring has not been demonstrated in DM2 patients with oral treatment.

Glycosylated hemoglobin A1c	< 7 %
Pre-prandial glycemias	70 - 130 mg/dl
Post-prandial glycemias	160 - 180 mg/dl

Table 3. Metabolic Goals

Target organ compromise

Retina. The fundus study should be performed at diagnosis of DM2. If normal, it should be repeated annually; if altered, the patient should be referred to a specialist.

Renal compromise. Assessment of plasma creatinine and calculation of glomerular filtration should be performed at diagnosis of DM2 and, if normal, should be repeated annually. Determination of proteinuria is performed at diagnosis of DM2; if negative, a microalbuminuria test is requested. Urinary albumin excretion (UAE) is quantified with the albumin/creatinine ratio in a random urine sample. UAE values between 30 and 300 mg/g should be repeated; microalbuminuria is diagnosed when 2 out of 3 samples continue to be altered. If the UAE values are <30 mg/g, the check-up can be performed annually.

Neuropathy and arteriosclerosis of the lower limbs. The clinical examination is conducted with exploration of feet and testing of tactile and vibratory sensitivity, reflexes and peripheral pulses. This examination is conducted at the patient's diagnosis; if no alterations exist, it should be systematically repeated once a year. In this examination, it is advisable to include the orthostatism test.

Detection and prevention of cardiovascular disease (CVD). DM in general is a risk factor for CVD and DM2 is associated with other factors which form part of the pre-diabetic status and which exert negative interrelations leading to a more precocious and severe CVD. Detection and control of these factors forms part of the treatment of DM; the most important are arterial hypertension and dyslipidemia.

Arterial hypertension. Diabetic patients have a high risk of CVD starting from the pre-hypertension stage, which also contributes to microvascular damage. Its optimized treatment reduces micro- and macrovascular complications of DM. It is essential to guarantee detection, control and treatment of hypertension. The goals to be achieved are < 130/ 80 mm Hg and, in nephropaths, < 125/75 mm Hg.

Dyslipidemia. Lipid alterations are a known risk factor for CVD and are more aterogenic in DM. The most important goal is to correct LDL cholesterol. Added to this is the so-called "aterogenic" dyslipidemia of the diabetic and pre-diabetic patient: elevated triglycerides, low HDL cholesterol and small, dense particles of LDL cholesterol. This explains why detection and treatment of lipid alterations is a main part of the check-up and follow-up of DM2. Lipid profiles should be included in the initial evaluation of DM2. If the result is normal, it should be repeated once a year. The goals to be achieved are: triglycerides <150 mg/dl, HDL >40 mg/dl in men, >50 in women and LDL <100 in primary CVD prevention and <70 in secondary CVD prevention.

With the aim of achieving an optimal metabolic control and prevention of micro- and macro-angiopathic complications, all patients should be encouraged to adhere to a healthy diet, low in cholesterol and saturated fatty acids and high in dietary fiber. Additionally, regular physical activity for 150 minutes per week, fractionated in 5 days, should be promoted.

3.2. Nutritional plan for DM2

Programmed diet (ADA, 2004) is one of the pillars of the treatment of DM2; without it, a proper metabolic control is not achieved, and the patient should permanently adhere to it. In some cases, together with exercise for some time, they both constitute sufficient total treatment for the disease.

Nutritional requirements. Nutritional requirements of persons with diabetes are similar to those of individuals without the disease. Calculation of total calories depends on the physical activity and the nutritional status of the patient. For an estimation of daily calories, the factors listed in **Table 4** are used.

In overweight or obese individuals, a weight loss of 5-10% of the present weight improves blood pressure and glycemic and lipid levels. Knowing the composition of the foods, the ingredients of kitchen recipes and the amounts that should be eaten, it is possible to design the dietary plan and apply the diet for the family group.

Nutritional status	Physical activity		
	Sedentary	Moderate	Intense
Obese (BMI >30 kg/m^2)	20-25	30	35
Overweight (BMI >25-29.9 kg/m^2)	26-29	28	30
Normal (BMI 20-24-9 kg/m^2)	30	35	40
Lean (BMI<20 kg/m^2)	35	40	45-50

Table 4. Caloric recommendations for adults. Calories/ kg of acceptable body weight

Carbohydrates (CH). The percentage of carbohydrate calories varies, it is individual and based on eating habits, targeted glycemia and lipids. The recommended range is between 55% and 60% of the total daily calories. Restriction of carbohydrates to less than 130 grams/day is not recommended, since the brain and the nervous system have an absolute requirement for glucose as a source of energy. In the dietary plan, it is advisable to leave out simple sugars (honey, panela, molasses, sugar) or lower them in well-controlled patients to <5 g per day.

Lipids. In the type 2 diabetic patient, elevations in very low density lipoprotein (VLDL) concentrations, reductions in high density lipoprotein (HDL) concentrations and elevations in the low density fraction (LDL) may be found. Type 2 diabetics may have an altered lipid profile, notwithstanding a good glycemic control.

The main goal in lipid intake is to reduce consumption of saturated fatty acids and trans fatty acids. Lipids should account for less than 30% of the total daily caloric intake. Foods containing monounsaturated and polyunsaturated fatty acids should be preferred in order to comply with the recommendations. Less than 7% of the calories provided by saturated (SFA) and *trans* fatty acids is recommended. SFAs are the main source of formation of LDL cholesterol and are found in fatty meats, dairy products and eggs. *Trans* fatty acids are produced by hydrogenating vegetable or fish oils in order to achieve a more solid texture.

Monounsaturated fatty acids (MFA) are recommended in a proportion of 13%, especially in the *cis* configuration, as found in olive oil, sesame, nuts and peanuts. MFAs may be beneficial in the control of blood lipids and of cardiovascular diseases. It is indicated that less than 10 % of the calories should be provided by polyunsaturated fatty acids (PFA), which are found in vegetable oils such as corn, sunflower, safflower and soybean oils. Omega 3 eicosapentenoic and docosahexenoic fatty acids (EPA and DHA) present in fish have a beneficial effect on triglycerides. It is recommended not to exceed an intake of 200 mg of cholesterol per day. Consumption of fish or fish oil containing omega-3 polyunsaturated fatty acids (PUFAs) reduce the risk of coronary heart disease, decrease mild hypertension, prevent certain cardiac arrhythmia and lower the incidence of diabetes. Omega-3 PUFAs play a vital role in the development and function of the nervous system and photoreception. Dietary lipids should be lowered if weight loss is desired; if this dietary scheme is maintained for a long term, it contributes to weight loss and to ameliorate dyslipidemia.

The recommended lipid composition in the diet of a type 2 diabetic patient is set forth in **Table 5.**

< 7% of the calories: saturated (SFA) and trans fatty acids
<10% of the calories: polyunsaturated fatty acids (PFA)
13% of the calories: monounsaturated fatty acids (MFA)
Omega 3 fatty acids (cis configuration) 0.15 g/day

Table 5. Contribution of dietary fatty acids in a DM2 patient

Proteins. Proteins should account for 15-20 % of total caloric intake, 0.8 – 1.0 g/Kg of body weight; dietary protein intake must be balanced and rich in essential amino acids. According to the dietary guidelines, the intake of protein in the usual range does not appear to be associated with the development of diabetic nephropathy, although it is advisable to avoid intakes over 20 % of the total daily energy.

The Recommended Dietary Allowance (RDA) indications for the general population of 0.8 g of proteins of high biological value, per kg of weight per day in the adult, are still followed. Proteins of high biological value provide all of the essential amino acids and in the amounts required by the body; they are the proteins of animal origin, all types of meat (beef, pork, fish, etc), milk and eggs. When the drop in glomerular filtration is initiated, proteins should not be restricted beyond 0.6 g/kg/day in order not to cause malnutrition. In the highly uncompensated type 2 diabetic patient, there could occasionally be a loss of body proteins.

Glycemic index. It is established as the incremental area under the glycemia curve produced by the intake of a standard amount of available CHs of a food (usually 50 g), in relation to the same amount of carbohydrates from a standard source (glucose or white bread). Recommendation is to prefer foods with low glycemic index (legumes, green vegetables).

Dietary fiber. Soluble fiber of vegetables, legumes and fruit (pectin) helps to control not only glycemia but also lipids, and should be accompanied by an increase in water intake. Fibers also help satiety. Processed foods tend to decrease the amount of available fiber. Complex carbohydrates, which also have a high percentage of soluble dietary fiber, are present in legumes, vegetables and fruits, and should be included in a healthy diet.

Sweeteners. Non-caloric sweeteners such as saccharin, aspartame, acesulfame K, sucralose, estevioside are accepted as safe, as long as their accepted daily intake is observed.

Sodium. Individuals differ in sensitivity to sodium intake, related to arterial pressure. Sodium recommendation is the same as for the general population: not more than 2.4 g/day, equivalent to 6.0 g/day of NaCl.

Alcohol. The same recommendations as for the general population are valid. Never to drink on an empty stomach and to prefer red wine due to its phenol (antioxidant) content; the maximal recommended portion is not more than 2 cups per day in men and not more than one in women. 100 ml of wine contain 9-13 g of alcohol, and one gram of alcohol provides 7 calories. Alcohol abstention is recommended during pregnancy, in hypertriglyceridemia, pancreatitis, arterial hypertension or neuropathy. If the individual with diabetes is abstemious, he/she will be advised not to initiate this practice. Fruit and vegetable intake provides a suitable amount of antioxidants.

Vitamins and Minerals. A suitable dietary intake provides vitamins and minerals in sufficient amounts and no supplementation is necessary. However, there are some exceptions: individuals on chronic hypocaloric diets, which should be supplemented with iron and B-Complex vitamins; iron, folate and calcium supplements are recommended to pregnant women; calcium supplement is recommended to women with osteoporosis; and undernourished subjects are advised to take supplements appropriate to the deficiency they present. Vitamin supplementation with antioxidants (vitamins E, C and A) is not advisable as a routine, due to lack of evidence and safety and long-term safety. Chromium, Selenium, Zinc and Manganese are contained in the usual diet, while supplements are recommended only when patients have a deficiency.

The nutritional plan detailed for DM2 is also recommended for individuals who are obese, insulin-resistant, pre-diabetic and carriers of metabolic syndrome, in order to prevent them from developing DM2.

To summarize, one of the key measures to achieve control targets in patients with diabetes is a diet plan, as there is ample evidence that the goals are not achieved if patients fail non-pharmacologic measures, diet and physical activity.

4. Nutrition and social behavior

The drastic and long-term changes in eating habits that are needed in order to prevent and control these diseases require a highly motivated and educated population with the economic means and a strong personal commitment to follow and maintain these indications. Changing dietary habits may be a very difficult task to accomplish and constant support is needed from health professionals who should develop individual therapeutic programs for each patient according to their personal lifestyle requirements, tastes or cultural backgrounds.

Why is it so difficult to achieve this change to healthy eating habits? In the first place it is important to understand that eating is not an isolated behavior, as in all societies it is part of the cultural context that defines what is considered edible or appropriate (or not) for each member of any particular group. Contreras & Grace (2005) suggest the presence of a food culture that accompanies any food system, which is defined as follows: "the set of representations, beliefs, knowledge and practices inherited and / or learned that are associated to food and that are shared by individuals of a given culture or a social group within a culture". In addition to keeping alive and avoiding overt hunger, food all over the world and in all possible settings is also used to keep and classify human relationships, indicate social status, enhance political, business and economic relations, provide praise and punishment, prevent and treat physical and mental disease, to indicate religious adherence or membership, to evidence emotions and even morals. As illustrated above, the underlying development of attitudes, from infancy to old age, in pregnancy and disease, for adolescents and adults influence food behavior and are determined by culture, economics, food technology, politics, the family and recently, by mass media. Consequently, to achieve significant impact, education in nutrition and dietetics also requires knowledge of the socio-cultural aspects of eating as well as its basic scientific aspects, and the professional providing nutrition services and education in the community needs an understanding of these facts (Bass *et al.*, 1979). Briefly, food and food consumption patterns underlie the social fabric in all societies and hence its cultural importance cannot be underestimated.

Second, the social act of eating has changed along the millennia of humankind; therefore it is of use to put the nutritional transitions into a historical context. From a long history of omnivorism of hunter-gatherers (mainly plants supplemented with occasional meat), that shaped our physiology to the present day, humans have moved through several important transitions in their nutrition. Omnivorism probably required cooperation between members of a species that is rather ill-equipped compared to other predators, possibly setting the stage for social patterns for providing and distributing food (Aguirre, 2010). These conditions selected among our ancestors those individuals endowed with genes that permitted the accumulation of calories in times of surplus, and survive in times of low access to food or starvation (Aguirre, 2010).

Later, approximately 15.000 to 10.000 B.P. a major nutritional transition occurs as an adaptation to the higher temperatures of the postglacial era (and the associated decrease of large prey for hunting) which leads to the development of agriculture (Smith & Munro, 2009). The introduction of staple food lead to the establishment of villages and an increase of the human population and a shift to meals based on cereals (i.e. carbohydrates) and a decrease of protein intake. As a result, on a global scale humans on average became approximately 20 cm shorter with a decreased life expectancy due to chronic malnutrition of micronutrients. Also, specific diseases related to agricultural labor and food processing appeared, such as arthritis, skeleton deformities and dental abrasion, particularly in women (Aguirre, 2010). The establishment of sedentary societies also set the stage for classes with differential foods, creating small well-fed upper classes with large, fat bodies and a majority of the population with the short and lean phenotype of poverty, fed a low variety of (or a single) cereal or tuber staple (Aguirre, 2010).

The next nutritional transition comes about with the industrial revolution, which initially causes a severe drop in the quality of life for the large majority of the population in the western world. The new technologies completely change the methods of producing, distributing and consuming foods. The modern relocation of edible plants throughout the world introduces the concept of plantations, and worldwide distribution of some edible products such as sugar, coffee, tea and potatoes, among others (Aguirre, 2010). The economic powers involved provoke colonial wars, and in the long run, create the industrial food production with large scale food transportation and storage, a panoply of additives (flavorings or dyes) and stabilizers, and the disappearance of seasonality of fruits and vegetables and local food production, that characterizes the modern food production of in our days.

The genetic makeup of our species has not changed at the pace of these nutritional transitions, so we are now faced with a large population, living in a largely industrial-urban setting that still maintains those biological features that constituted an advantage for survival in the past. Although there are 870 millions of people suffering hunger today (http://faostat3.fao.org/home/index.html), for the first time in human history, a large segment of the population has access to a large supply of calories in the form of carbohydrates and fats, albeit, not to a healthy diet with low fat proteins and micronutrients. Finally, this nutritional transition has happened so fast that the shift from undernourishment to obesity has occurred within just two generations. Indeed, in developing countries, it is not uncommon that an individual, who experienced undernourishment during childhood, is today an obese adult with overweight children. Therefore, in a completely different context, our genetic makeup in an era of surplus calories and changing lifestyles provides the basis for the worldwide epidemic of obesity and diabetes.

As pointed out at the beginning of this section, a highly motivated and educated population with the economic means and a strong personal commitment to follow and maintain the indications is needed to revert this situation. Low levels of education of mothers also tend to result in children that spent more time watching TV and eat a higher amount of fat and calorie-rich snacks and "junk food", highlighting the importance of enhancing school-based and community-based actions to promote healthy eating and physical activity addressed to children and young people (Aranceta *et al.*, 2003). Also, in the face of increasing food prices, many people with lower incomes do not have a realistic possibility of choosing an appropriate diet.

Since the general population in most developing countries such as Chile, is not able to keep these recommendations in the long term for any of the above reasons, several kinds of dietary interventions have been proposed. These include low calorie foods and foods containing high-quality ingredients such as peptides derived from fish. Some of these strategies include the replacement of red meat and its derivatives by fish and white meat, the reduction of the total fat intake (saturated fat) and replacement by the use of other oils (such as olive oil) and a higher intake of dietary fiber, replacing white bread with whole grain bread. Here we propose to include marine-derived proteins, specifically fish-derived protein hydrolysates as high biological value proteins of low cost as dietary supplements or ingredients, as a means of preventing obesity and diabetes.

5. Marine-derived protein

5.1. General aspects

Seafood and fish are sources of high biological value proteins, unsaturated essential fatty acids, vitamins and antioxidants, minerals or trace metals and physiological beneficial amino acids and peptides. Additional components in seafood may be of importance for the development of life style diseases like coronary heart disease. There is ample literature on marine-derived peptides (salmon and other fish) with biological activity against obesity, DM2 and cardiovascular disease, which leads to the proposal of using protein concentrates produced by enzymatic hydrolysis from co-products of the fish industry that may contain these peptides. Several research groups, including ourselves, are concentrated on generating an application or nutraceutical biological functionality of these products.

Different strategies have been studied for recovering protein from the marine products industry, as for example fish protein hydrolysates (FPHs, by its acronym in English). These treatments are obtained by solubilizing the raw protein, *via* peptide bond breaks which release smaller peptides and free amino acids, that can then be separated and recovered. In this type of application protein recovery by enzymatic hydrolysis is chosen, because this treatment gives rise to a final product of higher digestibility than untreated protein (Aurrekoetxea & Perera, 2002).

Several studies reveal that proteins derived from hydrolysis of marine products are of high nutritional value, rich in essential amino acids and even similar to proteins from beef (Kristinsson & Rasco, 2000). It has also been observed that hydrolysates, treated with commercial enzymes, exhibit functional characteristics (solubility, fat absorption, water absorption and stability of the emulsion) consistent with potential uses as emulsifying agents, and absorbing agents, being potentially competitive with existing protein hydrolysates, such as dairy products and vegetables, which are currently available on the market (Sathivel *et al.*, 2005).

Enzymatic digestion of proteins of marine origin results in FPH. Among the problems of obtaining the FPH, is the extreme susceptibility to oxidation of fats, and the presence of these oil residues which generate unpleasant odors and flavors from an organoleptic viewpoint (Hoyle & Merritt, 1994).

Protein hydrolysates also have non-food applications such as power supply for the growth of microorganisms such as yeast hydrolysates or casein. They can also be used eventually as plant fertilizers and also used in cosmetics for hair treatment (due to its suggested effect of strengthening of hair) (Vioque & Millan, 2005).

Enzymatic hydrolysis has clear advantages over traditional acid or alkaline chemical hydrolysis, for the following reasons (Guadix *et al.*, 2000):

- Selectivity. Enzymes are specific for a particular type of chemical bond, and the appearance of degradation products is not common. In contrast, the low selectivity of the acidic and basic treatments inevitably leads to the appearance of degradation products that are difficult to control and may be toxic.
- Moderate temperature and pH conditions. Enzymatic hydrolysis generally proceeds in the range of 40 to 60°C and pH of 4.0 to 8.0.
- No foreign substances are added. Chemical hydrolysis processes are carried out with strong acids or bases, which are then neutralized, thereby significantly raising the salt content of the product.
- Maintain the nutritional value. There is no degradation of the components, while alkaline hydrolysis destroys the amino acids arginine and cysteine, and acid hydrolysis removes tryptophan and deaminates serine and threonine.

As a result of biological hydrolysis, high-protein, low-fat FPHs can be obtained, which are completely soluble products (Aurrekoetxea & Perera, 2002).

5.2. Physiological effects of marine-derived peptides and aminoacids

Potent peptides with high anti-hypertensive activities (inhibitors of angiotensin I-converting enzyme or ACE) and peptides which may modulate central neuropeptide levels have been isolated from fish hydrolysates (Yoshikawa *et al.*, 2000; Sorensen *et al.*, 2004). Marine low molecular weight components antioxidants (tocopherols, CoQ10, selenium, taurine) have attracted special attention due to their possible prevention of low-density lipoprotein (LDL) oxidation. Fish proteins have also been shown to inhibit LDL oxidation in rat models (Kondo *et al.*, 2000).

It has been documented that peptides obtained from fish muscle digests possess potent inhibitory activity against ACE and antihypertensive properties (Galardy *et al.*, 1984; Kohama *et al.*, 1996). For assessment of relative antihypertensive activities of two peptides (LKPNM and LKP) derived from bonito fish to that of captopril, administered orally to SHR rats to monitor time-course changes of blood pressures (Fujita & Yoshikawa, 1999). Both LKPNM and captopril showed maximal decrease of blood pressure 4 h after oral administration and their efficacies lasted until 6 h post-administration. In sharp contrast, however, maximal reduction of blood pressure occurred as early as 2 h after administration of LKP. When compared on molar basis, antihypertensive activities of LKPNM and LKP accounted for 66% and 91% relative to that of captopril, respectively, whereas *in vitro* ACE-inhibitory activities of LKPNM and LKP were very low compared with that of captopril. It is of interest to note that both of these peptides exerted remarkably higher antihypertensive activities *in vivo* despite weaker *in vitro* ACE-inhibitory effects, using captopril as the reference drug (Fujita & Yoshikawa, 1999). Such peptides may be regarded as healthy components (through endogenous metabolism) of fish muscles and additionally may be produced as ingredients or diet supplements.

Amino acids (taurine) and peptides (ACE -inhibitors) are beneficial components from seafood and hence components in possible ingredients in functional foods. Seafood contains high levels of the amino acid taurine and the consumption of seafood has been shown to increase its serum concentration (Laidlaw *et al.*, 1990; Kim *et al.*, 1996). The suggestion of a possible association between fish intake and reduced cardiovascular risk through the beneficial effects of proteins and taurine, in addition to omega n-3 fatty acids, has been put forward (Mizushima *et al.*, 1997; Yamori *et al.*, 1994).

In humans, taurine is regarded to be a conditionally essential amino acid, as its physiological concentration can be partly regulated endogenously. Taurine is known to have several positive effects on the cardiovascular system, as described in a broad review by Niittynen *et al.* (1999). Firstly, taurine has antioxidant activity. This may reduce the production of proinflammatory products. Secondly, taurine has been shown to lower blood pressure in borderline hypertensive patients. It has also been reported that taurine can improve cardiac performance, reduce blood cholesterol values and suppress platelet aggregation (Niittynen *et al.*, 1999). A protective role from both taurine and ACE inhibitors has been found in age-related progressive renal sclerosis in 24 and 30 months old rats. Taking into account the antioxidant properties of taurine, these data suggest a role for ROS in age-related progressive renal fibrosis, perhaps through interactions with de TGF-β1 pathway (Iglesias-de la Cruz *et al.*, 2000). Although commonly used as a dietary supplement in the Far East, the potential advantages of dietary taurine consumption /supplementation have not been recognized in the Western World (Stapleton *et al.*, 1998).

Frozen-preserved commercial diets have been shown to maintain plasma taurine concentration, whereas the heat-processed diets do not (Kim *et al.*, 1996; Dragnes *et al.*, 2009). On the other hand, a significant correlation was found between the results of the biological assessment of the nutritional value of processed protein and of taurine content in the liver and urine of rats (Lipka *et al.*, 1993).

5.3. Improvement of FPHs through the use of enzymes

The functional properties of FPHs can be improved by the use of specific enzymes and by the choice of the hydrolysis conditions, such as time, temperature and pH. In this way partial hydrolysis can be achieved. There are a number of different commercial proteolytic enzymes that can be used to produce hydrolysates (Liceaga-Gesualdo & Li-Chan, 1999).

The addition of exogenous enzymes to the hydrolytic process makes it more controllable and reproducible. Consequently, different commercial proteolytic enzymes have been tested on a variety of marine substrates. The preferred commercial enzymes are proteases of bacterial origin, such as Alcalase, Neutrase, Protamex (bacterial proteases trade names), but also the plant proteases such as papain (commercially called Corolase L-10), present good yields in hydrolytic processes (Aspmo, 2005).

All enzymes used for hydrolyzing proteins of marine origin have to be of food grade, and if they are of bacterial origin, the production organism needs to be non-pathogenic. The choice of enzyme is usually determined by a combination of effectiveness and economy (Kristinsson & Rasco, 2000). Major factors in the choice of enzymes are the organoleptic and functional characteristics of the final food product.

5.4. Organoleptic properties of the hydrolysate

Although enzymatic hydrolysis of marine proteins produces peptides with desirable functional properties, it has the disadvantage of generating bitterness. This is a common problem with FPHs, and is the main reason for its low acceptance as a food ingredient. The mechanism for the development of bitterness is not yet clear, but it is widely accepted that the hydrophobic amino acids of the peptides are the main factor. The hydrolysis of proteins results in the exposure of internal hydrophobic peptides which are able to interact rapidly with the taste buds, resulting in the detection of bitter taste. However, extensive hydrolysis to produce free amino acids reduces the bitterness of peptides, because hydrophobic peptides are much bitterer compared with a blend of free amino acids, which are though, undesirable from a functional point of view. A strict control of the degree of hydrolysis in any experimental system is therefore desirable to prevent the development of bitter taste and also for the retention of functional properties (Kristinsson & Rasco, 2000; Liaset *et al.*, 2003; Benitez *et al.*, 2008).

Proteases have different specificity for the amino acids they cut, so the choice of the most appropriate enzyme or mixture of enzymes depends on the raw material subjected to hydrolysis, and may affect the degree of bitterness. For instance, enzymes with a high preference for hydrophobic amino acids, such as Alcalase, are often preferred and may yield products with low bitterness. The use of exopeptidases, instead of endoproteases, may also be useful in reducing the bitterness of the FPH, particularly if exopeptidases separating hydrophobic amino acids from bitter peptides are used. However, for an enzyme preparation to be effective in protein hydrolysis, both exopeptidases and endopeptidases are required. Many studies have shown that preparations containing proteolytic exopeptidases and endopeptidases produce less bitter peptides than single proteases. The addition of exopeptidases to the process often eliminates the bitter taste of the hydrolysates (FitzGerald & O`Cuinn, 2006).

The ideal method for the quantification of the bitterness of a hydrolysate is the use of a sensory evaluation panel. This is a time-consuming activity and requires an appropriate number of panelists trained to detect such bitterness, in order to obtain statistically relevant data (FitzGerald & O`Cuinn, 2006; Seo *et al.*, 2008).

5.5. Use of antioxidants in the hydrolysis

Oils and fatty products generally undergo oxidation during production and storage. A major problem of the preparation of FPHs is their extreme susceptibility to such oxidation fats (Hoyle & Merritt, 1994). This oxidation process in food causes a sequence of unfavorable changes, consisting mainly in deterioration of the sensory properties of the product such as rancidity, changes in color and texture and reduced nutritional value. It also increases health risks, along with economic losses and may even influence the development of bitter flavors (Palić & Lucan, 1995; Valenzuela *et al.*, 2003; Gramza & Korczak, 2005; Mendis *et al.*, 2005; Dong *et al.*, 2008).

Marine oils are rich in polyunsaturated fatty acids (PUFAs), especially of the ω3 family such as EPA and DHA, however diets containing these oils are more susceptible to oxidation than those containing other types of oils, because of their high concentrations of long chain PUFAs; the aforementioned examples are DHA and EPA (Gonzalez *et al.*, 1992; Fritsche & Johnston, 1988; Wanasundara & Shahidi, 1998).

PUFA degradation *via* chain reaction mechanisms of free radicals, results in changes of smell and taste (rancidity) of edible oils and oil-containing foods. The chemical reactions involved in oxidative processes require low activation energy, and do not significantly change their ranges at low storage temperatures; therefore, it is necessary to delay the onset of oxidation of the marine oil to maintain its flavor and odor (Wanasundara & Shahidi, 1998; Ahn *et al.*, 2007).

5.6. Antioxidants

Antioxidants, natural and synthetic, are commonly used by the food processing industry, to prolong the storage stability of food. The main commonly used synthetic antioxidants are butylhydroxybutilanisol, butylated hydroxytoluene, propyl gallate and tertiary butylhydroquinone (BHA, BHT, PG and TBHQ, respectively, for their acronyms in English). Natural antioxidants such as tocopherols, rosemary extracts (Herbalox, commercial product) and ascorbic acid are often preferred (Gramza & Korczak, 2005; Yu *et al.*, 2006).

5.7. Preliminary trials

Preliminary tests of the organoleptic properties of enzymatic hydrolysis of marine proteins with different commercial enzymes, among them Alcalase, and Colorasa Protamex (papain) and different commercial antioxidants, showed greater acceptability of the process than with the protease Colorasa L-10. These results were observed after organoleptic analysis of the obtained products in trials with healthy volunteers (unpublished results).

While the use of antioxidants improves the stability of the oil fraction obtained together with the protein fraction, products derived from an antioxidant-free process were more acceptable (organoleptic properties) than those obtained in a process in which antioxidants were are used, although the oil fraction underwent faster oxidation (unpublished results). These results suggest that the addition of antioxidants is not of vital importance in the course of an organoleptically suitable product with a high proportion of proteins of marine origin.

6. Concluding comments

In this chapter we present general data concerning the worldwide epidemic of obesity and diabetes and discuss the present day goals of metabolic control of affected patients. The current strategies used for prevention of the development of prediabetes and diabetes are discussed and a brief up-to-date review of summarizes the dietary strategies for the nutrition of diabetic patients.

In the following section we briefly describe the main impact of historic nutritional transitions and illustrate how the social impact of present day food production, distribution and consumption is exacting a high toll on public health (and also on the environment). To amend this general pattern, large changes of society on a global scale are needed. Since these do not seem realistic in the short term, alternative strategies to address particular problems are suggested, such as nutritional intervention with high quality nutrients of low economic value such as supplementing foods with marine-derived protein hydrolysates.

A discussion of the different procedures for obtaining fish derived protein hydrolysates is presented, centered on the advantages of enzymatic hydrolysis, with respect to chemical procedures. The use of antioxidants during the hydrolysis process is also analyzed and not found to be essential for obtaining a high quality product. The organoleptic properties of hydrolysates obtained by our group have proven acceptable in trials to healthy volunteers. In addition, fish derived protein hydrolysates may contain peptides and/or aminoacids which may bear additional beneficial effect.

To summarize, healthy dietary habits are part of the necessary lifestyle to prevent obesity and DM2; an increased intake of marine products is also recommended as a means to control risk factors of cardiovascular disease of DM2 patients.

Author details

Daniela Seelenfreund[1*], Pilar Durruty[2], Nicolas Palou[1], Sergio Lobos[1] and Rodrigo González[1]

1 Department of Biochemistry, Faculty of Chemical and Pharmaceutical Sciences, University of Chile, Providencia, Santiago, Chile

2 Diabetes Unit, Department of Medicine, Faculty of Medicine, University of Chile, Santiago, Chile

References

[1] Aguirre, P. (2010). Ricos flacos y gordos pobres: la alimentación en crisis. 1rst Ed. Capital Intelectual S.A., Buenos Aires, Argentina.

[2] Ahn, J, Grün, I, & Mustapha, A. (2007). Effects of plant extracts on microbial growth, color change, and lipid oxidation in cooked beef. Food Microbiol, , 24, 7-14.

[3] Alberti KGMZimmet P, Shaw J, (2007). International Diabetes Federation: a consensus on Type 2 diabetes prevention. Diabetic Medicine, , 24, 451-463.

[4] American Diabetes Association(2004). Nutrition Principles and Recommendations in Diabetes.. oi: 10.2337/diacare.27.2007.S36 Diabetes Care January 2004 no. suppl 1 s36., 27

[5] Aranceta, J, Pérez-rodrigo, C, & Ribas, L. Serra-Majem, Ll, (2003). Sociodemographic and lifestyle determinants of food patterns in Spanish children and adolescents: the enKid study. Eur J Clin Nutr, 57: Suppl 1, SS44., 40.

[6] Aspmo, S. (2005). Enzymatic hydrolysis of Atlantic cod (Gadusmorhua L.) viscera. Process Biochem, , 40, 1957-1966.

[7] Aurrekoetxea, G, & Pereira, M. (2002). Aprovechamiento de recursos pesqueros infrautilizados para la obtención de alimentos mejorados para el cultivo de peces. Boletín del Instituto Español de Oceanografía, , 18, 87-93.

[8] Bass, M. A, Wakefield, L, & Kolasa, K. (1979). Community nutrition and individual food behavior. Publisher Burgess Pub. Co., Minneapolis (USA).

[9] Benítez, R, Ibarz, A, & Pagan, J. (2008). Hidrolizados de proteína: procesos y aplicaciones. Acta Bioquímica Clínica Latinoamérica, , 42, 227-237.

[10] Contreras, J, & Gracia, M. (2005). Alimentación y Cultura: perspectivas antropológicas. Editorial Ariel. Barcelona, Spain. (Ibid. 2005: 96).

[11] Danescu, L. G, Levy, S, & Levy, J. and diabetes mellitus. Endocrine, , 35, 11-17.

[12] Diabetes Prevention Program Research Group(2002). Reduction in the incidence of type 2 diabetes with lifestyle intervention or metformin. N Engl J Med, , 346, 393-403.

[13] Dragnes, B. T, Larsen, R, Ernstsen, M. H, Mæhre, H, & Elvevoll, E. O. (2009). Impact of processing on the taurine content in processed seafood and their corresponding unprocessed raw materials. Int J Food Sci Nutr, , 60(2), 143-152.

[14] ENSMinisterio de Salud Chile. Encuesta Nacional, htpp:www.minsal.cl/portal/url/page/minsalcl/g_home/home.html, 2009-2010.

[15] FitzGerald RO`Cuinn G, (2006). Enzymatic debittering of food protein hydrolysates. Biotechnol Adv, , 24, 234-237.

[16] Fritsche, K, & Johnston, P. (1988). Rapid autoxidation of fish oil in diets without added antioxidants. J Nutrition, , 118-425.

[17] Fujita, H, & Yoshikawa, M. (1999). LKPNM: a prodrug-type ACE-inhibitory peptide derived from fish protein. Immunopharmacology, 44(1-2): 123-127.

[18] Galardy, R, Podhasky, P, & Olson, K. R. (1984). Angiotensin-converting enzyme activity in tissues of the rainbow trout. J Exp Zool, , 230(1), 155-158.

[19] González-torres, M, Betancourt-rule, M, & Ortiz, R. (2000). Daño oxidativo y antioxidantes. Bioquímica, , 25, 3-9.

[20] Gramza, A, & Korczak, J. (2005). Tea constituents (Camellia sinensis L.) as antioxidants in lipid systems. Trends in Food Science & Technology, , 16, 351-358.

[21] Guadix, A, Guadix, E, Páez-dueñas, M, González-tello, P, & Camacho, F. (2000). Procesos tecnológicos y métodos de control en la hidrólisis de proteínas. Ars Pharmaceutica, , 40, 79-89.

[22] Hoyle, N. T, & Merritt, J. H. (1994). Quality of Fish Protein Hydrolysates from Herring (Clupeaharengus). J Food Sci, , 59, 76-80.

[23] Iglesias de la Cruz CRuiz-Torres P, García del Moral R, Rodríguez-Puyol M, Rodríguez-Puyol D, (2000). Age-related progressive renal fibrosis in rats and its prevention with ACE inhibitors and taurine. Am J Physiol Renal Physiol, 278: FF129., 122.

[24] Iso, H, Date, C, Wakai, K, Fukui, M, & Tamakoshi, A. and the JACC Study Group, (2006). The relationship between green tea intake and type 2 diabetes in Japanese adults. Ann Inter Med, , 144, 554-562.

[25] Kim, S. W, Rogers, Q. R, & Morris, J. G. (1996). Maillard reaction products in purified diets induce taurine depletion in cats which is reversed by antibiotics. J Nutr, , 126(1), 195-201.

[26] Kohama, Y, Kuroda, T, Itoh, S, & Mimura, T. (1996). Tuna muscle peptide, PTHIKWGD, inhibits leukocyte-mediated injury and leukocyte adhesion to cultured endothelial cells. Biol Pharm Bull, , 19(1), 139-41.

[27] Kondo, K, Iwamoto, T, Hooda, K, Kamiyama, M, Hirano, R, Kidou, T, Matsumoto, A, Watanabe, S, & Itakura, H. (2000). Inhibition of low-density lipoprotein oxidation by fish protein and antioxidants. XIIth International Symposium on Atherosclerosis, Abstract W12: 113. June Stockholm, Sweden.(TuP18), 25-29.

[28] Kristinsson, H. G, & Rasco, B. A. (2000). Fish protein hydrolysates: production, biochemical, and functional properties, Crit Rev Food Sci Nutr, , 40, 43-81.

[29] Liaset, B, Julshamn, K, & Espe, M. (2003). Chemical composition and theoretical nutritional evaluation of the produced fractions from enzyme hydrolysis of salmon frames with Protamex. Process Biochemistry, , 38, 1747-1759.

[30] Liceaga-gesualdo, A, & Li-chan, E. (1999). Functional properties of fish protein hydrolysate from herring," J Food Sci, , 64-1000.

[31] Lindström, J, Ilanne-parikka, P, Peltonen, M, Aunola, S, Eriksson, J, & Hemio, K. (2006). Sustained reduction in the incidence of type 2 diabetes by lifestyle intervention: follow-up of the Finnish Diabetes Prevention Study. Lancet, , 368, 1673-1679.

[32] Lindström, J, & Tuomilehto, J. (2003). The Diabetes Risk Score. A practical tool to predict type 2 diabetes risk. Diabetes Care, , 26, 725-731.

[33] Mendis, E, Rajapakse, N, & Kim, S. (2005). Antioxidant properties of a radical-scavenging peptide purified from enzymatically prepared fish skin gelatin hydrolysate. J Agric Food Chem, , 53, 581-587.

[34] Nittynen, L, Nurminen, M. L, Korpela, R, & Vapaatalo, H. (1999). Role of arginine, taurine and homocysteine in cardiovascular diseases. Ann Med, , 31(5), 318-326.

[35] Palic, A, & Lucan, Ž. (1995). Antioxidative Effect of 'Herbalox' on Edible Oils. Lipid/Fett, , 97, 379-381.

[36] Redsalud(2006). www.redsalud.gov.cl/archivos/guiasges/diabetesGES.pdf http://www.fao.org/docrep/016/i3027e/i3027e03.pdf

[37] Rizzo, M. R, Abbatecola, A. M, Barbieri, M, et al. (2008). Evidence for anti-inflammatory effects of combined administration of vitamin E and C in older persons with impaired fasting glucose: impact on insulin action. J Am Coll Nutr, , 27, 505-11.

[38] Sathivel, S, & Smiley, S. (2005). Functional and nutritional properties of red salmon enzymatic hydrolysates. Journal of Food, , 70, 401-406.

[39] Smith, A, & Munro, N. D. (2009). A holistic approach to examining ancient agriculture. Curr Anthropol, , 50, 925-936.

[40] Valenzuela, A, Sanhueza, J, & Nieto, S. (2003). Natural antioxidants in functional foods: from food safety to health benefits. Grasas y aceites, , 104, 754-760.

[41] Van Dam, R, Willett, W, Manson, J, & Hu, F. (2006). Coffee, caffeine, and risk of type 2 diabetes. Diabetes Care, , 29, 398-403.

[42] Vioque, J, & Millán, F. (2005). Los hidrolizados proteicos en alimentación: Suplementos alimenticios de gran calidad funcional y nutricional. Agro CSIC, , 2-8.

[43] Wanasundara, U, & Shahidi, F. (1998). Antioxidant and pro-oxidant activity of green tea extracts in marine oils. Food Chemistry, , 63, 335-342.

[44] World Health Organization Prevalence of Diabetes(2010). htpp://www.who:int/diabetes/facts/world:figures/en/indexx2.html

[45] Yu, H-H, Liu, X, Xing, R, Liu, S, Guo, Z, Wang, P, Li, C, & Li, P. (2006). In vitro determination of antioxidant activity of proteins from jellyfish. Food Chemistry, , 95, 123-130.

Chapter 18

Beneficial Effects of Alternative Exercise in Patients with Diabetes Type II

Naruemon Leelayuwat

Additional information is available at the end of the chapter

http://dx.doi.org/10.5772/56610

1. Introduction

First of all, let's define the meaning of alternative exercise which means exercise activities aside from the ones that generally perform: running, walking, swimming, or biking [1]. This chapter provides reasons for encouraging alternative exercise to patients with diabetes type II. Moreover it provides knowledge of general modes of alternative exercise and their effects in diabetes and non-diabetes individuals. The exercise modes which are too difficult, aggressive, sports or normally performed such as swimming, cycling or running are not included. The clinical instruction such as indication or contraindication of the exercise is not described because it has already been mentioned elsewhere in this book. Moreover, other recommendation for these patients is well suggested in a previous study [2]. Finally, it described scientific knowledge of an alternative exercise i.e. Arm swing exercise (ASE) on improving glycaemic control and antioxidant activity in patients with diabetes type II. Further studies investigating the effects of ASE on other systems in patients with Diabetes Type II are needed.

2. Reasons for encouraging alternative exercise to patients with diabetes type II

Although moderate exercise (mostly are western style e.g. swimming, running or aerobic dance) at least 30 minutes of moderate-intensity exercise at least three days per week was recommended to prevent cardiovascular disease in diabetes patients [3], it is difficult to encourage them to these modes of exercise regularly. Alternative exercise is defined as various exercise modes performed alternatively e.g. Yoga, Martial Arts, TaeKwonDo and many others. Factors affecting the boring in exercise are intensity, equipment, complicated mode and duration. This alternative exercise should reduce boring and encourage people to do exercise regularly.

3. General modes of alternative exercise

This topic described many modes of alternative exercise which some of them are scientific proved in patients with diabetes type II but some are not proved.

3.1. Yoga

The word yoga means "union" in Sanskrit, the ancient Indian language [6].

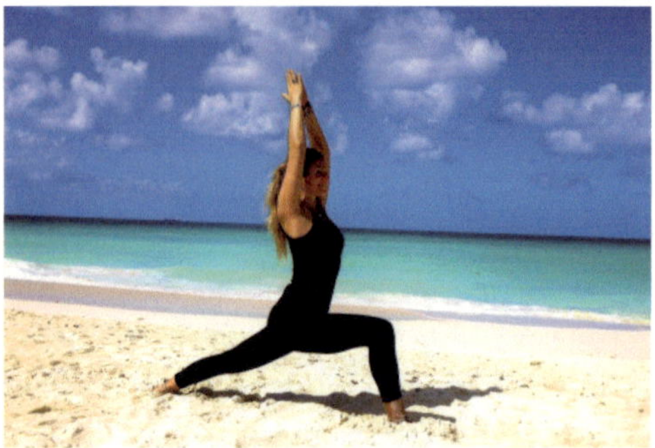

Figure 1. A posture of Warrior which is one of yoga positions [4]

Yoga is an old, traditional, Indian psychological, physical and spiritual exercise regimen that already has been known for its beneficial effects both the symptom and complication of patients with diabetes type 2 including;

- Decreasing reaction time [7]
- Improving lipid profile [7]
- Improving oxidative stress [8, 9],
- Can be incorporated along with the conventional medical therapy for improving cognitive brain functions in diabetes [8] and improve nerve function in mild to moderate Type 2 diabetes with sub-clinical neuropathy [10]
- Reducing Body mass index (BMI) and improving well-being [11]
- Reducing anxiety [8]
- Improving blood pressure, insulin, triglycerides and exercise self-efficacy indicated by small to large effect sizes. [12]

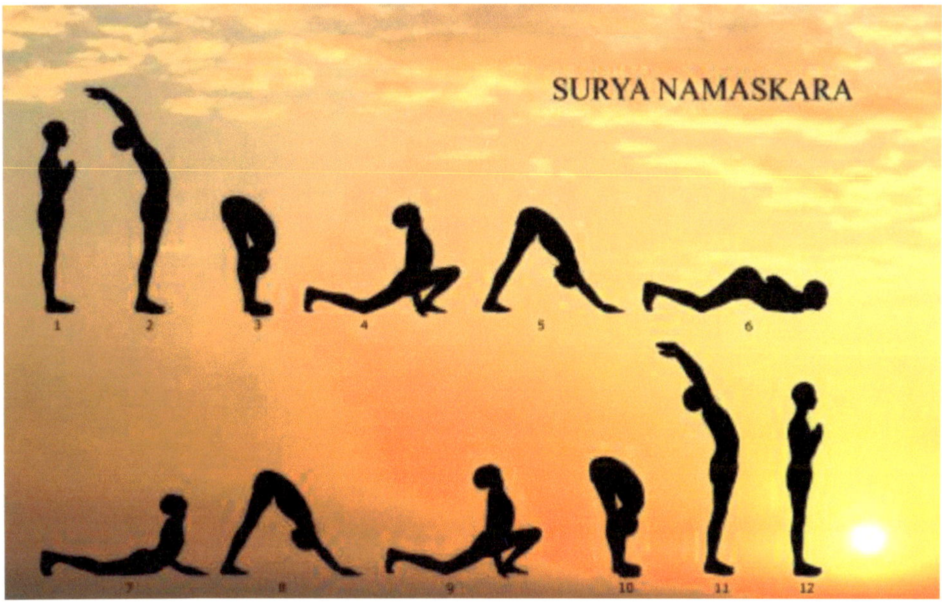

Figure 2. Postures of Surya Namaskara [5]

- Yoga-nidra with drug regimen had better control in their fluctuating blood glucose and symptoms associated with diabetes, compared to those were on oral hypoglycaemics alone. [13]
- Yoga asanas and pranayama improve glycaemic control and pulmonary functions [10].

Moreover, yoga practice was shown to improve pre-existing complication for those diabetic patients. Importantly, Yoga have a role even in prevention of diabetes. Yoga helps improving mind, body and spirit, leading to well-being and increased lovingly [15]. This may be due to mechanisms of reduction in stress and increase relaxations or noninvasive nature.

3.2. Bikram yoga

Bikram yoga is a system of yoga that Bikram Choudhury synthesized from traditional hatha yoga techniques [17] and popularized beginning in the early 1970s [18, 19]. Bikram Yoga sessions run for exactly 90 minutes and consist of a set series of 26 postures including 2 breathing exercises [20]. Bikram Yoga is ideally practiced in a room heated to 105°F (≈ 40.6°C) with a humidity of 40%,.

Bikram is a newer form of the practice that benefits blood circulation, improves cardiovascular conditioning and improves detoxification by increasing perspiration.

3.3. Koga

Koga combines the stretching and strengthening of Yoga with the cardiovascular workout of Kickboxing. Like yoga, Koga connects body with mind, and maintaining balance throughout.

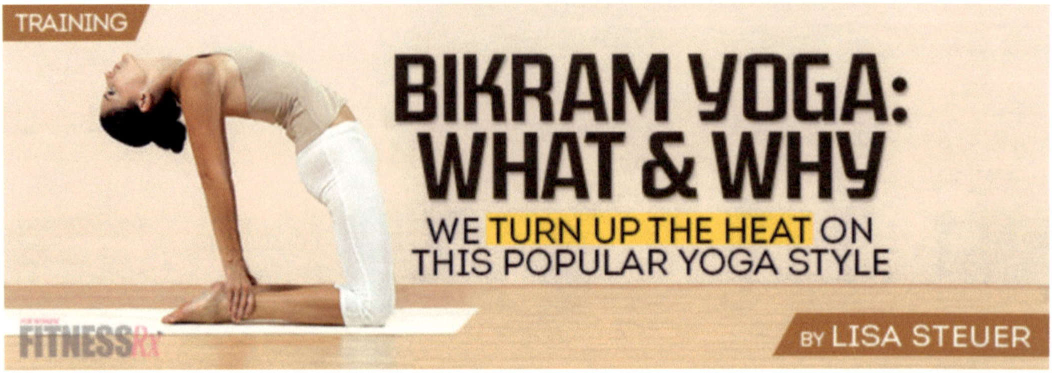

Figure 3. A posture of Bikram yoga [16]

Practicing Koga can help improve flexibility, increase muscle toning, relieve stress, increase lung capacity and decrease overall body fat.

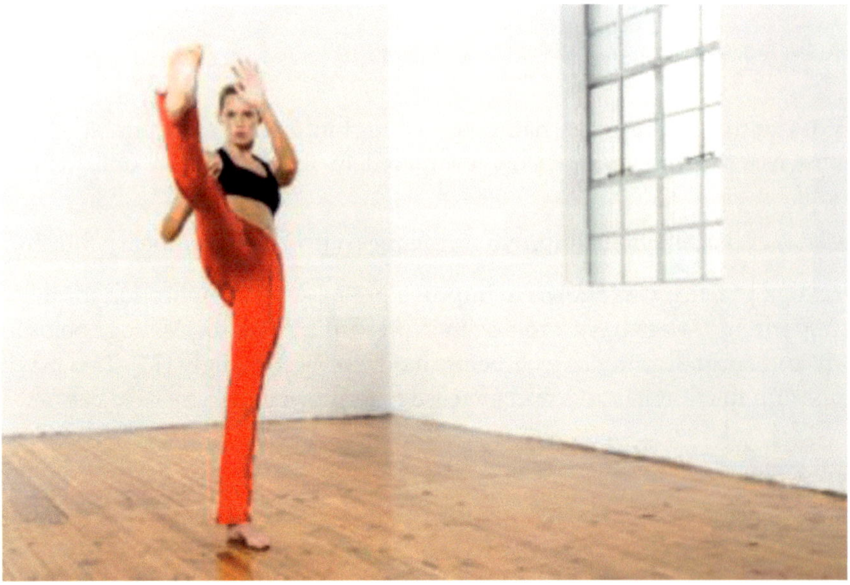

Figure 4. A posture of Koga [21]

3.4. Tai Chi

The Chinese characters for Tai Chi Chuan can be translated as the 'Supreme Ultimate Force' which is often associated with the Chinese concept of yin-yang, the notion that one can see a dynamic duality in all things. Tai Chi, can be thought of as a moving form of yoga and meditation combined. Many of these movements are originally derived from the martial arts although the way they are performed in Tai Chi is slowly, softly and gracefully with smooth and even transitions between them. Tai Chi is also situated in a wider philosophical context of Taoism. This is a reflective, mystical Chinese tradition first associated with the scholar and mystic Lao Tsu, an older contemporary of Confucius. He taught in the province of Honan in the 6th century B.C. and authored the seminal work of Taoism, the Tao Te Ching.

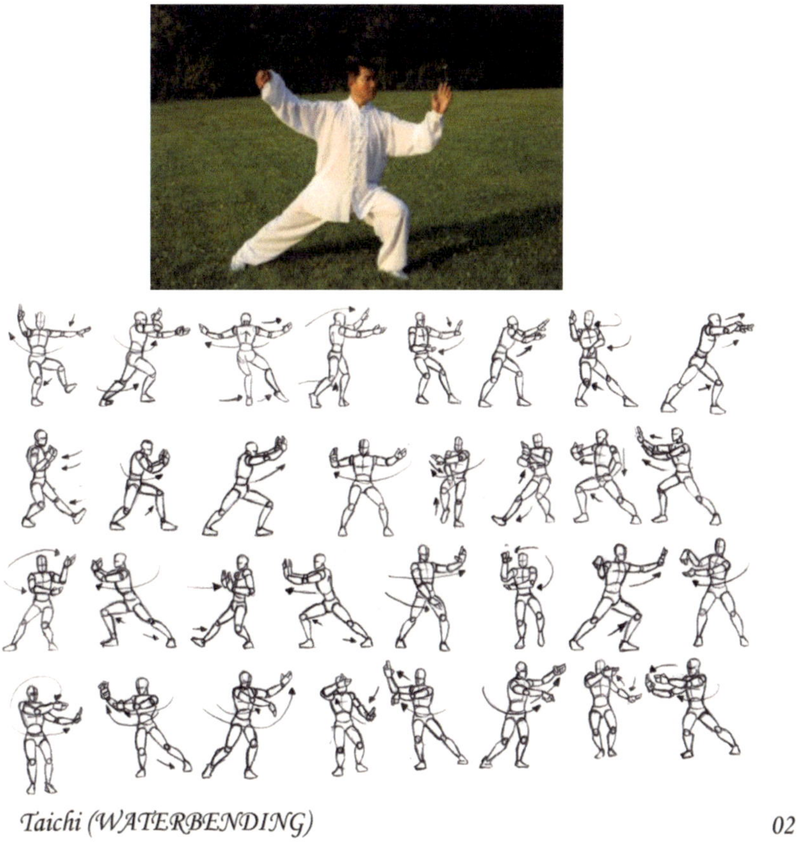

Figure 5. Postures and movements of Taichi [22]

Tai chi was shown to have many beneficial effects as the following;

- Improved indicators of health related quality of life (HR-QOL) including physical functioning, role physical, bodily pain and vitality in people with elevated blood glucose or diabetes who were not on diabetes medication [23]
- Improvements in fasting blood glucose and peripheral nerve conduction velocities [24].
- Improvements in physical and social functioning [25]
- Improvements in many parameters, such as BMI, lipid profile, C-reactive protein, and malondialdehyde [26]

- Preventing and improving psychological health and was associated with general health benefits for older people [27]
- Tai chi for those with type 2 diabetes could be an alternative exercise intervention to increase glucose control, diabetic self-care activities, and quality of life [28].

However, few studies did not support these beneficial effects of Tai chi [29]. Most of the studies are based on within group changes rather than attention control group comparisons [27].

3.5. Thai yoga (TY)

TY is a traditional form of exercise which appears to be a very light- to light-intensity exercise and have a low-impact alternative to jogging and walking for elderly individuals and requires no special equipment. TY may also have benefits in terms of stress management stemming from the meditation, relaxation and message aspects of the system. If individuals perform TY for longer duration especially standing position, they may gain benefits including reduction in cardiovascular mortality, reduction of symptoms, improvement in exercise tolerance and function capacity, and improvement in psychological well-being and quality of life [32].

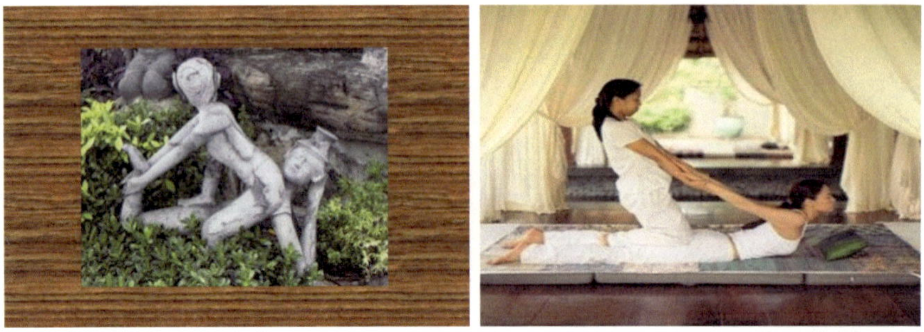

Figure 6. Postures of Thai yoga [30] [31]

3.6. Thai wand exercise

General health perceptions subscale of health related quality of life, functional capacity, body flexibility and obesity can be improved by Thai Wand Exercise training in older individuals [33]. This may partly reduce some cardiovascular disease risk factors. An advantage of this form of exercise is that this is a convenient, low impact on the joints and effective at home fitness program, with the only equipment need, a four feet long stick. But the major attraction is that it is also suited for the elderly who are not allegeable for the common training procedures.

3.7. Martial arts

Most people who are concerned with fitness often overlooked the martial arts. Besides learning to fight, it provides a true total body workout with improving core, upper and lower body strength. The core muscle generated the power in kicking and punching techniques. Impor-

http://dx.doi.org/10.5772/56610

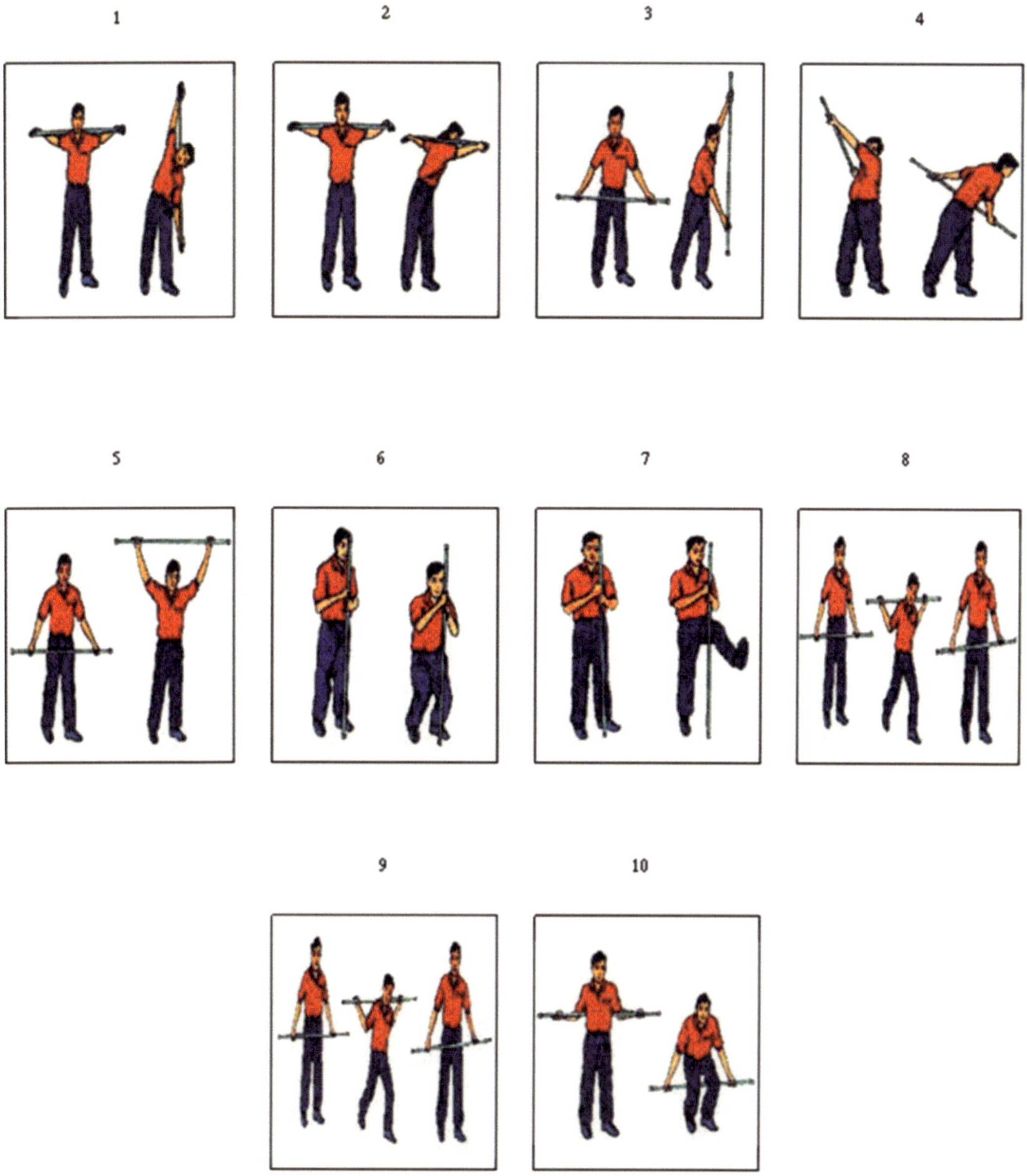

Figure 7. Postures and movements of Thai wand exercise

tantly, its training provides other benefits that are simply not found in an exercise class. First, it can help protecting someone from danger. It can also improve confidence and self-discipline which may change someone's life. Finally, it creates the friendships during training.

Example; Boxing-chaiya, Muay Thai, Chinese martial art, Judo, TaeKwonDo

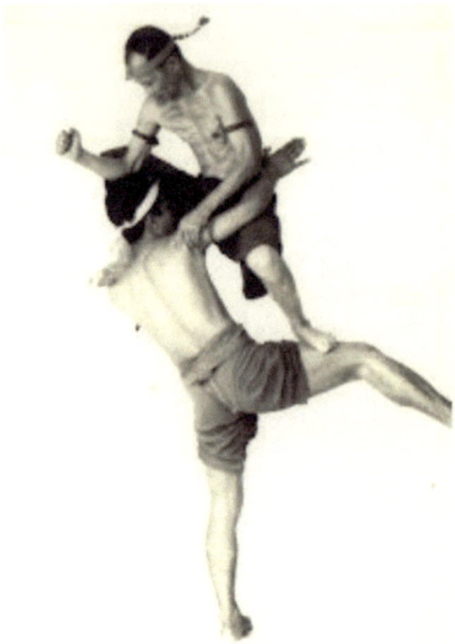

Figure 8. A posture of Boxing-chaiya [34]

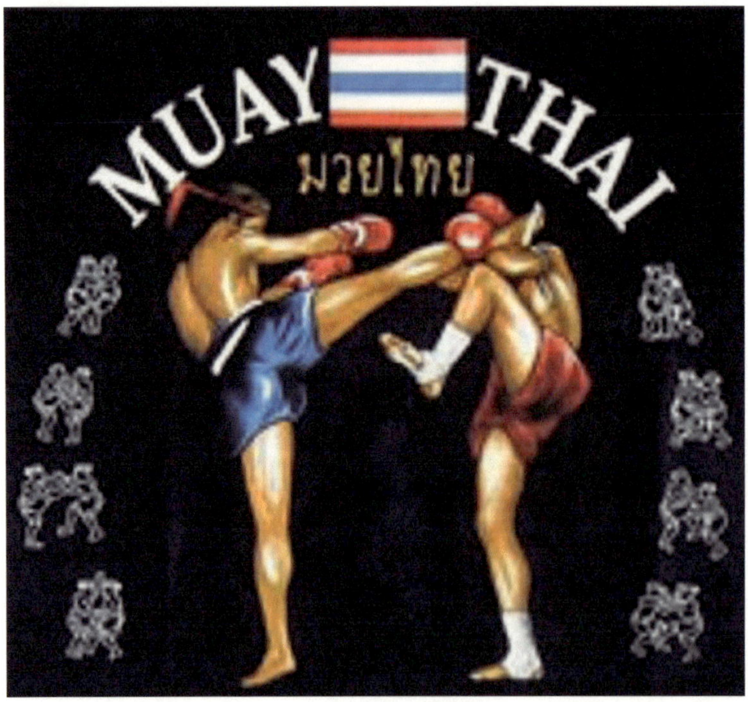

Figure 9. A posture of Muay Thai [35]

http://dx.doi.org/10.5772/56610

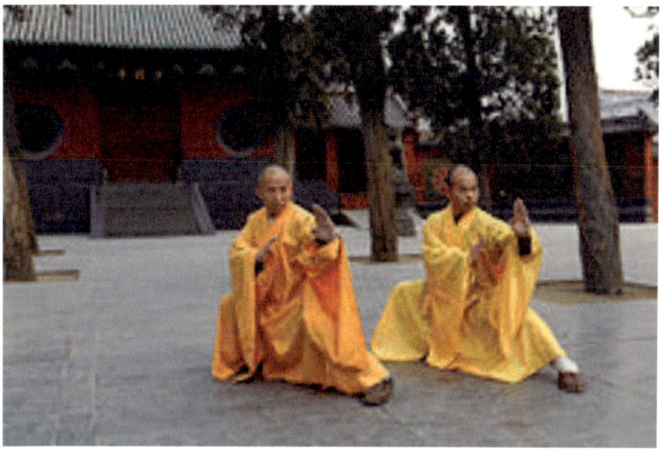

Figure 10. A posture of Chinese martial art [36]

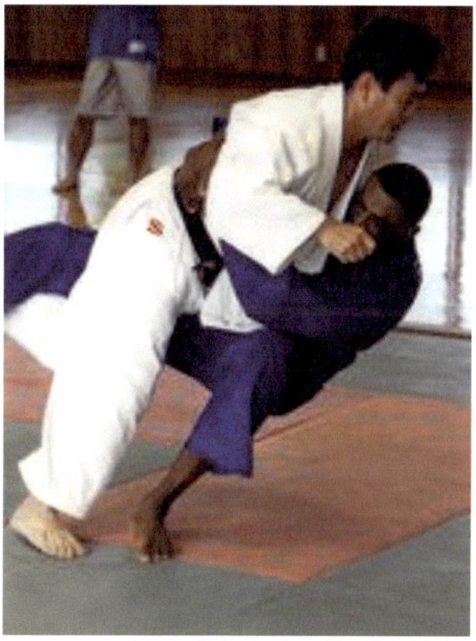

Figure 11. A posture of Judo [37]

3.8. Dancing

Dancing burns 2015 kilojoules an hour. It was shown to reduce risks for heart disease and diabetes in elementary school children [41]. Dancing 2 times per week for 12 weeks can reduce systolic BP and body fat in diabetes [42].

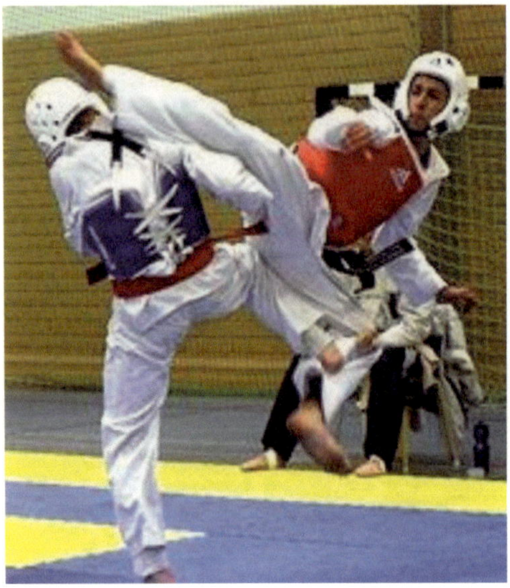

Figure 12. A posture of Taekwondo [38]

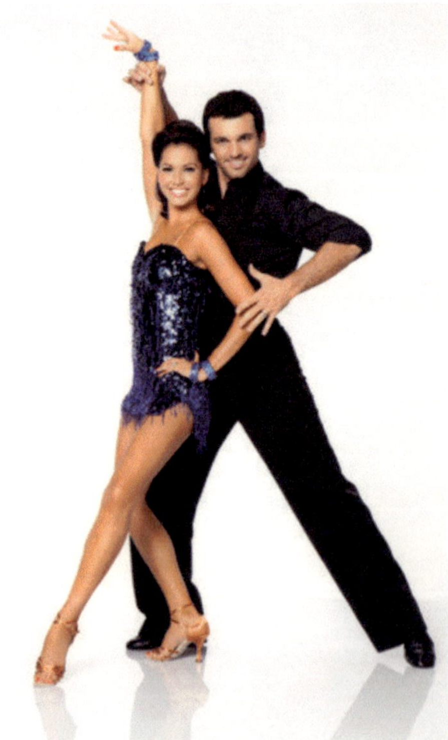

Figure 13. A posture of dancing [39]

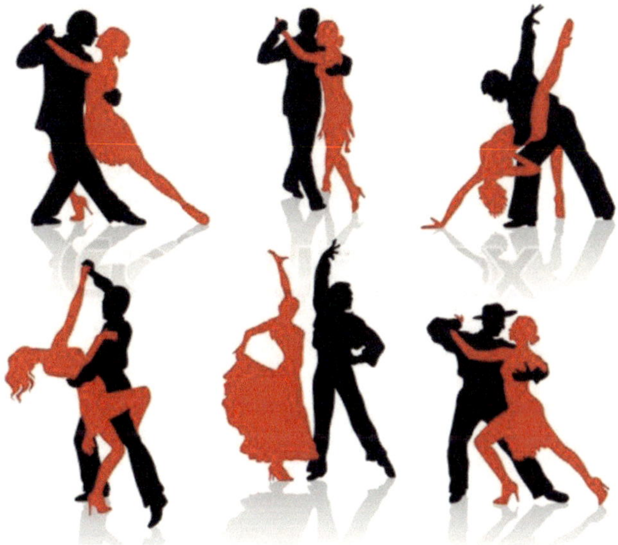

Figure 14. Postures of dancing [40]

3.9. Walking

Walking is recommended for preventing or treating diabetes patients [43]. However, walking with others can actually help patients stick with their health and fitness goals [44].

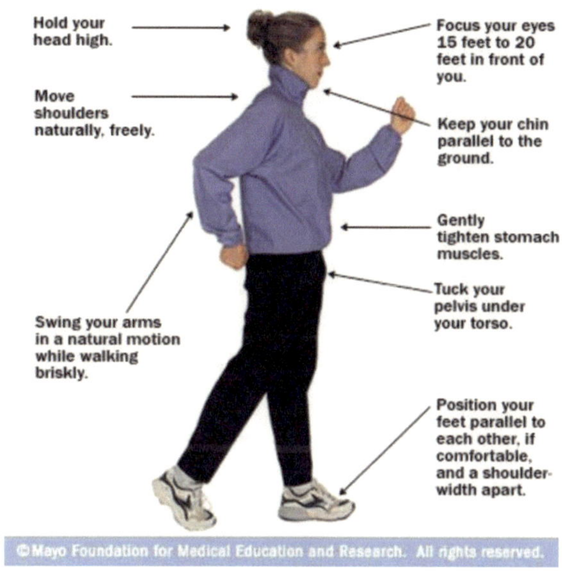

Figure 15. Detail of various postures and movements during walking

3.9.1. Brisk walking

The prescription of brisk walking represents an equally effective intervention to modulate glycaemic control and cardiovascular risk profile in type 2 diabetes patients when compared with more individualised medical fitness programmes. The Centers for Disease Control and Prevention (CDC) defined that brisk walking is at a pace of three miles per hour or more (but not race walking) or roughly 20 minutes per mile. This equates to about five kilometers per hour or 12 minutes per kilometer [45]. The exercise intensity of Brisk walking is moderate which heart rate is about 50-70% maximum heart rate or shouldn't be able to sing.

3.10. Go Ape

An exciting range of forest-based high-wire activities, comprise challenging courses that involve climbing, zip wires, balance beams and a whole range of fun-filled activities [47].

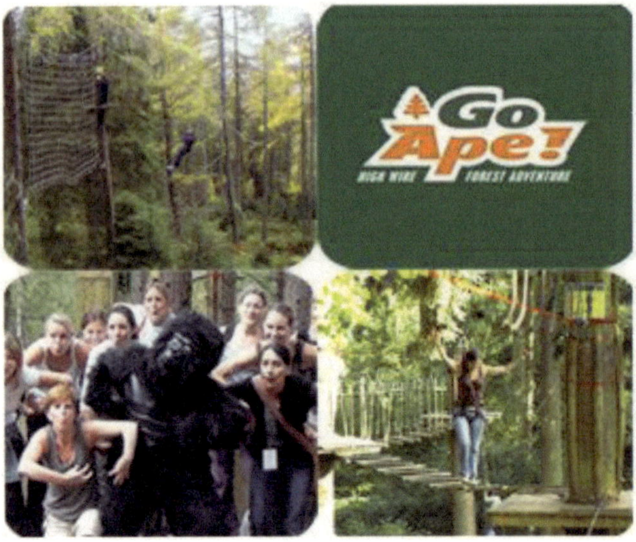

Figure 16. Different activities of Go Ape [46]

This activity lasts for 2 to 3 hours which some stamina to complete the course is needed. Upper body and legs will get benefit from this activity. Arm and leg flexibility will be maintained stretching and reaching for hand-holds along the course. Coordination will be definitely improved because of continually coordinating hands and feet as traverse the various obstacles.

3.11. Dinghy sailing

Dinghy sailing is the activity of sailing small boats by using five essential controls: [47]

- The sails

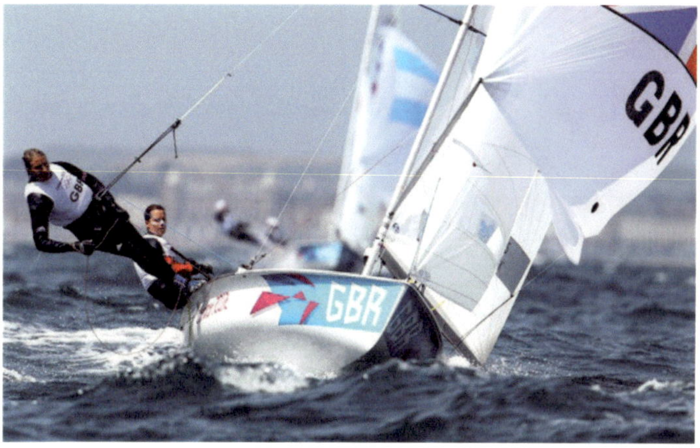

Figure 17. Movement of the crew during Dinghy sailing [48]

- The foils (i.e. the daggerboard or centreboard and rudder and sometimes lifting foils as found on the Moth).
- The trim (forward/rear angle of the boat in the water)
- Side to side balance of the dinghy by movement of the crew, particularly in windy weather ("move fast or swim").
- The choice of route (in terms of existing and anticipated wind shifts, possible obstacles, other water traffic, currents, tides etc.).

Dinghy sailing increases stamina because of the vigorous sailing especially shifting position to balance the boat. Rigging and de-rigging to hauling on the sheets increase upper body strength. Additionally, if there is a less stable boat situation abdominal and back muscles will be stimulated. Good flexibility is very necessary for dinghy sailing. Having a good range of movement and being able to stretch during balancing against the wind is vital. Successful small boat sailing requires because of frequently hauling on the sheets, tacking, shifting position and balancing all at the same time. This will certainly improve coordination.

3.12. Horse riding

Training of horse riding can increase insulin sensitivity in patients with diabetes type 2 [51, 52].

Generally, horse riding increases stamina according to maintaining an upright posture while continually controlling a moving horse at speed. It also strengthens core muscles in order to control horse's movements while maintaining an upright posture. However, there are few flexibility benefits from horse riding, but a good measure of all-round mobility to successfully riding is still needed. Coordination is important for marrying up small body movements with control of the reins — plus hand-to-eye coordination will be required during negotiating trails and obstacles [47].

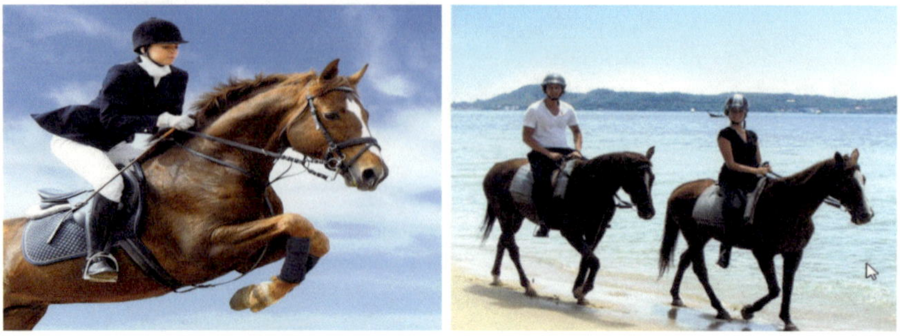

Figure 18. Upright postures during Horse riding [49] [50]

3.13. Fishing

During fishing, endurance is important for spending the best part of a day standing in a river, walking up and down a beach or fighting with a really big specimen for a few hours. Leg strength is increased from continually working a fly at full stretch. Casting a line is a skill that needs excellent arm and shoulder flexibility so upper body flexibility in particular will be improved by fishing. Casting the line and controlling the rod when reeling fish in requires good hand-to-eye coordination.

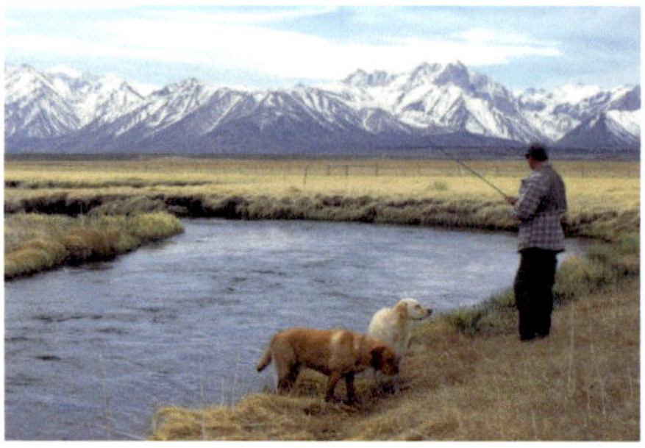

Figure 19. Standing posture during Fishing [53]

3.14. Lunge walking

The following is the movement of Lunge walking [54]:

- Stand upright, feet together, holding two light (5-8 pound) dumbbells at your sides (palms facing in).
- Take a controlled step forward with your left leg.
- Lower hips toward the floor and bend both knees (almost at 90 degree angles). The back knee should come close but never touch the ground. Your front knee should be directly over the ankle and the back knee should be pointing down toward the floor.

- Push off the weight with your right foot and bring it forward to starting position (#1). This completes one rep.
- Next step forward and repeat with the right leg.
- Do 2 sets of 15 reps.

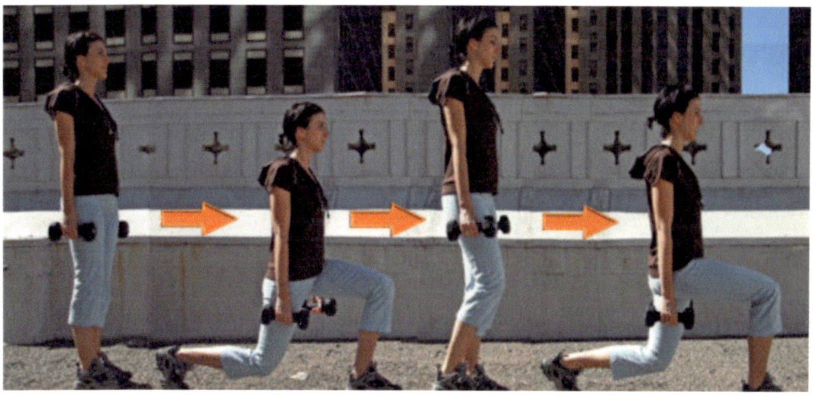

Figure 20. Series of movements of Lunge walking [54]

3.15. Make the most of the outdoors

Activities outdoors such as park benches, the kerb, and stairs for simple exercises are health benefit according to exposure to sun shine.

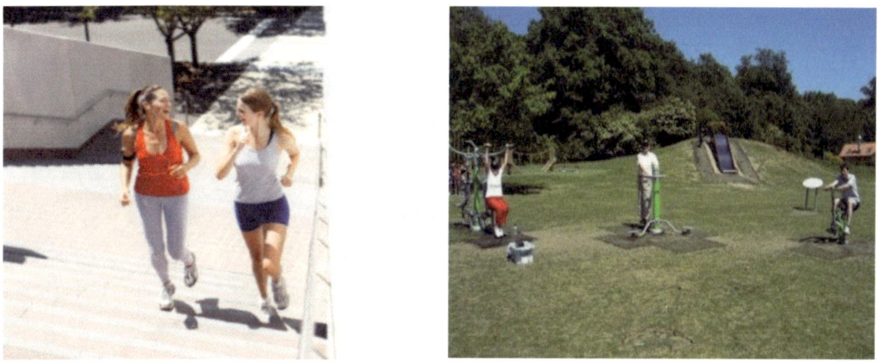

Figure 21. Activities outdoors such as park benches, and stairs [55] [56]

3.16. Surf

Feel the sun on your face and the thrill of catching waves along beautiful coastlines.

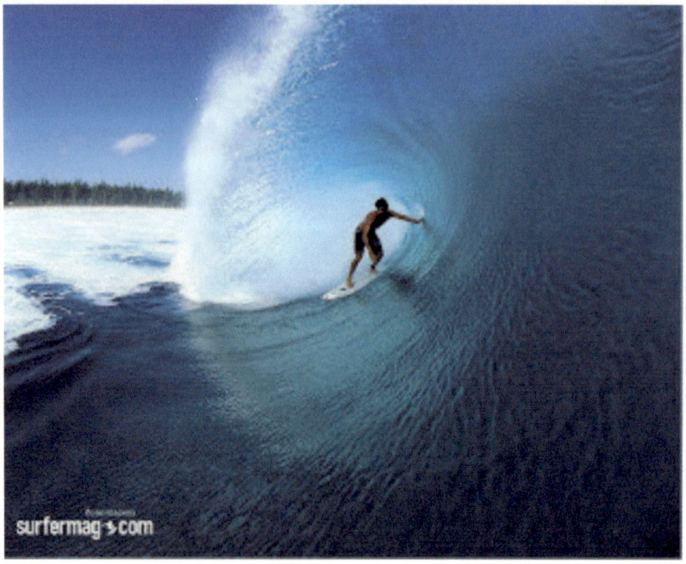

Figure 22. A posture under the wave during surfing [57]

3.17. Cardio tennis

Cardio Tennis is a new kind of group exercise that combines endurance with tennis skills. It includes thinking how to hit a backhand, followed by footwork exercises on a rope ladder and running drills. Then it's back to the volley line and hitting balls again. It was started in the US by the Tennis Industry Association as a way to get more people into tennis, but the programme has since rolled out to 1500 work-out sites in 25 countries.

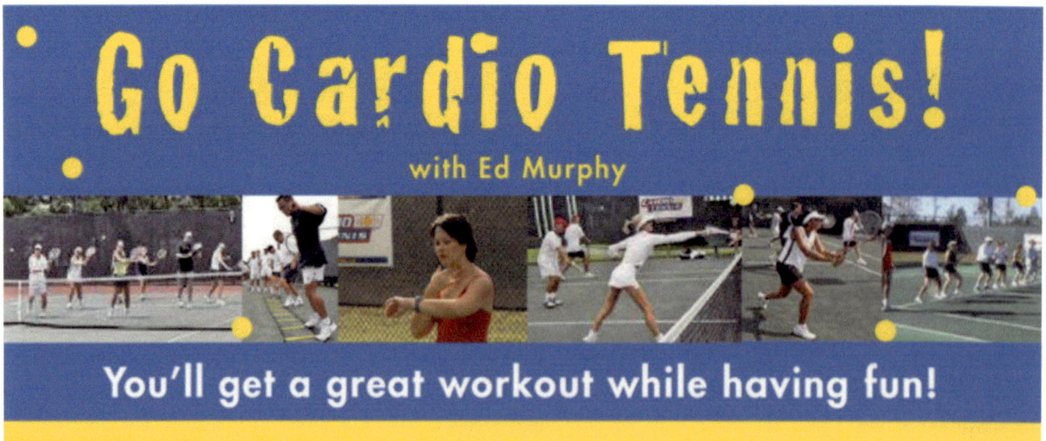

Figure 23. Activities of Cardio Tennis [58]

Each class includes 5-10 minutes warm-up segment including stretching and footwork drills and 50-55 minutes cardio segment including fun drills [58].

It provides:

- Much more fun than working out on a machine
- It's a fun group activity for advanced beginner and above players
- Elevate your heart rate into your aerobic training zone
- The focus is on getting a great workout while having fun!

3.18. Housework

Housework is so useful because it both increases energy expenditure, cardiovascular response and tidy a house. But if someone have balance problems, they must be careful going downstairs. It's very easy to fall, especially when carrying a vacuum cleaner. Whenever you see a set of stairs, use them. If there's time (and you're really enthusiastic), go back down and climb them again. If flexibility and balance aren't an issue, take two steps at a time.

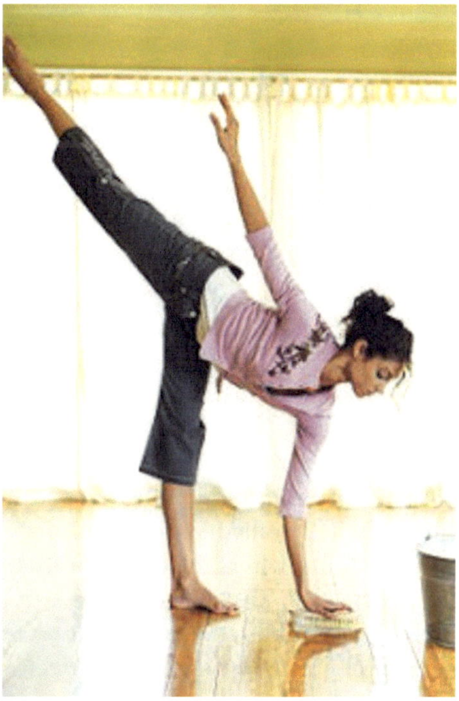

Figure 24. A posture of Housework [59]

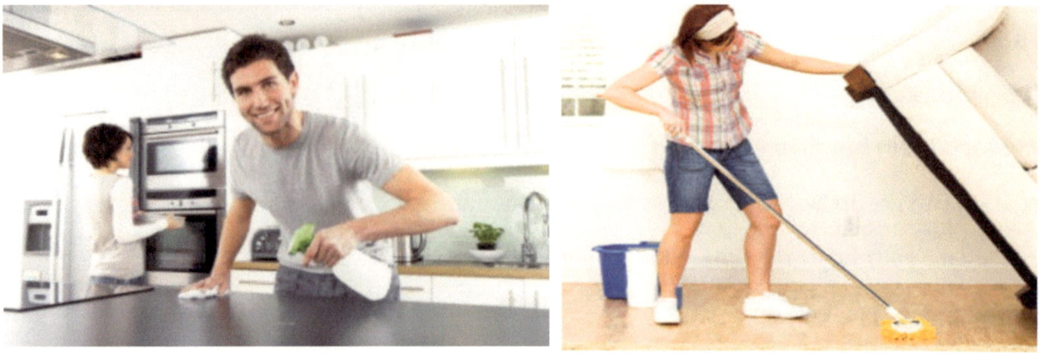

Figure 25. Activities of Housework [60] [61]

3.19. Alexander technique

Invented by an Australian in the 1890s, this technique helps to restore the body's capacity for ease by releasing tension, particularly in the head and neck. It aims to allow the body to reach its full potential.

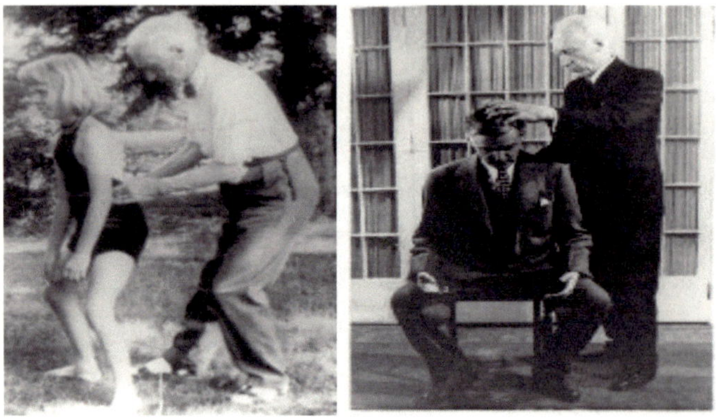

Figure 26. Alexander Technique [62]

"The Alexander Technique is a way of learning to move mindfully through life. The Alexander process shines a light on inefficient habits of movement and patterns of accumulated tension, which interferes with our innate ability to move easily and according to how we are designed. It's a simple yet powerful approach that offers the opportunity to take charge of one's own learning and healing process, because it's not a series of passive treatments but an active exploration that changes the way one thinks and responds in activity. It produces a skill set that can be applied in every situation. Lessons leave one feeling lighter, freer, and more grounded." [62]

The Alexander technique has been shown to be helpful for back pain and Parkinson's [63].

http://dx.doi.org/10.5772/56610

3.20. Feeldenkrais method

Developed in the 1940s, Moshé Feldenkrais (1904–1984) is a practical discipline to help develop awareness of body movement [65]. Feldenkrais aims to reduce pain or limitations in movement, to improve physical function, and to promote general wellbeing by increasing students' awareness of themselves and by expanding students' movement repertoire [66].

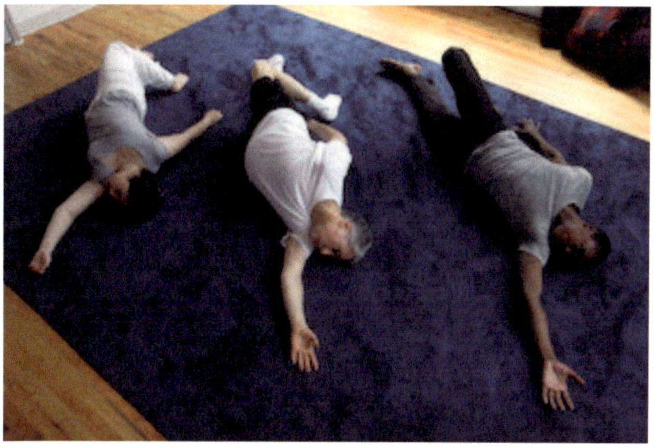

Figure 27. A posture of Feeldenkrais method [64]

3.21. Pilates

Invented in the early 20th century by Joseph Pilates, Pilates combines East and West, gymnastic and yogic principles, mind and body [70]. Pilates is a body conditioning routine that may help build flexibility, muscle strength, and endurance in the legs, abdominals, arms, hips, and back. It puts emphasis on spinal and pelvic alignment, breathing, and developing a strong core or center, and improving coordination and balance. Pilates' system allows for different exercises to be modified in range of difficulty from beginning to advance. Intensity can be increased over time as the body conditions and adapts to the exercises [71].

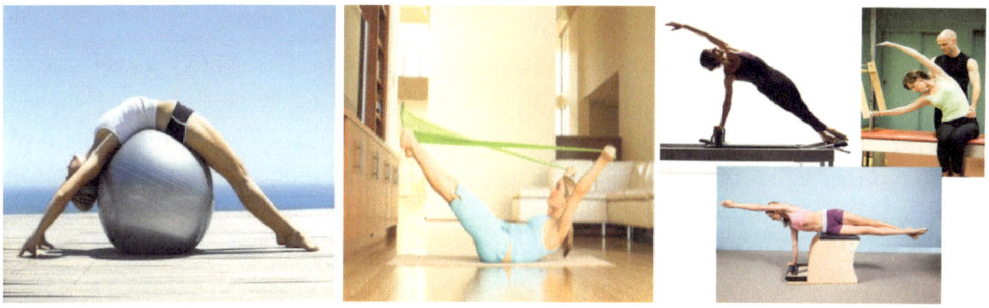

Figure 28. Postures of Pilates [67] [67] [68]

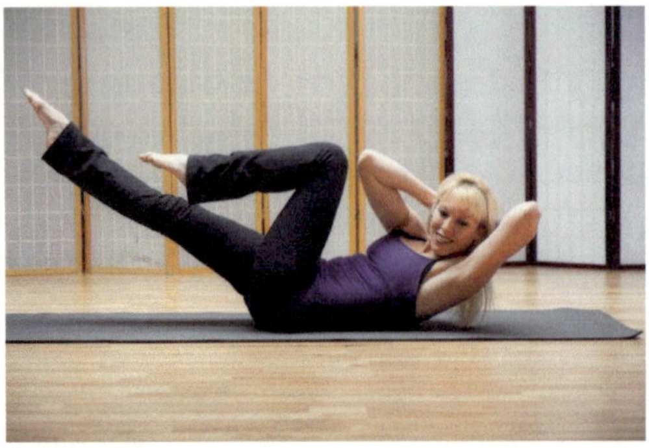

Figure 29. A posture of Pilates [69]

4. Beneficial effects of arm swing exercise on glycaemic control and oxidative stress in patients with diabetes type II [72]

4.1. Introduction

Although moderate exercise (mostly are western style e.g. swimming, running or aerobic dance) at least 30 minutes for five days per week was recommended to prevent cardiovascular disease in diabetes patients [2], it is difficult to encourage them to exercise regularly. Many Asian styles of exercise such as arm swing exercise seem to be more appropriate because of its simple, low impact to joint and easily accessible exercise.

Arm Swing Exercise (ASE) is a traditional Chinese exercise [73] which is convenient for diabetes patients to perform. It is believed to improve cardiovascular systems. However there were no scientific data concerning the beneficial effect and mechanism of this exercise on the glycaemic control. Therefore, this study aimed to investigate effects of the ASE training on blood glucose (glycated haemoglobin; HbA_{1c}), oxidant (determined by malondialdehyde; MDA) and antioxidant (determined by glutathione; GSH) in subjects with type 2 diabetes.

4.2. Experimental design and protocol

All subjects performed 2 study periods consecutively; i) maintaining daily life without regular exercise for 8 weeks (week 1-8) ii) performing 30-min ASE per day, 3 days per week for 8 weeks (week 9-16). Fasting blood glucose, HbA_{1c}, insulin, lipid profiles, C reactive protein (CRP), MDA and reduced GSH concentrations were analyzed using blood samples collected from the antecubetal vein. Anthropometry and body composition were also measured before and after of each study period. HbA_{1c} was used to determine glycaemic control because it is more stable throughout 2-3 months and related to the complications.

Insulin sensitivity was determined using Homeostatic Model Assessment – Insulin Resistance (HOMA-IR) [74]. Pharmacology, dietary and exercise treatment, were not modified during the study period. During the exercise period, patients performed the ASE program as prescribed. They were requested to record the 24-hour dietary composition and energy expenditure for 2 weekdays and 1 weekend day before the start and the last week of each period.

4.3. Arm Swing Exercise (ASE)

ASE is a traditional Chinese exercise which has been practiced for 50 years (Figure 1) and claimed for treatment of cancer and alimentary disorders by increasing blood flow [73]. The number of swing was 200 or 300 repetitions in the beginning and gradually increased to 1000-2000 repetitions or up to half an hour depending on the strength of the patients. The intensity of ASE is mild because it was around 23 percentage of maximal oxygen consumption and 45 percentage of maximal heart rate.

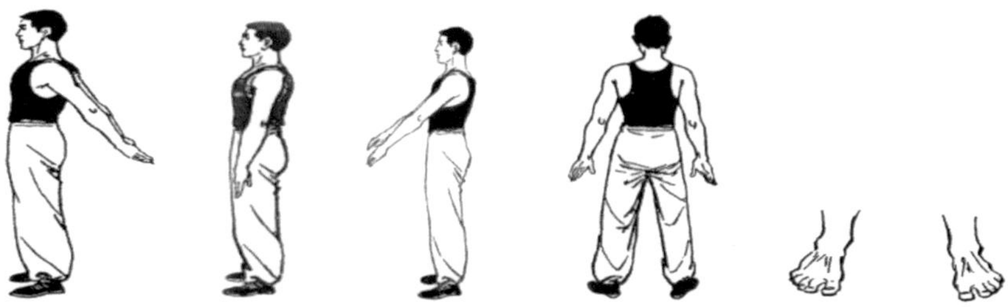

Figure 30. Postures and movements of body during the ASE

During ASE period participants learned to perform the ASE correctly on the first day of the experiment. For the next 8 weeks they performed the training at home via a video tape recording one session per day (30 minutes), 3 days/week. Each participant was telephoned every week to check their compliance to the program and to emphasize them to maintain their usual daily physical activity apart from the ASE program.

4.4. Statistical analysis

All dependent variables were analyzed using a two-way ANOVA with repeated measures (within subject factors were exercise and time) by Sigma Stat version 2 program. The Bonferroni method was used to adjust the multiple comparisons. A probability of $p<0.05$ was taken to indicate significance. Results are presented as means SE.

4.5. Results

Nine male and 33 female patients with type 2 diabetes mellitus completed the study. Before the experiment, they had high cardiovascular risks such as hyperglycaemia, overweight or obesity (based on criteria of World Health Organization Western Pasific region), high fasting blood glucose, haemoglobin A1c (HbA_{1c}), high sensitive C reactive protein (hsCRP), MDA and low reduced glutathione (GSH) concentrations. There were no differences in body mass, body mass index, fat mass, fat free mass, waist circumference, hip circumference, waist to hip circumference ratio, and physiological characteristics between the two periods. Mean daily dietary intakes were similar in both periods (1,468.6 ± 58.6 kJ and 1,462.2 ± 56.0 kJ; control and exercise periods, respectively). Mean energy expenditure in the exercise period was significantly higher than that in the control period (1,593.4 ± 54.6 and 1,472.7 ± 47.6 kJ, respectively; $p<0.05$).

4.6. Clinical chemistry

HbA_{1c} concentration was 0.2% lower after ASE training for 8 weeks compared with the control period ($p<0.05$, Table 1). However, there was no significant difference in fasting blood glucose between periods. There were no effect of ASE training on insulin sensitivity, hsCRP concentration and lipid profiles between periods

4.7. Oxidative stress

ASE training significantly reduced plasma MDA concentration ($p<0.05$) and increased antioxidant blood GSH concentration ($p<0.05$). No correlation between oxidative stress and HbA_{1c} at any periods was found.

4.8. Discussion

The results showed that the ASE training improves glycaemic control and oxidative stress in patients with type 2 diabetes. Thus, this simple and accessible exercise may have a potential effect on the prevention of complications of diabetes mellitus.

Previous studies also found the decreased HbA_{1c} after the arm exercise training [75-77]. Jeng et al (2002) have reported that arm exercise training for 10-40 min could induce a significant decrease in the HbA_{1c} concentration in patients with type 2 DM. Data from the United Kingdom Prospective Diabetes Study Group (UKPDS) have suggested that a 1% rise in HbA_{1c} concentration represents a 37% increased risk for microvascular complications (95% CI 33 to 41, $P < 0.0001$) [78]. Based on this information, a 0.2% decrease in HbA_{1c} after the ASE training detected in this study may reduce 7.4% of risk for microvascular complications.

Possible mechanisms that could explain for the benefit effect of the ASE training on improving glycaemic control include the reduced HbA_{1c} and the effect of exercise per se on improving the oxidative stress. The reduced HbA_{1c} may decrease many adverse effects of hyperglycaemia such as hyperglycaemia-induced glucose autoxidation, non-enzymatic glycation of proteins, and reactive oxygen species generation, in leading to the progression of diabetic vascular complications. These processes were shown to increase oxidant stress and decrease antioxidant agent [79-81]. The imbalance of oxidative stress with greater oxidant stress contributed to the cellular destruction and therefore vascular complications [82]. The decreased MDA found in this study indicated a reduction in lipid peroxidation, a process of oxidative stress, which then reflects an attenuation of the cellular damage in the patients. The increased level of non-enzymatic antioxidant GSH after the ASE training observed in the present study also supports the preventive effect of exercise on vascular complication. As found in the present study, the improved glycaemic control positively indicate a preventive action of ASE training in the vascular complications in type 2 diabetic patients via the improved oxidative stress [82].

The second mechanism is due to the effect of exercise per se on improving the oxidative stress. This is supported by the absence of relationship between HbA_{1c} and MDA and GSH at any periods in this study. Importantly, this may remind that only improvement of HbA_{1c} from medication or diet control may not be enough to prevent the complication. Previous studies in both animal and human also supports that low-intensity exercise could itself improve oxidative stress [83-86]. Moien-Afshari et al have confirmed that the low-intensity exercise could enhance antioxidant agent giving rise to less endothelial dysfunction independently on the improvement of hyperglycaemia.

The present study showed that ASE has no adverse effects such as exercise-related injury or hypoglycaemia. This was shown by the similar level of CRP in both periods. Therefore ASE is appropriate and safe for the patient with diabetes. The other strength of the present study is a study design which each subject performed both control and exercise periods. This eliminates the effect of inter-individual variation.

4.9. Conclusion

In conclusion, the present study showed that the ASE training, a low-intensity exercise contribute to protective effects on vascular complication which is a major problem of type 2 diabetic patients. This may attribute to an improved oxidative stress according to either improved glycaemic control or exercise per se. The major attraction is that it is suited for not only diabetic patients but also other people who are not allegeable for the common training procedures such as elderly adults and patients with lower limb disorders.

5. Beneficial mechanisms of exercise on type 2 diabetic patients

There are many possible mechanisms explaining the beneficial effects of exercise training on type 2 diabetic patients (T2D).

These are described based on their roles.

6. Improve glucose control

6.1. Insulin-independent mechanism

1. Exercise leads to an insulin independent increase in glucose transport, mediated in part by AMP activated protein kinase. Changes in protein expression may be related to increased signal transduction through the mitogen-activated protein kinase (MAPK) signaling cascades, a pathway known to regulate transcriptional activity [87].

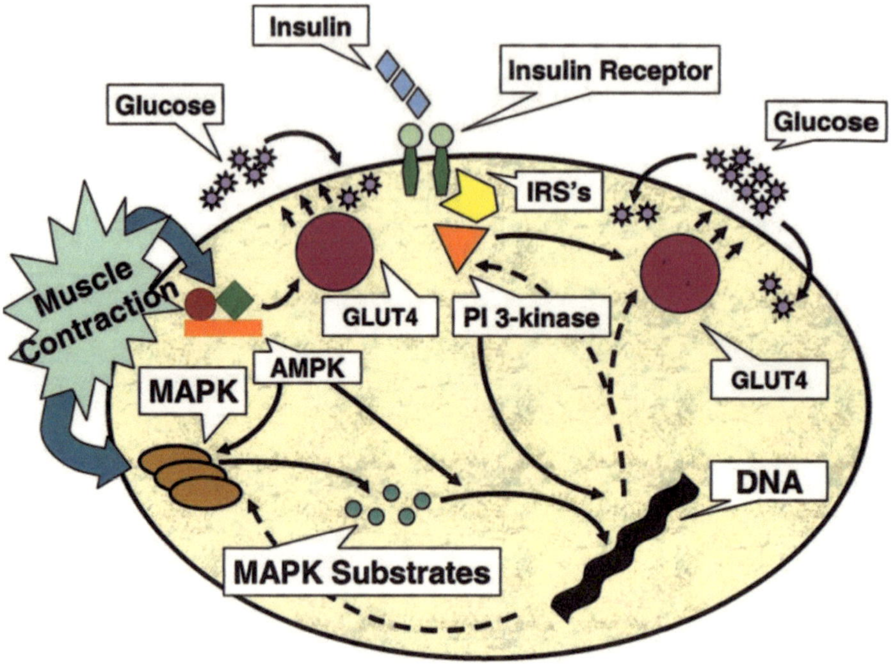

Figure 31. Exercise training-induced changes in insulin signaling via insulin-independent pathway in skeletal muscle [87].

2. Exercise increased skeletal muscle c-Jun N-terminal kinase (JNK) activity throughout the experiment, whereas insulin did not significantly increase JNK activity. The p38 activity was slightly stimulated by exercise and not by insulin [88]. However, the other previous study noted that exercise training improves basal glucose metabolism without a change in the stress kinases, JNK, the nuclear factor B (NF-B) pathway and Hsp72. Moreover, nuclear regulation of NF-B activity in diabetic muscle could be regulated independently of the cytosolic pathway [89].

3. The sodium-dependent glucose co-transporter system (hSGLT3), an insulin-independent glucose transporter, is activated by exercise and it may play a significant role in improving glycemic control [90].

4. Exercise training increases insulin-stimulated glucose disposal primarily by increasing GLUT4 protein expression without enhancing insulin-stimulated PI 3-kinase signaling, and that once the glucose enters the myocyte, increased glycogen synthase activity preferentially shunts it into glycogen synthesis [91].

6.2. Insulin dependent mechanism

The beneficial effect of exercise training on the control of glucose via insulin signaling has been reviewed by many previous studies [92-94]. In addition, many studies investigated the effects of exercise

1. More recent observations indicate that interactions exist at the distal signaling level of AS160 and atypical protein kinase C (aPKC) [95].

2. Acute exercise reverses TRB3 expression and insulin signaling restoration in muscle. Thus, these results provide new insights into the mechanism by which physical activity ameliorates whole body insulin sensitivity in type 2 diabetes [96]. TRB3 is an inducible gene whose expression is regulated by stress response and insulin and associated with insulin resistance and metabolic syndrome.

3. Exercise training increases skeletal muscle Nicotinamide phosphoribosyltransferase (NAMPT) which is known as pre-B-cell colony-enhancing factor 1 (PBEF1) or visfatin, is an enzyme belonging to the family of glycosyltransferases, to be specific, the pentosyltransferases. NAMPT was reported to be an activate insulin receptor and has insulin-mimetic effects, lowering blood glucose and improving insulin sensitivity [97].

4. Blood glucose concentration can be improved by exercise training-induced increases in muscle glycogen content. This could be regulated by multiple mechanisms, including enhanced insulin sensitivity, glycogen synthase expression, allosteric activation of glycogen synthase, and PP1 activity [98]. The increased muscle glycogen also plays important role in muscle strength [99]. This can improve glucose uptake and then glucose control.

5. Exercise overrules free fatty acid-mediated inhibition of pyruvate dehydrogenase (i.e., carbohydrate oxidation). This may improve carbohydrate oxidation although high fat was ingested [100]. The improved carbohydrate oxidation then enhances insulin sensitivity resulting in improved glucose control.

6. The metabolic outcomes were divided into six domains: glycogen, glucose facilitated transporter 4 (GLUT4) and insulin signaling, enzymes, markers of inflammation, lipids metabolism and so on. Beneficial adaptations to exercise were seen primarily in muscle fiber area and capillary density, glycogen, glycogen synthase and GLUT4 protein expressions [101]. This adaptation then play important role on improved glycaemic control.

7. Exercise training results in a persistent increase in insulin sensitivity in skeletal muscle from obese and insulin-resistant individuals [102]. Chronic exercise upregulated phosphorylation and expression of AMPK upstream kinase, LKB1. Particularly exercise reversed the changes in protein kinase C (PKC)ζ/λ phosphorylation, and PKCζ phosphorylation and expression. In addition, exercise also increased protein kinase B (PKB)/Akt1, Akt2 and GLUT4 expression, but AS160 protein expression was unchanged. Chronic exercise increased Akt (Thr (308)) and (Ser(473)) and AS160 phosphorylation. Finally, exercise increased peroxisome proliferator-activated receptor-γ coactivator 1 (PGC1) mRNA expression in the soleus of diabetic rats. These results indicate that both chronic and acute exercise influence the phosphorylation and expression of components of the AMPK and downstream to PIK3 (aPKC, Akt), and improve GLUT4 [103].

8. Exercise training reversed abnormality in subjects with type 2 diabetes i.e. increase in both IkappaB alpha and IkappaB beta protein, IkappaB alpha and IkappaB beta protein,

decrease in tumor necrosis factor alpha muscle content and an increase in insulin-stimulated glucose disposal [104].

9. Training significantly improved glucose tolerance in obese humans [105]. This may be benefit in control blood glucose concentration leading to prevention for patients diabetes type II.

10. Both moderate- and vigorous-intensity exercise training improved beta-cell function to the extent that the disposition index (DI) accurately reflects beta-cell function. Although through distinct mechanisms [106] were modeled from an intravenous glucose tolerance test. [DI = S(i) x AIRg (insulin sensitivity (S(i)), acute insulin response to glucose (AIRg)]

11. In diabetic rats, exendin-4 and exercise stimulate insulin receptor substrate (IRS)-2 expression [107, 108] through the activation of cAMP responding element binding protein in the islets [109]. This enhanced their insulin/insulin like growth factor-1 signaling. The potentiation of the signaling increased the expression of pancreas duodenum homeobox-1, involved in beta-cell proliferation. In conclusion, exendin-4 and exercise equivalently improved glucose homeostasis due to the induction of IRS-2 in the islets of diabetic rats through a cAMP dependent common pathway.

12. Exercise training substantially reduces the exposure of islets to exogenous lipid, thereby providing a potential mechanism by which exercise can prevent islet beta-cell failure leading to diabetes type 2 [110].

13. Exercise may have beneficial effects via monocyte since monocyte peroxisome proliferator activated receptors gamma (PPARγ) activation has been linked to beneficial antidiabetic effects. This is supported by the association between exercise-induced upregulation of monocytic PPARγ-controlled genes and reverse cholesterol transport and anti-inflammatory effects. Thus, exercise-induced monocyte PPARγ activation may contribute to rationale for prescribing exercise to type 2 diabetes patients [111].

14. High-intensity progressive resistance training, in combination with moderate weight loss, effectively improved glycemic control in older patients with type 2 diabetes. This may result from increased muscle mass leading to increased glucose uptake [112].

6.3. Weight reduction

Swim training can effectively prevent body weight gain, adiposity and lipid disorders caused by leptin receptor deficiency, in part through activation of UCPs in adipose tissue and skeletal muscle [113]. The training also increased carnitine palmitoyl transferase (CPT I) activity and became less sensitive to inhibition by malonyl-CoA, reduced both total ceramide content. In addition, it improved capacity for mitochondrial FA uptake and oxidation leads not only to a reduction in muscle lipid content but also to change in the saturation status of lipids [114]. These may contribute to alleviating weight reduction for patients with diabetes type 2.

6.4. Normalization of blood lipid profiles

Decreases in total cholesterol, increases in HDL, oxidized LDL (oxLDL), leukocyte mRNA expression for PPARgamma which was reinforced by increased PPARgamma DNA-binding activity and gene expression were observed for the oxLDL scavenger receptor CD36 LXRalpha. Two LXRalpha-regulated genes involved in RCT, namely, ATP-binding cassette transporters A1 and GI (ABCA1 and ABCG1, respectively), were significantly up-regulated post-exercise [115].

6.5. Improved nitric oxide-mediated skeletal muscle blood flow

1. Exercise training improves endothelium-dependent vasodilator function, not only as a localised phenomenon in the contracting muscle group, but also as a systemic response when a relatively large mass of muscle is activated regularly during an exercise training program. Shear stress-mediated improvement in endothelial function provides one plausible explanation for the cardioprotective benefits of exercise training [116].

2. In addition to being a possible modulator of blood flow, nitric oxide (NO) from skeletal muscle regulates muscle contraction and metabolism. Recently, human data indicate that NO plays a role in muscle glucose uptake during exercise independently of blood flow. Exercise training in healthy individuals increased NO bioavailability through a variety of mechanisms including increased NOS enzyme expression and activity. This contributed to increased exercise capacity and cardiovascular protection. Exercise training with high cardiovascular risk can increase NO bioavailability and may represent an important mechanism by which exercise training takes benefit in the prevention [117].

6.6. Improvement of nervous system function

Progressive exercise training significantly decreases diabetes-associated neuropathic pain, including thermal hyperalgesia and mechanical allodynia. In rats, this protective effect is related to the increase of Hsp72, but not TNF-α and IL-6, expression in the spinal cord and peripheral nerves of STZ-induced diabetes. [118]

6.7. Improved oxidative stress

Acute exercise was reported to elevate Ox LDL, SOD and GSH-Px levels which are associated with in type 2 diabetic patients [119]. Exercise training including low-intensity exercise can increase antioxidant and decrease oxidant [72]

6.8. Prevention of microangiopathy

Mitochondrial oxidative capacity appears to be involved in the overall mechanism by which exercise prevents microangiopathy in rats with type 2 diabetes. Luminal capillary diameter of the diabetic group was significantly lower than that of the control group, succinic dehydrogenase (SDH) activity was significantly higher in the diabetic with exercise group than in the control and diabetic groups [120].

6.9. Improve metabolic control

Exercise training results in an increase in the oxidative capacity of skeletal muscle by up-regulating lipid oxidation and the expression of proteins involved in mitochondrial biogenesis. This decreased liver triacylglycerol content [121].

Acknowledgements

This study was supported by a grant from Thailand Research Fund (TRF). The authors appreciate Associate Professor Jongonnee Wattanapermpool for her excellent assistance with critical commentary and suggestions. The authors thank Assistant Professor Dr. Thongchai Pratipanawatr for his invaluable assistance with data acquisition. The authors also thank Ms Saovanee Luangaram for her excellent measurement of oxidative stress. The authors appreciate all patients who participated in this study.

This chapter was supported by Exercise and Sport Sciences Research and Development Group.

Author details

Naruemon Leelayuwat*

Address all correspondence to: naruemon@kku.ac.th

Department of Physiology, Faculty of Medicine, Khon Kaen University, Thailand

References

[1] http://www.swfhealthandwellness.com/alternative-exercises-3-02

[2] Berry TR, Chan CB, Bell RC, Walker J. Collective knowledge: using a consensus conference approach to develop recommendations for physical activity and nutrition programs for persons with type 2 diabetes. Frontiers in Endocrinol (Lausanne) 2012;3:161. doi: 10.3389/fendo.2012.00161. Epub 2012 Dec 11.

[3] Buse JB, Ginsberg HN, Bakris GL, Clark NG, Costa F, Eckel R, et al. Primary prevention of cardiovascular diseases in people with diabetes mellitus: a scientific statement from the American Heart Association and the American Diabetes Association, Circulation 2007;115:114-126.

[4] http://ww1.prweb.com/prfiles/2011/12/19/10360439/Yoga%20Warrior%20Pose%202.jpg (accessed 22 February 2013).

[5] http://kateasana.wordpress.com/2012/07/02/announcing-the-great-108-challenge-and-august-yoga-in-the-park/ (accessed 25 February 2013)

[6] http://yoga.about.com/od/beginningyoga/a/whatisyoga.htm (accessed 25 February 2013)

[7] Madanmohan, Bhavanani AB, Dayanidy G, Sanjay Z, Basavaraddi IV. Effect of yoga therapy on reaction time, biochemical parameters and wellness score of peri and post-menopausal diabetic patients. International journal of yoga 2012;5(1):10-15. doi: 10.4103/0973-6131.91696.

[8] Kyizom T, Singh S, Singh KP, Tandon OP, Kumar R. Effect of pranayama & yoga-asana on cognitive brain functions in type 2 diabetes-P3 event related evoked potential (ERP). The Indian journal of medical research 2010;131:636-640.

[9] Hegde SV, Adhikari P, Kotian S, Pinto VJ, D'Souza S, D'Souza V. Effect of 3-month yoga on oxidative stress in type 2 diabetes with or without complications: a controlled clinical trial. Diabetes Care. 2011;34(10):2208-2210. doi: 10.2337/dc10-2430. Epub 2011 Aug 11.

[10] Malhotra V, Singh S, Tandon OP, Madhu SV, Prasad A, Sharma SB. Effect of Yoga asanas on nerve conduction in type 2 diabetes. Indian journal of physiology and pharmacology 2002;46(3):298-306.

[11] Kosuri M, Sridhar GR. Yoga practice in diabetes improves physical and psychological outcomes. Metabolic syndrome and related disorders 2009;7(6):515-517. doi: 10.1089/met.2009.0011.

[12] Yang K, Bernardo LM, Sereika SM, Conroy MB, Balk J, Burke LE. Utilization of 3-month yoga program for adults at high risk for type 2 diabetes: a pilot study. Evidence-based complementary and alternative medicine 2011;2011:257891. doi: 10.1093/ecam/nep117. Epub 2011 Jan 9.

[13] Amita S, Prabhakar S, Manoj I, Harminder S, Pavan T. Effect of yoga-nidra on blood glucose level in diabetic patients. Indian journal of physiology and pharmacology 2009;53(1):97-101.

[14] Malhotra V, Singh S, Singh KP, Gupta P, Sharma SB, Madhu SV, Tandon OP. Study of yoga asanas in assessment of pulmonary function in NIDDM patients. Indian journal of physiology and pharmacology 2002;46(3):313-320.

[15] Jyotsna VP, Joshi A, Ambekar S, Kumar N, Dhawan A, Sreenivas V. Comprehensive yogic breathing program improves quality of life in patients with diabetes. Indian journal of endocrinology and metabolism 2012;16(3):423-428. doi: 10.4103/2230-8210.95692.

[16] http://www.fitnessrxwomen.com/training/alternative-training/yoga/ (accessed 25 February 2013)

[17] "Bikram's Yoga College of India". Bikramyoga.com. Retrieved 2011-12-28.

[18] Corporate registration for "Bikram Choudhury Yoga, Inc." Number: C2288343

[19] Farrell, M. (September 3, 2009). "Bikram Yoga's New Twists". Forbes.com.

[20] Wilson, Cynthia. "Different types of yoga and their benefits". Womenio. Retrieved 26 September 2012.

[21] http://www.readersdigest.com.au/alternative-exercise-ideas (accessed 25 February 2013)

[22] http://universal-taichichuan.com/restoring-your-qi-with-tai-chi/ (accessed 25 February 2013)

[23] Liu X, Miller YD, Burton NW, Chang JH, Brown WJ. The effect of Tai Chi on health-related quality of life in people with elevated blood glucose or diabetes: a randomized controlled trial. Quality of life research 2012 Nov 10. [Epub ahead of print]

[24] Hung JW, Liou CW, Wang PW, Yeh SH, Lin LW, Lo SK, Tsai FM. Effect of 12-week tai chi chuan exercise on peripheral nerve modulation in patients with type 2 diabetes mellitus. Journal of rehabilitation medicine 2009;41(11):924-929. doi: 10.2340/16501977-0445.

[25] Lam P, Dennis SM, Diamond TH, Zwar N. Improving glycaemic and BP control in type 2 diabetes. The effectiveness of tai chi. Australian family physician 2008;37(10): 884-887.

[26] Chen SC, Ueng KC, Lee SH, Sun KT, Lee MC. Effect of t'ai chi exercise on biochemical profiles and oxidative stress indicators in obese patients with type 2diabetes. Journal of alternative and complementary medicine (New York, N.Y.) 2010;16(11): 1153-1159. doi: 10.1089/acm.2009.0560. Epub 2010 Oct 25.

[27] Field T. Tai Chi research review. Complementary therapies in clinical practice 2011 Aug;17(3):141-6. doi: 10.1016/j.ctcp.2010.10.002. Epub 2010 Oct 24.

[28] Song R, Ahn S, Roberts BL, Lee EO, Ahn YH. Adhering to a t'ai chi program to improve glucose control and quality of life for individuals with type 2 diabetes. Journal of alternative and complementary medicine (New York, N.Y.) 2009;15(6):627-632. doi: 10.1089/acm.2008.0330.

[29] Lee MS, Choi TY, Lim HJ, Ernst E. Tai chi for management of type 2 diabetes mellitus: A systematic review. Chinese journal of integrative medicine 2011 Jul 30. [Epub ahead of print]

[30] http://www.spirityogaonline.com/massage.html (accessed 25 February 2013)

[31] http://www.marycatherinestarr.com/2/post/2011/03/life-changing-discovery-thai-yoga-massage.html (accessed 25 February 2013)

[32] Buranruk O, La Grow S, Ladawan S, Makarawate P, Suwanich T, and Leelayuwat N. Thai Yoga as an Appropriate Alternative Physical Activity for Older Adults. Journal of Complementary and Integrative Medicine 2010;7:1-14.

[33] Puengsuwan P, Promdee K, Sruttabul W, Na Nagara R, Leelayuwat N. Effectiveness of Thai Wand Exercise training on health-related quality of life in sedentary older adults. Chulalongorn Medicine Journal 2008;52:120-122.

[34] http://www.kendimiz.com/tag/martial-arts-boxing-chaiya/ (accessed 25 February 2013)

[35] http://www.superprosamui.com/muay-thai/muay-thai-martial-arts.html (accessed 25 February 2013)

[36] http://en.wikipedia.org/wiki/Chinese_martial_arts (accessed 23 February 2013)

[37] http://en.wikipedia.org/wiki/Martial_arts (accessed 23 February 2013)

[38] http://en.wikipedia.org/wiki/Taekwondo (accessed 24 February 2013)

[39] http://www.eonline.com/news/355888/melissa-rycroft-released-from-hospital-after-dancing-with-the-stars-head-injury (accessed 24 February 2013)

[40] http://www.colourbox.com/vector/silhouettes-of-the-pairs-dancing-ballroom-dances-tango-vector-4335705 (accessed 24 February 2013)

[41] Hogg J, Diaz A, Del Cid M, Mueller C, Lipman EG, Cheruvu S, Chiu YL, Vogiatzi M, Nimkarn S. An after-school dance and lifestyle education program reduces risk factors for heart disease and diabetes in elementary school children. Journal of pediatric endocrinology & metabolism 2012;25(5-6):509-516.

[42] Murrock CJ, Higgins PA, Killion C. Dance and peer support to improve diabetes outcomes in African American women. Diabetes Education 2009;35(6):995-1003. doi: 10.1177/0145721709343322. Epub 2009 Sep 23.

[43] Tudor-Locke C, Schuna JM Jr. Steps to preventing type 2 diabetes: exercise, walk more, or sit less? Frontiers Endocrinology (Lausanne). 2012;3:142. doi: 10.3389/fendo.2012.00142. Epub 2012 Nov 19.

[44] http://www.mayoclinic.com/health/walking/SM00062_D (accessed 24 February 2013)

[45] http://walking.about.com/od/workouts/a/Brisk-Walking.htm (accessed 24 February 2013)

[46] http://www.worcestershiretouristguides.com/Articles/Article_168.asp (accessed 24 February 2013)

[47] http://www.realbuzz.com/articles/alternative-exercise-activities-gb-en/ (accessed 23 February 2013)

[48] http://www.telegraph.co.uk/sport/olympics/sailing/9463023/Saskia-Clark-and-Hannah-Mills-on-target-for-sailing-Olympic-gold.html (accessed 24 February 2013)

[49] http://www.horse-insurance.co.uk/blog/news/pioneering-new-therapy-offers-hope-for-spinal-injuries/attachment/horse-riding-spinal-injury/ (accessed 24 February 2013)

[50] http://www.globaltravelmate.com/asia/thailand/phuket/phuket-to-do/590-phuket-horse-riding-club.html (accessed 26 February 2013)

[51] Hosaka Y, Nagasaki M, Bajotto G, Shinomiya Y, Ozawa T, Sato Y. Effects of daily mechanical horseback riding on insulin sensitivity and resting metabolism in middle-aged type 2 diabetes mellitus patients. Nagoya journal of medical science 2010 Aug; 72(3-4):129-137.

[52] Kubota M, Nagasaki M, Tokudome M, Shinomiya Y, Ozawa T, Sato Y. Mechanical horseback riding improves insulin sensitivity in elder diabetic patients. Diabetes Research and Clinical Practice 2006;71(2):124-130. Epub 2005 Aug 18.

[53] http://californiaoutdoorsqas.com/2009/04/02/whereas-the-year-round-trout-fishing/ (accessed 26 February 2013)

[54] http://www.fitsugar.com/Back-Basics-Walking-Forward-Lunge-174913 (accessed 25 February 2013)

[55] http://www.chatelaine.com/tag/burn-calories/ (accessed 25 February 2013) (accessed 25 February 2013)

[56] http://www.huntingdonpeople.co.uk/sport/Fit-Huntingdon-s-Great-Outdoors/story-4529771-detail/story.html (accessed 26 February 2013)

[57] http://surfandlong.blogspot.com/ (accessed 25 February 2013)

[58] http://www.gocardiotennis.net/ (accessed 25 February 2013)

[59] http://sicefamily.blogspot.com/2012/03/make-change-learning-to-love-exercise.html (accessed 25 February 2013)

[60] http://images.yourdictionary.com/housework (accessed 25 February 2013)

[61] http://www.rodale.com/burn-calories-cleaning-house (accessed 25 February 2013)

[62] http://www.alexandertechnique.com/photos/ (accessed 25 February 2013)

[63] Woodman, J.P.; Moore, N.R. (2012). "Evidence for the effectiveness of Alexander Technique lessons in medical and health-related conditions: a systematic review". International Journal of Clinical Practice 66(1): 98–112. doi:10.1111/j.1742-1241.2011.02817.x. PMID 22171910

[64] http://wakeup-feldenkrais.blogspot.com/2007/03/new-version-what-is-feldenkrais-method.html (accessed 25 February 2013)

[65] http://en.wikipedia.org/wiki/Feldenkrais_Method (accessed 26 February 2013)

[66] Strauch R. An overview of the Feldenkrais Method. retrieved 14 May 2008

[67] http://www.muscle-fitness-tips.net/pilates-exercises.html (accessed 26 February 2013)

[68] http://pilates.about.com/od/intermediateadvexercises/ss/Side-Stretch-Pilates-Exercises_4.htm (accessed 26 February 2013)

[69] http://www.glamour.com/health-fitness/blogs/vitamin-g/2013/02/5-pilates-moves-thatll-blast-y.html (accessed 26 February 2013)

[70] http://en.wikipedia.org/wiki/Pilates (accessed 26 February 2013)

[71] Mayo Clinic Staff (2012). "Pilates for Beginners: Explore the Core of Pilates". Mayo Clinic. Retrieved 2012-11-04

[72] Leelayuwat N, Tunkumnerdthai O, Donsom M, Punyaek N, Manimanakorn A, Kukongviriyapan U, Kukongviriyapan V. An alternative exercise and its beneficial effects on glycaemic control and oxidative stress in subjects with type 2 diabetes. Diabetes Research and Clinical Practice 2008;82:e5–e8.

[73] Jwing-Ming Y. (2002). Swinging the Arms or Bai Bi. from. http://dactrung.net/truyen/noidung.aspx?BaiID=zlz3sRQzM57p%2Bhp8g9wOUg%3D%3D (accessed 18 Jun, 2008).

[74] Matthews MR, Hosker JP, Rudenski AS, Naylor BA, Treacher DF, Turner RC, Homeostasis model assessment: insulin resistance and beta-cell function from fasting plasma glucose and insulin concentrations in man, Diabetologia 28 (1985) 412-419.

[75] Jeng C, Chang WY, Chen SR, Tseng IJ. Effects of arm exercise on serum glucose response in type 2 DM patients. The journal of nursing research 2002;10:187-194.

[76] Maiorana A, O'Driscoll G, Goodman C, Taylor R, Green D. Combined aerobic and resistance exercise improves glycemic control and fitness in type 2 diabetes. Diabetes Research and Clinical Practice 2002;56:115-123.

[77] Tsujiuchi T, Kumano H, Yoshiuchi K, He D, Tsujiuchi Y, Kuboki T et al. The effect of Qi-gong relaxation exercise on the control of type 2 diabetes mellitus: a randomized controlled trial. Diabetes Care 2002;25: 241-242.

[78] Stratton IM, Adler AI, Neil HAW, Matthews DR, Manley SE, Cull CA et al. on behalf of the UK Prospective Diabetes Study Group. Association of glycaemia with macrovascular and microvascular complications of type 2 diabetes (UKPDS 35): prospective observational study. BMJ 2000;321:405-412.

[79] Ding Y, Kantarci A, Hasturk H, Trackman PC, Malabanan A, Van Dyke TE. Activation of RAGE induces elevated O^{2-} generation by mononuclear phagocytes in diabetes, Journal of leukocyte biology 2007;81:520-527.

[80] Ciuchi E, Odetti P, Prando R, Relationship between glutathione and sorbitol concentrations in erythrocytes from diabetic patients. Metabolism 1996;45:611-613.

[81] Sathiyapriya V, Selvaraj N, Nandeesha H, Bobby Z, Agrawal A, Pavithran P. Enhanced glycation of hemoglobin and plasma proteins is associated with increased lipid peroxide levels in non-diabetic hypertensive subjects. Archives of Medical Research 2007;38:822-826.

[82] Yamagishi S, Imaizumi T. Diabetic vascular complications: pathophysiology, biochemical basis and potential therapeutic strategy. Current Pharmaceutical Design 2005;11: 2279-2299.

[83] Kaczor JJ, Hall JE, Payne E, Tarnopolsky MA. Low intensity training decreases markers of oxidative stress in skeletal muscle of mdx mice. Free Radical Biology & Medicine 2007;43:145-154.

[84] Covas MI, Elosua R, Fitó M, Alcantara M, Coca L, Marrugat J. Relationship between physical activity and oxidative stress biomarkers in women. Medicine & Science in Sports & Exercise 2002;34:814-819.

[85] Heitcamp HC, Wegler S, Brehme U, Heinle H. Effect of an 8-week endurance training program on markers of antioxidant capacity in women. The Journal of Sports Medicine and Physical Fitness 2008;48:113-119.

[86] Moien-Afshari F, Ghosh S, Khazaei M, Kieffer TJ, Brownsey RW, Laher I. Exercise restores endothelial function independently of weight loss or hyperglycaemic status in db/db mice. Diabetologia 2008 Apr 25. [Epub ahead of print]

[87] Zierath, Juleen R. Invited Review: Exercise training-induced changes in insulin signaling in skeletal muscle. J Appl Physiol 93: 773–781, 2002;10.1152/japplphysiol. 00126.2002.

[88] Goodyear LJ, Chang PY, Sherwood DJ, Dufresne SD, Moller DE. Effects of exercise and insulin on mitogen-activated protein kinase signaling pathways in rat skeletal muscle. Am J Physiol. 1996 Aug;271(2 Pt 1):E403-8.

[89] Lee H, Chang H, Park JY, Kim SY, Choi KM, Song W. Exercise training improves basal blood glucose metabolism with no changes of cytosolic inhibitor B kinase or c-Jun N-terminal kinase activation in skeletal muscle of Otsuka Long-Evans Tokushima fatty rats. Exp Physiol. 2011 Jul;96(7):689-98. doi: 10.1113/expphysiol.2011.057737. Epub 2011 Apr 28.

[90] Castaneda F, Layne JE, Castaneda C. Skeletal muscle sodium glucose co-transporters in older adults with type 2 diabetes undergoing resistance training. Int J Med Sci. 2006;3(3):84-91. Epub 2006 May 17.

[91] Christ-Roberts CY, Pratipanawatr T, Pratipanawatr W, Berria R, Belfort R, Kashyap S, Mandarino LJ. Exercise training increases glycogen synthase activity and GLUT4

expression but not insulin signaling in overweight nondiabetic and type 2 diabetic subjects. Metabolism. 2004 Sep;53(9):1233-42.

[92] Thyfault JP, Cree MG, Zheng D, Zwetsloot JJ, Tapscott EB, Koves TR, Ilkayeva O, Wolfe RR, Muoio DM, Dohm GL. Contraction of insulin-resistant muscle normalizes insulin action in association with increased mitochondrial activity and fatty acid catabolism. Am J Physiol Cell Physiol. 2007 Feb;292(2):C729-39. Epub 2006 Oct 18.

[93] Hawley JA. Exercise as a therapeutic intervention for the prevention and treatment of insulin resistance. Diabetes Metab Res Rev. 2004 Sep-Oct;20(5):383-93.

[94] Ryder JW, Chibalin AV, Zierath JR. Intracellular mechanisms underlying increases in glucose uptake in response to insulin or exercise in skeletal muscle. Acta Physiol Scand. 2001 Mar;171(3):249-57.

[95] Frøsig C, Richter EA. Improved insulin sensitivity after exercise: focus on insulin signaling. Obesity (Silver Spring). 2009 Dec;17 Suppl 3:S15-20. doi: 10.1038/oby.2009.383.

[96] Matos A, Ropelle ER, Pauli JR, Frederico MJ, de Pinho RA, Velloso LA, De Souza CT. Acute exercise reverses TRB3 expression in the skeletal muscle and ameliorates whole body insulin sensitivity in diabetic mice. Acta Physiol (Oxf). 2010 Jan;198(1):61-9. doi: 10.1111/j.1748-1716.2009.02031.x. Epub 2009 Aug 12.

[97] Costford SR, Bajpeyi S, Pasarica M, Albarado DC, Thomas SC, Xie H, Church TS, Jubrias SA, Conley KE, Smith SR. Skeletal muscle NAMPT is induced by exercise in humans. Am J Physiol Endocrinol Metab. 2010 Jan;298(1):E117-26. doi: 10.1152/ajpendo.00318.2009. Epub 2009 Nov 3.

[98] Manabe Y, Gollisch KS, Holton L, Kim YB, Brandauer J, Fujii NL, Hirshman MF, Goodyear LJ. Exercise training-induced adaptations associated with increases in skeletal muscle glycogen content. FEBS J. 2013 Feb;280(3):916-26. doi: 10.1111/febs.12085. Epub 2013 Jan 7.

[99] Perseghin G, Price TB, Petersen KF, Roden M, Cline GW, Gerow K, Rothman DL, Shulman GI. Increased glucose transport-phosphorylation and muscle glycogen synthesis after exercise training in insulin-resistant subjects. N Engl J Med. 1996 Oct 31;335(18):1357-62.

[100] Kiilerich K, Gudmundsson M, Birk JB, Lundby C, Taudorf S, Plomgaard P, Saltin B, Pedersen PA, Wojtaszewski JF, Pilegaard HDiabetes. Low muscle glycogen and elevated plasma free fatty acid modify but do not prevent exercise-induced PDH activation in human skeletal muscle. 2010 Jan;59(1):26-32. doi: 10.2337/db09-1032. Epub 2009 Oct 15.

[101] Wang Y, Simar D, Fiatarone Singh MA. Adaptations to exercise training within skeletal muscle in adults with type 2 diabetes or impaired glucose tolerance: a systematic review. Diabetes Metab Res Rev. 2009 Jan;25(1):13-40. doi: 10.1002/dmrr.928.

[102] Hawley JA, Lessard SJ. Exercise training-induced improvements in insulin action. Acta Physiol (Oxf). 2008 Jan;192(1):127-35. doi: 10.1111/j.1748-1716.2007.01783.x.

[103] Cao S, Li B, Yi X, Chang B, Zhu B, Lian Z, Zhang Z, Zhao G, Liu H, Zhang H. Effects of exercise on AMPK signaling and downstream components to PI3K in rat with type 2 diabetes. PLoS One. 2012;7(12):e51709. doi: 10.1371/journal.pone.0051709. Epub 2012 Dec 13.

[104] Sriwijitkamol A, Christ-Roberts C, Berria R, Eagan P, Pratipanawatr T, DeFronzo RA, Mandarino LJ, Musi N. Reduced skeletal muscle inhibitor of kappaB beta content is associated with insulin resistance in subjects with type 2 diabetes: reversal by exercise training. Diabetes. 2006 Mar;55(3):760-7.

[105] Bruce CR, Thrush AB, Mertz VA, Bezaire V, Chabowski A, Heigenhauser GJ, Dyck DJ. Endurance training in obese humans improves glucose tolerance and mitochondrial fatty acid oxidation and alters muscle lipid content. Am J Physiol Endocrinol Metab. 2006 Jul;291(1):E99-E107. Epub 2006 Feb 7.

[106] Slentz CA, Tanner CJ, Bateman LA, Durheim MT, Huffman KM, Houmard JA, Kraus WE. Effects of exercise training intensity on pancreatic beta-cell function. Diabetes Care. 2009 Oct;32(10):1807-11. doi: 10.2337/dc09-0032. Epub 2009 Jul 10.

[107] Park S, Hong SM, Sung SR. Exendin-4 and exercise promotes beta-cell function and mass through IRS2 induction in islets of diabetic rats. Life Sci. 2008 Feb 27;82(9-10): 503-11. doi: 10.1016/j.lfs.2007.12.018. Epub 2007 Dec 31.

[108] Park S, Hong SM, Lee JE, Sung SR. Moreover, exercise improves glucose homeostasis that has been impaired by a high-fat diet by potentiating pancreatic beta-cell function and mass through IRS2 in diabetic rats. J Appl Physiol. 2007 Nov;103(5):1764-71. Epub 2007 Aug 30.

[109] Choi SB, Jang JS, Park S. Estrogen and exercise may enhance beta-cell function and mass via insulin receptor substrate 2 induction in ovariectomized diabetic rats. Endocrinology. 2005 Nov;146(11):4786-94. Epub 2005 Jul 21.

[110] Lamontagne J, Masiello P, Marcil M, Delghingaro-Augusto V, Burelle Y, Prentki M, Nolan CJ. Circulating lipids are lowered but pancreatic islet lipid metabolism and insulin secretion are unaltered in exercise-trained female rats. Appl Physiol Nutr Metab. 2007 Apr;32(2):241-8.

[111] Thomas AW, Davies NA, Moir H, Watkeys L, Ruffino JS, Isa SA, Butcher LR, Hughes MG, Morris K, Webb R. Exercise-associated generation of PPARγ ligands activates PPARγ signaling events and upregulates genes related to lipid metabolism. J Appl Physiol. 2012 Mar;112(5):806-15. doi: 10.1152/japplphysiol.00864.2011. Epub 2011 Dec 15.

[112] Dunstan DW, Daly RM, Owen N, Jolley D, De Courten M, Shaw J, Zimmet P. High-intensity resistance training improves glycemic control in older patients with type 2 diabetes. Diabetes Care. 2002 Oct;25(10):1729-36.

[113] Oh KS, Kim EY, Yoon M, Lee CM. Swim training improves leptin receptor deficiency-induced obesity and lipid disorder by activating uncoupling proteins. Exp Mol Med. 2007 Jun 30;39(3):385-94.

[114] Bruce CR, Thrush AB, Mertz VA, Bezaire V, Chabowski A, Heigenhauser GJ, Dyck DJ. Endurance training in obese humans improves glucose tolerance and mitochondrial fatty acid oxidation and alters muscle lipid content. Am J Physiol Endocrinol Metab. 2006 Jul;291(1):E99-E107. Epub 2006 Feb 7.

[115] Butcher LR, Thomas A, Backx K, Roberts A, Webb R, Morris K. Low-intensity exercise exerts beneficial effects on plasma lipids via PPARgamma. Med Sci Sports Exerc. 2008 Jul;40(7):1263-70. doi: 10.1249/MSS.0b013e31816c091d.

[116] J Appl Physiol. 2004 Nov;97(5):1823-9. Epub 2004 Jun 18. Exercise alters the profile of phospholipid molecular species in rat skeletal muscle. Mitchell TW, Turner N, Hulbert AJ, Else PL, Hawley JA, Lee JS, Bruce CR, Blanksby SJ.

[117] Kingwell BA. Nitric oxide-mediated metabolic regulation during exercise: effects of training in health and cardiovascular disease. FASEB J. 2000 Sep;14(12):1685-96.

[118] Chen YW, Hsieh PL, Chen YC, Hung CH, Cheng JT. Physical exercise induces excess hsp72 expression and delays the development of hyperalgesia and allodynia in painful diabetic neuropathy rats. Anesth Analg. 2013 Feb;116(2):482-90. doi: 10.1213/ANE.0b013e318274e4a0. Epub 2013 Jan 9.

[119] Vojnosanit Pregl. 2009 Jun;66(6):459-64. Clinical evaluation of oxidative stress in patients with diabetes mellitus type II -- impact of acute exercise. Kostić N, Caparević Z, Marina D, Ilić S, Radojković J, Cosić Z, Bakić-Celić V.

[120] Morifuji T, Murakami S, Fujita N, Kondo H, Fujino H. Exercise training prevents decrease in luminal capillary diameter of skeletal muscles in rats with type 2 diabetes. Scientific World Journal. 2012;2012:645891. doi: 10.1100/2012/645891. Epub 2012 Aug 13.

[121] Lessard SJ, Rivas DA, Chen ZP, Bonen A, Febbraio MA, Reeder DW, Kemp BE, Yaspelkis BB 3rd, Hawley JA. Tissue-specific effects of rosiglitazone and exercise in the treatment of lipid-induced insulin resistance. Diabetes. 2007 Jul;56(7):1856-64. Epub 2007 Apr 17.

Chapter 19

Understanding the Effects of Roux-en-Y Gastric Bypass (RYGB) Surgery on *Type 2* Diabetes Mellitus

Raymond G. Lau, Michael Radin,
Collin E. Brathwaite and Louis Ragolia

Additional information is available at the end of the chapter

http://dx.doi.org/10.5772/56398

1. Introduction

Obesity is a grave public health concern in the United States today. From 2007 to 2008, the prevalence of obesity was over one-third of the U.S. adult population [1]. It contributes to significant morbidity and mortality including heart disease, stroke, cancer, arthritis and sleep apnea. *Type 2* diabetes mellitus (T2DM) also has been shown to increase with increasing obesity. Findings from the National Health and Nutrition Examination Survey (NHANES) (1999 – 2006) showed that nearly half of individuals with a body mass index greater than 40 kg/m^2 have diabetes [2]. Results from various studies have shown that weight reduction significantly reduces the risk of developing T2DM in obese individuals [3], as well as improving glycemic control in those already with T2DM [4,5].

Long term medical therapy for obesity is often unsuccessful for the majority of patients in clinical practice. Bariatric weight loss surgery has remained the most effective means of achieving and maintaining weight loss. More significantly, it has been shown to decrease mortality [6]. The Roux-en-Y gastric bypass (RYGB) is a type of bariatric surgery that involves the creation of a smaller stomach with a connection to the middle portion of the small intestine, bypassing the duodenum and a portion of the jejunum (see figure 1). Two limbs are created after the surgery. One limb, referred to as the alimentary or *Roux limb*, is where nutrient boluses pass from the stomach pouch. The other limb, which is the bypassed portion of the gastrointestinal tract, is known as the biliopancreatic limb. This limb transports secretions from the pancreas, liver, and gastric remnant. Most remarkably, many obese *diabetic* patients who undergo RYGB are relieved of their anti-diabetic medications in a matter of days. This improvement in glycemic control occurs before any significant weight loss [7].

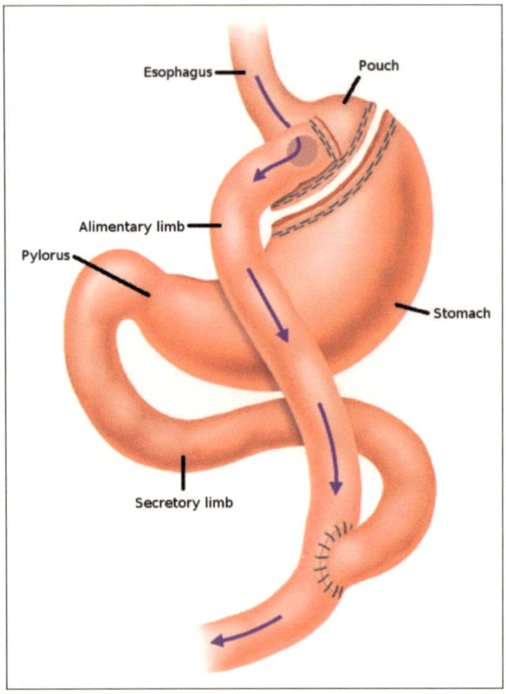

Dirksen C, Jorgensen NB, Bojsen-Moller KN et al. Mechanisms of improved glycemic control after Roux-en-Y Gastric Bypass. *Diabetologia. 2012*;55:1890-1901.

Figure 1. Roux-en-Y Gastric Bypass (RYGB)

This dramatic effect of gastric bypass on T2DM is not well understood. Improvement or remission of T2DM was thought to be due to weight loss in obese subjects [3, 5]. This was further supported by studies with gastric banding, a form of enforced caloric restriction [8]. However, clinicians began to observe that glucose levels were significantly lower in RYGB subjects as compared to weight matched controls [7]. Although malabsorption also likely contributes to the improved dysglycemia, there are other hormonal changes that are likely contributing to this effect. The most significant hormone changes occur in the secretion patterns of gut hormones. These are hormones that are secreted by enteroendocrine cells from the stomach, pancreas, and small intestine. A unique but significant post-prandial elevation of gut hormones is observed after RYGB. This is a well accepted phenomenon seen with RYGB subjects, and is believed to contribute significantly to this improvement of hyperglycemia in diabetics.

To better understand how RYGB affects those with *T2DM*, we will review the changes that occur with RYGB in key glucoregulatory organ systems within the body. In the ensuing sections, we will discuss in detail, the changes of *peripheral insulin sensitivity* and *insulin secretion* brought on by gastric bypass, and their effects on hyperglycemia. Identifying these changes will permit us to better understand how RYGB improves diabetes. We will also discuss the role that *caloric restriction* and *gut hormone elevation* may have in this process. Figure 2 demonstrates glucoregulatory variables that RYGB appears to modify. Cumulatively, this will permit the reader to develop an understanding of the relationship of how RYGB affects diabetes. We will begin our discussion describing the clinical potency of RYGB on T2DM.

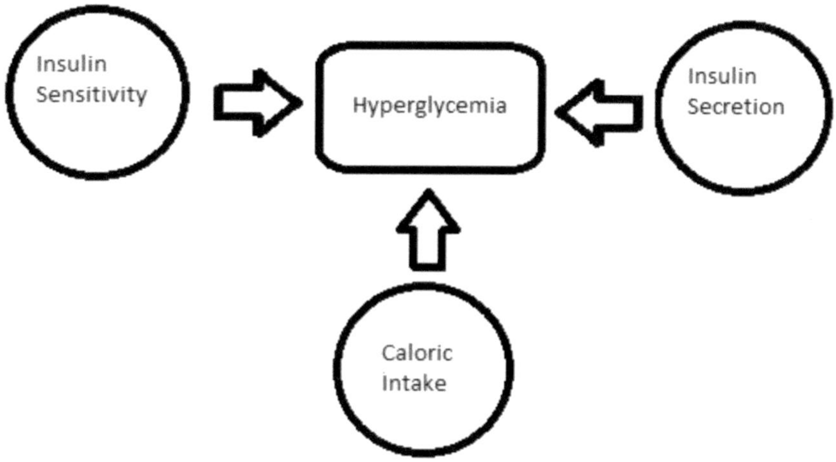

Figure 2. Glucoregulatory Variables

2. Problem statement: What is the effect of roux-en-Y gastric bypass on type 2 diabetes mellitus?

2.1. Roux-en-Y Gastric Bypass (RYGB) and its weight independent effect on T2DM

Since the early portion of the 21st century, there has been a growing interest in bariatric surgeries and their effect on ameliorating the diabetic state. Pories et al was arguably the first to describe remission of diabetes following gastric bypass. He reported gastric bypass not only caused weight loss, it also led to normalization of blood sugars in over 80% of his diabetic patients [9]. Initially, the normalization of blood sugars was thought to be directly caused by the weight loss. However, it has subsequently been noted that blood glucose control improves immediately following the surgery, prior to any significant weight loss. The concept that weight loss alone was not the reason for diabetes improvement after RYGB was a paradigm shift in the world of weight loss surgery, as well as the world of diabetes. This led to an explosion of research that attempts to understand how the surgery works.

There were few to no trials evaluating the efficacy of surgical treatment of obesity until the creation of the Swedish Obesity Study (SOS). The SOS trial is one of the largest prospective data collections to date that studies the clinical effects of various types of bariatric surgery. The SOS data demonstrates durable weight loss by as much 25% reduction at 10 years with various surgery types. The greatest weight loss is observed with RYGB [6] as compared to gastric

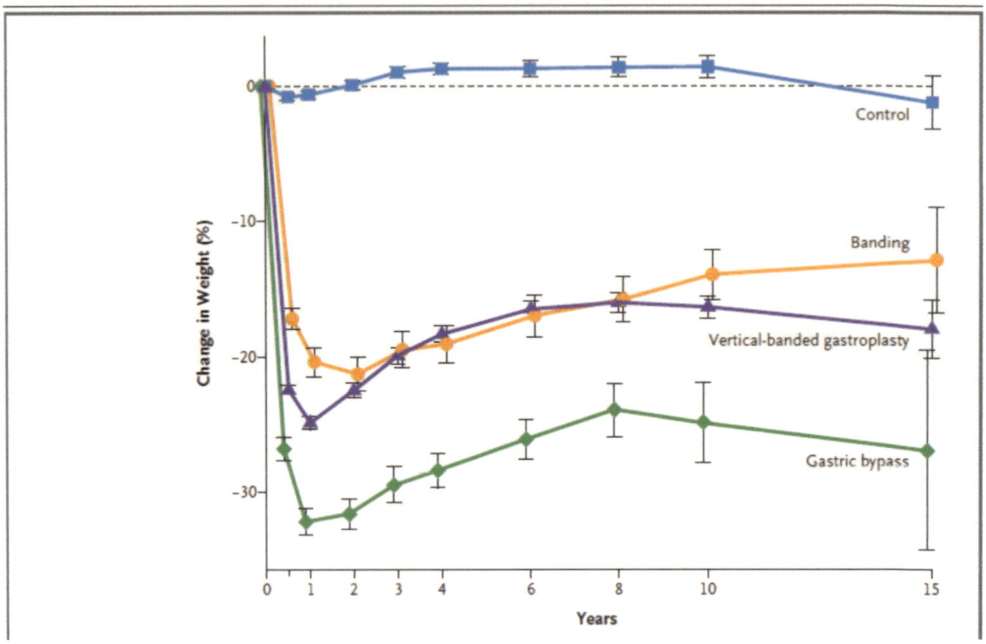

Sjostrom L, Narbro K, Sjostrom CD et al. Effects of bariatric surgery on mortality in Swedish obese subjects. *N Engl J Med*. 2007;357(8):741-52

Figure 3. Weight loss over 15 years between control groups (blue), gastric banding (orange), vertical banded gastroplasty (purple), and gastric bypass (green).

banding, and a modified restrictive surgery known as vertical banded gastroplasty, (see figure 3). Since SOS, additional studies of obese subjects that have undergone RYGB have verified that weight loss from the surgery is durable and long lasting [10, 11].

While durability of the surgery continues to be validated in ongoing trials, its weight independent effect on diabetes was initially uncertain during the infancy of bariatric surgery. This uncertainty was at least partially due to the absence of appropriate "control groups" in various studies. For instance, the SOS data demonstrated reduced incidence of diabetes in surgically treated groups, but this was compared to non-standardized medically treated groups [12]. Medical weight loss therapy can be difficult to implement effectively, and therefore, comparison to surgical subjects is often imbalanced. This begs the question that if we can implement a medical treatment that *is as effective at achieving weight loss as gastric bypass, would we see similar improvements in diabetes?* Are there available studies that compare effective calorie restriction versus RYGB in terms of diabetes improvement? There are published studies using strict low calorie diets as a comparator group [13-15]. One such study by Plum et al demonstrated greater improvement in diabetes in RYGB subjects when compared to low calorie diets over three months [13]. Both groups had similar amounts of weight loss, suggestive that RYGB has weight independent effects on diabetes.

The surgical obesity procedure known as the gastric band may be perceived as a superior "control group" to dietary weight loss. The gastric band is an anatomically enforced form of caloric restriction and can be difficult to "cheat." Diabetes remission in subjects who had the gastric band has been shown to be directly related to weight loss, and was superior to conventional therapy programs [8]. However, prospective longitudinal studies comparing RYGB to gastric banding have demonstrated that RYGB promotes greater insulin sensitivity along with superior weight loss at one year [16]. Additional other types of studies have validated the potency of RYGB on diabetes through the use of other controls. One such study by Adams et al [17] was a large retrospective study of several thousand, comparing RYGB subjects to weight matched controls. This study demonstrated a remarkable 92% reduction in diabetes. Despite the overall lack of prospectively randomized control trials, there has been compelling data to demonstrate RYGB effectively treats hyperglycemia and the diabetic state.

Only in 2012 were the first prospectively, randomized, non blinded controlled studies made available, comparing weight loss surgery to medical weight loss therapy. Schauer et al [18] compared the RYGB and gastric sleeve surgical procedures to medical therapy in the STAMPEDE study (Surgical Treatment and Medications Potentially Eradicate Diabetes Efficiently). Mingrone et al [19] compared RYGB and biliopancreatic diversion (BPD) procedures to medical therapy. The two studies had similar findings of greater "normalization" of glucose levels in the surgical patients as compared to medical therapy. However, there was still greater weight loss in the surgical groups, contributing to the greater glycemic improvement. Schauer et al [18] further demonstrated that the post-operative weight loss appeared to have no correlation with glucose control. This further highlights that RYGB has weight-independent effects on glucose control.

Both of the above discussed studies use *diabetes remission* as their endpoint. Before discussing the antidiabetic mechanisms behind RYGB, a further discussion of the meaning of *diabetes remission* will be explored. A seemingly simple concept, we wish to elaborate on the meaning of "diabetes remission," as well as discuss the associated complexities.

3. Application area: Can roux-en-Y gastric bypass be used to treat type 2 diabetes mellitus?

3.1. Roux-en-Y gastric bypass and remission of type 2 diabetes mellitus

Many subjects who undergo RYGB surgery and have T2DM observe a rapid normalization of their glucose levels, leading them to believe they have been "cured" of their diabetes. While these authors feel the term "cure" is incorrect, we cannot deny, and in fact pleasantly enjoy, watching the marked improvement in hyperglycemia following surgery. We agree that instead, the term *diabetes remission* should be used for these patients. Buse et al had [20] recently defined *prolonged diabetes remission* as hyperglycemia that is below the diagnostic threshold for diabetes for at least five years, while on no active pharmacologic therapy for diabetes. The increasing number of *diabetes remissions* after RYGB surgery has caused practitioners to revisit the definition.

Mingrone and Schauer's studies included similar definitions of *diabetes remission* in their trials, although their studies were less than five years in duration. Using diabetes remission as an endpoint acknowledges the potency of RYGB. But many questions come to mind amongst practitioners who manage diabetes. How does the surgery mediate such a potent effect? Should a reduced hemoglobin A1c be adequate for remission? Are the diabetic microvascular complications also reversed and should practitioners stop following these patients if they do go into remission? If there is complete reversal, why not use the term "cure?" Most important, has the characteristic pancreatic beta cell dysfunction reversed itself? These are questions proposed by these authors, some of which will be addressed in later sections.

Despite these questions, it is very hard to ignore the potent clinical effect the surgery has on diabetes. For those physicians and health care practitioners who struggle with uncontrolled diabetic patients, it is a seemingly effective and attractive solution. The metabolic potency of RYGB has even been addressed by the International Diabetes Federation (IDF) in a statement published in 2011 [21]. They discussed that bariatric surgery should be considered an option in those with a body mass index greater than 35 kg/m^2 and have T2DM. While a compelling argument can be made for this, we caution practitioners that not all RYGB subjects experience diabetes remission.

There are a small, but significant number of patients that have T2DM and undergo RYGB, but remain hyperglycemic post-operatively. In a retrospective review by DiGiorgi et al [22], as much as 24% of T2DM who had undergone RYGB had recurrence of their diabetes over a three year period, while a longer five year study demonstrated 31% recurrence [23]. Diabetes recurrence has also been seen as early three months following surgery [24]. These various studies demonstrated a number of factors that may contribute to recurrence. Higher BMI's, age, prior use of antidiabetic medications, and male gender were identified as factors associated with diabetes recurrence [23, 24]. A similar study in Chinese subjects demonstrated that diabetes duration, BMI, and fasting C-peptide were predictors for diabetes remission at one year. Based on this study by Dixon et al [25], suggestions of C-peptide above 2.9 ng/mL was a positive predictor for diabetes remission, which also implies residual good beta cell function within the diabetic group. These investigators were the first to suggest predictors and possible cutoffs in assessing the glycemic responses to RYGB.

Determining how to use RYGB in diabetes management is still in the early stages of development. Traditionally, this surgery was perceived only as a weight loss procedure. However, this has been an evolving paradigm within recent years. BMI alone is no longer the sole criteria for surgery in mildly obese subjects. Since 1991, the National Institutes of Health used both BMI and the presence of obesity-related comorbidities as the criteria for surgical weight loss. Even recent international guidelines still do not stray from these recommendations [26]. In the past, most studies looking at the effects of RYGB on diabetes have primarily focused on significantly obese subjects (BMI >35 kg/m^2), although this is now changing. We have already pointed out that post-operative weight loss does not always seem to correlate with glycemic control [18]. A recent study by Cohen et al [27] examined people who had a lower BMI (30-35 kg/m^2) and underwent bariatric surgery. They also demonstrated similar diabetes remission rates of 90%. Seeing such high rates of diabetes remission in a lower BMI range reinforces the concept of weight-independent effects of surgery on diabetes. As most obese individuals fall within this BMI range, clinicians may even consider recommending surgery at an earlier BMI.

Increasing evidence shows that BMI alone is not an adequate measure to predict successful health outcomes after RYGB. This is true for obese diabetics as well. We have mentioned that assessing for adequate beta cell function [25] could be used as criteria for successful diabetes remission. Additional evidence has suggested that those who have most benefited from surgery have elevated insulin levels, or insulin resistance [28, 29]. The simultaneous improved cardiovascular effects observed from the surgery [28] may also highlight the intrinsic relationship between insulin resistance and cardiovascular disease, often referred to as the metabolic syndrome. *As clinicians and scientists, it is critical for us to evaluate the effects of RYGB surgery beyond simple weight loss.* This may begin to help us stratify who best may benefit from the surgery. In the remaining portion of this chapter we will characterize the basic driving forces for T2DM and how the surgery brings about an improved glucose effect. This specifically will include *insulin sensitivity* and *insulin secretion*.

4. Observations and research: How does roux-en-Y gastric bypass improve Type 2 diabetes mellitus?

4.1. Effects of gastric bypass surgery on insulin resistance

Insulin action has a key role in regulating glucose homeostasis, facilitating glucose uptake in various tissue types. Its inability to cause glucose uptake is believed to be a key step in the pathogenesis of T2DM. This phenomenon is defined as insulin resistance. What mediates insulin resistance continues to be an active area of research. Glucose transport is maintained primarily through insulin-regulated glucose transporters, such as GLUT4. Commonly proposed theories that may mediate insulin resistance include impaired insulin signaling defects, GLUT transporter dysfunction, as well as increased availability of circulating free fatty acids. Both environmental and molecular factors may contribute to the development of insulin resistance. Obesity, as an environmental source, is believed to be a very common contributor.

Insulin resistance has been significantly observed at the level of the liver, skeletal muscle, adipose tissue, and pancreas. But it is skeletal muscle and adipose tissue that account for over 80% of total body glucose uptake. Because the reversal of diabetes immediately following gastric bypass is so profound, an alteration of peripheral tissue insulin sensitivity was thought to be the mechanism for achieving normoglycemia. With RYGB having superior weight loss, it has been well accepted that improved insulin sensitivity in surgical patients is also superior. However, the timing of when peripheral insulin sensitivity improves has been an area of uncertainty. Answering when peripheral insulin sensitivity begins after RYGB will also help to elucidate if it is a weight independent event.

The most frequently used measure of insulin resistance is the Homeostasis Model Assessment Insulin-Resistance (HOMA-IR). The ease of obtaining measurable glucose parameters have made this a popular method for quantifying insulin sensitivity. Several sources cite RYGB improves HOMA-IR from four days to two weeks following surgery in diabetic and non-diabetic subjects [30-31]. This is often before marked weight loss has taken place. In a non-weight controlled study, HOMA-IR was also decreased at three days following surgery [32]. However, these same sources demonstrate that HOMA-IR in RYGB subjects has comparable improvement to that of diet controlled subjects at similar time intervals while on calorie restriction [30-31]. Interestingly, there was minimal weight loss between the two study groups. *These findings are suggestive that immediate changes in HOMA-IR following RYGB are possibly related to caloric restriction alone.*

Besides HOMA-IR, there are other standard techniques for measuring insulin sensitivity. The gold standard remains the hyperinsulinemic euglycemic clamp. While most accurate in assessment of glucose uptake of *in vivo* systems, it requires experienced and skilled personnel often not readily available. The small body of literature that uses clamp data in gastric bypass subjects supports that insulin sensitivity in the post-operative period correlates with weight loss [31, 33], and therefore, is not a weight independent event in both diabetics and non-diabetics. Only Kashyap et al [34] demonstrated a slight increase of insulin sensitivity using clamp studies at one week following surgery for subjects that underwent gastric bypass as compared to gastric banding. However, as with all control groups, it is unclear if the oral intake of gastric band subjects was equivalent to the RYGB study group. Further molecular studies in rodent models that have undergone RYGB support the notion that insulin sensitivity is weight dependent. GLUT4 mRNA expression in skeletal muscle and adipose tissue of rodents that have undergone RYGB, does not increase until 28 days after surgery [35]. Therefore, the presence of adiposity reinforces the presence of insulin resistance. Because insulin clamp studies are the gold standard in assessment of peripheral insulin sensitivity, the *rapid glycemic improvement seen immediately following surgery appears not due to increased peripheral glucose uptake.*

Why there is this discordant finding between HOMA-IR measures and insulin clamp studies is unclear. Although HOMA-IR is an index of insulin sensitivity, it may also be used as a surrogate for hepatic insulin sensitivity. Therefore, one may observe there are more rapid improvements of hepatic insulin sensitivity than that seen with peripheral insulin sensitivity. However, there are only very few studies that intimately compare the two indices. HOMA-IR and peripheral insulin sensitivity were assessed through clamp studies, with individuals undergoing RYGB one month following surgery by Lima et al [36]. They demonstrated that there was no improvement of peripheral insulin resistance despite weight loss, although HOMA-IR did improve. Dunn et al used more dynamic and definitive methods for assessing hepatic insulin resistance using hyperinsulinemic euglycemic clamp studies with isotropic tracers, while also collecting data to asses for peripheral insulin resistance. They also demonstrated that there was also improvement in hepatic insulin sensitivity as compared to no improvement of peripheral insulin sensitivity at one month [37]. The reason for this requires further research.

Although RYGB and insulin secretion will be discussed in a later section, there are few studies that have measured hepatic glucose output in subjects that have undergone RYGB. Dunn et al [37] demonstrated decreased hepatic glucose production using clamp studies as described earlier. However, there was no appropriate dietary control group in this study. Contrary to these findings, Camastra et al [33] showed no improvement of endogenous glucose production one week following surgery against BMI matched controls. Because of these discrepant findings, the precise characterization of how RYGB affects hepatic glucose output also requires additional studies.

The clinical observation amongst practitioners in bariatric surgery is that in the immediate post-operative period after gastric bypass there is a rapid decrease of fasting glucose levels. However, dietary caloric restriction alone has been shown to decrease hepatic glucose output without affecting whole body glucose disposal [38-39]. People who undergo RYGB often have a post-operative decrease in appetite, anatomically imposed caloric restriction, and healing gastrointestinal anastomoses that require smaller nutrient boluses to allow for healing. In caloric restriction, the improvement of the endogenous glucose production (EGP) appears to be due to reduced glycogenolysis [40]. This finding is consistent with a study by Isbell et al [30] demonstrating comparable liver improvements (HOMA-IR) between RYGB subjects and calorie restricted subjects. Therefore, the rapid *alterations in hepatic metabolism seen immediately following gastric bypass may be from calorie reduction alone and not alterations brought on by the surgery itself.*

Further molecular studies have supported the notion that RYGB does not induce a weight independent effect on peripheral insulin sensitivity. Time-dependent GLUT4 expression in skeletal and adipose cells in rodents after RYGB and weight loss was discussed earlier [35]. Intramuscular lipid content has also been noted to decrease one year following surgery by as much as 44%, which also contributes to enhanced insulin action [41]. These observations alone suggest why peripheral insulin sensitivity is delayed and appears to be affected only by the presence of adiposity. Alteration in gut hormone levels have been strongly implicated as a cause for the metabolic improvement seen in RYGB subjects, but has not clearly been associated with the changes in altered insulin sensitivity. Glucagon-like peptide-1 (GLP-1) has been the most well studied of these gut hormones. The effect of GLP-1 on peripheral tissue has demonstrated some effect on glucose uptake in adipocytes and skeletal muscle cells [42-43]. However, the authors feel the effect of GLP-1 has more clinically significant effects on pancreatic function. The role of GLP-1 is discussed further in the section *"Identifying anti-diabetic factors of gastric bypass."*

It is of interest that RYGB and other weight loss surgeries have differential effects on insulin sensitivity and insulin secretion. The biliopancreatic diversion (BPD), a more malabsorptive surgery with a more extensive bypass, is often reserved for the super-obese population. However, this surgery been suggested to improve glycemia through normalization of insulin sensitivity [44]. This contrasts to RYGB, which we have discussed here, in that it does not appear to rely on insulin sensitivity for rapid improvement of hyperglycemia. We have demonstrated here that peripheral insulin sensitivity improves as a function of weight loss, independent of RYGB, whereas hepatic insulin sensitivity improves as a function of caloric restriction. Neural based mechanisms have also been implied as contributors to the glycemic improvement, although much is still not understood. This will be further discussed later in *"Other contributing factors to the anti-diabetic effect of RYGB."* We now will discuss how RYGB may affect pancreatic beta cell function, an essential hormonal regulator of glucose control.

4.2. Effects of gastric bypass surgery on pancreatic function

T2DM is characterized by both peripheral insulin resistance, as well as pancreatic beta cell dysfunction. For this reason, understanding how RYGB affects the pancreas may allow us to better understand why diabetes improves after the surgery. The majority of available studies involve dynamic biochemical measurements involving nutrient challenges. The impetus for study of these nutrient challenges, such as mixed meal testing, is based on the link between RYGB and postprandial gut hormone hypersecretion [45]. Exaggerated gut hormone secretion appears to occur because of the altered transit of nutrient boluses caused by the gastric bypass, and is a well accepted phenomenon. Several gut hormones have been suggested to also alter insulin secretion, and are termed "incretins." The *incretin* effect relates to the ability of an oral glucose load to result in an enhanced insulin response as compared to a similar intraveous glucose load. The distal gut hormone GLP-1 has been shown to be primarily responsible for mediating this effect, although other possible contributing anti-diabetic factors have yet to be characterized. There have been surprisingly few studies that have addressed the impact of RYGB on the release of insulin secretion and its relation to other gut hormones. We will first characterize the pancreatic secretory alterations brought on by the surgery, and then further explain associated hormonal and pancreatic cellular changes.

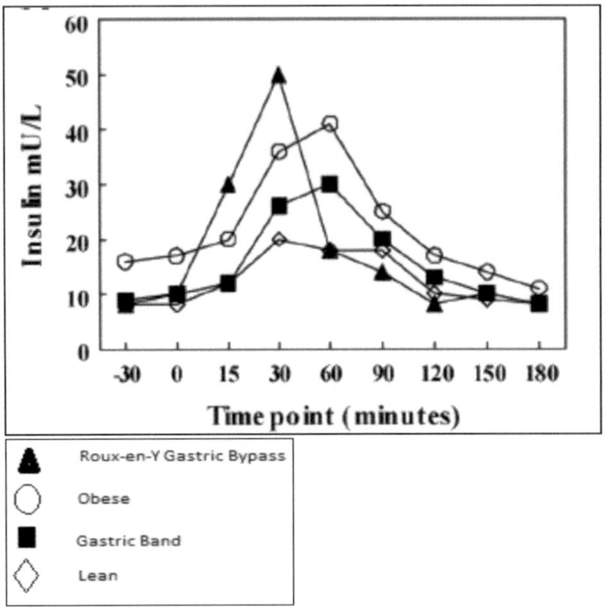

Le Roux CW, Aylwin SJ, Batterham RL et al. Gut Hormone Profiles following bariatric surgery favor an anorectic state, facilitate weight loss, and improve metabolic parameters. *Ann Surg*. 2006;243(1):108-14.

Figure 4. Roux-en-Y Gastric Bypass Insulin levels in Response to a Test Meal Le Roux C et al

Review of the descriptive studies of insulin secretion following RYGB suggest that fasting insulin levels appear to decrease within one week following RYGB in both diabetics and non-diabetics [32-34], which may be more of a function of improved hepatic insulin sensitivity. The majority of studies also demonstrate *a postprandial rise of insulin concentration that has a higher and earlier peak than seen pre-operatively* [32-34, 46-48]. While this suggests a possible restoration of the first phase of insulin secretion, this remains unclear. It also does not explain the exaggerated postprandial peak of insulin. The insulin peak also does not appear to be as marked as the postprandial GLP-1 elevations. The insulin peak is typically followed by a rapid decrease of insulin and glucose levels following the peak. This rapid decrease in levels is also not well explained. However, the insulin area under the curve (AUC), based on these prior studies, is either unchanged or decreased as compared to pre-operative measurements. Figure 4 demonstrates an example of post-prandial insulin levels in subjects that underwent gastric band and RYGB, as compared to control obese and lean subjects. The control obese subjects were matched to the pre-operative BMI of the surgical patients, and the subjects that underwent either operation had an equivalent post-operative BMI. Here, RYGB subjects exhibit the largest post-prandial insulin peak as compared to the gastric band and the remaining non-surgical subjects. Obese subjects likely have elevated insulin levels due to insulin resistance.

Decreased insulin levels following RYGB was generally believed to be the case with the perceived notion that insulin sensitivity was improved. However, as mounting evidence shows that peripheral insulin sensitivity is not immediately improved, these alterations in insulin secretion may hold more significance. Potential changes in alpha cell secretion of glucagon was then investigated to see if that had a possible role in these glycemic changes, namely if levels were decreased. However, they also had unexpected post-prandial elevations [48]. Why hyperglucagonemia would be present during the glycemic improvement seen after RYGB is unclear, and needs further studies to validate these findings.

Based on the postprandial insulin concentration profile demonstrated in figure 4, the glycemic effects do not clearly show why there would be an improvement of hyperglycemia. Available studies do not demonstrate consistently how postprandial glucose levels behave in response to these insulin secretory changes. Some have demonstrated significantly elevated postprandial glucose levels with a subsequent decrease [32], while others mostly show the postprandial decrease [8]. Inconsistency may have to do with varying nutritional content of test meals and timing after the surgery. Using other methods in assessment of glycemic changes with RYGB, continuous glucose monitoring (CGM) has revealed unusual patterns. In a group of RYGB subjects, CGM revealed increased glycemic variability using a calculation parameter known as "mean amplitude of glycemic excursions" (MAGE) [49]. The *increased glucose variability* may reflect an *altered postprandial insulin profile* that has been observed following RYGB, although this variability has only been identified in those afflicted with the condition known as *post-gastric bypass hypoglycemia* (*see Anti-diabetic effect gone too far? Postgastric bypass hypoglycemia* for further discussion). Studies into those RYGB patients without symptoms or documented hypoglycemia are ongoing. It is possible glycemic variability is a precursor to the metabolic complication *post-gastric bypass hypoglycemia.* Our laboratory is involved in trials studying this effect.

There are a greater number of studies examining the changes of insulin resistance in those that undergo RYGB and caloric restriction. There are far fewer studies comparing these two groups and assessing for differences in beta cell function. One study by Hofso D et al [50] compared RYGB to "intensive lifestyle intervention" as the nearest appropriate control. However, as expected, RYGB achieved superior weight loss, with significantly improved beta cell function. There are no available or appropriate weight matched trials to compare diet to RYGB on beta cell function.

The anatomic and histologic changes brought on by RYGB on the pancreas are also not well studied, due to the inability to easily access pancreatic tissue. The body of literature of known histologic or molecular changes within the pancreas that have been observed are restricted to rodent models, or those afflicted with post-gastric bypass hypoglycemia. One may expect hyperinsulinemia, especially in the setting of a marked peak in the postprandial insulin level. However, if the AUC of postprandial insulin levels are unchanged from prior to surgery, it is difficult to assess what cellular changes would occur if the same quantity of insulin was made by the beta cell. In rodents that have undergone RYGB, there has been a demonstrated increase in pancreatic beta cell area [51], less beta cell apoptosis [52], and increased beta cell proliferation [53]. This suggests that RYGB surgery enhances insulin secretion and insulin activity. However, as with all studies, appropriate controls are needed.

Much may also be learned of how RYGB affects the pancreas by the associated complication known as post-gastric bypass hypoglycemia (*reviewed further in"Antidiabetic effect gone too far? Post gastric bypass hypoglycemia*). Meier et al [54] demonstrated in human subjects who are afflicted with hyperinsulinemic post-gastric bypass hypoglycemia, the pancreatic beta cell area was not increased as compared to obese or even lean control subjects. They did demonstrate increased beta cell nuclear diameter in those afflicted with post-gastric bypass hypoglycemia compared to BMI-matched controls, suggestive of altered insulin production and secretion. One may therefore hypothesize that the decreased weight in response to the elevated insulin levels in RYGB subjects may be the responsible factor that improves glycemic control.

Despite these studies, further characterization is needed to understand how the pancreas responds to RYGB in T2DM independent of weight loss. Beta cell dysfunction is considered a hallmark of T2DM, often with hyperinsulinemia and gradual insulinopenia. This prompts the question of whether RYGB induces a reversal of these states. The altered post-prandial insulin profile seen after RYGB suggests beta cell function has only been altered, and not necessarily restored to appropriate physiologic function.

4.3. Identifying anti-diabetic factors of gastric bypass

Alterations of insulin secretion itself is a contributing factor that ameliorates the diabetic state in RYGB. Other contributing anti-diabetic factors brought on by RYGB are still being identified. Several investigators have proposed various intestinal mediators that may induce euglycemia, none of which have fully explained the clinical potency of RYGB.

Earlier studies suggested that exclusion of the proximal gut was responsible for the improvement of hyperglycemia, implying a potential "diabetogenic factor." Rubino et al [55] was the first to support this concept, by performing a duodenal-jejunal exclusion in diabetic rodents known as Goto-Kakizaki rodents. This was a surgery that led to preservation of gastric volume, with a pure exclusion of proximal intestinal absorptive surfaces. The initial excitement of his findings surrounded the premise that there was greater glycemic control as compared to calorie restricted rodents, simply by removing a portion of the intestine without creating caloric restriction. Born from this procedure was the concept of the *"foregut theory."* From this, it was perceived that there was a "diabetogenic factor" in this region of the intestine. However, this concept was later challenged by the *"hindgut theory."*

The *"hindgut theory,"* perhaps more popular, operated on the premise that there were factors in the distal intestine that became elevated and had potent anti-diabetogenic effects. It is the author's opinion that this is the more likely theory. Further support for this are studies performed with feeding tubes placed in the gastric remnant of the intestine following RYGB. Hansen et al [56] demonstrated that using gastric feeding tubes led to increased gut hormones, as well as via oral (jejunal) routes. The similar alterations in insulin sensitivity between the two nutrient routes suggest the exclusion of nutrients from the foregut is not significant. Instead, distal gut factors such as GLP-1 may more likely be the cause.

GLP-1 physiology will not be covered here in depth. Its anti-diabetic effect in gastric bypass has been demonstrated in rodent models that underwent RYGB [57]. Research into GLP-1 led to drug development of GLP-1 receptor agonists. These agents are now in clinical use for the treatment of hyperglycemia. Its usage operates on the premise of augmenting beta cell function. Use of GLP-1 agonists or GLP-1 continuous infusions increased basal insulin secretion, often leading to an improved second phase of insulin secretion [58, 59]. Because fasting GLP-1 levels do not increase following surgery, many questions remain regarding its postprandial effects. Perhaps the most important evidence that there are other factors besides GLP-1 in RYGB that contribute to the anti-diabetic effect, is that the pharmacologic use of GLP-1 agonists have not led to the equivalent potency of RYGB surgery alone. This suggests there continues to be factors of the surgery that have still yet to be identified.

4.4. Other contributing factors to the anti-diabetic effect of RYGB

4.4.1. Roux-en-Y gastric bypass, satiety, and the central nervous system

The importance in assessment of decreased caloric intake with diabetes remission has already been discussed, in particular those that undergo gastric banding [8]. Similarly, the RYGB involves creation of a small stomach size, causing similar restriction. It is remarkable that subjects that undergo RYGB actually appear to have a markedly decreased appetite as compared to their gastric band counterparts. Because postprandial elevation of gut hormones is a distinguishing factor of RYGB from gastric banding, investigation of their orexogenic and anorexogenic tendencies have recently begun to be characterized. Earlier prospective studies generally demonstrated RYGB induced altered satiety [45, 60-62], although the field appears to be lacking trials that are appropriately controlled.

The evidence continues to mount for this gut brain communication effect, with several biochemical mechanisms that affect neural signaling of hunger and satiety being discovered.

Therefore, RYGB has effects on satiety that are *independent* of the physical limitations imposed by the formation of the gastric pouch. The effect gut hormones have on the neural circuitry are most studied specifically within the hypothalamus [63], with the balance of orexogenic and anorexogenic hormones. Prime hormonal candidates for these changes include insulin, leptin, GLP-1, peptide YY (PYY), and ghrelin [61-62, 64-65]. While findings with ghrelin have been mixed, there is growing evidence that the other aforementioned hormones may play a significant role. PYY [66-67] and GLP-1 [68-69] are currently being studied in great detail. Origins of these mediators come from multiple different organ systems, which subsequently affect neurons within the arcuate nucleus and other hypothalamic regions. These lead to alterations in food intake and body fat mass. Research into these anti-obesity mechanisms for pharmacologic uses are still being investigated.

4.4.2. Roux-en-Y gastric bypass, type 2 diabetes mellitus, and the central nervous system

Autonomic nerve regulation has often been the target for pharmacologic weight loss therapy. Therefore, there has been renewed interest in the role of the vagus nerve within bariatric surgical procedures to determine its role in weight loss. Preservation of the vagus nerve is a common practice by many bariatric surgeons. An intact vagus nerve with RYGB appears to have a significant and improved effect on food intake and weight loss [70]. However, the beneficial effect appears to carry over to improved glucose metabolism that also appears to be weight independent.

Obese and diabetic rodent models studies have demonstrated that hepatic vagotomy will worsen glucose metabolism [71-72]. This further highlights the necessary role of the vagus for helping attain euglycemia via hepatic-mediated mechanisms. This is not without some conflicting studies such as by Shin et al [73], although their focus was on food intake, body weight, and energy expenditure. Vagal signaling to the liver is mediated predominantly by parasympathetic fibers. These parasympathetic fibers are derived from the medio-basal hypothalamus. The source of this neuroendocrine regulation may suggest that hepatic glucose metabolism is uniquely regulated by a hypothalamic source.

Pocai A et al [74] demonstrated that activation of potassium-ATP channels within the hypothalamus appears to lower blood glucose through hepatic gluconeogenesis. This was a significant advance in better understanding the mechanisms that may mediate hepatic gluconeogenesis. Similarly, insulin presence near the hypothalamus has also been demonstrated to suppress lipolysis [75], which directly affects insulin resistance and T2DM. Additional characterization of the hypothalamic and vagal mediated effects may also help us to better understand the role of the nervous system in glucose and lipid regulation. Besides insulin, other hormonal candidates that were discussed earlier (e.g. PYY) may not only have anorexogenic effects that modify caloric intake, but they may also directly mediate glucose regulation via central nervous system mechanisms. Further identification of where gut hormone receptors exist are needed to better understand this potentially significant glucose-governing mechanism.

4.5. Anti-diabetic effect gone too far? Postgastric bypass hypoglycemia

Perhaps best described by the title of the article by Patti ME et al "*Hypoglycemia following gastric bypass surgery-diabetes remission in the extreme*?"[76] the condition of post-gastric bypass hypoglycemia has been an increasingly observed phenomenon. Contrasting mechanisms of how this occurs have been proposed, with the initial reports suggesting islet cell hyperplasia [77]. However, follow up studies suggested there was no change in beta cell mass, although there was an increase in beta cell nuclear diameter [54]. The increase in beta cell diameter may be more of a function of increased nuclear transcriptional activity of insulin production. This would coincide with those afflicted with this condition may have hypersecretion of insulin.

Hypersecretion of insulin at disproportionate levels to the decreased BMI following surgery may potentially lead to clinically significant hypoglycemia. This has been demonstrated in weight matched individuals by Goldfine AB et al [78]. If we recall the changes in peak of insulin secretion discussed earlier brought on by RYGB [32-34, 46-48], a comparison to BMI-matched subjects afflicted with hypoglycemia demonstrated a greater post prandial peak of insulin secretion [78]. This may lead to increased glycemic variability, which has been demonstrated in subjects who are afflicted with post-gastric bypass hypoglycemia [40].

While this is suggestive that RYGB may induce hypoglycemia via pancreatic mediated mechanisms, the question of the contribution of peripheral insulin sensitivity to hypoglycemia was answered by Kim et al [79]. Using intravenous glucose infusions in BMI matched controls, Kim et al [80] showed that those who are afflicted with hypoglycemia demonstrated appropriate insulin secretion rates in response to intravenous glucose challenges. Therefore, it appears the hypoglycemia is only brought on by ingestion of nutrient boluses which elicits an abnormal insulin response. While the response may be effective in mediating improved glucose control, it is unclear why some subjects develop hypoglycemia and others do not. Possible causes may have to do with prior history of diabetes and residual insulin resistance.

Because of the increasing number of bariatric surgeries being performed, this is an area that is in urgent need of further study. Understanding how this condition develops will also likely shed light on how the surgery helps improve hyperglycemia. Currently, our laboratory is involved with ongoing clinical trials to better understand the mechanisms behind this clinically significant phenomena.

5. Further Research: Can other weight loss surgeries help type 2 diabetes mellitus?

5.1. Sleeve gastrectomy: The future?

The growing popularity of the bariatric weight loss surgery known as the sleeve gastrectomy is worthy of discussion. The procedure involves the removal of the antrum of the stomach, with a creation of a sleeve-like structure. The potency of the sleeve gastrectomy on diabetes has been demonstrated by Schauer et al [18]. While the improvement of hemoglobin A1c reduction was greater in those that underwent RYGB, the sleeve gastrectomy had a similar reduction of almost 3% at one year following surgery. There was also a comparable reduction in BMI between the two surgeries. The question remains if there is a weight-independent effect of diabetes improvement with this surgery?

Earlier prospective studies of the sleeve gastrectomy, as compared to the RYGB, demonstrated that weight loss and glucose homeostasis was also similarly improved between the two [80-81]. However, they also demonstrated increased postprandial elevation of GLP-1, PYY, and insulin levels, although generally slightly less than RYGB. Short term (6 weeks) and long term (1 year) follow up demonstrated comparable GLP-1 responses to mixed meal challenges [82-83]. The alterations of GLP-1 and PYY secretion is confusing and remains not well explained within the literature. RYGB has been associated with earlier transit of nutrients to the distal intestine, stimulating an elevation of the "hindgut hormones." These elevations may potentially explain the glycemic improvement. However, these observations do not explain why the postprandial hormone elevation with the sleeve gastrectomy occurs. The literature still lacks a satisfactory mechanism of the stimulating mechanism for these elevations.

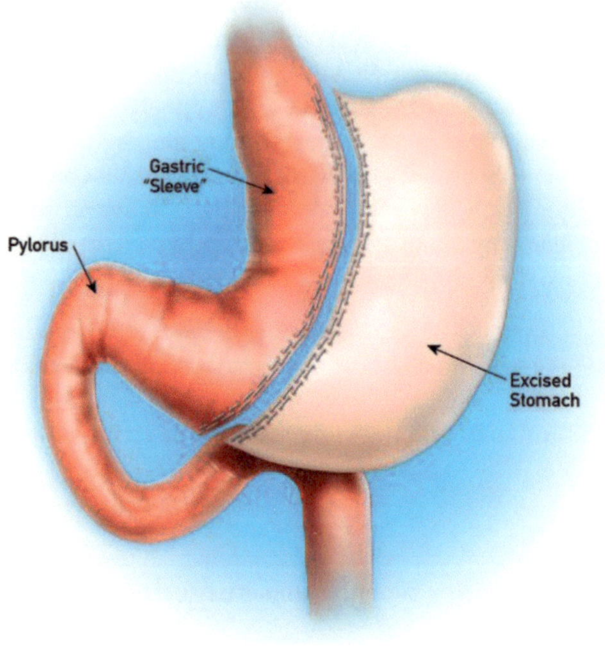

http://www.google.com/imgres?um=1&hl=en&client=tablet-android-asus-nexus&sa=N&rlz=1Y3NDUG_enUS499&biw=1280&bih=699&tbm=isch&tbnid=MwIS5kgaHvl2BM:&imgrefurl=http://www.ct-obesitysurgery.com/index.cfm/PageID/6424&docid=uP3rjSe-Kv1fMM&imgurl=http://ct-obesitysurgery.com//images_content/sleeve%252520gastrectomy.jpg&w=628&h=568&ei=DOyNUMC2NOPs0QHIzI-CABQ&zoom=1&iact=hc&vpx=184&vpy=183&dur=122&hovh=213&hovw=236&tx=127&ty=142&sig=110329031745694344091&page=1&tbnh=148&tbnw=164&start=0&ndsp=20&ved=1t:429,r:0,s:0,i:112

Figure 5. Sleeve Gastrectomy

http://dx.doi.org/10.5772/56398

It should be noted that most of these studies had small samples sizes and lacked appropriate controls. However, the clinical effects of the sleeve gastrectomy on diabetes remains difficult to ignore. The mechanism remains elusive, and many questions remain about the effects of the sleeve gastrectomy. Why do the post-prandial gut hormone elevations occur? What is the biologic mechanism? Is the surgery susceptible to the same post-surgery hypoglycemia seen with the RYGB? The increasing popularity of the procedure is for various reasons. The intact nature of the pylorus prevents the dumping phenomenon. The lack of an intestinal bypass prevents associated malabsorption and the plethora of micronutrient deficiencies. Lastly, the hypoglycemia phenomenon has not yet been reported with this procedure.

Despite these appealing features, we would advise practitioners to evaluate their patients carefully when considering a bariatric surgical method for weight loss. Little to no long-term studies are currently available on their clinical potency, and the lack of understanding how the surgery affects diabetes should give practitioners pause. However, the surgery is still very promising with apparently little metabolic complications. The authors are excited about the growing role of the sleeve gastrectomy in weight loss procedures.

6. Conclusion

RYGB unquestionably ameliorates the hyperglycemic state in many of those with T2DM. Many who undergo the surgery gain significant health benefits, and achieve remission of their diabetes. Investigators are attempting to understand the clinical impact of diabetes remission on RYGB patients, as well as the mechanism of how this is achieved. The improvement of peripheral insulin sensitivity appears to be weight dependent, while hepatic insulin sensitivity seems to be a function of caloric restriction. However, alterations in pancreatic function are reflected in the robust postprandial insulin secretion profile, and appear to be a direct result of RYGB. Understanding the condition of the pancreas' endogenous insulin producing ability and the whole body insulin resistance may allow us to predict who will achieve diabetic remission.

The increasing clinical phenomenon of post-gastric bypass hypoglycemia may be a result of an undesired overenhancement of the alterations brought on by surgery. This condition needs further study to better aide those afflicted with this potentially debilitating condition. As a possible alternative, the sleeve gastrectomy may potentially be an alternative weight loss surgery that appears to have lesser metabolic complications than are associated with RYGB. However, understanding of how it mediates its effect on diabetes is still not understood, and also is in great need of additional research.

Acknowledgements

We would like to thank Winthrop University Hospital for their support.

Author details

Raymond G. Lau[1], Michael Radin[2], Collin E. Brathwaite[1] and Louis Ragolia[3*]

*Address all correspondence to: lragolia@winthrop.org

1 Department of Bariatric Surgery, Winthrop University Hospital, Mineola, New York, USA

2 Department of Endocrinology and Metabolism, Winthrop University Hospital, Mineola, New York, USA

3 Department of Vascular Biology, Winthrop University Hospital, Mineola, New York, USA

References

[1] Flegal KM, Carroll MD, Ogden CL, Curtin LR. Prevalence and trends in obesity among US adults,1999-2008. *JAMA*. 2010;303(3):235-41.

[2] Nguyen NT, Nguyen XM, Lane J, Wang P. Relationship Between Obesity and Diabetes in a US Adult Population Findings from the National Health and Nutrition Examination Survey, 1996-2006. *Obes Surg*. 2011; 21(3): 351-5.

[3] Knowler W, Barrett-Connor E, Fowler SE et al. Reduction in the incidence of type 2 diabetes with lifestyle intervention or metformin. *N Engl J Med*. 2002; 346(6):393-403.

[4] Ross SA, Dzida GVJ, Khunti K, Kaiser M, and Ligthelm RJ. Impact of Weight Gain on Outcomes in type 2 diabetes. *Curr Med Res Opin*. 2011; 27(7):1431-8.

[5] Pi-Sunyer X, Blackburn G, Brancati FL et al. Reduction in Weight and Cardiovascular Disease Risk Factors in Individuals with type 2 diabetes: one year results of the look AHEAD trial. *Diabetes Care*. 2007;30(6):1374-83.

[6] Sjostrom L, Narbro K, Sjostrom CD et al. Effects of bariatric surgery on mortality in Swedish obese subjects. *N Engl J Med*. 2007;357(8):741-52

[7] Pories WJ. Diabetes: the evolution of a new paradigm. *Ann Surg*. 2004;239(1):12-13.

[8] Dixon JB, O'Brien PE, Playfair J et al. Adjustable gastric banding and Conventional Therapy for Type 2 Diabetes. *JAMA*. 2008;299(3):316-323.

[9] Pories WJ, Swanson MS, MacDonald KG et al. Who would have thought it? An operation proves to be the most effective therapy for adult-onset diabetes mellitus. *Ann Surg*. 1995;222(3):339-350.

[10] Edholm D, Svensson F, Naslund I et al. Long Term results 11 years after primary gastric bypass in 384 patients. *Surg for Obes and Relat Diseases*. 2012; [Epub ahead of print].

[11] Attiah MA, Halpern CH, Balmuri U et al. Durability of Roux-en-Y Gastric Bypass Surgery A Meta-Regression Study. *Annals of Surg*. 2012; 256(2):251-4.

[12] Sjostrom L, Lindroos AK, Peltonen M et al. Lifestyle, Diabetes, and Cardiovascular Risk Factors 10 Years after Bariatric Surgery. *N Engl J Med*. 2004;351(26): 2683-93.

[13] Plum L, Ahmed L, FebresG et al. Comparison of Glucostatic Pamaeters After Hypocaloric Diet or Bariatric Surgery and Equivalent Weight Loss. *Obesity*. 2011.; 19(11): 2149-57.

[14] Laferrere B. Effect of gastric bypass surgery on the incretins. *Diabetes Metab*. 2009;35(6 Pt 2): 513-517.

[15] Laferrere B, Teixeira J, McGinty J et al. Effect of Weight Loss by Gastric bypass Surgery Versus Hypocaloric Diet on Glucose and Incretin Levels in Patients with Type 2 Diabetes. *J Clin Endocrinol Metab*. 2008; 93:2479-2485.

[16] Korner J, Inabnet W, Febres G et al. Propsective Study Of Gut Hormone and Metabolic Changes after Adjsutable Gastric Banding and Roux-en-Y Gastric Bypass. *Int J Obes*. 2009;33(7):786-795.

[17] Adams TD, Gress RE, Smith SC et al. Long Term Mortality after Gastric Bypass Surgery. *N Engl J Med* . 2007;357:753-61

[18] Schauer PR, Kashyap SR, Wolski K et al. Bariatric surgery versus intensive medical therapy in obese patients with diabetes. *N Engl J Med*, 2012;366(17):1567-76.

[19] Mingrone G, Panunzi S, De Gaetano A et al. Bariatric surgery versus conventional medical therapy for type 2 diabetes. *N Engl J Med*. 2012;366(17):1577-85.

[20] Buse JB, Caprio S, Cefalu WT et al. How Do We Define Cure of Diabetes? *Diabetes Care*. 2009;32(11):2133-5.

[21] Dixon JB et al. Bariatric Surgery: an IDF statement for obese Type 2 diabetes. *Surg Obes Relat Dis*. 2011;7(4):433-47.

[22] DiGiorgi M et al. Re-emergence of diabetes after gastric bypass after gastric bypass in patients with mid to long term follow up. *Surg Obes Relat Dis*. 2010;6(3):249-53.

[23] Yamaguchi CM, Faintuch J, Hayashi Sy et al. Refractory and new-onset diabetes more than 5 years after gastric bypass for morbid obesity. *Surg Endo*. 2012;26(10): 2843-7

[24] Jurowich C et al. Improvement of Type 2 Diabetes Mellitus After Bariatric Surgery- Who Fails in the Early Postoperative Course? *Obes Surg*. 2012;22(10):1521-6.

[25] Dixon JB, Chuang LM, Chong K et al. Predicting the Glycemic Response to Gastric Bypass Surgery in Patients with Type 2 Diabetes. *Diabetes Care*.2012; [Epub ahead of print].

[26] Dixon AB, Zimmet P, Alberti KG et al. Bariatric Surgery: An IDF statement for obese Type 2 Diabetes. *Arq Bras Endocrinol Metab*. 2011;28 (6):628-642.

[27] Cohen RV, Pinheiro JC, Schiavon CA et al. Effects of Gastric Bypass Surgery in Patients with Type 2 Diabetes and Only Mild Obesity. *Diabetes Care*. 2012; 35:1420-1428.

[28] Sjostrom L, Peltonen M, Jacobsen P et al. Bariatric Surgery and Long Term Cardiovascular Events. *JAMA*. 2012; 307(1)56-65.

[29] Carlsson LM, Peltonen M, Ahlin S et al. Bariatric Surgery and Prevention of Type 2 Diabetes in Swedish Obese Subjects. *N Engl J Med*. 2012; 367:695-704.

[30] Isbell JM, Tamboli RA, Hansen RE et al. The Importance of Caloric Restriction in the Early Improvements in Insulin Sensitivity after Roux-en-Y Gastric Bypass Surgery. *Diabetes Care*. 2010;33(7):1438-1442.

[31] Campos GM, Rabl C, Peeva S et al. Improvement in peripheral glucose uptake after gastric bypass surgery is observed only after substantial weight loss has occurred and correlates with the magnitude of weight lost. *J Gastrointest Surg*. 2010;14(1):15-23.

[32] Falken Y, Hellstrom PM, Holst JJ et al. Changes in Glucose Homeostasis after Roux-en-Y Gastric Bypass Surgery for Obesity at Day Three, Two Months, and One Year After Surgery: Role of Gut Peptides. *J Clin Endocrinol Metab*. 2011; 96:2227-2235.

[33] Camastra S, Gastaldelli A, Mari A et al. Early and longer term effects of gastric bypass surgery on tissue-specific insulin sensitivity and beta cell function in morbidly obese patients with and without type 2 diabetes. *Diabetologia*. 2011;454:2093-2102.

[34] Kashyap SR, Daud S, Kelly KR et al. Acute effects of gastric bypass versus gastric restrictive surgery on B-cell function and insulinotropic hormones in severely obese patients with type 2 diabetes. *Int J Obes*. 2010;34(3):462-471.

[35] Bonhomme S, Guijarro A, Keslacy S et al. Gastric Bypass up-regulates insulin signalling pathway. *Nutrition*. 2011;27(1):73-80.

[36] Lima MM, Pareja JC, Alegre SM et al. Acute effect of roux-en-y gastric bypass on whole body insulin sensitivity: a study with the euglycemic hyperinsulinemic clamp. *J Clin Endocrinol Metab*. 2010;95(8):3871-5.

[37] Dunn JP, Abumrad NN, Breitman J et al. Hepatic and Peripheral Insulin sensitivity and Diabetes Remissionss at 1 Month afte ROux-en-Y Gastric Bypass Surgery in Patients Randomized to Omentectomy. *Diabetes Care*. 2012; 35(1):137-42.

[38] Jazet IM, Pijl H, Frolich M et al. Two days of a very low calorie diet reduces endogenous glucose production in obese type 2 diabetic patients despite the withdarwal of blood glucose lowering therapies including insulin. *Metabolism*. 2005;52:705-712.

[39] Kirk E, Reeds DN, Finck BN et al. Dietary fat and carbohydrates differentially alter insulin sensitivity during caloric restriction. *Gastroenterology*. 2009;136:1552-1560.

[40] Christiansen MP, Linfoot PA, Neese RA, and Hellerstein MK. . Effect of dietary energy restriciton on glucose production and substrate utilization in type 2 diabetes. *Diabetes* 2000;49(10):1691-1699

[41] Gray RE, Tanner CJ, Pories WJ et al. Effect of weight loss on muscle lipid content in morbidly obese subjects. *Am J Physiol Endocrinol.* 2003;284(4):E726-32.

[42] Villanueva-Penacarillo ML et al. Characteristics of GLP-1 effects on glucose metabolism in human skeletal muscle from obese patients. *Regul Pept.* 2011;168(1-3);39-44.

[43] Sancho V, Nuche B, Arnes L et al. The Action of GLP-1 and exendins upon glucose transport in normal human adipocytes, and on kinase activity as compared to morbidly obese patients. *Int J Mol Med.* 2007;19(6):961-6.

[44] Castagneto M, and Mingrone G. The Effect of Gastrointestinal Surgery on Insulin Resistance and Insulin Secretion. *Curr Atheroscler Rep.* 2012; 14(6):624-630.

[45] Borg CM, Le Roux CW, Ghaeti MA et al. Progressive rise in gut hormone levels after Roux-en-Y gastric bypass suggests gut adaptation and explains altered satiety. *Br J Surg.* 2006;93(2):210-5.

[46] Korner J, Bessler M, Inabnet W et al. Exaggerated GLP-1 and Blunted GIP Secretion are Associated with Roux-en-Y Gastric Bypass but not Adjustable Gastric Banding. *Surg Obes Relat Dis.* 2007;3(6):597-601.

[47] Laferrere B, Teixeira J, McGinty J et al . Effect of Weight Loss by Gastric Bypass Surgery Versus Hypocaloric Diet on Glucose and Incretin Levels in Patients with Type 2 Diabetes. *J Clin Endocrinol Metab.* 2008;93(7):2479-2485.

[48] Dirksen C, Jorgensen NB, Bojsen-Moller KN et al. Mechanisms of improved glycemic control after Roux-en-Y Gastric Bypass. *Diabetologia.* 2012;55:1890-1901.

[49] Hanaire H, Bertrand M, Guerci B et al. High Glycemic Variability Assessed by Continuous Glucose Monitoring After Surgical Treatment of Obesity by Gastric Bypass. *Diabetes Technology & Therapuetics.* 2011;13(6):625-30.

[50] Hofso D, Jenssen T, Bollerslev J et al. Beta Cell Function after Weight Loss: A clinical trial comparing gastric bypass surgery and intensive lifestyle intervention. *Eur J Endocrin.* 2011;164(2):231-8.

[51] Speck M, Cho YM, Asadi A et al. Duodenal Jejunal bypass protects GK rats from B-cell loss and aggravation of hyperglcyemia and increases enteroendocrine cells coexpressing GIP and GLP-1. *Am J Physiol Endocrinol Metab.* 2011;300(5):E923-32.

[52] Chai F, Wang Y, Zhou Y et al. Adiponectin Downregulates Hyperglycemia and Reduces Pancreatic Islet Apoptosis after Roux-en-Y Gastric Bypass Surgery. *Obes Surg.* 2011;21:768-773.

[53] Li Z, Zhang HY et al. Roux-en-Y gastric bypass promotes expression of PDX01 and regeneration of B-0cells in Goto-Kakizaki rats. *World J Gastro.* 2010;16(18):2244-2251

[54] Meier JJ, Butler AE, Galasso R et al. Hyperinsulinemic Hypoglycemia After Gastric Bypass Surgery Is Not Accompanied by Islet Hyperplasia or Increased B-cell Turnover. *Diabetes Care.* 2006;29:1554-1559.

[55] Rubino F, Marescaux J. Effect of Duodenal-Jejunal Exclusion in a Non-obese Animal Model of Type 2 Diabetes: A New Perspective for an Old Disease. *Annals of Surg.* 2004;239(1):1-11.

[56] Hansen EN, Tamboli RA, Isbell JM et al. Role of the foregut in the early improvement in glucose tolerance and insulin sensitivity following Roux-en-Y gastric bypass surgery. *Am J Physiol Gastrointest Liver Physiol.* 2011;300:G795-G802.

[57] Chambers P, Jessen L, Ryan KK et al. Weight Independent Changes in Blood Glucose Homeostasis After Gastric Bypass or Vertical Sleeve Gastrectomy in Rats. *Gastroenterology.* 2011;141(3):950-58.

[58] Nauck MA, Kleine N, Orskov C et al. Normalization of Fasting Hyperglycemia by Exogenous Glucagon-Like Peptide 1 (7-36) in Type 2 (non-insulin-dependent) Diabetic Patients. *Diabetologia.* 1993;36(8):741-4.

[59] Hojberg PV, Vilsboll T, Rabol R et al. Four Weeks of Normalization of Blood Glucose Improves the Insulin Response to Glucagon-Like Peptide-1 and Glucose-Dependent Insulinotropic Polypeptide in Patients with Type 2 Diabetes. *Diabetologia.* 2009;52(2): 199-207.

[60] Morinigio R, Moize V, Musri M et al. Glucagon-like peptide-1, peptide YY, hunger, and satiety after gastric bypass in morbidly obese subjects. *J Clin Endocrinol Metab.* 2006;91(5):1735-1740.

[61] Le Roux CW, Aylwin SJ, Batterham RL et al. Gut Hormone Profiles following bariatric surgery favor an anorectic state, facilitate weight loss, and improve metabolic parameters. *Ann Surg.* 2006;243(1):108-14.

[62] Le Roux CW, Welbourn R, Werling M et al. Gut Hormone as mediators of appetite and weight loss after Roux-en-Y gastric bypass. *Ann Surg.* 2007; 246(5):780-5.

[63] Korner J and Leibel RL. To eat or not to eat – how the gut talks to the brain. *N Engl J Med.* 2003;349(10):926-8.

[64] De Silva A, Bloom SR. Gut hormones and Appetite Control: A Focus on PYY and GLP-1 as Therapuetic Targets in Obesity. *Gut and Liver.* 2012;6(1):10-20.

[65] Korner J, Inabnet W, Conwell IM et al. Differential effects of gastric bypass and banding on circulating gut hormone and leptin levels. *Obesity.* 2006;14(9):1553-61.

[66] Chan JL, Mun EC, Stoyneva VA et al. Peptide YY levels are elevated after gastric bypass surgery. *Obesity.* 2006;14(2):194-8.

[67] Batterham RL, Cohen MA, Ellis SM et al. Inhibition of food intake in obese subjects by peptide YY 3-36. *N Engl J Med.* 2003;349(10)941-8.

[68] Gallwitz B. Anorexogenic effects of GLP-1 and its analogues. *Handb Exp Pharmcol.* 2012;209:185-207.

[69] Kanoski SE, Fortin SM, Arnold M et al. Peripheral and Central GLP-1 receptor populations mediate the anorectic effects of peripherally administered GLP-1 receptor agonists , liraglutide and exendin-4. *Endocrinology.* 2011;152(8):3103-12.

[70] Bueter M, Lowenstein C, Ashrafian H et al. Vagal Sparing surgical tehcnique but not stoma size affects body weight loss in rodent model of gastric bypass. *Obes Surg.* 2010;20(5):616-22.

[71] Milanski M, Arruda AP, Coope A et al. Inhibition of Hypothalamic Inflammation Reverses Diet-Induced Insulin Resistance in the Liver. *Diabetes.* 2012;61(6):1455-1462.

[72] Li X, Wu X, Camacho R et al. Intracerebroventricular Leptin Infusion Improves Glucose Homeostasis in Lean Type 2 Diabetic MKR Mice via Hepatic Vagal and Non-Vagal Mechanisms. *PLoS ONE.* 2011;6(2):1-7.

[73] Shin AC, Zheng H, Brethoud HR. Vagal innervation of the hepatic portal vein is not necessary for Roux-en-Y gastric bypass surgery-inducing hypophagia, weight loss, and hypermetabolism. *Ann Surg.* 2012:255(2):294-301.

[74] Pocai A, Lam TK, Gutierrez-Juarez R et al. Hypothalamic K(ATP) channels control hepatic glucose production. *Nature.* 2005; 434(7036):1026-31.

[75] Scherer T, O'Hare J, Diggs-Andrews K et al. Brain insulin controls adipose tissue lipolysis and lipogenesis. *Cell Metabolism.* 2011;13(2):183-94.

[76] Patti ME, Goldfine AB . Hypoglycemia following gastric bypass surgery—diabetes remission in the extreme? *Diabetologia.* 2010;53(11)2276-9.

[77] Service GJ, Thompson GB, Service FJ et al. Hyperinsulinemic hypoglycemia with nesidioblastosis after gastric bypass surgery. *N Engl J Med.* 2005;353:249-54.

[78] Goldfine AB, Mun EC, Devine E et al. Patients with Neuroglycopenia after Gastric Bypass Surgery Have Exaggerated Incretin and Insulin Secretory Responses to a Mixed Meal. *J Clin Endocrinol Metab.* 2007;92(12):4678-4685.

[79] Kim SH, Abbasi F, Lamendola C et al. Glucose-Stimulated Insulin Secretion in Gastric Bypass Patients with Hypoglycemic Syndrome: No Evidence for Inappropriate Pancreatic B-cell Function. *Obes Surg.* 2010;20:1110-1116.

[80] Peterli R, Wolnerhanssen B, Peters T et al. Improvement in Glucose Metabolism After Bariatric Surgery: Comparison of Laparascopic Roux-en-Y Gastric Bypass and Laparascopic Sleeve Gastrectomy: A Prospective Randomized Trial. *Annals of Surg.* 2009;250(2):234-41.

[81] Karamanakos SN, Vagenas K, Kalfarentzos F et al. Weight Loss, Appetite Supression, and Changes in Fasting and Postprandial Ghrelin and Peptide YY Levels afte Roux-

en-Y Gastric Bypass and Sleeve Gastrectomy: A prospective, Double Blind Study. *Annals of Surg*. 2008;247(3):401-7.

[82] Romero F, Nicolau J, Flores L et al. Comparable early changes in gastrointestinal hormones after sleeve gastrectomy and Roux-en-Y gastric bypass surgery for morbidly obese type 2 diabetic subjects. *Surg Endosc*. 2012;26(8):2231-9.

[83] Jimenez A, Casamitjana R, Flores L et al. Long-Term Effects of Sleeve Gastrectomy and Roux-en-Y Gastric Bypass Surgery on Type 2 Diabetes in Morbidly Obese Subjects. *Ann of Surg*. 2012;256(6):1023-9.

Chapter 20

Pharmacological Treatments for Type 2 Diabetes

Roberto Pontarolo,
Andréia Cristina Conegero Sanches, Astrid Wiens,
Helena Hiemisch Lobo Borba, Luana Lenzi and
Suelem Tavares da Silva Penteado

Additional information is available at the end of the chapter

http://dx.doi.org/10.5772/56456

1. Introduction

Type 2 diabetes mellitus (T2DM) results from relative defects in insulin secretion and action. T2DM may be associated with metabolic syndrome, and it is characterized by insulin resistance, android obesity, dyslipidemia and hypertension. Furthermore, it is responsible for increased morbidity and mortality related to cardiovascular diseases.

In Latin America, diabetes is a major health problem, where the prevalence has reached more than 19 million people [1], many of whom are at the productive age for work. This phenomenon has resulted in an increased burden on social security, thereby fueling the continuation of the vicious cycle of poverty and social exclusion.

In terms of morbidity, diabetes mellitus currently represents one of the major chronic diseases affecting people today, including individuals in countries at all stages of economic and social development. Even developed countries, which, despite scientific advances and easy access to health care, are affected by the increasing prevalence of diabetes. Thus, it is assumed that interventions aimed at preventing this disease, such as physical activity and diet, are underutilized [2].

The relevance of diabetes has increased in recent decades as a result of various factors, such as a high urbanization rate, increased life expectancy, industrialization, hypercaloric diets rich in carbohydrates, displacement of populations to urban areas, changes in lifestyle, physical inactivity and obesity. It is estimated that by 2020, two-thirds of the disease burden will be attributed to chronic, noncommunicable diseases [3]. High-calorie diets and sedentary lifestyles are the major factors contributing to the increased prevalence of obesity, representing additional major risk factors for T2DM [4].

Diabetes is the seventh leading cause of death in the United States. Among adults diagnosed with either type 1 or type 2 diabetes,12 percent take insulin only, 14 percent take both insulin and oral medication, 58 percent take oral medication only, and 16 percent do not take either insulin or oral medication [5].

The treatment of diabetes is aimed predominantly at glycemic control. The treatment objectives are to relieve the symptoms, improve the quality of life, prevent acute and chronic complications, reduce mortality and treat the disease. The basic strategies for treatment and disease control of type 1 and 2 diabetes consist primarily of a specific diet, physical activity and the appropriate use of medication (oral agents and / or insulin). The outcome of the treatment depends on providing diabetic patients with education and ensuring that they adopt specific behavioral measures and practices.

Currently, there is a tendency to use unconventional measures of care for patients with chronic diseases, such as methods involving nonpharmacological treatment [6], emphasizing continued practice and frequent daily exercise and walks. These approaches also emphasize proper nutrition, which is now regarded more as a benefit than as a punishment. The use of medications is indicated for T2DM, together with diet and increased physical activity [7, 8].

Because it is not always possible to establish a full behavioral change in the high-risk population, and even trying to improve the prevention of T2DM can be difficult, a number of drugs have been tested with the intention of preventing this disease. Several drugs have been used, and some of the key studies are summarized here, including drugs such as oral anti-diabetic agents and other oral medications.

In obese patients with T2DM, the priority is weight loss. If glycemic control is not achieved after 4 to 6 weeks, drugs that sensitize the action of insulin (biguanide and thiazolidinedione) may be indicated, either in combination or not with anti-obesity drugs. If satisfactory glycemic control is not achieved, drugs that reduce the intestinal absorption of glucose (acarbose or miglitol) or that enhance insulin secretion (sulfonylurea, repaglinide or netaglinida) may be used.

In type 2 diabetic normal weight or overweight (body mass index <30 kg/m^2) individuals, sulfonylureas, repaglinide or nateglinide can be tried initially. If adequate glycemic control is not achieved after 2 to 4 weeks, biguanide, thiazolidinedione or an inhibitor of intestinal absorption of glucose can be added [7, 8].

Often, the effectiveness of the chosen pharmacological treatment cannot be predicted. Pharmacotherapeutic failure or undesired effects that lead to other health problems, such as adverse reactions and toxicities, may arise. These events are regarded as a negative outcomes associated with the medication use.

In some cases, negative results associated with the use of a medication are inevitable, as in the case of some adverse reactions. However, negative reactions can sometimes be avoided, such as those that result from the inappropriate use of a drug or problems with the monitoring of a drug's effects. The occurrence of these avoidable outcomes could be reduced by adequate follow-up of patients [9].

Non-effective treatment of T2DM leads to a significant increase in the values of glycated hemoglobin, which leads to a decreased quality of life for patients and a significant economic impact [10, 11]. The consequences of diabetes on health systems reflect only a fraction of the damage that is caused to individuals, their families and society.

In recent years, great progress in the treatment of T2DM has been observed. Different classes of drugs are used for this purpose, including analog and human insulin, drugs that act by reducing insulin resistance (biguanides and thiazolidinediones), secretagogues and their analogs (sulfonylureas, metglinides, inhibitors of DPP-4 or GLP-1 agonists) and drugs that reduce the rate of degradation of carbohydrates (alfaglicosidase inhibitors). Some treatments have been used for several decades, such as human insulin, which was first isolated in the 1930s. Other drugs have been developed over the last century, including metformin, which is the most used oral antidiabetic in the U.S. today, and liraglutide, an analog of GLP-1.

The current treatments aim to reduce insulin resistance and maintain adequate glycemic control to prevent or reduce microvascular and macrovascular complications by improving the function of the pancreatic beta cells through interventions involving diet, exercise, oral hypoglycemic agents, anti-hyperglycemic agents and / or anti-obesity drugs. There are currently several types of treatments, which may be used alone or in combination.

Among the class of biguanides, which sensitize the action of insulin, are metformin and phenformin. Metformin is used more frequently than phenformin and has fewer side effects (diarrhea, metallic taste and nausea - which may decrease with continued use). Among the advantages of this class of drugs is its anorectic effect, which aids in weight loss, and the fact that it does not cause hypoglycemia (it does not stimulate insulin secretion).

In the United States and some European countries, other classes of antidiabetic thiazolidinedione derivatives are available, such as rosiglitazone and pioglitazone, which act by increasing the sensitivity of the liver, muscles and adipocytes to insulin, resulting in a decrease in peripheral resistance. The use of troglitazone, which belongs to this therapeutic class, was suspended due to hepatotoxicity. Rosiglitazone is more potent and has lower liver toxicity and fewer interactions with other drugs because it does not induce metabolism by cytochrome P450 (CYP) 3A4. The side effects include upper respiratory tract infections, headache, elevated transaminases, edema, weight gain and anemia. Pioglitazone is also associated with less liver toxicity and has the same mechanism of action and side effects as rosiglitazone. However, pioglitazone interacts with some medications.

The competitive alpha-glucosidase inhibitors, such as acarbose, miglitol and voglibose, act as antagonists of sucrase and amylase, and they also decrease the intestinal absorption of glucose. The most frequent side effects of alpha-glucosidase inhibitors are bloating, diarrhea, abdominal pain and elevated transaminases, and they are contraindicated in cases of inflammatory bowel disease, pregnancy and lactation, hepatic or renal impairment.

Another class of drugs used to treat T2DM is the class of sulfonylureas, including chlorpropamide (first generation), glibenclamide, gliclazide and glipizide (the second generation) and glimepiride (third generation). These drugs act as insulin secretagogues, and the side effects are hypoglycaemia, hematological (leukopenia, agranulocytosis, thrombocytopenia and hemolytic anemia) and gastrointestinal (nausea, vomiting, more rarely cholestatic jaundice) complications and allergic reactions. They may also cause an increase in weight as a result of binding to the plasma proteins, and their effects can be enhanced by the use of other drugs concomitantly, causing hypoglycemia.

Additional insulin secretagogues include repaglinide, nateglinide and meglitinida. Derivatives of benzoic acid and the amino acid D-phenylalanine increase insulin secretion through an action similar to that of the sulfonylureas. Due to their rapid absorption, this action begins approximately 30 minutes after administration. These drugs do not have interactions with other medications and are not contraindicated during pregnancy, lactation or in the presence of other pathologies.

In many diabetic patients, a hypocaloric diet aimed at weight reduction alone is able to control glucose levels. The anti-obesity effects of catecholaminergic (amfepramone, fenproporex, mazindol), serotonergic (fluoxetine, sertraline) and mixed action catecholaminergic and serotonergic (such as sibutramine) drugs that affect appetite and the induction of satiety may be used. In addition to these, orlistat or tetrahydrolipstatin, which inhibit intestinal lipase and fat absorption, may allow a reduction of the dose of hypoglycemic medications.

The use of insulin in the treatment of T2DM reverses diabetes symptoms and may be used in those with severe hyperglycemia with ketonemia or ketonuria, newly diagnosed patients, or in diabetics who do not respond to treatment with diet, exercise and / or treatments with oral hypoglycemic agents with anti-hyperglycemic or insulin-sensitizing action. Initially, human insulin in association with porcine insulin and regular or single insulin were used. There is a high chance of developing hypoglycemia as a result of the use of interprandial insulin analogous, which have faster action than human insulin. Currently, several types of insulin analogs have been synthesized: lispro, aspart and glargine. These analogs differ in their speed of action and duration of effect due to structural changes in the position of the amino acid chains of insulin. There are multiple options for the rout of administration, and they can be used in combination with oral hypoglycemic agents.

New drugs for the treatment of diabetes are emerging, making multiple therapeutic options possible. Furthermore, the use of insulin by inhalation has been studied to reduce the difficulties associated with subcutaneous administration.

The aim of this chapter was to evaluate all of the available treatments for T2DM, their mechanisms of action and side effects, and also to describe the emerging drugs and trends that are anticipated in the coming years. A better understanding of the mechanisms of action of drugs and the adverse reactions associated with them is important for health professionals and caregivers of patients with T2DM.

2. Treatments

2.1. Biguanides

Metformin and phenformin are oral antidiabetic drugs of the biguanide class. Metformin is the drug of choice for treatment of adults with T2DM due to its low frequency of side effects. It is currently used by nearly one-third of diabetic patients in Italy and is prescribed in the U.S. (> 40 m million prescriptions in 2008). Phenformin is no longer marketed in many countries, although it is still available in Italy [12, 13].

Both metformin and phenformin facilitate weight loss in obese nondiabetic patients without appreciably reducing glucose levels in the blood of such individuals. This weight loss is attributed to the anorectic effect and the slight reduction in the gastrointestinal absorption of carbohydrates [14].

2.1.1. Metformin

Metformin is marketed in tablets of 500 or 850 mg, and the maximum dose is 2.5 g/day, although there are no reports in the literature on the use of metformin at doses up to 3 g when administered after meals to minimize gastrointestinal side effects [15]. It has been reported that this drug increases the number and improves the affinity of insulin receptors in adipocytes and muscle. In the muscle, metformin increases glucose uptake by 15 to 40% and stimulates glycogenolysis. In adipocytes, metformin inhibits lipolysis and the availability of free fatty acids (FFA). Moreover, metformin improves insulin action in the liver, decreasing hepatic production of glucose by 10 to 30% and, at the cellular level, it increases the tyrosine kinase activity of the insulin receptor, stimulating translocation of GLUT4 and the activity of glycogen synthase [16].

The use of metformin also improves the lipid profile, resulting in a decrease in the triglyceride levels by 20 to 25%, a decrease in LDL-cholesterol by as much as 10%, an increase in HDL-cholesterol by 17%, and a decrease in the level of factor plasminogen activator inhibitor (PAI-1) by 20-30 %. Insulin secretion in response to stimuli may remain unchanged or decrease as a result of the anorectic effect, which helps with weight loss. In addition to being associated with weight reduction, its effectiveness in glycemic control is similar to that of sulfonylurea [17]. Another advantage of metformin is that it does not induce hypoglycemia or stimulate insulin secretion [18].

The isolated use of metformin in T2DM lowers blood glucose by approximately 25%, or 60 to 70 mg / dl, and glycosylated hemoglobin is reduced by 1.5 to 2% [16]. The intensive glucose control resulting from the use of metformin significantly decreases the risk of cardiovascular disease and mortality related to diabetes and patients presented less weight gain compared to other medications including insulin. Metformin also avoids the inconvenience of hypoglycemia induced by treatment with insulin or sulfonylureas [19].

Metformin is absorbed in the intestine and excreted by the kidneys. It is minimally metabolized by the liver, has a low affinity for mitochondrial membranes, and it does not interfere with oxidative phosphorylation. Metformin is indicated as a monotherapy in obese diabetic or glucose intolerant patients. Approximately 5 to 10% of patients each year will not have an appropriate response to the drug. In these cases, to achieve satisfactory control, metformin can be used in combination with sulfonylureas, acarbose, thiazolidinedione, repaglinide and / or insulin [7, 20-24].

The most frequent side effects are diarrhea (15%), a metallic taste and nausea, and these often decrease with continued use of the medication. The occurrence of lactic acidosis is rare (0.03 to 0.4 / 1000/year), occurring most often in people who have a contraindication to metformin, such as chronic liver disease (elevated transaminase 2 to 3 times normal values), heart failure, respiratory or renal failure (creatinine clearance <70 ml / min or serum creatinine ≥ 1.5 mg / dl). Metformin is not advisable for use in people over age 80, pregnant women, infants or alcoholics. In patients with proteinuria or those who are subjected to radiological examination containing iodine, it is prudent to provide adequate hydration and discontinue the medication a few days before [18]. Metformin shows synergistic effects with cimetidine and may decrease the absorption of vitamin B12 [15].

2.1.2. Phenformin

Phenformin presents a hypoglycemic action based on its insulin-sensitizing properties, similar to metformin. Approximately 30% of phenformin has hepatic metabolism and shows a high affinity for mitochondrial membranes, and it may also interfere with oxidative phosphorylation [18].

Due to its greater propensity to cause serious and fatal adverse events such as lactic acidosis, this drug was withdrawn from clinical practice in the 1970s. These effects are attributed to inhibition of Complex I of the mitochondrial respiratory chain. However, though no longer in clinical use, phenformin remains a widely used research tool to help delineate the cellular and molecular mechanisms that underlie the action of biguanides [25].

2.2. Thiazolidinediones

The thiazolidinediones (TZD) are popularly known as glitazones. Among the representatives of TZD are troglitazone (withdrawn from the market due to liver toxicity), rosiglitazone and pioglitazone (second generation thiazolidinediones).

Widely used in the treatment of T2DM, these drugs exert their effect by increasing and sensitizing insulin action in the liver, muscle and fat cells, decreasing peripheral resistance. They activate the intracellular nuclear receptors (PPAR-gamma, peroxisome proliferator activated receptor), which regulate the expression of genes involved in the metabolism of glucose and lipids, genes that are responsible for glucose uptake mediated by insulin in the peripheral tissues and genes that participated in the differentiation of preadipocytes into adipocytes. Moreover, these drugs inhibit peripheral lipolysis in adipocytes and assist in reducing the levels of free fatty acids and visceral adiposity, resulting in improvement of glycemic and metabolic parameters in these patients. They show good results in maintaining long-term glycemic control compared with other therapeutic options such as sulfonylureas and metformin [26-28].

Thiazolidinediones decrease glucose levels by approximately 20%, but no increase insulin secretion is observed. These drugs inhibit oxidation of long chain fatty acids in the liver, and they decrease gluconeogenesis and the availability of free fatty acids. Although they induce a decrease of triglycerides by 15 to 20% and an increase of HDL-cholesterol of 5 to 10%, the total cholesterol and LDL-cholesterol levels may not change or they may increase by 10 to 15% [18]. When compared to metformin, it has been observed that troglitazone has a greater potentiating effect for peripheral insulin action and less of an effect for reducing the hepatic glucose output. The association of thiazolidinedione with metformin is interesting because these drugs have additive effects [22].

Thiazolidinediones also increase the expression of the glucose transporter (GLUT4) and lipoprotein lipase, and they reduce the expression of leptin and tumor necrosis factor (TNF-alpha). These results make this drug class the most widely prescribed for the treatment of T2DM [18, 29].

Side effects occur in less than 5% of patients, consisting of upper respiratory tract infections, headache, elevated transaminases, edema, weight gain and anemia. Hypoglycemia can occur when the use of thiazolidinediones is concomitant with secretagogues or insulin. Their use is contraindicated in children, pregnant women, or in individuals with elevated transaminase levels that are 2-3 times the values of reference [18].

2.2.1. *Troglitazone*

In mice subjected to arterial injury, troglitazone inhibited the growth of vascular smooth muscle cells and intimal hyperplasia, suggesting that thiazolidinediones decrease the progression of atherosclerosis. In diabetic patients treated with troglitazone, decreases were observed in platelet aggregation, factor plasminogen activator inhibitor (PAI-1) and blood pressure levels. These multiple effects strengthen its indication for the treatment of metabolic syndrome. However, caution is recommended with the indication because of the possibility of hepatic complications, including reports of fatalities associated with the use of troglitazone. Additionally, this drug should be administered with caution in cardiac patients due to the possibility of edema [18, 30, 31].

2.2.2. *Pioglitazone*

Pioglitazone can be used as monotherapy or in combination with metformin, which has anti-hyperglycemic effects, or with sulfonylurea, meglitinida, or even insulin, especially in diabetic patients with metabolic syndrome. The dose varies from 15 to 45 mg, and it may be administered once a day. This drug displays mechanism of action and similar side effects to rosiglitazone, and it causes less liver toxicity than troglitazone. However, pioglitazone may interact with other drugs metabolized by P450 enzymes through changing their serum levels. An example is a decrease by approximately 30% of the contraceptive effect of ethinyl estradiol and norethindrone. Accordingly, the dose of the contraceptive must be increased in diabetic women who do not wish to become pregnant. The pharmacokinetics of pioglitazone are not altered by mild to moderate renal insufficiency [32].

2.2.3. *Rosiglitazone*

Rosiglitazone is more potent and has lower hepatotoxicity than troglitazone. Furthermore, it stimulates metabolism by cytochrome P450 (CYP) 3A4 without interacting with oral contraceptives, digoxin, ranitidine or nifedipine. Rosiglitazone dosage varies from 4 to 8 mg, and it may be given once a day. Similar to pioglitazone, rosiglitazone's pharmacokinetics are not altered by mild to moderate renal insufficiency, and dose modification is not required [33].

Recently published safety data prompted concerns about a possible association between the chronic use of rosiglitazone and an increased risk of cardiovascular events, leading to some parsimony in the use of TZDs in clinical practice. Furthermore, studies have recently shown bone loss and increased fracture among users of these medications in [27, 29, 34].

2.3. Alpha-glucosidase inhibitors

The competitive inhibitors of alpha-glucosidase, such as acarbose, miglitol and voglibose, act as enzymatic antagonists of oligosaccharide (e.g. amylase, maltase and sucrase) and decrease the intestinal absorption of glucose, particularly postprandial absorption, thereby modulating the insulin secretion [35]. These inhibitors present the advantage of lowering the incidence of cardiovascular events, and they have no systemic absorption [36].

More specifically, alpha-glucosidase is inhibited competitively, and its availability for oligosaccharides derived from the diet is reduced. Thus, the formation of monosaccharide decreases, and less insulin is required for metabolism, which leads to a reduction of glucose (because it is not absorbed) as well as postprandial insulin-induced increases [37]. These effects reflect a significant decrease in glycated hemoglobin [38, 39], which is more evident in highly hyperglycemic patients. Hyperglycemia in patients with mild or moderate glycemic control is less common than in those using other oral antidiabetic agents. In such cases, competitive inhibitors of alpha-glucosidase can be used in combination with insulin or any other oral hypoglycemic agents.

2.3.1. *Acarbose*

Acarbose has microbial origin and is structurally similar to natural oligosaccharides, having an affinity 104-105 times higher than drugs of the same class of alpha-glucosidases. With regard to the pharmacokinetic aspects, acarbose is poorly absorbed in the intestine (less than 2%). The products produced by bacterial enzymes cleave acarbose, yielding intermediate 4-metipirogalol, which is conjugated and excreted as sulfates or glucuronidate [39].

In a prospective, randomized, double-blind, placebo-controlled trial [40], there was a satisfactory control of fasting and postprandial glucose with acarbose in T2DM. In a multicenter, randomized, double-blind, placebo-controlled clinical trial [41] conducted in patients with T2DM who were subjected to a specific diet and use of insulin, the patients showed decreased levels of blood glucose and glycated hemoglobin as well as a reduced daily requirement for insulin.

In a systematic review [42], it was concluded that acarbose inhibits postprandial hyperglycemia by lowering insulin levels after a glucose overload. However, it presents no advantages with respect to corporal weight or lipid metabolism, and there are no statistically significant effects on mortality, morbidity and quality of life in patients with T2DM. Compared with placebo, acarbose reduces HbA1c and fasting plasma glucose and postprandial glucose. Compared with sulfonylureas, it reduces glycemic control and has major adverse effects, particularly gastrointestinal.

2.3.2. Voglibose

Voglibose also has a microbial origin, and only 3-5% of the drug is absorbed at the intestinal level. It is a potent inhibitor of alpha-glucosidase, but it is weaker than acarbose in the inhibition of sucrase and has little effect on pancreatic alpha-amylase [39].

2.3.3. Miglitol

Miglitol has a synthetic origin. It is absorbed rapidly through a transport mechanism in the jejunum that is partly identical to glucose, and it is quantitatively excreted unchanged by the kidney. Miglitol differs from acarbose, as it does not inhibit alpha-amylase, but rather it inhibits intestinal isomaltase [39].

The most frequent side effects of alpha-glucosidase inhibitors are seen at the intestinal level: flatulence, diarrhea, abdominal pain and elevated transaminases. The occurrence of hypoglycemia and an increase in body weight are rare because the agent does not stimulate insulin release or hypersecretion. These effects are only observed when miglitol is combined with other therapies. Its use is contraindicated in cases of inflammatory bowel disease, pregnancy and lactation, and hepatic or renal impairment.

2.4. Sulfonylureas

Another class of drugs used in the treatment of T2DM is the class of sulfonylureas, chlorpropamide and tolbultamide (first generation), glibenclamide, glipizide and gliclazide (second generation) and glimepiride (third generation). This class was introduced commercially in the 1950s and has since been recognized as first-line therapy and as a monotherapy or in combination [43]. The sulfonylureas are the drugs of choice for type 2 diabetics who do not benefit exclusively from diet and exercise [44].

These drugs act as insulin secretagogues and exert their main action on islet B cells, stimulating insulin secretion and thereby reducing the plasma glucose concentration [45]. The mechanism of action involves binding of the drug to a subunit of the ATP-sensitive potassium channels in the plasma membranes of B cells. The channels are closed, leading to a change in the membrane voltage, calcium influx and exocytosis of insulin granules [46, 47].

The basal secretion and insulin secretory response to various stimuli are intensified in the early days of treatment with sulfonylureas. With longer-term treatment, insulin secretion continues to increase, and tissue sensitivity to insulin also improves by an unknown mechanism [45].

The sulphonylureas are well absorbed after oral administration, and most reach peak plasma concentrations in 2-4 hours. The duration of the effect varies. All of these drugs bind tightly to plasma albumin and are involved in interactions with other drugs (e.g., salicylates and sulfonamides) such that there is competition for binding sites. The sulfonylureas (or their active metabolites) are mostly excreted in the urine; thus, their action is increased in elderly patients or those with renal disease [45].

2.4.1. *First-generation sulfonylureas*

The action of chlorpropamide and tolbultamide is long lasting, with substantial excretion in urine. Therefore, these drugs can cause severe hypoglycemia in elderly patients where there is a progressive decline in glomerular filtration. They cause flushing after alcohol consumption and exert similar effects to the diuretic hormone on the distal nephron, producing hyponatremia and water intoxication [45].

2.4.2. *Second-generation sulfonylureas*

The second-generation sulfonylureas (glibenclamide, glipizide and gliclazide) are more potent, but their hypoglycemic effects are not much greater, and failure to control blood glucose is as commonly observed as that with tolbutamide. All of these drugs contain the sulfonylurea molecule, but different substitutions result in pharmacokinetic differences, and thus differences in the duration of action. Glibenclamide should be avoided in the elderly and in patients with mild renal impairment because of the risk of hypoglycemia, as several of its metabolites are excreted in the urine and are moderately active [45].

The sulfonylureas cross the placenta and stimulate insulin release by fetal B cells, causing severe hypoglycemia at birth. Consequently, their use is contraindicated during pregnancy, and gestational diabetes is treated by diet supplemented where necessary with insulin [45].

In general, sulfonylureas are well tolerated. The observed side effects are hypoglycemia, hematological (leukopenia, agranulocytosis, thrombocytopenia, and hemolytic anemia) and gastrointestinal (nausea, vomiting, more rarely cholestatic jaundice) problems and allergic reactions. Sulfonylureas may also cause weight gain, and binding to plasma proteins can be potentiated by other drugs used concomitantly, causing hypoglycemia. This condition is the most worrisome adverse event observed and may be prolonged, which can have severe consequences in elderly patients, patients treated with multiple drugs and those with impaired renal function. Moreover, sulfonylureas stimulate appetite and can occasionally cause allergic rashes and bone marrow injury [45].

2.4.3. *Glimepiride*

The United States Food and Drug Administration (FDA) approved glimepiride in 1995 for the treatment of T2DM alone and in combination with metformin or insulin. It has prolonged action, lasting over 24 hours. Glimepiride has advantages with respect to its clinical and pharmacological profile, and it has also been shown to cause a lower incidence of severe hypoglycemia compared to other representatives of their class [48, 49].

Regarding hypoglycemia, the findings observed in some studies differ. In a systematic review and meta-analysis [50], we concluded that glimepiride caused more hypoglycemia compared to other sulfonylureas, and even more than other secretagogues. In other studies, the long-acting sulfonylureas, such as chlorpropamide and glibenclamide, have been shown to be more likely to cause hypoglycemia [51-53]. In a UK survey, the rate of diagnosis of hypoglycemia was higher for glibenclamide compared to other representatives of the same class [51].

With regard to weight gain, in the United Kingdom Prospective Diabetes Study (UKPDS), the mean weight change after 10 years of follow up ranged from a minimum of 1.7 kg as a result of glibenclamide use to a maximum 2.6 kg with chlorpropamide use [19]. Glimepiride was claimed to be at least neutral with respect to body weight, and weight reduction has been observed by some authors [54, 55].

Sulfonylureas have different cross reactivities with cardiovascular ATP-dependent potassium channels. The closing of these channels by ischemic preconditioning can lead to cardiovascular mortality [56].

Several compounds increase the hypoglycemic effect of sulfonylureas, and several of these interactions are potentially important from a clinical standpoint. The non-steroidal anti-inflammatory agents (including azapropazone, phenylbutazone and salicylates), coumarin, some uricosuric agents (e.g., sulfinpyrazone), alcohol, monoamine oxidase inhibitors, some antibacterials (including sulfonamides, and chloramphenicol trimethropim) and some antifungal agents (including miconazole and possibelmente, fluconazole) produce severe hypoglycemia when administered with sulfonylureas. The probable basis for these interactions is the competition for metabolizing enzymes, but interference in the plasma protein binding or excretion may also exert some effect. The agents that reduce the action of sulfonylureas include diuretics (thiazides and loop diuretics) and corticosteroids [45].

2.5. Glinides

Other insulin secretagogues drugs include repaglinide, nateglinide and mitiglinide. Derivatives of benzoic acid and the amino acid D-phenylalanine increase insulin secretion through an action similar to the sulfonylureas. Due to their rapid absorption, the action begins approximately 30 minutes after administration. These drugs have no interactions with other medication and are not contraindicated in pregnancy, lactation or in the presence of other pathologies

Repaglinide and nateglinide are insulin secretagogues with short action, with a half-life equivalent to 1 hour for the repaglinide and 1.5 h for nateglinide. Both of these secretagogues act by triggering an insulin peak during the postprandial period when administered before meals [57].

2.5.1. *Repaglinide*

Repaglinide ((S) - (+)-2-ethoxy-4-[2 - (3-methyl-1-[2 - (piperidin-1-yl) phenyl] Butylamino)-2-oxoethyl] benzoic acid) was the first representative of the class of glinides, which differs from other classes of anti-hyperglycemic drugs due to its distinct molecular structure, mechanism of action and mechanism excretion [58].

This drug acts as a short-acting insulin secretagogue that targets the postprandial-released glucose. It significantly reduces the levels of plasma glucose in individuals with T2DM [59].

The mechanism of action of repaglinide involves blocking potassium efflux from pancreatic β cells. This action depolarizes the cells by opening voltage-gated calcium channels. This process results in increased calcium influx into the B cells, which stimulates the exocytosis of insulin-containing secretory granules [60, 61]. Regarding the pharmacokinetics, this drug has rapid absorption and rapid elimination, with a plasma half-life of up to 1 hour [61]. Repaglinide is primarily metabolized in the liver, and 90% of the drug is excreted through the gut and 8% through the urine [62]. Because the action of this drug is rapid and the time of effect is relatively short, it carries a low risk of hypoglycemia [63]. Repaglinide may be used as a monotherapy or in combination with other antidiabetic agents, such as metformin and glitazone [62].

2.5.2. *Nateglinide*

Nateglinide (3-phenyl-2-[(4-propan-2-ylcyclohexanecarbonyl) amino] propanoic acid) as well as repaglinide acts by inhibiting potassium channels that are sensitive to ATP, causing depolarization of the plasma membrane of the β cell. This processes culminates in the influx of calcium ions into the cell and subsequent insulin secretion [64]. Nateglinide is thus an insulinotropic agent that is capable of restoring the physiological pattern of insulin secretion, which is not regulated in diabetic patients [65].

Potassium channels are known to be ATP-dependent in cardiac cells as well as in pancreatic β cells. Thus, a reasonable degree of concern exists regarding the influence of therapeutic agents that act on these channels on heart function. Nateglinide has a high selectivity for pancreatic potassium channels and is more reliable in relation to repaglinide and glibenclamide with regard to the possible onset of cardiovascular events [65].

Nateglinide induces rapid and transient insulin secretion in a glucose-dependent manner. The response of potassium channels to nateglinide is remarkably lower during periods of euglycemia compared to periods when the glucose levels are high. Thus, the minimum total insulin exposure generated by this drug protects against hypoglycemia attacks, allowing the patient some flexibility regarding the intervals between meals [62].

The effects of nateglinide are specific to prandial insulin release, allowing for the observed reduction in glycated hemoglobin (HbA1c) without the risk of hypoglycemia between meals [65].

With regard to the pharmacokinetic properties, nateglinide is rapidly absorbed, and the peak plasma concentration is reached in 1 hour. The drug metabolism occurs in the liver, and approximately 10% is excreted unchanged via the kidneys [62].

As with repaglinide, nateglinide can be used as a monotherapy or in combination with other agents, such as metformin or glitazone. Both repaglinide and nateglinide have similar efficacy for reducing the fasting blood glucose levels and postprandial plasma glucose, and during early insulin secretion, they contribute to an improvement of insulin sensitivity and pancreatic β cell function. However, repaglinide was shown to be more effective with regard to reducing HbA1c [65].

2.5.3. Mitiglinide

Mitiglinide is also an analogue of the meglitinides, and it has a mechanism of action that has been previously elucidated for other substances [60]. However, mitiglinide is not yet approved by the FDA for the treatment of T2DM.

2.6. Treatment based on the effects of incretin hormones

The use of incretin hormones in the treatment of type 2 diabetes is the subject of extensive investigations that have culminated in the development of new classes of drugs that have been recently approved for the treatment of the disease. The intensification of the action of incretin, especially GLP-1, is the basis of numerous new options for the metabolic control of T2DM.

Incretin mimetics, such as exenatide, as well as inhibitors of the enzyme DPP-4, such as sitagliptin and vildagliptin, have been developed. In general, these agents reduce the blood glucose levels to a level similar to that induced by other oral hypoglycemic agents with minimal risk of hypoglycemia. Furthermore, they have potential preventive effects and may promote disease regression. They may also have possible protective effects and promote growth in pancreatic β cells.

2.7. Antagonists of GLP-1R

2.7.1. Exenatide

Exenatide is an exendin-4 GLP-1 mimetic with ~53% homology to endogenous GLP-1. It is currently approved for use as a monotherapy or in combination with metformin and/or sulphonylureas [66]. Exenatide is administered subcutaneously at a dose of 5 or 10 mg, twice a day. It binds to the GLP-1 receptor and has a longer lasting action because it presents greater resistance to the action of DPP-4 [67, 68].

In phase III studies, exenatide improved glycemic control in patients with type 2 diabetes for whom glycemic control was not achieved with metformin and / or sulfonylurea. These studies were double-blind, placebo-controlled, 30-week trials. The initial HA1c ranged from 8.2% to 8.7% and was reduced by approximately 1% when exenatide was compared with placebo. There was a mean weight loss of approximately 2 Kg. In the clinical trials that have been performed to date, the drop-out rate due to side effects of exenatide was less than 5% [69, 70]

The main adverse effects of exenatide are nausea, vomiting and diarrhea. Most episodes of nausea are mild to moderate and dose dependent, and they decrease in frequency with continued treatment [71].

2.8. GLP-1 analogs

2.8.1. Liraglutide

Liraglutide is a long-acting human GLP-1 analogue that shares 97% amino acid sequence identity with human GLP-1 and is resistant to dipeptidyl peptidase-IV. Native GLP-1 has a short elimination half-life of 1-2 min, whereas liraglutide has a long half-life of approximately 13 hours and can be administered once a day [67, 72]. When administered once daily, liraglutide enables significantly superior glycemic control compared to that obtained with the administration of exenatide 2 times per day and is generally well tolerated [69].

Other GLP-1 analogs, taspoglutide and albiglutide are currently in phase III clinical trials. Albiglutide has a long half-life, allowing administration once per week.

2.9. DPP-4 inhibitors

2.9.1. Vildagliptin

Vildagliptin is a DPP-4 inhibitor that prolongs the activity of endogenous GLP-1. A study that compared vildagliptin with metformin showed a smaller decrease in HA1c after one year with vildagliptin, but fewer gastrointestinal side effects. Comparison of vildagliptin and pioglitazone showed similar reductions in HA1c [73].

Vildagliptin is used in several countries, but it has not been approved by the FDA because of the occurrence of elevated enzyme levels in patients taking higher doses of vildagliptin.

2.9.2. Sitagliptin

Sitagliptin is a DPP-4 inhibitor that was approved by the FDA in October 2006 to improve glycemic control in patients with type 2 diabetes. It is approved for use as a monotherapy or in combination with other oral hypoglycemic agents. It is administered at a dose of 100 mg per day [74]. Treatment with this DPP-4 inhibitor is generally well tolerated. Sitagliptin monotherapy or in combination was shown to have a neutral effect on body weight. The incidence of hypoglycemia and gastrointestinal effects, such as abdominal pain, diarrhea, nausea and vomiting, was not significantly different between the groups treated with sitagliptin and placebo [75].

Sitagliptin displays a relatively low effectiveness in reducing HA1c and plasma glucose compared to other antidiabetic agents that have been utilized clinically for many years. Additionally, sitagliptin does not have beneficial effects beyond its effects on glycemic control, such as reduction in body weight [76].

Alogliptina and saxagliptin are still under investigation, and they have not been approved for use by the FDA.

2.10. Anti-obesity drugs

Many clinical studies have reported the significant influence of excess body fat on metabolic disorders, such as T2DM. Notably, patients with T2DM who are significantly overweight (20% to 40%) have a higher mortality rate compared with patients with the same disease but who are within the proper range of weight. In many diabetic patients, a reduced calorie diet aimed at weight reduction alone is able to control blood glucose levels. However, for these individuals, body weight control is more complicated, both due to a mechanism of disease and for the treatment of disease. Thus, many doctors resort to drugs that are capable of inducing weight loss in patients with metabolic disorders [77].

In patients whose body mass index (BMI) is above 30 kg/m2 or those with morbid conditions associated with overweight for whom non-pharmacological weight loss methods (diet, exercise) have failed, the use of antiobesity drugs is recommended [78]. These drugs may include medications with catecholaminergic action (amfepramone, femproporex, mazindol), serotonergic action (fluoxetine, sertraline) and mixed catecholaminergic and serotonergic action (such as sibutramine), which promote appetite control and induction of satiety. In addition to these drugs, tetrahydrolipstatin or orlistat may be used to inhibit lipase reducing intestinal fat absorption, allowing for a reduction of the dose of the hypoglycemic drug.

Amfepramone (diethylpropion), femproporex and mazindol are amphetamine derivatives. They work by stimulating the central nervous system, prompting the release of noradrenaline in the central and peripheral synapses. Through this mechanism, these drugs cause appetite suppression [79]. Amfepramone has been available in the market for weight loss since the 1960s [80]. It has been demonstrated in clinical trials with animals that mazindol stimulates the consumption of oxygen by increasing the stimulation of noradrenaline in the brown adipose tissue. Through this thermogenic effect, mazindol is capable of inducing weight loss [78].

The anorectic catecholaminergic drugs usually have good gastrointestinal absorption and are able to reach peak plasma levels within 2 hours of administration, and their metabolism is mainly hepatic. The catecholaminergic drugs have serious side effects, such as increased heart rate and blood pressure [78]. Generally, the use of amphetamine derivatives is accompanied by a remarkable pharmacodynamic tolerance, and their anorectic actions over the long term are not known [79].

Catecholaminergic and serotonergic medications have different effects on food intake. The former delay the start of ingestion, and the latter anticipate the completion of food intake [78].

Sibutramine acts by inhibition of noradrenaline and serotonin receptors, elevating the levels of these neurotransmitters in the hypothalamus and brainstem regions associated with energy homeostasis. This mechanism induces satiety and therefore the reduction of food intake. In addition to generating weight loss, sibutramine significantly reduces triglyceride and HDL-cholesterol levels, its therapeutic action may be accompanied by some adverse effects, such as constipation, headache, and insomnia, which are usually mild [81]. However, cardiovascular events associated with the use of this substance, such as an increased heart rate and elevated blood pressure, are of concern [82, 83].

Orlistat is a reversible inhibitor of pancreatic and gastric lipase that induces weight loss by preventing the absorption of a significant amount of fat digested in the intestine [82]. It inactivates fat hydrolyzing, thereby reducing the absorption of calories by the patient [84]. The effect of orlistat on body weight reduction corresponds to benefits for other cardiometabolic parameters, such as blood pressure, waist circumference, and blood glucose. Among the most common adverse side effects of orlistat are diarrhea, flatulence, bloating and dyspepsia [81].

Although the weight loss caused by these drugs is generally not very significant, there is an improvement in insulin sensitivity and glycemic control in overweight patients who use these substances [84]. This effect emphasizes the importance of aid in the pharmacological management of obesity in patients with T2DM and other metabolic disorders; it is insufficient to only change the patient's lifestyle.

2.11. Insulin

The classification of insulin is based on the preparation. Namely, the duration of its action as short-acting, intermediate or basal insulin determines the classification. The latter two are the result of changes in crystalline insulin (short-acting). The addition of protamine and zinc result in Neutral Protamine Hagedorn (NPH) with intermediate and basal action, respectively.

The change in amino acid sequence allowed for the development of insulin analogues. The fast-acting insulin analogues lispro and aspart are available for clinical use and show similar pharmacokinetic and pharmacodynamic properties. The formulations glargine and detemir represent similar groups that may have either basal or long-term action (24 hours) [85].

2.11.1. Short or ultra-rapid-acting insulin

This group includes regular insulin and the analogues lispro, aspart and glulisine.

Regular insulin is usually administered by the subcutaneous route, often in combination with an intermediate-acting or long-duration insulin. Specific buffers are used to prevent crystallization due to its slow infusion. With this type of insulin, the monomers are presented in an associated hexamer form, which reduces the rate of absorption. Generally, regular insulin is indicated for the treatment of diabetic ketoacidosis, and it is also associated with human insulin intermediate-acting or basal analogs before meals [86]. This insulin must be given 30-45 minutes before meals to reduce the postprandial glycemia peak, and the activity lasts between 2 and 4 hours. However, patients tend to apply it at mealtime, which contributes to postprandial hyperglycemia and hypoglycemia in the period between meals because the regular insulin will peak at the time that the food has been metabolized. The first rapid-acting insulin analogue became available in 1996, and other rapid-acting analogs have been developed since. These analogues were produced by different modifications of the chemical structure of the human insulin protein, substituting various amino acids at different positions to shorten the onset and duration of action when compared to regular/ soluble insulin.

Insulin lispro is an analogue of human insulin developed using genetic engineering to reverse the amino acids proline and lysine in positions 28 and 29 of the beta chain, resulting in a sequence of Lys (B28) Pro (B29). This insulin in pharmaceutical preparations with phenol and zinc forms stable hexamers [86]. It has a lower tendency to self-aggregate at the site of subcutaneous injection, it is absorbed faster than regular human insulin, and it mimics the physiological insulin profile in response to a meal. Lispro begins to take effect within 5 - 15 minutes, and the duration of action is 1-2 hours [87]. During the use of these analogs, an additional dose is required in the afternoon to compensate for hyperglycemia that may result from an afternoon snack. There is evidence that compared with regular insulin, lispro insulin reduces the postprandial hyperglycemic peaks as well as the risk of hypoglycemia, especially at night [86].

In insulin aspart, a proline residue is replaced with a negatively charged aspartic acid at position 28 of the beta chain, producing electrical repulsion among the insulin molecules, which reduces their tendency for self-association. In vials or cartridges, the drug is present in the form of hexamers that rapidly dissociate into monomers and dimers in the subcutaneous tissue, ensuring rapid absorption. The pharmacokinetic profile includes the onset of action within 5 - 15 minutes and a duration of action of 1-2 hours [86].

The insulin glulisine is another insulin analogue with ultra-rapid action that is obtained by the exchange of asparagine for lysine at position 3 of the beta chain and lysine for glutamic acid at position 29 of the same chain. To date, there are few studies with glulisine, which seems to be similar to lispro and aspart with regard to its efficacy and the occurrence of hypoglycemic events. Due to its faster absorption, glulisine should be administered 5-10 minutes before a meal, ensuring greater flexibility for the patient and thus improving his/her quality of life. The short half-life reduces the need to eat food 2-3 hours after its administration, which is necessary with regular insulin, for which the greater half-life causes postprandial hypoglycemia. Although chemical structures of glulisine and insulin are different, no significant difference in time or duration of action was reported between them.

2.11.2. Intermediate-acting insulin

NPH insulin was introduced in 1946. It is a suspension of insulin in a complex with zinc and protamine in a phosphate buffer. Generally, a dose is given once a day before breakfast or twice daily. NPH has an absorption peak at approximately 4.6 hours after subcutaneous administration, followed by a steady decline in the level of plasma insulin [88]. This insulin can be mixed with regular insulin in the same syringe to increase patient compliance, especially in the case of children. However, the zinc present in the slow-acting insulin can prolong the effect of regular insulin [86].

The profiles of action of intermediate-acting insulin make them suitable for systems in which basal insulin is given one to three times daily. A rigid daily feeding programming is required, including a relatively fixed schedule for meals and snacks with consistent indices of carbohydrate meals / snacks. The major disadvantages of NPH are the wide variations in the daily timing and duration of the peaks within and between individuals, which, when compared to long-acting analogs, may result in non-optimal metabolic control and an increased risk for nocturnal hypoglycemia. The slow-acting insulin was used for many years as an intermediate-acting insulin with a profile of action similar to that of NPH.

2.11.3. Basal insulin analogs (long-action insulin analogs)

The insulins glargine and detemir belong to a group referred to as long-acting or basal insulin analogs [86].

Insulin detemir is produced by recombinant DNA technology, with expression in *Saccharomyces cerevisiae* followed by chemical modification [89]. A fatty acid (myristic acid) is attached to the lysine at position 29, which binds to circulating albumin, forming a complex that dissociates slowly, thus prolonging the duration of its action [79]. The insulin detemir is soluble at neutral pH; however, it can be mixed with rapid analogs. Insulin detemir has shown potential benefits for body weight, with weight loss or decreased weight gain in adults, in children and in adolescents [90].

Insulin glargine is synthesized by introducing changes into the amino acid chain of human insulin, including a substitution of asparagine with glycine at position A21 and the addition of two arginines at position B30. These changes result in a standard single release from the injection site. That is, this analog precipitates in the subcutaneous tissue, allowing a gradual absorption into the bloodstream [91].

Basal insulin was developed to promote basal levels within 24 hours, and it may be administered once a day or at bedtime. When comparing conventional long-acting insulin with insulin glargine, it can be observed that insulin has a similar profile at a constant concentration without prominent peaks [92]. It has an onset of action between 1 and 2 hours, reaching the plateau of biological action between 4 and 6 hours with termination of the effect between 20 and 24 hours. Due to a slightly acidic pH, glargine cannot be mixed with any other insulin in the same syringe; accordingly, some children complain of a burning sensation at the application site [86]. The timing of administration of glargine seems to have no impact on its efficacy for glycemic control, but the dose should be given at approximately the same time each day to maintain its efficacy as a free insulin peak action. If a dose is omitted, 50% of the daily insulin will be missed on that day.

2.11.4. Inhalable insulin

The benefits of injectable insulin are often limited, considering the difficulty of persuading patients to comply with the requirements for adequate treatment due to the need for multiple injections [93].

Aiming to alleviate this discomfort, the first US-approved inhaled insulin (Exubera ®) Pfizer / Nektar became available in January 2006. This product consisted of a dry powder formulation containing 1-3 g of human insulin administered via a single inhaler dose [94]. A polyethylene glycol inhalable dry powder that releases the equivalent of 3 to 8 UI of short-acting insulin subcutaneously [95] was developed for this product. Although Exubera has demonstrated efficacy and a low risk of hypoglycemia, there was a poor acceptance by the prescriber and the patient, and in April 2008, the first clinical evidence that it may cause cancer emerged, with 6 cases diagnosed with lung cancer. There were also cases of primary lung malignancy in patients who had a history of smoking. Other important aspects include coughing, pulmonary function deterioration and an increase of anti-insulin antibodies [96].

AERx insulin was developed by Aradigm Corporation and Novo Nordisk. This system generates aerosol droplets from liquid insulin. The device guides the user to inhale reproducibly. It also offers the ability to download data related to the patient's insulin use, such as the frequency of inhalation, allowing for the monitoring of the treatment. Because of the experiences reported in the Exubera studies, their studies have been discontinued [97].

Technosphere Insulin (TI) is another system involving inhaled dry powder blends of recombinant human insulin (MannKind Corp.) using a MedTone ® (Pharmaceutical Discovery Corp.) inhaler. This system is currently in phase II clinical research, and the partners have developed a placebo for inhalation, allowing for controlled and double-blind studies in patients with diabetes mellitus [95, 97].

2.11.5. Insulin and cancer risk

Studies report that chronic hyperinsulinemia is associated with the pathogenesis of colon cancer and also with breast, pancreas and endometrium cancer [98]. One possible mechanism that explains this relationship is that insulin resistance and hyperinsulinemia, which are characteristic of diabetic patients, or even increased levels of therapies based on endogenous insulin secretagogues or insulin, may increase the level of growth factor 1 of insulin, which plays an essential role in carcinogenesis [99]. Insulin receptors are present in (pre)-neoplastic cells, and insulin can stimulate growth. Furthermore, these cells may be susceptible to mechanisms that cause insulin resistance, such as subclinical chronic inflammation with increased TNF-alpha, which act as promoters of tumor growth. Obesity is associated with an increased risk of developing cancer due to factors such as the endocrine and metabolic effects and the consequent changes that they induce in the production of peptide and steroid hormones [98]. The results of a meta-analysis published in 2012 reported an increase of 28% in the risk of developing cancer in patients using insulin compared to non-users. Thus, there is growing that we are experiencing a worldwide epidemic of diabetes mellitus due to a large aging population and the increasing number of obese people who develop insulin resistance and hyperinsulinemia, which may further contribute to the number of patients with cancer [99].

The results of recently published meta-analyses indicate that some cancers develop most frequently in patients with diabetes, especially type 2 diabetes, although prostate cancer was shown to be less frequent in men with diabetes. Thus, preventive measures should be encouraged among the population to prevent these diseases [99].

3. Conclusion

Despite the clear benefits of achieving and maintaining glycemic goals and the availability of newer and potentially more effective drugs for the management of T2DM, the number of patients with poor glycemic control has not substantially decreased over the past 10 years.

The progressive nature of T2DM has been a significant challenge for achieving adequate glycemic control. The inability of classical oral antidiabetic agents to prevent the disease and maintain good metabolic control over the long term has motivated research on new physiological pathways involved in glucose homeostasis. The use of agents based on the effect of incretin hormones for the treatment of T2DM is quite promising. These treatments act through a mechanism that is distinct from that of drugs that have been commonly used in the treatment of this pathology. Furthermore, these agents reduce blood glucose levels to a level similar to other oral hypoglycemic agents with a minimal risk of hypoglycemia, they have few side effects, and they have no immediate need for dose titration.

However, although some of these agents have already been approved for the treatment of type 2 diabetes by regulatory authorities, phase IV studies and clinical experience are necessary to establish their actual benefits with greater certainty. The extra-glycemic effects, safety profiles and advantages and disadvantages compared to classically used oral antidiabetics remain to be fully characterized.

The increasing availability of numerous classes of medications has given clinicians and patients more therapeutic choices and perhaps an improved ability to achieve glycemic goals.

Author details

Roberto Pontarolo[1*], Andréia Cristina Conegero Sanches[2], Astrid Wiens[1], Helena Hiemisch Lobo Borba[1], Luana Lenzi[1] and Suelem Tavares da Silva Penteado[1]

*Address all correspondence to: pontarolo@ufpr.br

1 Department of Pharmacy – Federal University of Paraná, Curitiba, Paraná, Brazil

2 Department of Medical and Pharmaceutical Sciences - State University of West of Paraná, Cascavel, Paraná, Brazil

References

[1] World Health Organization. http://www.who.int/en/. (acessed 5 november 2012).

[2] George PM, Valabhji J, Dawood M, Henry JA. Screening for Type 2 diabetes in the accident and emergency department. Diabet Med 2005;22(12):1766-9.

[3] Chopra M, Galbraith S, Darnton-Hill I. A global response to a global problem: the epidemic of overnutrition. Bull World Health Organ 2002;80(12):952-8.

[4] Zimmet P, Shaw J, Alberti KG. Preventing Type 2 diabetes and the dysmetabolic syndrome in the real world: a realistic view. Diabet Med 2003;20(9):693-702.

[5] U.S. Department of Health and Human Services. NDIC: National Diabetes Statistics. http://diabetesniddknihgov/dm/pubs/statistics/#fast 2011. acessed in 12 november 2012.

[6] Boog M, Magrini V. Relato de experiência: reeducação alimentar por meio de abordagem interdisciplinar envolvendo as áreas de Nutrição e Saúde Mental. Revista da Sociedade de Cardiologia do Estado de São Paulo 1999;9(3):1-8.

[7] Hirsch I, Riddle M. Current therapies for diabetes. Endocr Clin North Am 1997 1997;26:3.

[8] Pan XR, Li GW, Hu YH, Wang JX, Yang WY, An ZX, et al. Effects of diet and exercise in preventing NIDDM in people with impaired glucose tolerance. The Da Qing IGT and Diabetes Study. Diabetes Care 1997;20(4):537-44.

[9] Hepler CD, Strand LM. Opportunities and responsibilities in pharmaceutical care. Am J Hosp Pharm 1990;47(3):533-43.

[10] American Diabetes Association. Economic consequences of diabetes mellitus in the U.S. in 1997. American Diabetes Association. Diabetes Care 1998;21(2):296-309.

[11] Donovan JL, Blake DR. Patient non-compliance: deviance or reasoned decision-making? Soc Sci Med 1992;34(5):507-13.

[12] Association AD. Standards of medical care in diabetes--2008. Diabetes Care 2008;31 Suppl 1:S12-54.

[13] Farmaco AId. L'uso dei farmaci in Italia - Rapporto nazionale anno 2007. 2007.

[14] Anderson J. Obesity. Br Med J 1972;1(5799):560-3.

[15] Cusi K, DeFronzo R. Metformin: a review of its metabolic effects. Diabetes Rev 1998;6:89-131.

[16] Santos RF, Nomizo R, Wajhenberg BL, Reaven GM, Azhar S. Changes in insulin receptor tyrosine kinase activity associated with metformin treatment of type 2 diabetes. Diabete Metab 1995;21(4):274-80.

[17] Johansen K. Efficacy of metformin in the treatment of NIDDM. Meta-analysis. Diabetes Care 1999;22(1):33-7.

[18] Araújo L, Britto MdS, Cruz T. Tratamento do Diabetes Mellitns do Tipo 2: Novas Opções. Arq Bras Endocrinol Metab 2000;44(6):509-18.

[19] Group U. Effect of intensive blood-glucose control with metformin on complications in overweight patients with type 2 diabetes (UKPDS 34). UK Prospective Diabetes Study (UKPDS) Group. Lancet 1998;352(9131):854-65.

[20] Chiasson JL, Josse RG, Hunt JA, Palmason C, Rodger NW, Ross SA, et al. The efficacy of acarbose in the treatment of patients with non-insulin-dependent diabetes mellitus. A multicenter controlled clinical trial. Ann Intern Med 1994;121(12):928-35.

[21] DeFronzo R, Goodman A. The multicenter metformin study group: efficacy of metformin in NIDDM patients poorly controlled on diet done or diet plus sulfonylurea. N Engl J Med 1995;333:541-9.

[22] Inzucchi SE, Maggs DG, Spollett GR, Page SL, Rife FS, Walton V, et al. Efficacy and metabolic effects of metformin and troglitazone in type II diabetes mellitus. N Engl J Med 1998;338(13):867-72.

[23] Moses R, Slobodniuk R, Boyages S, Colagiuri S, Kidson W, Carter J, et al. Effect of repaglinide addition to metformin monotherapy on glycemic control in patients with type 2 diabetes. Diabetes Care 1999;22(1):119-24.

[24] Hirsch IB. Metformin added to insulin therapy in poorly controlled type 2 diabetes. Diabetes Care 1999;22(5):854.

[25] Turban S, Stretton C, Drouin O, Green CJ, Watson ML, Gray A, et al. Defining the contribution of AMP-activated protein kinase (AMPK) and protein kinase C (PKC) in regulation of glucose uptake by metformin in skeletal muscle cells. J Biol Chem 2012;287(24):20088-99.

[26] Flier JS. Diabetes. The missing link with obesity? Nature 2001;409(6818):292-3.

[27] Kahn SE, Haffner SM, Heise MA, Herman WH, Holman RR, Jones NP, et al. Glycemic durability of rosiglitazone, metformin, or glyburide monotherapy. N Engl J Med 2006;355(23):2427-43.

[28] Olokoba AB, Obateru OA, Olokoba LB. Type 2 diabetes mellitus: a review of current trends. Oman Med J 2012;27(4):269-73.

[29] Silva A, Lazaretti-Castro M. Diabetes melito, tiazolidinedionas e fraturas: uma história inacabada. Arq Bras Endocrinol Metab 2010;54(4):345-51.

[30] Horton ES, Whitehouse F, Ghazzi MN, Venable TC, Whitcomb RW. Troglitazone in combination with sulfonylurea restores glycemic control in patients with type 2 diabetes. The Troglitazone Study Group. Diabetes Care 1998;21(9):1462-9.

[31] Iwamoto Y, Kosaka K, Kuzuya T, Akanuma Y, Shigeta Y, Kaneko T. Effect of combination therapy of troglitazone and sulphonylureas in patients with Type 2 diabetes who were poorly controlled by sulphonylurea therapy alone. Diabet Med 1996;13(4): 365-70.

[32] Day C. Thiazolidinediones: a new class of antidiabetic drugs. Diabet Med 1999;16(3): 179-92.

[33] Balfour JA, Plosker GL. Rosiglitazone. Drugs 1999;57(6):921-30; discussion 31-2.

[34] Grey A. Skeletal consequences of thiazolidinedione therapy. Osteoporos Int 2008;19(2):129-37.

[35] van de Laar FA. Alpha-glucosidase inhibitors in the early treatment of type 2 diabetes. Vasc Health Risk Manag 2008;4(6):1189-95.

[36] Inzucchi SE, Bergenstal RM, Buse JB, Diamant M, Ferrannini E, Nauck M, et al. Management of hyperglycemia in type 2 diabetes: a patient-centered approach: position statement of the American Diabetes Association (ADA) and the European Association for the Study of Diabetes (EASD). Diabetes Care 2012;35(6):1364-79.

[37] Rosak C, Mertes G. Critical evaluation of the role of acarbose in the treatment of diabetes: patient considerations. Diabetes Metab Syndr Obes 2012;5:357-67.

[38] Coniff R, Krol A. Acarbose: a review of US clinical experience. Clin Ther 1997;19(1): 16-26; discussion 2-3.

[39] Lebovitz HE. alpha-Glucosidase inhibitors. Endocrinol Metab Clin North Am 1997;26(3):539-51.

[40] Braun D, Schönherr U, Mitzkat H. Efficacy of acarbose monotherapy in patients with type 2 diabetes: a double-blind study conducted in general practice. Endocrinol Metabol 1996;3:275-80.

[41] Coniff RF, Shapiro JA, Seaton TB, Hoogwerf BJ, Hunt JA. A double-blind placebo-controlled trial evaluating the safety and efficacy of acarbose for the treatment of patients with insulin-requiring type II diabetes. Diabetes Care 1995;18(7):928-32.

[42] van de Laar FA, Lucassen PL, Akkermans RP, van de Lisdonk EH, Rutten GE, van Weel C. Alpha-glucosidase inhibitors for patients with type 2 diabetes: results from a Cochrane systematic review and meta-analysis. Diabetes Care 2005;28(1):154-63.

[43] Holman RR. Long-term efficacy of sulfonylureas: a United Kingdom Prospective Diabetes Study perspective. Metabolism 2006;55(5 Suppl 1):S2-5.

[44] Wannmacher L. Antidiabéticos orais: comparação entre diferentes intervenções. Uso Racional de medicamentos: temas relacionados - Organização Pan-Americana da Saúde/Organização Mundial da Saúde 2005;2(11).

[45] Rang H, Dale M, Ritter J. Farmacologia. 4 ed. Rio de Janeiro: Guanabara Koogan; 2001.

[46] Akalin S, Berntorp K, Ceriello A, Das AK, Kilpatrick ES, Koblik T, et al. Intensive glucose therapy and clinical implications of recent data: a consensus statement from the Global Task Force on Glycaemic Control. Int J Clin Pract 2009;63(10):1421-5.

[47] Lee SJ, Eng C. Goals of glycemic control in frail older patients with diabetes. Jama 2011;305(13):1350-1.

[48] Basit A, Riaz M, Fawwad A. Glimepiride: evidence-based facts, trends, and observations. Vasc Health Risk Manag 2012;8:463-72.

[49] Holstein A, Plaschke A, Egberts EH. Lower incidence of severe hypoglycaemia in patients with type 2 diabetes treated with glimepiride versus glibenclamide. Diabetes Metab Res Rev 2001;17(6):467-73.

[50] Gangji AS, Cukierman T, Gerstein HC, Goldsmith CH, Clase CM. A systematic review and meta-analysis of hypoglycemia and cardiovascular events: a comparison of glyburide with other secretagogues and with insulin. Diabetes Care 2007;30(2): 389-94.

[51] Ben-Ami H, Nagachandran P, Mendelson A, Edoute Y. Drug-induced hypoglycemic coma in 102 diabetic patients. Arch Intern Med 1999;159(3):281-4.

[52] Ferner RE, Neil HA. Sulphonylureas and hypoglycaemia. Br Med J (Clin Res Ed) 1988;296(6627):949-50.

[53] Shorr RI, Ray WA, Daugherty JR, Griffin MR. Individual sulfonylureas and serious hypoglycemia in older people. J Am Geriatr Soc 1996;44(7):751-5.

[54] Bugos C, Austin M, Atherton T, Viereck C. Long-term treatment of type 2 diabetes mellitus with glimepiride is weight neutral: a meta-analysis. Diabetes Res Clin Pract 2000;50(1):S47.

[55] Martin S, Kolb H, Beuth J, van Leendert R, Schneider B, Scherbaum WA. Change in patients' body weight after 12 months of treatment with glimepiride or glibenclamide in Type 2 diabetes: a multicentre retrospective cohort study. Diabetologia 2003;46(12):1611-7.

[56] Lazdunski M. Ion channel effects of antidiabetic sulfonylureas. Horm Metab Res 1996;28(9):488-95.

[57] Rosenstock J, Hassman DR, Madder RD, Brazinsky SA, Farrell J, Khutoryansky N, et al. Repaglinide versus nateglinide monotherapy: a randomized, multicenter study. Diabetes Care 2004;27(6):1265-70.

[58] Derosa G, Mugellini A, Ciccarelli L, Crescenzi G, Fogari R. Comparison between repaglinide and glimepiride in patients with type 2 diabetes mellitus: a one-year, randomized, double-blind assessment of metabolic parameters and cardiovascular risk factors. Clin Ther 2003;25(2):472-84.

[59] Stephens JW, Bodvarsdottir TB, Wareham K, Prior SL, Bracken RM, Lowe GD, et al. Effects of short-term therapy with glibenclamide and repaglinide on incretin hormones and oxidative damage associated with postprandial hyperglycaemia in people with type 2 diabetes mellitus. Diabetes Res Clin Pract 2011;94(2):199-206.

[60] Reimann F, Proks P, Ashcroft FM. Effects of mitiglinide (S 21403) on Kir6.2/SUR1, Kir6.2/SUR2A and Kir6.2/SUR2B types of ATP-sensitive potassium channel. Br J Pharmacol 2001;132(7):1542-8.

[61] Wolffenbuttel BH, Nijst L, Sels JP, Menheere PP, Muller PG, Kruseman AC. Effects of a new oral hypoglycaemic agent, repaglinide, on metabolic control in sulphonylurea-treated patients with NIDDM. Eur J Clin Pharmacol 1993;45(2):113-6.

[62] Dornhorst A. Insulinotropic meglitinide analogues. Lancet 2001;358(9294):1709-16.

[63] Papa G, Fedele V, Rizzo MR, Fioravanti M, Leotta C, Solerte SB, et al. Safety of type 2 diabetes treatment with repaglinide compared with glibenclamide in elderly people: A randomized, open-label, two-period, cross-over trial. Diabetes Care 2006;29(8): 1918-20.

[64] Keilson L, Mather S, Walter YH, Subramanian S, McLeod JF. Synergistic effects of nateglinide and meal administration on insulin secretion in patients with type 2 diabetes mellitus. J Clin Endocrinol Metab 2000;85(3):1081-6.

[65] Tentolouris N, Voulgari C, Katsilambros N. A review of nateglinide in the management of patients with type 2 diabetes. Vasc Health Risk Manag 2007;3(6):797-807.

[66] Fehse F, Trautmann M, Holst JJ, Halseth AE, Nanayakkara N, Nielsen LL, et al. Exenatide augments first- and second-phase insulin secretion in response to intravenous glucose in subjects with type 2 diabetes. J Clin Endocrinol Metab 2005;90(11):5991-7.

[67] Brown DX, Evans M. Choosing between GLP-1 Receptor Agonists and DPP-4 Inhibitors: A Pharmacological Perspective. J Nutr Metab 2012;2012:381713.

[68] Holst JJ, Deacon CF, Vilsboll T, Krarup T, Madsbad S. Glucagon-like peptide-1, glucose homeostasis and diabetes. Trends Mol Med 2008;14(4):161-8.

[69] Buse JB, Rosenstock J, Sesti G, Schmidt WE, Montanya E, Brett JH, et al. Liraglutide once a day versus exenatide twice a day for type 2 diabetes: a 26-week randomised, parallel-group, multinational, open-label trial (LEAD-6). Lancet 2009;374(9683):39-47.

[70] Kendall DM, Riddle MC, Rosenstock J, Zhuang D, Kim DD, Fineman MS, et al. Effects of exenatide (exendin-4) on glycemic control over 30 weeks in patients with type 2 diabetes treated with metformin and a sulfonylurea. Diabetes Care 2005;28(5): 1083-91.

[71] Iltz JL, Baker DE, Setter SM, Keith Campbell R. Exenatide: an incretin mimetic for the treatment of type 2 diabetes mellitus. Clin Ther 2006;28(5):652-65.

[72] Inoue K, Maeda N, Kashine S, Fujishima Y, Kozawa J, Hiuge-Shimizu A, et al. Short-term effects of liraglutide on visceral fat adiposity, appetite, and food preference: a pilot study of obese Japanese patients with type 2 diabetes. Cardiovasc Diabetol 2012;10:109.

[73] Bloomgarden Z, Drexler A. What role will 'gliptins' play in glycemic control? Cleve Clin J Med 2008;75(4):305-10.

[74] Zerilli T, Pyon EY. Sitagliptin phosphate: a DPP-4 inhibitor for the treatment of type 2 diabetes mellitus. Clin Ther 2007;29(12):2614-34.

[75] Gallwitz B. Review of sitagliptin phosphate: a novel treatment for type 2 diabetes. Vasc Health Risk Manag 2007;3(2):203-10.

[76] Nathan DM. Finding new treatments for diabetes--how many, how fast... how good? N Engl J Med 2007;356(5):437-40.

[77] Ye Z, Chen L, Yang Z, Li Q, Huang Y, He M, et al. Metabolic effects of fluoxetine in adults with type 2 diabetes mellitus: a meta-analysis of randomized placebo-controlled trials. PLoS One 2011;6(7):e21551.

[78] Mancini MC, Halpern A. Pharmacological treatment of obesity. Arq Bras Endocrinol Metabol 2006;50(2):377-89.

[79] Fuchs F, Wannmacher L, Ferreira M. Farmacologia clínica: fundamentos da terapêutica racional. Rio de Janeiro: Guanabara Koogan; 2004.

[80] Ioannides-Demos LL, Piccenna L, McNeil JJ. Pharmacotherapies for obesity: past, current, and future therapies. J Obes 2011;2011:179674.

[81] Kang JG, Park CY. Anti-Obesity Drugs: A Review about Their Effects and Safety. Diabetes Metab J 2012;36(1):13-25.

[82] Heal DJ, Gosden J, Smith SL. Regulatory challenges for new drugs to treat obesity and comorbid metabolic disorders. Br J Clin Pharmacol 2009;68(6):861-74.

[83] Sargent BJ, Moore NA. New central targets for the treatment of obesity. Br J Clin Pharmacol 2009;68(6):852-60.

[84] Li M, Cheung BM. Pharmacotherapy for obesity. Br J Clin Pharmacol 2009;68(6): 804-10.

[85] Maia F, Melo F. Substituição da insulina NPH por insulina glargina em uma coorte de pacientes diabéticos: estudo observacional. Arquivos Brasileiros de Endocrinologia & Metabologia 2007;51(3):426-30.

[86] Pires A, Chacra A. A evolução da insulinoterapia no diabetes melito tipo 1. Endocrinol Metab 2008;52(2):268-78.

[87] Wajchenberg B, Forti A, Ferreira S, Oliveira O, Lopes C, Lerário A, et al. Menor incidência de hipoglicemia noturna com o uso de insulina lispro comparada à insulina humana regular no tratamento de pacientes com diabetes do tipo 1. Arq Bras Endocrinol Metab 2000;44(2):133-8.

[88] Home PD, Rosskamp R, Forjanic-Klapproth J, Dressler A. A randomized multicentre trial of insulin glargine compared with NPH insulin in people with type 1 diabetes. Diabetes Metab Res Rev 2005;21(6):545-53.

[89] Kurtzhals P. Pharmacology of insulin detemir. Endocrinol Metab Clin North Am 2007;36 Suppl 1:14-20.

[90] Soran H, Younis N. Insulin detemir: a new basal insulin analogue. Diabetes Obes Metab 2006;8(1):26-30.

[91] Rollin G, Punales N. Utilização da insulina glargina em crianças menores de oito anos de idade. Arq Bras Endocrinol Metab 2009;53(6):721-25.

[92] Vazquez-Carrera M, Silvestre JS. Insulin analogues in the management of diabetes. Methods Find Exp Clin Pharmacol 2004;26(6):445-61.

[93] Bailey CJ, Barnett AH. Inhaled insulin: new formulation, new trial. Lancet 2010;375(9733):2199-201.

[94] Siekmeier R, Scheuch G. Inhaled insulin--does it become reality? J Physiol Pharmacol 2008;59 Suppl 6:81-113.

[95] Mastrandrea LD. Inhaled insulin: overview of a novel route of insulin administration. Vasc Health Risk Manag 2010;6:47-58.

[96] Arnolds S, Heise T. Inhaled insulin. Best Pract Res Clin Endocrinol Metab 2007;21(4): 555-71.

[97] Tibaldi JM. Evolution of insulin development: focus on key parameters. Adv Ther 2012;29(7):590-619.

[98] Carvalheira J, Saad M. Insulin resistance/hyperinsulinemia associated diseases not included in the metabolic syndrome. Arq bras endocrinol metab 2006;50(2):360-7.

[99] Janghorbani M, Dehghani M, Salehi-Marzijarani M. Systematic review and meta-analysis of insulin therapy and risk of cancer. Horm Cancer 2012;3(4):137-46.

Chapter 21

Insulin Therapy for Diabetes

Shara S. Azad, Esma R. Isenovic,
Subhashini Yaturu and Shaker A. Mousa

Additional information is available at the end of the chapter

http://dx.doi.org/10.5772/56379

1. Introduction

Diabetes affects 25.8 million people, or 8.3% of the U.S. population. Among people with diabetes, 26% are insulin users.[1] Therapy with insulin is effective at lowering blood glucose in patients with diabetes. Insulin is a key player in the control of diabetes for patients with type 1, and it is required at later stages by patients with type 2. Hyperglycemia in type 1 diabetes is a result of the deficiency of insulin, and in type 2 diabetes hyperglycemia is due to impaired tissue response to insulin.

The discovery of insulin is hailed as one of the most dramatic events in the history of the treatment of disease. It was isolated in 1921, with its first clinical use in 1922.[2] The major advances achieved in this area include the human insulin analogue synthesis. Insulin delivery systems currently available for insulin administration include syringes, infusion pumps, jet injectors, and pens. The traditional and most predictable method for insulin administration is by subcutaneous injections. The major drawback of current forms of insulin therapy is their invasive nature. In type 1 diabetes, good glycemic control usually requires at least two, three, or more daily insulin injections. To decrease the suffering, the use of supersonic injectors, infusion pumps, sharp needles, and pens has been adopted.

Such invasive and intensive techniques have spurred the search for alternative, more pleasant methods for administering insulin. Several non-invasive approaches for insulin delivery are being pursued. The ultimate goal is to eliminate the need to deliver insulin exogenously and for patients to regain the ability to produce and use their own insulin. The success of the administration route is measured by its ability to elicit effective and predictable lowering of blood glucose level, therefore minimizing the risk of diabetic complications. Newer methods explored include the artificial pancreas with a closed-loop system, transdermal insulin, and buccal, oral, pulmonary, nasal, ocular, and rectal routes. This chapter focuses on the new methods that are being explored for use in the future.

2. Current methods in insulin therapy

Current methods of insulin delivery include using syringes, continuous subcutaneous insulin infusion (CSII), and insulin pens. Use of syringes is the most common method, and there is a wide choice of products that are easy to read and operate. CSII, also referred to as an insulin pump system, is designed to provide a continuous supply of insulin infusion around the clock and can be individualized and adjusted as per the specific needs of the patient. CSII is a way to simulate the physiology of daily insulin secretion where an appropriate level of insulin is delivered. The use of an insulin pump is superior to multi-dose insulin injections because it is easier to use and therefore provides the patient with more flexibility. A disadvantage is that insulin pump therapy is expensive compared to the use of traditional syringes and vials.

Insulin pen devices offer an alternative method for insulin delivery that is more accurate and less painful versus vials and syringes.[3] Reusable insulin pens offer a number of advantages including durability and flexibility in carrying a multiple days' supply.

3. Future trends (Table 1)

Injectable insulin: Two promising new insulin preparations include a long-acting basal insulin analogue called insulin degludec and an ultrafast-acting insulin analogue, human insulin Linjeta™ (formally called VIAject®).

Insulin degludec is novel, ultra-long-acting basal insulin.[4] Insulin degludec is almost identical to human insulin in structure except for the last amino acid deleted from the B-chain and addition of a glutamyl link from LysB29 to a hexadecandioic fatty acid.[4] It forms soluble multi-hexamers after subcutaneous injection, resulting in an ultra-long action profile with a half life of more than 24 hours.

Insulin degludec has proven to be non-inferior to currently available, long-acting insulin analogue insulin glargine in trials carried out in both type 1 and type 2 diabetes.[5-6] In an exploratory phase 2 trial in subjects with type 1 diabetes, insulin degludec was found to be safe and well tolerated and had comparable glycemic control to insulin glargine, but with reduced rates of hypoglycemia.[7] In a multicenter phase 3 clinical trial in adults with type 1 diabetes, at one year, compared to insulin glargine, glycemic control was similar to glycemic control using glargine with decreased nocturnal hypoglycemia.[6] Similarly, in an open-label phase 3 non-inferiority trial in type 2 diabetes patients, improvement in glycemic control was comparable to insulin glargine at one year follow-up (drop in HbA1C by 1.1% in the degludec group and 1.2% in the glargine group) with fewer hypoglycemic episodes in insulin degludec users.[5] Insulin degludec is not yet approved by the FDA.

Linjeta™, formally called VIAject®, is recombinant human insulin with a fast onset of action. In a study of pharmacodynamics and pharmacokinetic properties of an ultrafast insulin, it was found to have an earlier onset of action and shorter time to maximal plasma insulin concentration. VIAject®, compared to human insulin, had less within-subject variability of plasma insulin.[8] In a double blind, three-way crossover study with VIAject® compared to lispro insulin, VIAject® was found to be bioequivalent to the previously used formulation and had a faster absorption/onset of action than insulin lispro.[9] VIAject® is currently undergoing two pivotal phase 3 clinical studies for both type 1 and type 2 diabetes. Since the VIAject® pharmacodynamics mimic 1st phase release insulin and the amount of insulin circulating several hours after a meal, it leads to possible reduction in hypoglycemia, and it is predicted to possibly prevent weight gain.[8]

Artificial pancreas: Closed-loop insulin delivery is an emerging therapeutic approach for people with type 1 diabetes. [10] Even with the use of continuous glucose monitors and insulin pumps, most people with type 1 diabetes do not achieve glycemic goals and continue to have unacceptable rates of hypoglycemia. The goal of closed-loop therapy is to achieve good glycemic control with the use of a control algorithm that directs insulin delivery according to glucose levels while reducing the risk of hypoglycemia. Insulin delivery in the closed-loop system is modulated at intervals of 1-15 minutes, depending on interstitial glucose levels. The uniqueness of this approach is the real-time response of insulin delivery to the glucose levels, similar to that of the beta-cell. The algorithms that are most relevant include the proportional-integral-derivative control (PID) and the model-predictive control (MPC).[11]

Several areas need improvement to have a near normal closed-loop system. First and foremost is the rapid onset of action. The lag period of current fast-acting insulin analogs is 90-120 minutes. Current trials show promise. In a phase 2 study with or without recombinant human hyaluronidase (rHuPH20) that accelerates insulin absorption in healthy volunteers, both lispro and recombinant human insulin with rHuPH20 produced earlier and greater peak insulin concentrations, improved postprandial glycemic control, and reduced hypoglycemia.[12]

Rapid acting insulins are being developed that use monomeric insulins that cannot form hexamers.[13] As mentioned earlier, ultrafast insulin VIAject®, a formulation of human soluble insulin, improves the rate of insulin absorption. It has been reported in a study to evaluate its pharmacodynamics and pharmacokinetic properties that VIAject® has higher metabolic activity in the first two hours after injection.[14] True closed-loop systems, which determine minute-to-minute insulin delivery based on continuous glucose sensor data in real time, have shown promise in small inpatient feasibility studies using a variety of algorithmic and hormonal approaches.

Buccal delivery of insulin: The buccal delivery system for insulin delivers insulin through an aerosol spray into the oral cavity and hence differs from inhalers. The insulin is absorbed through the inside of the cheeks and in the back of the mouth instead of the lungs. In vivo studies performed on diabetic rats showed promising results with stable blood glucose profile with a significant hypoglycemic response after 7 hours using buccal insulin.[15] Similar studies in the rabbit and rat have shown that buccal spray of insulin is an effective insulin delivery system, which is promising for clinical trial and future clinical application.[16] Though promising in rat models, they are not appropriate models because rats have a keratinized buccal mucosa. The only animal models with comparable human buccal permeability are pigs.

Oral-lynTM: Generex Biotechnology Corporation (Toronto, Canada) is developing a buccal insulin formulation based on RapidMistTM, an advanced buccal drug delivery technology.[17] Oral-lynTM is a liquid formulation of human regular insulin with a spray propellant for prandial insulin therapy. The formulation results in an aerosol with relatively large micelles where the majority of the particles have a mean size >10 μm and therefore cannot go into the lungs. Each puff is claimed to deliver 10 U of insulin. The absorption rate of administered insulin as a puff is 10%, and that corresponds to 1 U when 1 puff of 10 U is delivered, which means 10 puffs will deliver 10 U insulin for a meal.[17]

Clinical studies in healthy volunteers and subjects with type 1 and type 2 diabetes have shown that the oral insulin spray was absorbed in direct relation to the amount given, and it had a rapid onset and a shorter duration compared with regular insulin given subcutaneously. In all of the studies conducted, the oral insulin spray was generally well tolerated. The only side effects included mild episodes of transient dizziness in some healthy volunteers and subjects with type 1 diabetes.[18] The product is on the market in a number of countries (e.g., Ecuador and India).[17] Without appropriately designed and performed phase 3 trials at hand, it is not possible to make any clear statement about the benefits/risk ratio of the different buccal insulins.[17]

Oral insulin: Oral insulin has benefits in terms of compliance among patients, as well as physiological advantages because oral insulin can mimic the physiological fate of insulin through first pass to the liver, directly and effectively inhibiting hepatic glucose production.[19] Since the initial discovery of insulin by Banting and Best in 1922, the oral form of insulin has been the elusive goal. Difficulties encountered for oral insulin delivery, since it is a protein, include degradation by the low pH of the stomach and the digestive enzymes in the stomach and small intestine. The major barrier for insulin absorption is the intestinal epithelium. All these factors lead to low bioavailability, and that leads to significant inter- and intra-subject variability.

Nanotechnologies have brought some hope for improved delivery of insulin. Nanotechnology applications for delivery of hydrophilic drugs such as insulin might be achieved using biodegradable polymers such as chitosan, which has been extensively exploited for the preparation of nanoparticles for oral controlled delivery of several therapeutic agents.[20-24] In recent years, chitosan cross-linked to various hydrophobic polymers has been utilized for the preparation of orally delivered drugs because of improved permeation and sustained release characteristics.[25-26]

The newer products that are being tried include water-soluble, long-acting insulin derivative, [(2-sulfo)-9-fluorenylmethoxycarbonyl]3-insulin,[27] vitamin B12-dextran nano particles,[28] lipid nanoparticles,[29] and PEGylated calcium phosphate nanoparticles as oral carriers for insulin.[30] Protection of insulin from the gastric environment has been achieved by coating the nanoparticles with a pH-sensitive polymer that dissolves in the intestine at mild alkaline pH. In rats, oral insulin nanoformulation significantly ($P<0.05$) reduced blood glucose in normal and diabetic rats.[31]

Biocon (Bangalore, India) is manufacturing IN-105, which is in late phase 3.[17] IN-105 is a human recombinant insulin conjugated with polyethylene glycol via an acetyl chain. It is orally bioavailable and stable at ambient conditions. Preclinical studies in different species have shown acceptable efficacy and safety. Its maximal circulating insulin levels after oral administration of 5 mg were observed after 20 minutes, and the maximum drop in glucose occurred at 40 minutes after oral administration. Phase 1 and phase 2 trials demonstrated that the absorption of IN-105 and the reduction in blood glucose levels were proportional to the dose administered.[32]

Inhaled insulin: The inhaled products fall into two main groups: the dry powder formulations and solution, which are delivered through different inhaler systems. Exubera®, containing rapid-acting insulin in powder form, was studied in patients with type 1 and type 2 diabetes mellitus.[33-34] The results of a patient preference study, using a comparison of utility scores, showed a greater preference for the inhaled route over insulin injection.[35] However, issues like cost, the bulkiness of the device, and the small number of studies in subjects with underlying respiratory disease prevented widespread use of this new mode of delivery.[36-37] Exubera® was available for less than one year, and then Pfizer took it off the market in 2007 because the drug failed to gain market acceptance.

Afrezza®: (MannKind Corporation, Valencia, CA, USA) is recombinant human insulin, using the Technosphere® concept and administered using a next-generation inhaler called Dreamboat®. Technosphere® is a drug delivery system created by micro particles (2-3 μm) that form microspheres, which are then lyophilized into a dry powder for inhalation.[38]

Transdermal insulin: Transdermal insulin delivery is a needle-free alternative and avoids the disadvantages associated with other alternative routes such as the pulmonary and nasal routes. Permeation of compounds is limited to small, lipophilic molecules. The stratum corneum, the outermost layer of the skin, constitutes the major barrier for insulin permeation to reach useful levels. Several chemical and physical enhancement techniques such as iontophoresis, ultrasound/sonophoresis, micro-needles, electroporation, laser ablation, and chemical enhancers have been explored to overcome the stratum corneum barrier to increase skin permeability.

Methods to improve transdermal delivery:

1. Chemical enhancers, which alter the lipid structure of the stratum.

2. Iontophoresis, which enhances the transdermal delivery of compounds via the use of a small electric current.[39]

3. Micro-needle technology, which involves the creation of micron-sized channels in the skin, thereby disrupting the stratum corneum barrier[40] and delivering the drug into the epidermis without disruption of nerve endings.[41]

4. Sonophoresis, which uses ultrasound and has been shown to increase skin permeability of insulin. It is still being evaluated.[42]

4. Conclusions

Effective glycemic control remains an important clinical goal. Patient barriers to accepting insulin initiation include fear of hypoglycemia, weight gain, and the inflexible timing of scheduled insulin doses, leading to adherence issues. Additionally, the invasive nature of the insulin syringe, pump, and pen remains an obstacle for patients. Of the alternatives to subcutaneous and injected insulin, intranasal, inhalable, and oral insulin could prove to be the most cost-effective ones. Oral insulin in particular could prove to be promising, especially since as a therapy it seems to have progressed with nanotechnology research, allowing for several types of encapsulations to bypass the gastric acidic environment. Artificial pancreas or closing the loop with insulin pumps that deliver insulin in response to sensors also appears to be promising.

Method	Mechanism
Artificial pancreas	Insulin pump controlled by algorithm with glucose monitor
Buccal insulin	Insulin through an aerosol spray
Oral insulin	Various nanoparticle encasings bound to insulin
Inhalable insulin	Insulin absorbed through alveolar membranes
Transdermal insulin (patches)	Insulin absorbed through pores in skin opened with ultrasound energy, microdermabrasion, etc.
Intranasal insulin	Absorbed through nasal mucosae

Table 1. Methods for Future Types of Insulin Therapy

Author details

Shara S. Azad[1], Esma R. Isenovic[2], Subhashini Yaturu[3] and Shaker A. Mousa[1*]

*Address all correspondence to: Shaker.Mousa@acphs.edu

1 Pharmaceutical Research Institute, Albany College of Pharmacy and Health Sciences, 1 Discovery Drive, Rensselaer, NY, USA

2 Vinca Institute, University of Belgrade, Department for Molecular Genetics and Radiobiology, Belgrade, Serbia

3 Stratton Veterans Affairs Medical Center /Albany Medical College, Albany, NY, USA

References

[1] National Diabetes Statistics, 2011. U.S. Department of Health and Human Services; 2011. http://diabetes.niddk.nih.gov/dm/pubs/statistics/#fast. Accessed 15 November, 2012.

[2] Rosenfeld L. Insulin: discovery and controversy. Clin Chem. 2002;48(12) 2270-88.

[3] Magwire ML. Addressing barriers to insulin therapy: the role of insulin pens. Am J Ther. 2011;18(5) 392-402.

[4] Danne T, Bolinder J. New insulins and insulin therapy. Int J Clin Pract Suppl. 2011;65(Suppl 170) 26-30.

[5] Garber AJ, King AB, Del Prato S, Sreenan S, Balci MK, Munoz-Torres M, et al. Insulin degludec, an ultra-longacting basal insulin, versus insulin glargine in basal-bolus treatment with mealtime insulin aspart in type 2 diabetes (BEGIN Basal-Bolus Type 2): a phase 3, randomised, open-label, treat-to-target non-inferiority trial. Lancet. 2012;379(9825) 1498-507.

[6] Heller S, Buse J, Fisher M, Garg S, Marre M, Merker L, et al. Insulin degludec, an ultra-longacting basal insulin, versus insulin glargine in basal-bolus treatment with mealtime insulin aspart in type 1 diabetes (BEGIN Basal-Bolus Type 1): a phase 3, randomised, open-label, treat-to-target non-inferiority trial. Lancet. 2012;379(9825) 1489-97.

[7] Birkeland KI, Home PD, Wendisch U, Ratner RE, Johansen T, Endahl LA, et al. Insulin degludec in type 1 diabetes: a randomized controlled trial of a new-generation ultra-long-acting insulin compared with insulin glargine. Diabetes Care. 2011;34(3) 661-5.

[8] Hompesch M, McManus L, Pohl R, Simms P, Pfutzner A, Bulow E, et al. Intra-individual variability of the metabolic effect of a novel rapid-acting insulin (VIAject) in comparison to regular human insulin. J Diabetes Sci Technol. 2008;2(4) 568-71.

[9] Heinemann L, Nosek L, Flacke F, Albus K, Krasner A, Pichotta P, et al. U-100, pH-Neutral formulation of VIAject(®) : faster onset of action than insulin lispro in patients with type 1 diabetes. Diabetes Obes Metab. 2012;14(3) 222-7.

[10] Elleri D, Dunger DB, Hovorka R. Closed-loop insulin delivery for treatment of type 1 diabetes. BMC Med. 2011;9 120.

[11] Radziuk J. The artificial pancreas. Diabetes. 2012;61(9) 2221-4.

[12] Hompesch M, Muchmore DB, Morrow L, Vaughn DE. Accelerated insulin pharmacokinetics and improved postprandial glycemic control in patients with type 1 diabetes after coadministration of prandial insulins with hyaluronidase. Diabetes Care. 2011;34(3) 666-8.

[13] Brange J, Owens DR, Kang S, Volund A. Monomeric insulins and their experimental and clinical implications. Diabetes Care. 1990;13(9) 923-54.

[14] Steiner S, Hompesch M, Pohl R, Simms P, Flacke F, Mohr T, et al. A novel insulin formulation with a more rapid onset of action. Diabetologia. 2008;51(9) 1602-6.

[15] Venugopalan P, Sapre A, Venkatesan N, Vyas SP. Pelleted bioadhesive polymeric nanoparticles for buccal delivery of insulin: preparation and characterization. Pharmazie. 2001;56(3) 217-9.

[16] Xu HB, Huang KX, Zhu YS, Gao QH, Wu QZ, Tian WQ, et al. Hypoglycaemic effect of a novel insulin buccal formulation on rabbits. Pharmacol Res. 2002;46(5) 459-67.

[17] Heinemann L, Jacques Y. Oral insulin and buccal insulin: a critical reappraisal. J Diabetes Sci Technol. 2009;3(3) 568-84.

[18] Pozzilli P, Raskin P, Parkin CG. Review of clinical trials: update on oral insulin spray formulation. Diabetes Obes Metab. 2010;12(2) 91-6.

[19] Arbit E, Kidron M. Oral insulin: the rationale for this approach and current developments. J Diabetes Sci Technol. 2009;3(3) 562-7.

[20] Trapani A, Lopedota A, Franco M, Cioffi N, Ieva E, Garcia-Fuentes M, et al. A comparative study of chitosan and chitosan/cyclodextrin nanoparticles as potential carriers for the oral delivery of small peptides. Eur J Pharm Biopharm. 2010;75(1) 26-32.

[21] Cui F, Qian F, Zhao Z, Yin L, Tang C, Yin C. Preparation, characterization, and oral delivery of insulin loaded carboxylated chitosan grafted poly(methyl methacrylate) nanoparticles. Biomacromolecules. 2009;10(5) 1253-8.

[22] Li T, Shi XW, Du YM, Tang YF. Quaternized chitosan/alginate nanoparticles for protein delivery. J Biomed Mater Res A. 2007;83(2) 383-90.

[23] Pan Y, Li YJ, Zhao HY, Zheng JM, Xu H, Wei G, et al. Bioadhesive polysaccharide in protein delivery system: chitosan nanoparticles improve the intestinal absorption of insulin in vivo. Int J Pharm. 2002;249(1-2) 139-47.

[24] Ma Z, Yeoh HH, Lim LY. Formulation pH modulates the interaction of insulin with chitosan nanoparticles. J Pharm Sci. 2002;91(6) 1396-404.

[25] Jose S, Fangueiro JF, Smitha J, Cinu TA, Chacko AJ, Premaletha K, et al. Cross-linked chitosan microspheres for oral delivery of insulin: Taguchi design and in vivo testing. Colloids Surf B Biointerfaces. 2012;92 175-9.

[26] Chaudhury A, Das S. Recent advancement of chitosan-based nanoparticles for oral controlled delivery of insulin and other therapeutic agents. AAPS PharmSciTech. 2011;12(1) 10-20.

[27] Sung HW, Sonaje K, Feng SS. Nanomedicine for diabetes treatment. Nanomedicine (Lond). 2011;6(8) 1297-300.

[28] Chalasani KB, Russell-Jones GJ, Jain AK, Diwan PV, Jain SK. Effective oral delivery of insulin in animal models using vitamin B12-coated dextran nanoparticles. J Control Release. 2007;122(2) 141-50.

[29] Severino P, Andreani T, Macedo AS, Fangueiro JF, Santana MH, Silva AM, et al. Current state-of-art and new trends on lipid nanoparticles (SLN and NLC) for oral drug delivery. J Drug Delivery. 2012;2012 750891.

[30] Ramachandran R, Paul W, Sharma CP. Synthesis and characterization of PEGylated calcium phosphate nanoparticles for oral insulin delivery. J Biomed Mater Res B Appl Biomater. 2009;88(1) 41-8.

[31] Najafzadeh H, Kooshapur H, Kianidehkordi F. Evaluation of an oral insulin formulation in normal and diabetic rats. Indian J Pharmacol. 2012;44(1) 103-5.

[32] Khedkar A, Iyer H, Anand A, Verma M, Krishnamurthy S, Savale S, et al. A dose range finding study of novel oral insulin (IN-105) under fed conditions in type 2 diabetes mellitus subjects. Diabetes Obes Metab. 2010;12(8) 659-64.

[33] Fineberg SE. Diabetes therapy trials with inhaled insulin. Expert Opin Investig Drugs. 2006;15(7) 743-62.

[34] Barnett AH. Exubera inhaled insulin: a review. Int J Clin Pract. 2004;58(4) 394-401.

[35] Chancellor J, Aballea S, Lawrence A, Sheldon R, Cure S, Plun-Favreau J, et al. Preferences of patients with diabetes mellitus for inhaled versus injectable insulin regimens. Pharmacoeconomics. 2008;26(3) 217-34.

[36] Zarogoulidis P, Papanas N, Kouliatsis G, Spyratos D, Zarogoulidis K, Maltezos E. Inhaled insulin: too soon to be forgotten? J Aerosol Med Pulm Drug Deliv. 2011;24(5) 213-23.

[37] Hegewald M, Crapo RO, Jensen RL. Pulmonary function changes related to acute and chronic administration of inhaled insulin. Diabetes Technol Ther. 2007;9 Suppl 1 S93-S101.

[38] Steiner S, Pfutzner A, Wilson BR, Harzer O, Heinemann L, Rave K. Technosphere/Insulin--proof of concept study with a new insulin formulation for pulmonary delivery. Exp Clin Endocrinol Diabetes. 2002;110(1) 17-21.

[39] Batheja P, Thakur R, Michniak B. Transdermal iontophoresis. Expert Opin Drug Deliv. 2006;3(1) 127-38.

[40] Chen H, Zhu H, Zheng J, Mou D, Wan J, Zhang J, et al. Iontophoresis-driven penetration of nanovesicles through microneedle-induced skin microchannels for enhancing transdermal delivery of insulin. J Control Release. 2009;139(1) 63-72.

[41] Bariya SH, Gohel MC, Mehta TA, Sharma OP. Microneedles: an emerging transdermal drug delivery system. J Pharm Pharmacol. 2012;64(1) 11-29.

[42] Rao R, Nanda S. Sonophoresis: recent advancements and future trends. J Pharm Pharmacol. 2009;61(6) 689-705.

Chapter 22

Psychodiabetic Kit and Its Application in Clinical Practice and Research

Andrzej Kokoszka, Aleksandra Jodko-Modlińska, Marcin Obrębski, Joanna Ostasz-Ważny and Rafał Radzio

Additional information is available at the end of the chapter

http://dx.doi.org/10.5772/56468

1. Introduction

A patient-centered approach is recommended for the management of diabetes type 2 by the American Diabetes Association and the European Association for the Study of Diabetes [1] "These recommendations should be considered within the context of the needs, preferences, and tolerances of each patient; individualization of treatment is the cornerstone of success. (…). The implementation of these guidelines will require thoughtful clinicians to integrate current evidence with other constraints and imperatives in the context of patient-specific factors" [1. p. 1364]. It includes taking into consideration the variable and progressive nature of type 2 diabetes, the specific role of each drug, the patient and disease factors that drive clinical decision making, and the constraints imposed by age and comorbidity. This implies diagnosis of psychosocial factors in regular medical practice. This is justified by sterling data indicating that psychosocial factors have meaningful impact on the management of diabetes. There is extensive literature suggesting that the patient's mental state has a profound impact on adherence to medical recommendations [2] and influences the course of the disease. Major diabetic problems are more widespread among patients with clinical depression, than those with subthreshold depression [3]. On the other hand, depression is more common among people with diabetes than in general population [4], and even in its subclinical form, it increases the risk of complications [5]. Research points to a link between the intensity of diabetes treatment and the occurrence of depressive mood [2]. It also indicates that the course of the disease affects the patient's ability to cope with stressful situations [6] and sense of control over the disease [7]. Many conducted studies reveal the importance of psychosocial factors in diabetes self-care. Diabetes-related emotional distress is connected with difficulties with diabetes self-management and poor glycemic control [8]. Self-efficacy and problem solving were associated with self-management behaviors like healthy eating and physical activity [9]. It is known that patients understand the importance of diabetes management and the consequences of bad metabolic control. Their poor control results not from a lack of knowledge but on the way diabetes is prioritised in their lives [10]. There is evidence that diabetes management is strongly influenced by psychosocial factors [11]. This implies the necessity of inclusion of diagnosis of psychological and psychotherapeutic factors during a routine visit of patients with diabetes. Team approach in this management, including diabetologist, nurse, psychologist, educator, and social worker is optimal. However, in many countries significant rates of outpatient clinics can offer their patients therapeutic interventions made only by doctors and the nurses. Working in such setting they need diagnositic and therapeutic tools helpful in management of psychosocial problems related with diabetes. However, the number of tolls that are useful in such conditions is limited. The computerized assessment tool "Monitoring of Individual Needs in persons with Diabetes" (MIND) [12,13] includes World Health Organization's Five Well-being index (WHO-5) [14,15], Problem Areas In Diabetes (PAID) [16-18], life events and patient's agenda, can be used for diagnosis of psychosocial factors connected to diabetes management. Analysis of data from the cross-national Diabetes Attitudes Wishes and Needs (DAWN) MIND study, conducted in 8 countries, also in our center in Poland, confirmed that "MIND" computer procedure is feasible as a part of ongoing diabetes care and helps to identify unmet psychosocial needs in diabetes patients. However it does not help in psychotherapeutic diagnosis that is needed for the basic psychotherapeutic interventions that can be made by doctors during a regular visit[12,13]. The psychodiabetic KIT was elaborated in response to such needs. The analysis of literature in MEDLINE and PUBMED indicates that there are no concise comprehensive diagnostic tools for supporting psychotherapeutic diagnosis during the regular medical visit of patients with diabetes and there are no simple psychotherapeutic strategies of interventions in such a setting. Psychodiabetic KIT supports a diagnosis of coping styles, perception of self-influence on diabetes course and a more reliable diagnosis of depression and anxiety, than the one WHO-5 and PAID used as screening tools for depression. In this chapter we describe: a theoretical rationale of the Psychodiabetic Kit, three tools that it comprises together with "The Practical Schema of Psychotherapeutic Management within a Regular Medical Visit" as well as a review of research confirming its usefulness both in research and clinical practice.

2. Rationale of psychodiabetic KIT

Improvement of patients' adherence to the optimum management of diabetes may be considered as the target of psychotherapeutic interventions during medical visits, when education about the diabetes is not efficient. The theoretical framework of psychotherapeutic diagnosis and interventions should be easy to understand for both therapists and patients. It was presumed that due to the common time constrains the diagnostic tools should:

1. be brief
2. compromise goals of enhancing psychological thinking and psychometric proprieties
3. rather support the clinical psychological diagnosis, than replace it

4. promote psychological understanding both of the patient and of the therapist
5. integrate the psychological diagnosis and interventions with the regular clinical management

Eventually the concept of coping with stress was chosen as theoretical background for the diagnosis. Whereas the practical interventions following the recommendations of the International Diabetes Association [19] are based on philosophy of empowerment, and rule self-management [19,20], that applies elements of behavioral therapy.

The concept of coping with stress related with diabetes and perception of self-influence on the diabetes course

Coping is defined as 'constantly changing cognitive and behavioral efforts to manage specific external and/or internal demands that are appraised as taxing or exceeding the resources of the person [21]. Coping is an adaptation activity that involves effort and aims to diminish the physical, emotional, and psychological burden linked to stressful life events [22]. However, the outcome of the coping process can also be maladaptation. The dispositional traits that influence how stressful events are assessed and that consequently determine the strategies a person uses to manage or address a stressor, may be described as coping strategies. Endler and Parker [23] offered simple classification of coping styles: task-oriented, emotion-oriented and avoidance-oriented. Patients utilizing an emotion- oriented strategy try to process reactions to stressor(s) by acting and thinking and in this scenario the person is focused on the emotion evoked by the stressor; overall, efforts are directed at altering the emotional responses. Patients who use a task-oriented strategy believe that they can prevail the situation caused by their disease or that they can adapt their resources to manage the situation, which often involves taking direct action to alter the situation itself. An avoidance-oriented coping style includes strategies such as avoiding a situation, denying its existence, or losing hope, via conscious and/or unconscious mechanisms; when using this coping style, the person also uses indirect efforts to adjust to stressors by distancing them, evading the problem, or engaging in unrelated activities to reduce feelings of stress. In addition to emotion-, task-, and avoidance-orientated, "the best solution oriented coping" style has been described [24]. When engaging in the 'identifying the best solution' coping style, the person actively searches for the most effective solutions, taking into account that they may be more "expensive" and risky than the standard ones. The classification of coping styles into just four main categories simplifies the understanding of these behaviors for both doctors and their patients. The concept of stress introduced by Seyle [25,26] is commonly known, unlike its most important developments dealing with the intensity of reactions to stressful events, that depends on [27] :

1. How the challenge is evaluated, what's its meaning for the individual
2. Which coping style is used
3. What the level of social support is

Analysis of literature reveals a close relationship between an individual's overall psychological disposition and the cognitive and emotional aspects of their illness-coping strategies, which indirectly affect health-seeking behaviors [28]. According to the goodness of fit hypothesis, the effectiveness of problem- versus emotion-focused coping is moderated by appraisal of control over the stressful event [21,29]. The application of a problem-oriented coping style requires a feeling of control over the stressor, while in situations where there is an actual or perceived lack of control, an emotion-oriented or avoidance oriented coping style is applied. This concept has received some empirical support in a study involving patients with type 2 diabetes mellitus (T2DM) [30].

Indeed, among the variety of psychological factors described, the coping style and the perception of control over the disease course seem to have an important effect on outcomes in patients with diabetes [31,32]. Thus it is also likely that, in terms of coping strategies used to deal with diabetes, the individual's appraisal of illness as controllable or uncontrollable plays a role in the choice of strategy and therefore, ultimately, also in illness-associated outcomes.

In long-term progressive diseases, the concept of control is misleading because, in the majority of cases, even total adherence to the recommended treatment regimen can not guarantee restraining of either disease progress or recurrence of acute symptoms [7]. Perception of self-influence on a disease course can be defined as the extent of belief about one's own abilities to shape the disease course. It was formulated in response to data indicating that the coping style applied in response to a particular stressor is dependent on the perceived degree of control over that stressor [7]. As such, the concept of perceived self-influence on the disease course may be a more appropriate notion than control, when considering long-term progressive diseases, as even with chronic diseases, adherence to the recommended treatment and management plan can modify the disease course. Self influence also differs from perceived self-efficacy, which is defined as beliefs about the capabilities to produce designated levels of performance that exercise influence over events that affect lives. More specifically, self-efficacy beliefs determine how people feel, think, behave and motivate themselves [28], while perception of self-influence is related to disease management and is therefore more precise. Indeed, perceived control of diabetes was found to be a significant predictor of engagement in diabetes-specific health behaviors and positive perception of quality of life [31,32].

2.1. Depression and anxiety

Research analysis points to a high prevalence of depressive symptoms in a population of patients with diabetes [4,33]. Depression and its subclinical forms are connected to a negative course of diabetes. Depression is linked with poorer glicemic control [34]. Research confirms higher mortality in those groups of patients, in which major or moderate depression was diagnosed, when compared to a group in which depression was not found [35]. Moreover, patients reporting higher intensity of depressive symptoms are less willing to talk to their doctor about self-care [36]. Authors of the recent study, point that doctors need to be careful for depressive symptoms in their patients, and suggests the usefulness of brief diagnostic tools that may be used during a routine visit.

A higher prevalence of anxiety disorders and significant intensity of anxiety symptoms can also be observed among patients with diabetes [37,38]. The occurrence of those symptoms is connected to a poorer quality of life in diabetes patients [39]. The referred studies justify the purposefulness of evaluating depression and anxiety in patients with diabetes.

2.2. Description of the psychodiabetic KIT

Psychodiabetic KIT is a concise method of psychotherapeutic diagnosis and interventions aiming at improving the patient's adherence to therapeutic regimen. It was comprehensively described in a series of manuals [40-44] widely distributed among Polish diabetologists. Its application was discussed during many workshops. The Psychodiabetic Kit consists of:

1. Brief Methods of Evaluating Coping with Disease;
2. Brief Measure to Assess Perception of Self-Influence on the Disease Course: Version for Diabetes;
3. Brief Self-Rating Scale of Depression and Anxiety;
4. The Practical Schema of Psychotherapeutic Management within a Regular Medical Visit

The Brief Method of Evaluating Coping with Disease (BMECD; published in the appendix) [24] was created to assess the main four coping styles factors, which were mentioned above. This questionnaire consists of four questions with a choice of four behaviors. Each response relates to one of four distinguished coping styles related to aspects of life that are important for patients with diabetes (interpersonal, social, economic, and health related matters). The four BMECD questions are an outcome of a focus group interview with patients with T2DM who, in the opinion of their doctors, had developed either adaptive or maladaptive styles in order to cope with their disease. Data from the focus group were used by psychology students working on their Masters theses to generate 16 questions that related to typical methods of dealing with stressful situations according to each of the four main established coping styles. These 16 questions were correlated with the scores of the Coping Inventory for Stressful Situations (CISS) [45], the choice of the final four items was based on these results and on the opinion of two experienced clinical psychologists from the Medical University of Warsaw. Due to clinical observations indicating gender difficulties in perception and interpretation of some examples used in the questionnaire, which resulted in the reliability not being as satisfying as expected, the final version of BMECD [6] was elaborated. The changes included the descriptions of stressful situations adjusted to gender and to Polish language spelling by creating separate versions for males and females, and to making the test easier to read. The gender adjusted version has a relatively good reliability, as for an only four item questionnaire, designed for screening for maladaptive coping and as for an educational tool. Cronbach's alpha= 0.67 for avoidance oriented coping style; 0.68 for emotion oriented style; 0.75 for task oriented style; 0.59 for the best solution oriented style in the male version and respectively: 0.65; 0.67; 0.71; 0.55 in female version. The validity of the BMECD was assessed with the Polish version of the CISS questionnaire [45] among 125 women and 104 men only. The strongest correlations were found between: found between task-oriented coping style in CISS and combined results for the task oriented and the best-solution oriented coping style in BMECD among women ($r = 0.42$; $p < 0.001$) among men ($r = 0.41$; $p < 0.001$) and between scores in the emotion oriented coping ($r=0.29$; $p < 0.001$ both for men and women). There were no significant correlations between scores in avoidance oriented coping styles in both measures, both in group men and women. Those correlations indicate that the coping styles identified in BMECD have some similarities with those differentiated by CISS, but measure different modes of reaction to stressful events.

The Brief Measure to Assess Perception of Self-Influence on the Disease Course: Version for Diabetes (BMAPS-IDC, published in the appendix)[7]. The BMAPS-IDC questions were developed based on methodology that was discussed during a focus group interview with patients with T2DM who, in the opinion of their doctors, had developed either adaptive or maladaptive styles in order to cope with their disease. This led to the originating of 50 items, each using a 5-point Likert scale to assess outcomes. These 50 items were then modified following a discussion with two persons with diabetes. To further validate the 50-item version of the BMAPS-IDC, the questionnaire was used among 170 patients, in whom their doctor, using clinical judgment, rated the patient's perception of self-influence on the diabetes course.

Statistical analysis (Wald test and logistic regression) identified six items that optimally differentiated the group in terms of high and low perception of self-influence on the disease course; thus, the final BMAPS-IDC questionnaire consisted of six items, each presented using a 5-point Likert scale. Higher BMAPS-IDC scores denote a greater perception of self-influence over the disease course.

The BMAPS-IDC has good reliability (Cronbach's alpha, 0.75) and acceptable validity (Kendall tau, 0.54), as well as a standardized ten scale for the assessment of results, which was created to describe clinically significant differences. According to the ten scale, low raw scores of 0–11 scores correspond with <5 on the ten scale, average raw scores of 12–15 correspond to ten scale scores of 5–6, and high raw scores of 16–24 of translate to 7–10 on the ten scale. There were no meaningful gender differences in scores on this scale. In a study among 655 females and 544 males the mean score in BMAPS-IDC was 14.88 (SD= 4.332) and 14.11 (SD = 4.348) respectively. This difference was statistically significant t = - 3.04, df=1193, p = 0.002, but was not clinically significant [46].

A Brief Self-Rating Scale of Depression and Anxiety (BS-RSDA) [47]. It is a short method for evaluating the intensity of depression and anxiety symptoms, developed with norms for patients with diabetes. It consists of 10 items with an 11 degree Likert scale (from 0 to 10). The overall score therefore falls somewhere between 0 to 100. 5 questions fall in the depression category, 5 into the anxiety one (the result is from 0 to 50 for each of the scales). Construction of these scales was based on most significant psychopathological symptoms characteristic for depression in both classifications – DSM-IV and ICD 10. In the depression scale the following factors were developed: mood, intensity of energy, strength of interests, ability to feel pleasure, speed of thought and action. They constitute elements of depression episode and might appear in other depressive disorders. In case of anxiety there are many categories of anxiety disorders. For the evaluation of anxiety symptoms, the following factors were included: 1. worry, tension, uneasiness; 2. anxiety or fear of specific threat; 3. apprehension, distress; 4. physical tension; 5. desire to avoid situations that cause anxiety.

The tool has good psychometric properties, evaluated on the basis of a study conducted on 240 respondents – patients with diabetes. Both scales proved to have good reliability, the Cronbach's alpha was 0.95 for depression and 0.94 for anxiety. Both scales were also found to be valid. The depression scale correlated with the results of Beck Depression Inventory (r=0.809) and the HADS Depression Scale (r=0.797). The anxiety scale correlated with the results of HADS Anxiety Scale (r=0.805). Reliability of the entire scale was also high (Cronbach's alpha=0.956). Because of the lack of a reference tool, the validity of the whole scale was not measured. High reliability of the subscales was replicated in a study among 101 persons with diabetes: Cronbach's alpha was 0.92 for the depression scale and 0.91 for the anxiety scale. In the study among 133 persons with cardiologic and orthopedic disease in the test-retest reliability measurement, after 30 minutes, the correlation of subscale scores for depression was r=0.845, and for the subscale of anxiety r=0.814

A temporary ten norm scales were developed, and the analysis of relations of the BS-RSDA scores and diagnosis of depression with structured interview indicated that results of depression subscale >11 have sensitivity for detection of depression that is 0.886 and specificity that is 0.727.

2.3. The practical schema of psychotherapeutic management within a regular medical visit [40,44,48]

The schema was created in order to help doctors in making basic psychotherapeutic interventions during the regular visit. Its application was encouraged by series of workshops for doctors treating diabetes in Poland, however it may be used without the training. The main goals of this intervention is helping patients in the stressful problems related with diabetes. The diagnosis focuses on the assessment and practical teaching patients about coping mechanisms, perception of self-influence on the diabetes course and development of patient abilities of problem-solving and use of coping task oriented and "the best solution oriented" coping styles. It eventually broadens the range of behaviors aiming at problem solving. This is congruent with self-management with diabetes based on empowerment. The study [49] shows that a mere transfer of information between the doctor and the patient (regarding the disease and the proposed treatment) does not ensure satisfactory results in terms of the outcome of treatment and the patient's adherence to medical recommendations. An improvement on the doctor-patient relationship has been suggested, basing on the tenets of cognitive behavioral therapy. The traditional model in which the health-care provider is the 'expert' to be consulted by the 'patient' has been replaced by a partnership in which both parties cooperate to achieve best results. In this approach, the patient is the central figure and – acknowledged to be an expert in his/her problematic symptoms - becomes an active member of his/her disease management team. The role of the therapist, on the other hand, is to assist the patient in this process. One of the methods which can be employed by the therapist is the Socratic method in the form of Socratic dialog that enables the patient to determine the problem areas and to guide them to make decisions regarding the course of treatment. Instead of offering ready solutions the therapist is required to guide the patient to work out the solutions to their problems. Thus the patients are empowered to use their own initiative, which shifts the locus of control closer to them and motivates them to effectively manage their own care leading to significant improvements in healthy behavior. In order to achieve this, cognitive behavioral therapy recommends the method of "small steps" whereby the patient is encouraged to make gradual alterations in their habits rather than introduce radical changes. Even modest results serve as positive reinforcement and motivate further efforts. The Schema consists of the following steps:

1. Welcoming and establishing contact.

– doctor's warm attitude towards the patient

– giving the patient a chance to say what he/she really wants to say

– It is crucial that the doctor establishes good contact with the patient so that the patient feels comfortable enough to confide in the doctor.

2. Discussing the implementation of the last homework.

– realistic estimation of achievements

– realistic estimation of difficulties

When assessing the degree to which the patient succeeded in complying with the doctor's recommendations it is important to ask open questions so as not to exert pressure on the patient or make them feel examined. In order to empower the patient, the doctor needs to appreciate any effort on the part of the patient and analyze any difficulties with which they may be struggling.

3. Setting the goals of the present visit

– asking the patient what he/she would most like to discuss

– in case of problems with making the choices:

- placing the possible goals in order,
- dividing very difficult goals into smaller ones ("step-by-step" approach)

– in case of serious problems in everyday life - adjusting the therapeutic goals to the to this circumstances

The goal which the patient is to pursue, ought to be realistic, specific (clearly defined) and measurable. In establishing the goal, the patient's current problems need to be considered, including non-medical ones, and assess their impact on the illness. If it is needed, the doctor is recommended to suggest taking small steps, which means breaking the goal down into smaller, more achievable goals. This will enhance the chances of success.

4. Medical examination

– adjustment of the set up goals to an outcome of the medical examination and conducting the required diagnostic procedure

The goals need to be established in the context of the patient's general condition. Only after examining the patient appropriate steps can be set.

5. A brief medical psychotherapeutic diagnosis

– screening for depression and anxiety

It may be made with A Brief Self-Rating Scale of Depression and Anxiety or any other diagnostic tool. The patients identified with risk of depressive disorders or anxiety disorders should be referred for a psychiatric consultation.

– dominating style of coping with stress related with the disease

– the feeling of the influence on the course of the disease

The coping style and perception of self-influence on the diabetes course may be made with use of aforementioned. The physician needs to assess how ready the patient is to introduce changes in his/her lifestyle, how strongly he/she believes in the positive outcome of the changes and to what degree the patient feels he/she has the perception of self-influence on a particular problem.

6. Socratic dialog leading to a realistic evaluation of the main problem's source and its possible solutions

– assessment of the problem in the context of general life situation

–formulation of possible solutions

– assessment of advantages and disadvantages of possible solutions

Asking the patient a series of questions enables him/her to determine the source of the problem and to seek the most suitable solution. Since the patient is encouraged to use their own initiative, they will more strongly believe in their ability to achieve their goals.

7. Setting the realistic homework for the period prior to the next visit.

– "small steps" that have good chance for successful outcomes

– defining the criteria of the outcome estimation

– formulating actions that will be taken in case of serious problems with conducting homework

On the basis of the information gathered during the visit, the doctor is recommended to work out a list of recommendations to be implemented by the patient after the visit. It is important to consider any foreseeable difficulties and discuss the means to overcome them.

8. Recapitulation of the visit by the patient

– what are the conclusions of the discussion

– what is the homework to be conducted prior to the following appointment

It is good if the physician asks the patient to recapitulate briefly to make sure that the patient understands the arrangements discussed during the visit

3. Discussion

The Psychodiabetic KIT was created in order to encourage doctors to make psychotherapeutic diagnoses and basic psychotherapeutic interventions that will improve their patients' coping with diabetes. Realistically, it may be helpful during a yearly follow up visit, that according to International Diabetes Federation guidelines [19] should include assessment of psychological functioning of patients with diabetes type 2 or when screening tools or clinical assessment indicate a risk of psychological problems related to diabetes, including comorbid depression or anxiety disorders. The diagnostic tools can be used together or separately. However, it is recommended that the doctor or the nurse using the KIT become familiar with the details of The Brief Method of Evaluating Coping with Disease and are able to use examples of situations and reactions specific for the four main coping styles, in the process of educating the patient about his/her coping styles and, if needed, possibilities of its improvement. It may also be helpful for the patient to get a copy of the questionnaire with the key. It is crucial to explain to the patient that his/her perception of self-influence on the disease course, explain the need for the development by him/her the task oriented coping and the best solution oriented coping for dealing with diabetes related stressful problem. The patients with low level of the perception of self-influence on the disease course need interventions increasing this aspect of illness perception. It includes the "step-by-step" approach to the diabetes related problem together with self-monitoring effects of activity by making written records or self-rating scales. Otherwise, nonadherence to many of therapeutic recommendations among patients with a low perception of self-influence on diabetes course is very likely. Brief Self-Rating Scale of Depression and Anxiety needs specific norms for each language. However, the Polish sten norms can be helpful in a preliminary assessment of the intensity of symptoms of depression and anxiety(detailed ten norms are available from the first author).

They may also be used for the comparison of those symptoms in time. The version of the Psychodiabetic KIT tools included in the Appendix followed the rules of back-translation as it is a commonly accepted methodology in such cases. Still, their psychometric proprieties should be assessed in English speaking countries. Translations into other languages need back-translation procedures and assessment of their psychometric proprieties, before application in research. The main idea of the Psychodiabetic KIT is to facilitate clinical diagnosis, psycho-education of the patient considering coping, perception of self-influence as well as the need for monitoring depression and anxiety. Even non-validated translations of the KIT may be helpful in reaching these goals.

4. Application of the components of psychodiabetic KIT in research

Components of Psychodiabetic KIT were used in several research. This review presents only those which were published, including two cross-sectional, national studies. However, the results of other studies that resulted in on Ph. Thesis, and more than 10 M.A. thesis are currently in process of preparation for publications.

The national, cross- sectional study "Relationship between psychological coping style and insulin pen choice in patients with T2DM" [50] was aiming at assessment of relationship among coping styles and a choice of one of four available pens – insulin injectors that differed in technological complexity, size and accuracy:

- InnoLet – big and disposable, filled with insulin
- NovoLet – small and disposable; filled with insulin
- NovoPen 3 – durable, for multiple use, and filled each time by the patient

Innovo – durable, for multiple use, compact size, that make discretely injection in social situations possible, as well as record of the dosage and time of injection. The study was conducted by general practitioners with subsequent patients and only included a single visit during which treatment with insulin was initiated and when the patient chose an insulin injector. The style of coping was assessed at the same time with the working version of The Brief Method of Evaluating Coping with Disease (BMECD)[24], that had worst psychometric proprieties, assessed on smaller group that final one). The study involved 945 patients (553 females [59.1%]; 382 males [40.9%] – gender data were missing for 10 patients) aged 18–90 years (mean [SD]: 61.7 [11.7] years) who were beginning insulin therapy after a period of treatment for T2DM ranging from several months to 61 years (mean [SD]: 8.3 [5.9] years). The number (proportion) of patients in this study choosing each type of pen was: 460 (48.7%) NovoPen® 3; 269 (28.5%) NovoLet®; 25 (2.6%) Innovo®; 176 (18.6%) InnoLet®; data were missing for 15 (1.6%) patients. Statistically significant differences between mean BMECD scores were found among patients who chose one of four types of insulin pens. The results indicated that an avoidance-oriented coping style was associated with choosing the simplest insulin pen, an emotion-oriented coping style with a more complicated insulin pen, a task-oriented coping style with a modern pen, and the 'the best solution oriented' coping style with the technologically most advanced pen. In spite of many methodological limitations of this study its results encouraged the elaboration of the final version of the BMECD and supported its usefulness in clinical practice.

Another cross-sectional national study [46] involved 480 physicians and 1199 patients (655 females [54.6%]; 544 males [45.4%]) aged 4–93 years (mean [SD]: 62.0 [11.6] years) who were beginning insulin therapy after a period of treatment for diabetes ranging from several months to 36 years (mean [SD]: 8.0 [5.5] years). The study was conducted with consecutive patients and only included a single visit during which treatment with insulin was initiated and when the patient made their choice of insulin injector. Analysis of the relationship between the perception of self-influence on the disease course and choice of insulin pen was possible for 1184 (98.7%) persons enrolled in the study. The Brief Measure to Assess Perception of Self-Influence on the Disease Course: Version for Diabetes (BMAPS-IDC) was applied. The number (proportion) of patients in this study choosing each type of pen was: 538 (44.9%) NovoPen® 3; 383 (31.9%) NovoLet®; 220 (18.4%) InnoLet®; data were missing for 58 (4.8%) patients. In the group that chose the simplest disposable injector – InnoLet® – the mean BMAPS-IDC score (12.23) was significantly lower than in group that chose the smaller and more complicated type of injector (NovoPen® 3, 15.72). The mean BMAPS-IDC score in the group that chose the intermediate injector (NovoLet®, 13.88) lay between, and was statistically different from, the means of the other two groups.

Of the 395 patients in this study with data from relevant assessments, mean HbA_{1c} levels were ≤6.5% (low risk of cardiovascular [CV] complications) in 10 (2.5%) patients; between 6.6 and 7.5% (risk of arterial complications) in 38 (9.6%) patients; and >7.5% in 347 (87.8%) patients. Mean (SD) BMAPS-IDC scores in the groups with low risk of CV complications, risk of arterial complications, and risk of microvascular complications were: 18.20 (2.97), 16.55 (4.38), 14.43 (4.35), respectively. The difference in BMAPS-IDC scores between the group at low risk of CV complications (HbA_{1c} ≤6.5%) and the group at risk of microvascular complications (HbA_{1c} >7.5%) was statistically significant ($p<0.01$).

A correlation analysis suggested that the perception of self-influence on the course of diabetes has an increasing impact on the effectiveness of the treatment, as assessed by HbA_{1c} levels following long-term treatment. In total, 72 patients had been treated for less than 3 years, 72 for 3 years or more, and 249 for more than 5 years. The correlations were not significant in the group treated for diabetes for less than 3 years. Weak, but statistically significant correlations were found in the group treated for more than 3 years for diabetes ($r=-0.18$; $p<0.05$) and for those with a disease length over 5 years ($r=-0.2$; $p<0.05$).

Limitations of both of these studies include the observational design, which meant that participating doctors were not blinded to the results and could potentially influence patients' results. Due to the cross-sectional design the data presented in this paper only describe a relationship between coping styles or the perception of self-influence on the disease course and the type of device used at the beginning of insulin therapy, but cannot prove a cause and effect relationship, which may be worthy of further investigation.

Studies, which were presented above, revealed that the coping style and perception of self-influence on the course of diabetes have an important role in the process of the treatment choice. The relationship between the perception of self-influence on the disease course and the effectiveness of the treatment manifested by HbA1c level is also noteworthy.

Overall, the results of these studies indicate that psychological intervention aimed at developing task-oriented and 'the best solution-oriented' coping styles may result in the choice of more precise treatment, allowing more accurate glycemic control. Therefore, helping patients understand and believe that they can control the outcome of their diabetes is of value.

Conversely, clinicians may wish to use these findings to help them identify the coping style and the level of belief in self influence for a particular patient, which could enable further individualization of the treatment plan.

Comparing coping styles, occurrence of depressive and anxiety symptoms, and locus of control among patients with diabetes type 1 and type 2 in groups of 30 with type 1 and 27 with type 2 [51]. In the group of patients with diabetes type 2 there were found significantly higher, than in diabetes type 1: emotion oriented coping style ($M = 0.4$; $SD = 0.814$ vs. $M = 0.93$; $SD = 0.958$; $p = 0.029$), avoidance oriented coping style ($M = 0.63$; $SD = 0.809$ vs. $M = 1.22$; $SD = 0.892$; $p = 0.011$); level of depression ($M = 4.13$; $SD = 2.662$ vs. $M = 5.63$; $SD = 2.911$; $p = 0.047$), attribution of the health control to a chance ($M = 19.03$; $SD = 6.672$ vs. $M = 24.26$; $p = 0.004$) and also lower task-oriented coping style. ($M = 1.8$; $SD = 1.095$ vs. $M = 1.07$; $SD = 0.829$; $p = 0.007$).

What was also found, were the significant relations among the best solution-oriented coping style, emotion oriented style and the level of anxiety (respectively $r = -0.373$; $r = 0.37$) and level of depression (respectively $r = -0.352$ i $r = 0.476$); solution-oriented coping style, emotion-oriented coping style, level of anxiety and with the attribution of the health control to a chance (respectively $r = 0.341$; $r = 0.271$; $r = 0.301$); level of depression and locus of control ($r = 0{,}322$), i.e.: higher level of depression is correlated with more external locus of control; attribution of the health control to a chance and the older age ($r = 0.407$). The results of this preliminary study suggests that patients with diabetes type 2 use more maladaptive coping styles (emotion and avoidance oriented) than patients with diabetes type 1, and that use of specific coping styles is related with depression and anxiety

5. Assessment of psychodiabetic kit by doctors

In a survey conducted during a series of educational conferences in 2006, out of 217 doctors treating patients with diabetes, approximately half of them were acquainted with the BMECD and one-third with the BMAPS-IDC. In addition, 52.6% of doctors familiar with the BMECD, reported using it in everyday practice, and the majority were keen to further develop their experience with psychological tools used for the support of diabetic patients. [52]

6. Conclusions

1. Current guidelines of the International Diabetes Federation [19] and American Diabetes Association [20] as well as consensus statement of the American Diabetes Association and Europeans Association for Study of Diabetes, in respect to current knowledge, recommend individualized patient–centered approach in treatment and management of diabetes type.

2. A team approach, including variety of medical professionals, is recommended by IDF [19] on the "comprehensive" and "recommended" levels of care. However, these guidelines also describe a kind of "limited" care in respect to existence of "settings with very limited resources – drugs, personnel, technologies and procedures" [19].

3. The Psychodiabetic KIT facilitates, brief psychotherapeutic diagnosis and education of patients dealing with coping with diabetes related stressors as well as simply therapeutic interventions based on currently recommended rules of self-management and empowerment aiming at increasing the patients' perception of self-influence on the diabetes course and at the development of task related and "the best solution oriented" coping with stressful problems. It also may be used for depressive disorders and anxiety disorders screening.

4. The results of research indicate that the Brief Method of Evaluating Coping with Disease and the Brief Measure To Assess Perception Of Self- Influence On The Disease Course are useful in research. Their results confirm that coping styles and perception of self-influence on the disease course are related with the choice of treatment modality, i.e. insuline injector. The difference of the level of perception of self- influence on diabetes course was statistically significantly higher in between the group at low risk of CV complications (HbA_{1c} ≤6.5%) than in the group at risk of microvascular complications (HbA_{1c} >7.5%). There were also week, but statistically significant correlations between the perception of self-influence on the course of diabetes, the effectiveness of the treatment, as assessed by HbA_{1c} levels in groups of treated patients. The results of the preliminary study suggest that patients with diabetes type 2 use more maladaptive coping styles (emotion and avoidance oriented) than patients with diabetes type 1, and that a use of specific coping styles is related with depression and anxiety.

5. The results of anonymous survey among Polish doctors treating diabetes indicate that Psychodiabetic KIT may by useful in everyday practice.

Appendix

Brief method of evaluating coping with disease[1]: Version for men (Kokoszka, Radzio, Kot, 2008)

Name...Date.................................

Please circle one answer to each of the four questions:

1. If you found yourself in a group of people having to deal with a serious problem (among people shamed by a building society authorities or a service company not meeting its obligations), you would most probably:

- **a.** Do nothing and count on someone else to take care of it or would figure out that its pointless and dealing with it is a waste of time
- **b.** Look for others who were harmed and, together with them, try to protect my rights
- **c.** Try to influence the people who got engaged in solving the problem, so that I could get the best outcome
- **d.** Be mainly angry and upset and would not feel like doing anything

2. When you notice longer-lasting swerves in your health (minor pain, weakness), you usually:

- **a.** Not worry for a while and wait for them to pass
- **b.** Worry that it might be a beginning of a serious illness, which may potentially cause problems
- **c.** Look for information in a health-guide, ask acquaintances who have had similar problems or contact a doctor
- **d.** Contact a doctor as soon as possible and want to do everything possible to prevent the development of the disorder or at least assuage its course

3. If you had a chance to inherit, but it required a long-drawn participation in a trial, you would probably:

- **a.** Decline participation as not being sure about the success you wouldn't want to waste time on unpleasant activities
- **b.** Lodge a lawsuit yourself
- **c.** Hire a lawyer to best represent your interest
- **d.** Be irritated by the situation and ask relatives or friends to take care of it

4. When there is a serious conflict between your close-ones, you usually:

- **a.** Try talking to them in order to resolve the conflict
- **b.** Do nothing and try to avoid thinking about it
- **c.** Feel upset and worries because I don't like situations like that
- **d.** Try to link them to others who had similar problems or talk to them about how others handled similar situations

---

1 The authors gratefully acknowledge permission to translate this method to Via Medica, that published paper: Kokoszka A, Radzio R, Kot W. Krótka Metoda Ocena Radzenia Sobie z Chorobą: wersja dla mężczyzn i kobiet (Brief Method of Evaluating Coping with Disease: versions for men and women). Diabetologia Praktyczna 2008;9(1) 1-11.

http://dx.doi.org/10.5772/56468

Brief method of evaluating coping with disease: Version for women (Kokoszka, Radzio, Kot, 2008)

Name…………………………………………..Date……………………………..

Please circle one answer to each of the four questions:

1. If you found yourself in a group of people having to deal with a serious problem (with young people disturbing peace in your community, with your superior at work or with the authorities of a building company), you would most probably:

- **a.** I would try to engage in some other activity and wait patiently, believing that that the problem will be solved
- **b.** Engage in the activities of the group trying to solve the problem
- **c.** Try to influence the people who got engaged or lead them myself, but mainly I would try to solve the problem in the best option for me
- **d.** Be mainly angry and upset and would not feel like doing anything

2. When you notice longer-lasting swerves in your health (minor pain, weakness), you usually:

- **a.** Hope, they are not serious and wait for them to pass
- **b.** Worry and are afraid of different possible illnesses
- **c.** Look for information in a health-guide, ask acquaintances who have had similar problems or contact a doctor
- **d.** Contact a doctor as soon as possible and want to do everything possible to prevent the development of the disorder or at least assuage its course

3. If you had a chance to inherit, but it required a long-drawn participation in a trial, you would probably:

- **a.** Resign your participation
- **b.** Lodge a lawsuit yourself
- **c.** Hire a lawyer to best represent your interest
- **d.** Be worried by the need of participating in the procedure and rely on my relatives' opinions

4. When there is a serious, prolonged conflict between your close-ones, you usually:

- **a.** Try talking to them in order to resolve the conflict
- **b.** Do nothing and try to avoid thinking about it
- **c.** Feel upset and worried and want them to solve it as quickly as possible
- **d.** Try to assess whether they need help and what I could do to offer best possible support

Key for interpreting answers

Versions for both gender

Find each of the patient's answer on the list below then calculate the number of the responses characteristic for each of four coping styles. This result can be discussed with the patient and the answers characteristic for each of the coping style can be used for the patient education on coping styles. In research, row results are used.

Task-oriented coping style

1. b) look for others who were harmed and, together with them, try to protect my rights/ engage in the activities of the group trying to solve the problem
2. c) look for information in a health-guide, ask acquaintances who have had similar problems or contact a doctor
3. b) lodge a lawsuit yourself;
4. a) try talking to them in order to resolve the conflict

Best solution-oriented coping style

1. c) try to influence the people who got engaged in solving the problem, so that I could get the best outcome/ try to influence the people who got engaged or lead them myself, but mainly I would try to solve the problem in the best option for me
2. d) contact a doctor as soon as possible and want to do everything possible to prevent the development of the disorder or at least assuage its course
3. c) hire a lawyer to best represent your interest
4. d) try to link them to others who had similar problems or talk to them about how others handled similar situations/ try to assess whether they need help and what I could do to offer best possible support

Emotion-oriented coping style

1. d) be mainly angry and upset and would not feel like doing anything
2. b) worry that it might be a beginning of a serious illness, which may potentially cause problems/ worry and are afraid of different possible illnesses
3. d) be irritated by the situation and ask relatives or friends to take care of it/ be worried by the need of participating in the procedure and rely on my relatives' opinions
4. c) feel upset and worries because I don't like situations like that/ feel upset and worried and want them to solve it as quickly as possible

Avoidance-oriented coping style

1. a) do nothing and count on someone else to take care of it or would figure out that its pointless and dealing with it is a waste of time/ I would try to engage in some other activity and wait patiently, believing that that the problem will be solved
2. a) not worry for a while and wait for them to pass/ hope, they are not serious and wait for them to pass
3. a) decline participation as not being sure about the success you wouldn't want to waste time on unpleasant activities/ resign your participation
4. b) do nothing and try to avoid thinking about it

The sum of given answers

Task-oriented coping style – ….
Best-solution oriented coping style –....
Emotion-oriented coping style –....
Avoidance-oriented coping style –....

http://dx.doi.org/10.5772/56468

Brief measure to assess perception of self- influence on the disease course (Kokoszka, 2005)[2]

Name...Date...................................

Please circle your personal opinion on each of the following questions:

1. If I take care of myself, I will have a better health

I fully agree — I rather agree — It is hard to say — I rather disagree — I disagree

2. If I accomplish all my plans related to the management of diabetes (treatment, diet, physical activity) I generally feel relief

I fully agree — I rather agree — It is hard to say — I rather disagree — I disagree

3. I spend a lot of time preventing possible future complications of my illness

I fully agree — I rather agree — It is hard to say — I rather disagree — I disagree

4. Diet and lifestyle do not influence my health, because the most important is medication (and insulin)

I fully agree — I rather agree — It is hard to say — I rather disagree — I disagree

5. The course of my illness depends mostly on fate

I fully agree — I rather agree — It is hard to say — I rather disagree — I disagree

6. The experience gained during therapy helps me to better cope with other problems in my life

I fully agree — I rather agree — It is hard to say — I rather disagree — I disagree

---

2 The authors gratefully acknowledge permission to translate this method to Wydawnictwo Przegląd Lekarski that published the paper: Kokoszka A. Krótka metoda oceny poczucia wpływu na przebieg choroby: opis wersji dla osób z cukrzycą (Brief measure to assess perception of self-influence on the disease course. Version for diabetes).Przegląd Lekarski 2005;62(8) 742-745

Key

Questions 1, 2 ,3, 6

I fully agree – 4

I rather agree – 3

It is hard to say – 2

I rather disagree –1

I disagree – 0

Questions 4, 5 – inverted score

I fully agree – 0

I rather agree – 1

It is hard to say – 2

I rather disagree – 3

I disagree – 4

Interpretation according to standardized ten scale:

Low scores 0-11(< 5 sten)

Average scores 12-15 (5-6 sten)

High scores 16-24 (> 6 sten)

Brief Self- rating scale of depression and anxiety (Kokoszka, 2008) [3]

Name...Date..................................

Please assess your well-being on the following scales by putting an X in a chosen place of the scale.

You should compare your current well-being with previous feeling of comfort.

Number 10 stands for an intensity of the assessed feature that is the highest that you can imagine.

1. Mood

0 1 2 3 4 5 6 7 8 9 10

good — moderate sadness — sadness — intense sadness — severe sadness

2. Intensity of energy

0 1 2 3 4 5 6 7 8 9 10

good intensity of energy — moderate lack of energy — considerable lack of energy — great lack of energy — complete lack of energy

3 The authors gratefully acknowledge permission to translate this method to Termedia, that published, the paper: Kokoszka A. Krótka Skala Samooceny Depresji i Lęku: opis konstrukcji oraz właściwości psychometrycznych dla osób z cukrzycą (Brief Self-Rating Scale of Depression and Anxiety: description of the scale construction and psychometric proprieties for persons with diabetes). Przewodnik Lekarza 2008;11(6) 74-81

3. Power of interests

0 1 2 3 4 5 6 7 8 9 10

normal | moderately weakened | considerably weakened | highly weakened | severely weakened

4. The capacity to feel pleasure

0 1 2 3 4 5 6 7 8 9 10

normal | moderately weakened | considerably weakened | highly weakened | severely weakened

5. Speed of thought and action

0 1 2 3 4 5 6 7 8 9 10

normal | moderately weakened | considerably weakened | highly weakened | severely weakened

6. Worry, tenseness, nervousness

0 1 2 3 4 5 6 7 8 9 10

none | moderate | strong | very strong | severe

7. Anxiety (feeling of fear without a certain reason), fear of a specified threat

0 1 2 3 4 5 6 7 8 9 10

none | moderate | strong | very strong | severe

8. Apprehension and distress about something that might happen

0 1 2 3 4 5 6 7 8 9 10

none | moderate | strong | very strong | severe

9. Feeling of physical tension in a body (intense muscle tension, trembling hands, aches)

0 1 2 3 4 5 6 7 8 9 10

none | moderate | strong | very strong | severe

10. Desire to avoid situations that cause anxiety (hiding, withdrawing)

0 1 2 3 4 5 6 7 8 9 10

none | moderate | strong | very strong | severe

Key — Adding the scores 1-5 depression subscale; 6-10 anxiety subscale

Reliability: depression scale α Cronbacha= 0,95; anxiety scale α Cronbacha= 0,94, entire scale α Cronbacha=0,956.

Interpretation according to standardized ten scale:

Depression scale:

Low scores 0-2 (1–4 sten)
Average scores 3-12 (5–6 sten)
High scores 13-50 (7–10 sten)

Anxiety scale:
Low scores 0-4 (1–4 sten)
Average scores 5-14 (5–6sten)
High scores 15-50 (7–10 sten)

Entire scale:
Low scores 0-8 (1–4 sten)
Average scores 9-27 (5–6 sten)
High scores 28-100 (7–10 sten)

Author details

Andrzej Kokoszka[1*], Aleksandra Jodko-Modlińska[2], Marcin Obrębski[2], Joanna Ostasz-Ważny[1] and Rafał Radzio[2]

*Address all correspondence to: andrzej.kokoszka@wum.edu.pl

1 II Department of Psychiatry, Medical University of Warsaw, Warsaw, Poland

2 University of Social Sciences and Humanities, Warsaw, Poland

References

[1] Inzucchi SE, Bergenstal RM, Buse JB, Diamant M, Ferrannini E, Nauck M, Peters AL, Tsapas A, Wender R, Matthewset DR. American Diabetes Association (ADA)European Association for the Study of Diabetes (EASD). Management of hyperglycemia in type 2 diabetes: a patient-centered approach. Position statement of the American Diabetes Association (ADA) and the European Association for the Study of Diabetes (EASD). Diabetes Care 2012;35(6) 1364–1379.

[2] Kokoszka A, Sieradzki J. Poczucie wpływu na przebieg choroby a sposób leczenia cukrzycy (Relationship between the feeling of influence on the course of disease and the management with diabetes). Diabetologia Praktyczna 2005;6(1) 1-5.

[3] Kokoszka A, Szmalec M. Relationships of eating disorders with psychological problems in the course of diabetes type 2: cross-sectional study. The 14th Scientific Meeting of the PSAD Psycho Social Aspects of Diabetes Study (PSAD) Group at the European Association for the Study of Diabetes, Dubrovnik, 2009.

[4] Ali S, Stone MA, Peters JL, Davies MJ, Khunti K. The prevalence of co-morbid depression in adults with Type 2 diabetes: a systematic review and meta-analysis. Diabetic Medicine 2006;23(11) 1165-1173.

[5] Cuijpers P, Smith F. Subthreshold depression is a risk factor for major depressive disorder. A systematic review of prospective studies. Acta Psychiatrica Scandinavica 2004;109(5) 325-331.

[6] Kokoszka A, Radzio R, Kot W. Krótka Metoda Oceny Radzenia Sobie z Chorobą: wersja dla mężczyzn i kobiet (Brief Method of Evaluating Coping with Disease: versions for men and women). Diabetologia Praktyczna 2008;9(1) 1-11.

[7] Kokoszka A. Krótka metoda oceny poczucia wpływu na przebieg choroby: opis wersji dla osób z cukrzycą (Brief measure to assess perception of self-influence on the disease course. Version for diabetes). Przegląd Lekarski 2005;62(8) 742-745.

[8] Zulman DM, Rosland AM, Choi H, Langa KM, Heisler M. The influence of diabetes psychosocial attributes and self-management practices on change in diabetes status. Patient Education And Counseling 2012;87(1) 74-80.

[9] King DK, Glasgow RE, Toobert DJ, Strycker LA, Estabrooks PA, Osuna D, Faber AJ. Self-efficacy, problem solving, and social-environmental support are associated with diabetes self-management behaviors. Diabetes Care 2010;33(4) 751-753.

[10] Greenfield C, Gilles M, Porter C, Shaw P, Willis K. It's not just about the HbA1c, Doc! Understanding the psychosocial is also important in managing diabetes? The Australian Journal Of Rural Health 2011;19(1) 15-19.

[11] Peyrot M, Rubin RR, Lauritzen T, Snoek FJ, Matthews DR, Skovlund SE. Psychosocial problems and barriers to improved diabetes management: results of the Cross-National Diabetes Attitudes, Wishes and Needs (DAWN) Study. Diabetic Medicine 2005;22(10) 1379-1385.

[12] Snoek FJ, Kersch NYA, Eldrup E, Harman-Boehm I, Hermanns N, Kokoszka A, Matthews DR, McGuire BE, Pibernik-Okanovic M, Singer J, de Wit M, Skovlund SE. Monitoring of Individual Needs in Diabetes (MIND)-2: Follow-up data from the cross-national Diabetes Attitudes, Wishes, and Needs (DAWN) MIND study. Diabetes Care 2012;35(11) 2128-2132.

[13] Snoek FJ, Kersch NYA, Eldrup E, Harman-Boehm I, Hermanns N, Kokoszka A, Matthews DR, McGuire BE, Pibernik-Okanovic M, Singer J, de Wit M, Skovlund SE. Monitoring of Individual Needs in Diabetes (MIND): baseline data from the Cross-National Diabetes Attitudes, Wishes, and Needs (DAWN) MIND study. Diabetes Care 2011;34(3) 601–603.

[14] Bech P, Olsen RL, Kjoller M, Rasmussen NK. Measuring well-being rather than the absence of distress symptoms: a comparison of the SF-36 Mental Health subscale and the WHO-Five Well-Being Scale. International Journal Of Methods In Psychiatric Research 2003;12(2) 85-91.

[15] Bech P. Measuring the dimensions of psychological general well-being by the WHO-5. Quality of Life Newsletter 2004;32 15-16.

[16] Snoek FJ, Pouwer F, Welch G, Polonsky WH. Diabetes- related emotional distress in Dutch and U.S. diabetic patients. Cross- cultural validity of the Problem Areas in Diabetes Scale (PAID). Diabetes Care 2000;23(9) 1305-1309.

[17] Welch GW, Jacobson AM, Polonsky WH. The problem areas in diabetes scale. An evaluation of its clinical utility. Diabetes Care 1997;20(5) 760-766.

[18] Polonsky WH, Anderson BJ, Lohrer PA, Welch G, Jacobson AM, Aponte JE, Schwartz CE: Assessment of diabetes- related distress. Diabetes care 1995;18(6) 754-760.

[19] International Diabetes Federation, Global Guideline for Type 2 Diabetes, International Diabetes Federation. Brussels, 2012.

[20] Standards of Medical Care in Diabetes—2011. Diabetes Care 2011;34(Suppl. 1) 11-61.

[21] Lazarus RS. Folkman S. Stress, Appraisal and Coping. New York: Springer; 1984.

[22] Tuncay T, Musabak I, Gok DE, Kutlu M. The relationship between anxiety, coping strategies and characteristics of patients with diabetes. Health and Quality of Life Outcomes 2008;6:79 http://www.hqlo.com/content/6/1/79 (accessed 13 October 2008).

[23] Endler N.S., Parkeri.D"A.: Multidimensional assessment of coping: A critical evaluation. Journal Of Personality And Social Psychology1990;58(5) 844-854.

[24] Kokoszka A, Jodko A, Radzio R. Krótka metoda radzenia sobie z chorobą – geneza i opis roboczej wersji metody [Brief Method of Evaluating Coping with Disease – description of the preliminary version]. Przewodnik Lekarza 2003;6(10) 39–46.

[25] Selye H. Stress of life. New York: McGraw-Hill; 1956.

[26] Selye H. Stress in health and disease. Massachusetts: Butterworth's Reading; 1976.

[27] Everly GS, Rosenfeld R. The Nature and Treatment of the Stress Response. New York: Plenum; 1981.

[28] Bandura A. Self-efficacy. In: Ramachaudran V.S. (ed.) Encyclopedia of Human Behavior, Vol. 4. New York: Academic Press 1994. p71–81.

[29] Conway VJ, Terry DJ. Appraised controllability as a moderator of the effectiveness of different coping strategies: A test of the goodness of fit hypothesis. Australian Journal of Psychology 1992;44(1) 1–7.

[30] Macrodimitris SD, Endler NS. Coping, control and adjustment in type 2 diabetes. Health Psychology 2001;20(3) 208–216.

[31] Rubin RR, Peyrot M. Quality of life and diabetes. Diabetes/Metabolism Research And Reviews 1999;15(3) 205–218.

[32] Watkins KW, Connell CM, Fitzgerald JT, Klem L, Hickey T, Ingersoll-Dayton B. Effect of adults' self-regulation of diabetes on quality-of-life outcomes. Diabetes Care 2000;23(10) 1511–1515.

[33] Anderson RJ, Freedland KE, Clouse RE, Lustman PJ. The prevalence of comorbid depression in adults with diabetes: a meta-analysis. Diabetes Care 2001;24(6) 1069-1078.

[34] Lustman PJ, Anderson RJ, Freedland KE, de Groot M, Carney RM, Clouse RE. Depression and poor glycemic control: a meta-analytic review of the literature. Diabetes Care 2000;23(7) 934-942.

[35] Katon WJ, Rutter C, Simon G, Lin EH, Ludman E, Ciechanowski P, Kinder L, Young B, Von Korff M. The association of comorbid depression with mortality in patients with type 2 diabetes. Diabetes Care 2005;28(11) 2668-2672.

[36] Beverly EA, Ganda OP, Ritholz MD, Lee Y, Brooks KM, Lewis-Schroeder NF, Hirose M, Weinger K. Look who's (not) talking: diabetic patients' willingness to discuss self-care with physicians. Diabetes Care 2012;35(7) 1466-1472.

[37] Fisher L, Skaff MM, Mullan JT, Arean P, Glasgow R, Masharani U. A longitudinal study of affective and anxiety disorders, depressive affect and diabetes distress in adults with Type 2 diabetes. Diabetic Medicine 2008;25(9) 1096-1101.

[38] Collins MM, Corcoran P, Perry IJ. Anxiety and depression symptoms in patients with diabetes. Diabetes Care 2009;26(2) 153-161.

[39] Lewko J, Zarzycki W, Krajewska-Kulak E. Relationship between the occurrence of symptoms of anxiety and depression, quality of life, and level of acceptance of illness in patients with type 2 diabetes. Saudi Medical Journal 2012;33(8) 887-894.

[40] Kokoszka A, Santorski J. Psychodiabetologia dla lekarzy: postępowanie psychoterapeutyczne w cukrzycy (Psychodiabetology for physicians. Psychotherapeutic management in diabetes). Warszawa: Marketing and Media; 2003.

[41] Kokoszka A. Psychodiabetologia dla lekarzy. Część II: Ocena i kształtowanie poczucia wpływu na przebieg choroby u osób z cukrzycą (Psychodiabetology for physi-

cians. Part II: The assessment and shaping of perception of an influence on the course of disease in diabetes). Warszawa: Pracownia; 2005.

[42] Kokoszka A. Psychodiabetologia dla lekarzy. Cześć III: Zaburzenia depresyjne w przebiegu cukrzycy (Psychodiabetology for physicians. Part III: Depressive disorders in the course of diabetes). Warszawa: Medical Communications; 2007.

[43] Kokoszka A. Psychodiabetologia dla lekarzy. Część IV. Zaburzenia depresyjne i lęk w cukrzycy: Postępowanie w praktyce klinicznej (Psychodiabetology for physicians. Part IV: Anxiety and Depression in clinical practice). Warszawa: Medical Communications; 2010.

[44] Kokoszka A. Diagnoza i postępowanie psychoterapeutyczne w cukrzycy: Zestaw Psychodiabetologiczny (Psychotherapeutic diagnosis and management in diabetes: Psycho-Diabetic Kit). Psychiatria w Praktyce Ogólnolekarskiej 2005;5(4) 146-152.

[45] Endler NS, Parker JDA. Assessment of multidimensional coping: Task, emotion and avoidance strategies. Psychological Assessment 1994;6(1) 50–60.

[46] Kokoszka A, Sieradzki J. Poczucie wpływu na przebieg choroby a sposób leczenia cukrzycy (Relationship between the feeling of influence on the course of disease and the management with diabetes). Diabetologia Praktyczna 2005;6(1) 1–5.

[47] Kokoszka A. Krótka Skala Samooceny Depresji i Lęku: opis konstrukcji oraz właściwości psychometrycznych dla osób z cukrzycą (Brief Self-Rating Scale of Depression and Anxiety: description of the scale construction and psychometric proprieties for persons with diabetes). Przewodnik Lekarza 2008;11(6) 74-81.

[48] Kokoszka A. Schemat psychoterapeutycznej diagnozy i interwencji psychoterapeutycznych w praktyce ogólnolekarskiej (Schema of psychotherapeutic diagnosis and of psychotherapeutic interventions in general medical practice). Przewodnik Lekarza 2004;7(5) 60–69.

[49] Anderson R., Funnell M., Carlson A., Saleh-Statin N., Cradock S., Skinner T.C. Facilitating self-care through empowerment. In: Snoek FJ, Skinner TC (ed.) Psychology in Diabetes Care. Chichester: John Wiley & Sons; 2000. p69–97.

[50] Kokoszka A, Sieradzki J. Styl radzenia sobie z chorobą a wybór rodzaju wstrzykiwacza insuliny u chorych na cukrzycę typu 2 rozpoczynających insulinoterapię (The relationship of style of coping and choice of pen type at the beginning of insulinotherapy in type 2 diabetes). Diabetologia Praktyczna 2004;5(2) 67–74.

[51] Mućko P, Kokoszka A, Skłodowska Z. Porównanie stylów radzenia sobie z chorobą, występowania objawów depresyjnych i lękowych oraz lokalizacji poczucia kontroli u chorych na cukrzycę typu 1 i 2 (The comparison of coping styles, occurrence of depressive and anxiety symptoms, and locus of control among patients with diabetes type 1 and type 2). Diabetologia Praktyczna 2005;6 (5) 240-246.

[52] Kot W, Kokoszka A, Sieradzki J. Ocena zestawu psychodiabetolgicznego oraz potrzeb szkoleniowych z psychodiabetologii wśród lekarzy zajmujących się leczeniem cukrzycy (Assessment of psychodiabetologic kit and psychodiabetology training needs of doctors treating patients with diabetes). Diabetologia Praktyczna 2006;7(6) 405–408.